W9-CEH-130

MARTIN FROBISHER, Sc.D.

Formerly, Special Consultant,
Laboratory Branch, Communicable Disease Center,
United States Public Health Service;
Associate Professor of Bacteriology,
Johns Hopkins University, Baltimore, and
Emory University Medical School, Atlanta;
Professor and Head, Department of Bacteriology,
University of Georgia, Athens

ROBERT FUERST, Ph.D.

Professor of Biology,
Head of Microbiology Research Laboratory,
Texas Woman's University,
Denton, Texas

Microbiology

in

Health

and

Disease

THIRTEENTH
EDITION

1973

W. B. SAUNDERS COMPANY

PHILADELPHIA
LONDON
TORONTO

W. B. Saunders Company: West Washington Square
Philadelphia, Pa. 19105

12 Dyott Street
London, WC1A 1DB

833 Oxford Street
Toronto 18, Ontario

Microbiology in Health and Disease   ISBN 0-7216-3938-0

Print No.: 9   8   7   6   5   4   3   2   1

PREFACE

For the thirteenth edition, this book has been extensively revised, corrected and updated; a number of parts have been rearranged and largely rewritten. Because of extensive growth in the field of microbiology and its relations to individual and community health, the authors have been forced to make difficult choices between what they considered absolutely necessary and what, while valuable, must be treated briefly or left out entirely because of space limitations. The scope of most discussions has been widened and new data added to replace older or obsolete material.

Much time and effort have been expended in selection and preparation of new illustrative and tabular materials, and it is believed that these aspects of the book are much improved. For many of the beautiful photographs and diagrams we are indebted to numerous scientists whose contributions to the book are individually acknowledged in the legends to the illustrations. Some valuable photography was performed through the courtesy of Rabbi Stephen E. Fisch and Ben R. Fisch, M.D.

Other specific betterments are found in the discussions of asepsis and sanitation, especially in the hospital, which have been reviewed by Jan F. Fuerst, M.D., son of Robert Fuerst, Ph.D., and by Gesine A. Franke, R.N., Assistant to the Dean, College of Nursing, Texas Woman's University. Notable new features are the Proposed (or interim) Outline of the Classification and Nomenclature of Bacteria (our Appendix A) from the forthcoming eighth edition of *Bergey's Manual of Determinative Bacteriology*, and certain manuscript pages of that volume from which we have rearranged our descriptions of the Enterobacteriaceae—all of which were generously made available to us by Dr. Norman E. Gibbons, Editor-in-Chief of the eighth edition of *Bergey's Manual;* Dr. Erwin F. Lessel, Curator of Bacteria, American Type Culture Collection; and Miss Sara A. Finnegan, Editor at The Williams & Wilkins Co., publishers of the book for the Bergey Trust.

A helpful ancillary volume is a Laboratory Manual prepared especially for this book by Robert Fuerst, Ph.D.

A serious loss to this edition is the name of Lucille Sommermeyer, R.N., Ed.M., for many years one of the coauthors of this book. Prolonged illness has made it impossible for her to continue her valuable contributions to the volume. The loss is deeply felt and sincerely regretted by all concerned.

For any shortcomings of the text the present authors take full responsibility. Applause, if any, they accept with a bow. In any case they make an appreciatory gesture toward Mr. Robert E. Wright, of the W. B. Saunders Company, and to the traditional expertise, know-how and craftsmanship that for decades have been characteristic of the entire W. B. Saunders organization.

MARTIN FROBISHER, Sc.D.

ROBERT FUERST, PH.D.

CONTENTS

SECTION FOUR   INFECTION, IMMUNITY, AND ALLERGY

SECTION FIVE   PATHOGENIC MICROORGANISMS

Microbiology
in
Health
and
Disease

General Introduction

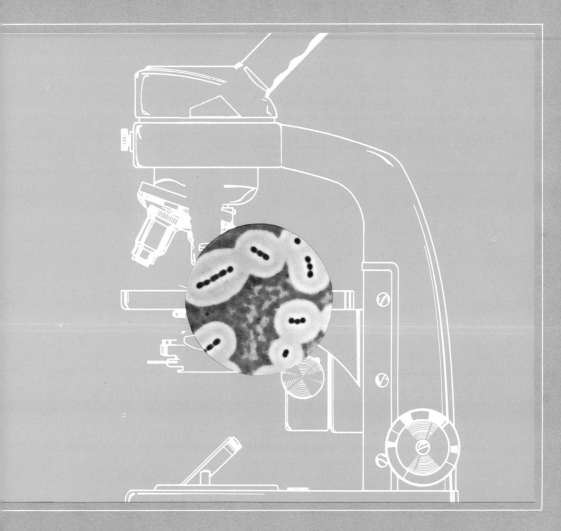

Section One

An Introduction To The Study of Microorganisms

Microbiology is the study of microorganisms. These are living organisms that are so small as to be visible only through microscopes. Some are so minute that they require yet greater magnification, which can be obtained only by using a powerful instrument called the electron microscope. Groups of plants and animals that are included in the term microorganisms are yeasts, molds, bacteria [including rickettsias, chlamydias, and mycoplasmas (PPLO)], viruses and protozoa.

WHY MICROBIOLOGY? In this century alone, owing in large part to the application of discoveries in microbiology, your life expectancy has been increased by approximately 50 per cent. You have inherited a healthier world without fear of epidemics of smallpox, typhus, polio, plague, diphtheria, rubella, measles or mumps. We know how to protect our children against tuberculosis and we give them more wholesome foods. Because of microbiology we know how to preserve better our food and we eat and we live cleaner in better houses under more sanitary conditions. Due in part to advances in microbiology, you, the people living in the twentieth to the twenty-first century, are the tallest, brightest, healthiest, and best looking generation ever to inhabit this planet.

On July 20, 1969, Neil Armstrong, standing on the moon, uttered the historic words: "One small step for a man, one giant leap for mankind." Yet space technology is only in its infancy; the universe is vast and is here to be conquered by man — let us hope, in peace! What life exists on other planets? What microorganisms will the space traveler meet? What benefit will we derive and what dangers will we encounter? Our astronauts were kept in quarantine after their return to earth to make relatively certain that they were not infected with some strange organism. The progress of mankind never stops for long. We must ask what bacteria, protozoa, or virus we shall encounter as man moves farther and farther out into space. Yes, microbiology and medicine must be ready to face the challenges of the future, as they have faced them during this turbulent century, nearly three-fourths completed. Will you be ready for the year 2000 and beyond?

The science of microbiology is essential to members of the health professions and, in fact, to everyone who is interested in maintaining health

4

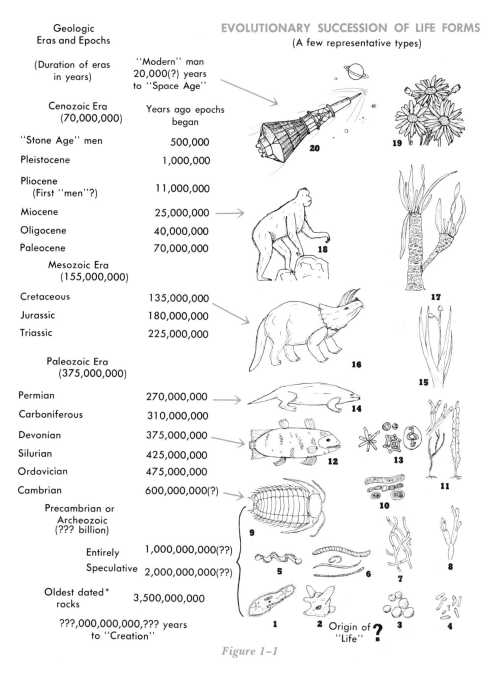

Geologic Eras and Epochs	EVOLUTIONARY SUCCESSION OF LIFE FORMS (A few representative types)

(Duration of eras in years)	"Modern" man 20,000(?) years to "Space Age"
Cenozoic Era (70,000,000)	Years ago epochs began
"Stone Age" men	500,000
Pleistocene	1,000,000
Pliocene (First "men"?)	11,000,000
Miocene	25,000,000
Oligocene	40,000,000
Paleocene	70,000,000
Mesozoic Era (155,000,000)	
Cretaceous	135,000,000
Jurassic	180,000,000
Triassic	225,000,000
Paleozoic Era (375,000,000)	
Permian	270,000,000
Carboniferous	310,000,000
Devonian	375,000,000
Silurian	425,000,000
Ordovician	475,000,000
Cambrian	600,000,000(?)
Precambrian or Archeozoic (??? billion)	
Entirely	1,000,000,000(??)
Speculative	2,000,000,000(??)
Oldest dated* rocks	3,500,000,000
???,000,000,000,??? years to "Creation"	

Figure 1–1

Geologic time scale (left) showing ancient origin of bacteria and other microorganisms in Precambrian times (entirely speculative) at foot of evolutionary scale. Pictures: 1, 2, protozoa; 3, 4, bacteria; 5, spirochete (protozoa-like bacterium); 6, marine worms; 7, mold-like bacteria; 8, aquatic fungus (*Saprolegnia*); 9, trilobite (fossil marine arthropod); 10, 13, bacteria-like algae (Cyanophyceae), desmids); 11, higher algae; 12, fossil fish; 14, cotylosaur (fossil reptile); 15, *Psilopsida*, first vascular land plants (Silurian); 16, *Triceratops*, a dinosaur; 17, cycad tree (Jurassic); 18, fossil man-like ape; 19, hybrid (1964) daisies; 20, man in space. *Oldest rocks dated by modern measurements of radioactivity.

and preventing disease. For example: knowledge of the method of transfer of microorganisms from one person to another can reduce the number of "colds" and incidents of "flu" that you and your family suffer; knowledge of sterilization and disinfection will teach you precautions to take in bandaging minor cuts and care to take in handling food; knowledge of immunity will help you understand the importance of immunization injections to prevent smallpox, typhoid fever, and influenza; and knowledge of the relation of microbiology to health and disease is both broadening and useful and may encourage some to embark on careers in microbiological research.

These are only a few simple examples of how you will apply microbiology every day of your life. Fortunately, health procedures today are based upon principles of microbiology so that health workers can not only assist in the prevention of disease but help to promote recovery when disease does occur. It is obvious that everyone in the health professions should understand the underlying principles of the maintenance of health and prevention of disease so that they will know the "why" of preventive procedures, can make intelligent adaptations of them, and can teach auxiliary personnel (attendants, orderlies, maids, technicians, and others) how to proceed correctly.

Is the study of microbiology difficult? Not excessively so. It is a very logical science and certainly one of the most fascinating. It explains why we refrigerate food, how to avoid certain kinds of infectious diseases, why penicillin and the "sulfas" are effective in treating certain diseases but ineffective in others, and much about some seemingly peculiar but really very sensible and intelligent activities of members of the health professions.

EVOLUTIONARY SUCCESSION OF LIFE FORMS. All available evidence shows that the various types of organisms existing today have slowly evolved from older species. For example, some of the present-day species of plants and animals have evolved, through millions of generations, from more primitive ancestors (Fig. 1–1). Many ancient types such as trilobites have long since perished from the earth, though animals that evolved from them may be common species today. In reviewing the ancestors of present-day living things, it is noted that the farther back we go in point of time, the simpler and more lowly were plants and animals. It may be inferred, then, that the simplest and most lowly creatures alive today would be descendants of those that existed in the earliest ages, probably more than four billion years ago. Although we do not actually know what the first plants or animals were like, it seems reasonable to suppose that they may have been something like bacteria or other microorganisms, possibly viruses, possibly protozoa. Many scientists regard present-day microorganisms as more or less direct descendants of some of the earliest forms of life on earth. Others even speculate on the origin of cellular organelles, called mitochondria and chloroplasts. These components of cells in higher forms of life superficially resemble bacteria and may have descended from free-living bacteria-like organisms by evolutionary processes of endosymbiosis.

A more recent theory proposes that the mitochondria and other organelles of eucaryons, instead of being derived from phagocytized procaryons, evolved from the procaryons themselves by intracellular metamorphoses of already existing parts of the procaryons, especially the cytoplasmic membrane.

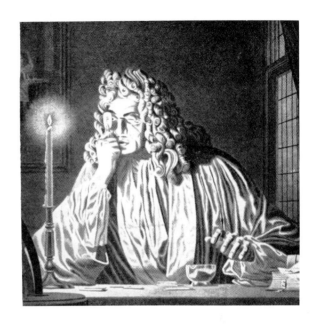

Figure 1–2

Antony van Leeuwenhoek. A fanciful delineation based on a famous portrait. The picture shows accurately the size and shape of the first microscopes and the manner in which they were used. (Courtesy of Lambert Pharm. Co.)

DISCOVERIES THROUGH THE MICROSCOPE

Ancient though the lineage of microorganisms may be, they were not discovered until fairly recent times (about 1680); because of their minuteness, a knowledge of their existence had to await the invention of the microscope. Although Zacharias Janssen devised the first compound microscope in 1590, the first person to see and also describe microorganisms was *Antony van Leeuwenhoek* (1632–1723), a Dutch dry goods merchant of Delft who wanted to observe the weave of fine cloth (Fig. 1–2). His microscopes, which he made himself, consisted of a biconvex lens held in a metal frame (sometimes gold and silver!). These lenses magnified up to 270 diameters. With such crude instruments he examined water from pools, the tartar from his teeth, feces from a case of dysentery, and

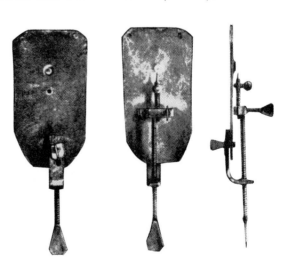

Figure 1–3

One of van Leeuwenhoek's original microscopes exists at the University of Utrecht. The single minute lens was mounted in the perforated metal plate and held close to the eye. The two vertical screws surmounted by a fine point were used to hold the object before the lens and adjust its position.

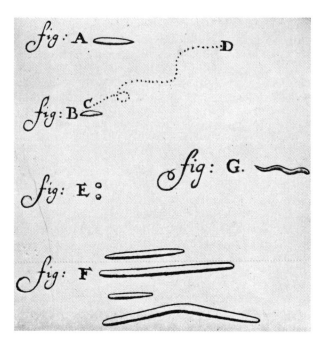

Figure 1–4

Drawings of bacteria made by van Leeuwenhoek in 1684.

many other substances and fluids (Fig. 1–3). He was amazed to see in all these substances what he called "animalcules"—tiny organisms, spherical, cigarette-shaped, or spiral in form, some of which were in rapid motion. The drawings that he made are still in existence and prove that what he

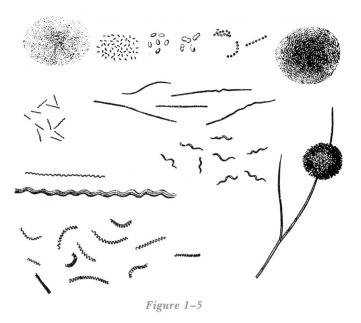

Figure 1–5

Otto Frederik Müller (1730–1784) published the first standard treatise on microorganisms entitled "*Animalcula infusoria fluriatilia et marina.*" In it he supplied generic and specific names for his organisms, arranged in systematic order. This figure shows one plate from Müller's book (1786). (about 800×). (From Ford, W. W.: Bacteriology. New York, Paul B. Hoeber, Inc., 1939.)

Figure 1-6

Ignaz Philipp Semmelweis, pioneer of asepsis in obstetrics. Because of his work on childbed fever, childbirth has lost most of its dangers. This portrait is based on a commemorative Austrian postage stamp honoring Semmelweis.

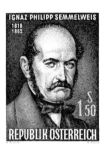

saw actually were bacteria and protozoa and other microorganisms (Fig. 1–4). It is fortunate that he described his findings to the Royal Society of London and that he left twenty-six of his microscopes to the Society after his death. Later on these heirlooms were lost, but not before Baker[1] left us with exact descriptions of all of them. Van Leeuwenhoek's discoveries opened up a whole new world to investigators that followed him (Fig. 1–5) and one that can be explored by all who learn to use our present-day microscopes.

EARLY HISTORY OF MICROBIOLOGY. Some of our present methods of preventing disease originated before very much was known of microorganisms. For example, in 1796 smallpox could be prevented by vaccination with cowpox, and Semmelweis (1818–1865) had fought the spread of disease in the maternity wards of hospitals with chemical disinfectants (Fig. 1–6). The rules and methods of the new science of preventive medicine, however, are to a considerable degree the result of the life work of two men, Louis Pasteur (1822–1895) and Robert Koch (1843–1910) (Figs. 1–7 and 1–8).

---

[1]Henry Baker, in his work *The Microscope Made Easy* (1742).

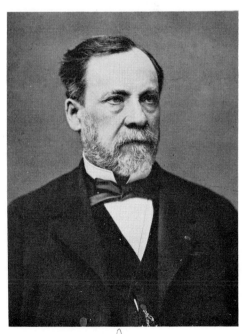

Figure 1-7

Louis Pasteur, 1822–1895. "Chance favors the prepared mind." (From Carpenter: Microbiology, 3rd ed. Philadelphia, W. B. Saunders Company, 1972.)

GREAT ADVANCES IN THE SCIENCE OF MICROBIOLOGY.   Shortly after the middle of the last century, the French chemist Pasteur, famous for founding the science of polarimetry, proved that fermentation and putrefaction were caused by living microorganisms and suggested the similarity between these processes and infectious diseases. He spoke of spoilage of wines and beer as "diseases" of those beverages. It was still generally believed by many scientists that living forms may arise spontaneously from dead matter. Spallanzani had disproved the "doctrine of spontaneous generation" almost a century earlier; however, it was Pasteur who devised a simple experiment to show that, so far as was known on the basis of data then available, living organisms originated only from living organisms. Although the question of spontaneous generation had thus seemingly been resolved in the nineteenth century, it was raised again in the twentieth century with infinitely more sophistication under the heading "chemical evolution." Today biochemists and microbiologists, using simple, naturally occurring substances and electric sparks, gases, and steam under high temperature and pressure, can synthesize many complex organic compounds that formerly had been found only in living cells. In fact it is now possible to build genelike structures as they may have occurred originally some two billion or more years ago. Yet the fanciful eighteenth century "doctrine of spontaneous generation" is dead: bacteria come only from existing bacteria.

After studying fermentation of wine, Pasteur investigated a communicable disease in silkworms; as a result he formulated the *germ theory* of disease. In dealing with diseases in humans, he insisted that bandages

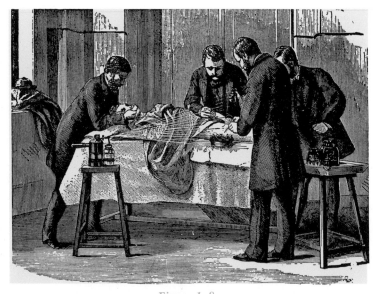

Figure 1–8

Lister operating with carbolic spray. The illustration represents the general arrangement of surgeon, assistants, towels, and spray in an operation performed with (supposed) complete aseptic precautions (1882). Note the carbolic spray playing over the field of operation. Also note the coats. (W. Watson Cheyne).

should be cleaned and instruments in the hospital boiled. Joseph Lister (1827–1912), an English surgeon, applied Pasteur's discoveries to surgery even before the actual bacteria that cause surgical infections had been discovered. Lister's work is the basis of present-day aseptic surgical technique (Fig. 1–8).

In clever experiments Pasteur protected sheep against anthrax by vaccinating them with a preparation of attenuated anthrax organisms. The Pasteur "treatment" of rabies was developed to protect against the disease by injections of dried material from the spinal cords of animals that had died from rabies. Joseph Meister, a small boy bitten by a mad dog, was the first human whose life was saved by this method and who did not get the disease hydrophobia (rabies) because he was protected by Pasteur's injections. It is an irony of history that half a century later Joseph Meister, who was then the gatekeeper of the Pasteur Institute, killed himself when ordered by curious German soldiers to open Pasteur's crypt.

At the time of Pasteur's discoveries, Ferdinand Cohn (1828–1898) was one of the foremost microbiologists in Germany. He extended Pasteur's findings in his own laboratory, where he worked with algae and fungi. Cohn became so interested in bacteriology that he wrote some of the earliest books about bacteria. In them, following Müller, he classified bacteria into genera and species. Cohn was of great help to Robert Koch and encouraged him to publish his paper on anthrax.

Although 200 years before the days of bacteriology Boyle suggested that some diseases are caused by some action of living microorganisms and in 1839 Schönlein made the admirable discovery of the infectious nature of ringworm, it was Henle, the gifted anatomist, who proposed that infectious diseases might be directly caused by microorganisms. His considerations, however, were deficient in experimental data. One of Henle's students was Robert Koch, who became a famous physician and supplied all the evidence needed to prove further the "germ theory of disease," as formulated in the meantime by the great Pasteur and others.

PURE CULTURE STUDY AND THE ETIOLOGY OF INFECTIOUS DISEASES.   The development of methods for isolating bacteria in pure culture (see the following paragraph) was among the most important early advances in microbiological techniques and was largely the work of Robert Koch. A pure culture of microorganisms is one in which only one kind of organism is actively growing in test tubes, plates, or flasks on substances that are appropriate as food.[2] Under natural conditions many microorganisms of different species usually exist together in the same environment. In the feces of a typhoid patient, for example, there may be typhoid bacilli, but they are mixed with billions of cells of other species of bacteria and other forms of microorganisms. It is part of the work of the medical diagnostic microbiologist to isolate a pure culture of the typhoid bacillus from the feces of the patient.

In 1876 Koch isolated in "pure culture" the bacterium causing anthrax from the spleens of infected cattle and was able to infect mice with the culture. Previously, in 1850, C. J. Davaine had observed little threadlike bodies in the blood of animals that had died of anthrax.

Having become involved in questions concerning the true etiology of infectious diseases, Koch summarized what he believed to be the evidence necessary to prove an organism to be the cause of a disease. The evidence

[2]Such a nutrient preparation is called a *culture medium.*

consists of four postulates, generally called _Koch's postulates_. Essentially, they are as follows:

1. The organism must be found in all observed cases of a given disease in pathological relationship to its symptoms and lesions.

2. The organism must be isolated from these victims of the disease into pure culture for study in the laboratory.

3. When the pure culture is inoculated into a susceptible animal, possibly man, it must reproduce the disease or, as later modified, engender specific antibodies in the new host.

4. The organism must be isolated again into pure culture from such experimentally caused infections.

Using these rules and techniques, Koch discovered the tubercle bacillus, the cholera bacillus, and modes of transmissions of numerous other diseases. Discovery after discovery was made in Koch's laboratory by himself, his pupils, and his assistants, among them Gaffky, Kitasato, others shown in Figure 1–9, and also Ehrlich and von Behring.

The discoveries and work of van Leeuwenhoek, Pasteur, Koch, and many other dedicated pioneer investigators were the beginnings of the sciences of bacteriology and other areas of microbiology (mycology, virology, parasitology, immunology, and so forth) and they opened up a new world to preventive medicine (Fig. 1–9). Within the 15 years following 1880 the organisms causing many important infectious diseases were dis-

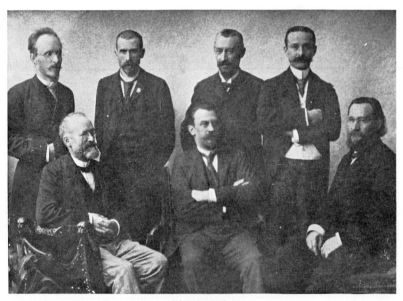

Figure 1–9

One of the groups of famous scientists who studied microbiology under Koch. Standing, left to right: Alphonse Laveran (1845–1922), discoverer of the malarial parasite; Émile Roux (1853–1933), codiscoverer of diphtheria toxin; Edmund Étienne Nocard (1850–1903), French veterinarian and mycologist; George H. F. Nuttall (1862–1937), British microbiologist. Sitting, left to right: Robert A. Koch (1843–1910), discoverer of the tubercle bacillus and pioneer microbiologist; Karl Joseph Eberth (?) (1835–1926), discoverer of the typhoid bacillus; Elie Metchnikoff (1845–1916), Russian zoologist and discoverer of phagocytes and phagocytosis. (Courtesy of Wiley A. Penn, Director of Laboratories, Department of Health, Savannah, Georgia.)

covered and isolated in pure cultures in which each could be studied as a single, living entity.

THE HEALTH PROFESSIONS AND EARLY MICROBIOLOGY. It is interesting to note the historical relationships between the health professions and the field of microbiology. Although nursing in some form has existed from the beginning of man's life on earth, the beginning of professional nursing is usually credited to Florence Nightingale (1820–1910), who began her work more than 100 years ago during the war in the Crimea (1854–1856). Microbiology was then in its infancy.

Subsequent discoveries concerning the relationships of microorganisms to disease necessitated the development of nursing procedures far more complex and refined than those used by "The Angel of the Crimea." In her time little was known about the transfer of infections from person to person. The development of aseptic surgery after Lister's discoveries (about 1865) opened the whole field of operating room technique to the surgeon and the professional nurse.

The earlier discovery of preventive measures such as smallpox vaccine (Edward Jenner, 1796), and later of diphtheria and tetanus toxoids and antitoxins, or immune sera (von Behring, Fränkel, and Kitasato, 1890) (Fig. 1–10), to say nothing of polio and measles vaccines (Enders, Weller, and Robbins, 1949; Salk, 1954; Sabin and others, 1954–1967), and gamma globulins[3] for prevention of measles, rabies, pertussis, and some other diseases has necessitated the development of new concepts and education in the principles of preparation of these substances and of procedures to administer them.

---

[3]Protective proteins (antibodies, Chapter 19) derived from the blood serum of immune persons or animals.

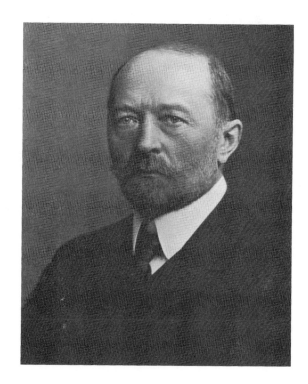

Figure 1–10

Emil von Behring (1854–1917), discoverer with Kitasato of tetanus toxin and of tetanus antitoxin. In emergency rooms 250 to 500 units of human hyperimmune tetanus gamma globulin are commonly used for prophylaxis after injury in nonimmunized persons. Hyperimmune human gamma globulin eliminates problems of hypersensitivity, it is retained longer and it is more effective than horse antitoxin for prophylaxis or treatment.

The discovery of diagnostic tests in the field of microbiology by hundreds of scientists has necessitated more advanced microbiologic training of medical technologists, doctors, nurses, and other health professionals in methods for collecting specimens and the importance of reporting specific laboratory findings immediately so that therapy can be started early. The discoveries of specific chemicals (chemotherapeutic agents such as sulfonamides) and antibiotic substances (such as penicillin, streptomycin, the tetracyclines, and chloramphenicol) have altered medical care and presented new problems and new opportunities for the health team.

Discoveries of means by which infections are transmitted led to the development of effective methods to prevent the spread of disease. For example, the transmission of some diseases through the bites of arthropods (insects, arachnids, and so forth) was demonstrated in 1893 by Theobald Smith in connection with Texas fever, a disease of cattle transmitted by ticks. In 1895, Sir Ronald Ross (1857–1932), an army physician in India, demonstrated the transmission of malarial protozoa by mosquitoes. The parasite had, however, been seen in human red blood cells as early as 1881 by Laveran (Fig. 1–9), a French army surgeon in Algeria. In 1900, the transmission of yellow fever virus by a particular species of mosquito (*Aedes aegypti*) was demonstrated in Cuba by Drs. Walter Reed (1851–1902), James Carroll (1854–1907), Aristides Agramonte (1868–1931), and Jesse Lazear (1866–1900) of the United States Army. The discoveries of the modes of transmission of malaria and yellow fever are among the most brilliant in medicine and have been epoch-making in their results.

THE HEALTH PROFESSIONS AND MODERN MICROBIOLOGY. Modern surgical procedures would be impossible without applications of principles of disinfection and sterilization. The present-day dairy, frozen and packaged food, and canning industries are dependent on the knowledge of microbiology. Sanitation of water supplies and reclamation of polluted waters (previously called sewage disposal) are possible only because of knowledge gained from microbiology in the past 100 years. The life span of man has been extended partly because of what is now known about prevention of deadly transmissible diseases. In many ways every health profession is dependent upon basic knowledge, understanding, and utilization of information from microbiology.

Thanks to the efforts of many scientists, the incidence of certain microbial diseases has been decreased. Only constant vigilance on the part of all members of the health professions, however, will continue this downward trend in preventable diseases. The registered medical technologist, the practicing physician, and the professional nurse need to apply knowledge from microbiology to the everyday practice of their profession. Although certain techniques and skills could be learned by rote, the truly professional person performs these techniques by use of knowledge and understanding of the underlying scientific facts and principles. This basic knowledge permits the professional person to make judgments and to function in aberrant situations. The person who has only technical competency, without knowledge of basic principles, cannot make these necessary judgments, but must mechanically follow procedures, without deviation, exactly as directed or taught him or her by others.

The well-qualified person has a fundamental knowledge of the principles of microbiology and knows what techniques must be used to protect all people from infectious diseases; what modifications need to be made for certain kinds of patients (e.g., patients who have had cardiac surgery, or patients with certain debilitating conditions); what techniques must be used in the operating room, the delivery room, and the nursery, and how these can be safely modified in emergency conditions (e.g., war or other disaster); and why patients, families, and the general public should be informed about immunizing agents that are available, such as polio vaccines.

A qualified member of the health team who is knowledgeable about microbiology can easily differentiate the truth from misinformation or misinterpretation of medical literature written for the laity and can recognize error in popularized versions of health practices that are widely circulated through mass communications of radio and television media, magazines, and daily newspapers.

As the health worker learns more about this profession, he or she will find that there is rarely a duty or act performed in ordinary living that does not involve knowledge of principles learned in the course in microbiology. The clever student soon realizes that the fundamental information in this course is essential to first-rate professional practice and the health of each individual, family and community.

Supplementary Reading

Asimov, A.: Asimov's Biographical Encyclopedia of Science and Technology. 1964, Garden City, Doubleday & Co., Inc.

Bulloch, W.: The History of Bacteriology. 1938, New York, Oxford University Press.

Demain, A. L.: Application of the microbe to the benefit of mankind: Challenges and opportunities. *Amer. Soc. Microbiol. News*, 1972, *38*:237.

Dobell, C.: Antonj van Leeuwenhoek and his Little Animals. 1958, New York, Russell & Russell Publishers.

Dolan J. A.: History of Nursing, 12th Ed. 1968, Philadelphia, W. B. Saunders Co.

Fox, S. W. (Editor): The Origins of Prebiological Systems and of Their Molecular Matrices. 1965, New York, Academic Press, Inc.

Kummel, B.: History of the Earth. 1961, San Francisco, W. H. Freeman & Co.

Lechevalier, H. A., and Solotorovsky, M.: Three Centuries of Microbiology. 1965, New York, McGraw-Hill Book Co., Inc.

Marquardt, M.: Paul Ehrlich. 1951, New York, Henry Schuman, Inc.

Microbiology Training Committee (R. D. DeMoss, Chairman): Microbiology for the future. *Amer. Soc. Microbiol. News*, 1972, *38*:33.

Newerla, G. J.: Medical History in Philately. 1964, Milwaukee, Wisconsin, American Topical Association, Publisher.

Raff, R. A., and Mahler, H. R.: The non symbiotic origin of mitochondria. *Science*, 1972, *177*:575.

Schierbeek, A., and Swart, J. J.: The Collected Letters of Antonj van Leeuwenhoek. 1961, Amsterdam, The Netherlands, Swets & Zeitlinger.

Stewart, I. M., and Austin, A. L.: A History of Nursing from Ancient to Modern Times: A World View. 5th Ed. 1962, New York, G. P. Putnam's Sons.

Vallery-Radot, R.: The Life of Pasteur. 1926, New York, Doubleday-Doran & Co.

General Classification of Microorganisms; Cells and Cell Structures

2

GENERAL INTRODUCTION

Microorganisms may be found in four groups of living forms: algae, protozoa, fungi, and viruses. To many biologists it is quite clear that in the two kingdoms, animals and plants, the bacteria, other fungi (molds), and the algae, belong to the plants, while protozoa (primitive animals) obviously are in the animal kingdom. Because there are many organisms that are not so "obviously" either protozoa (animals) or algae (plants) the trend is now again to place all unicellular organisms in a third kingdom, the Protista as suggested by Haeckel in 1868. (See also Fig. 2–1.)

The principal[1] groups that contain *unicellular* organisms may be listed as follows:

1. Algae—green or blue-green plants: various seaweeds, many microscopic species.
2. Protozoa[2]—microscopic animals: amebas, malarial parasites, and so forth.
3. Fungi—true fungi or Eumycetes: yeasts, molds, "mushrooms," and so forth.

> Fission fungi or Schizomycetes (the bacteria), including rickettsias[3] (cause of Rocky Mountain spotted fever and other diseases); chlamydias[4] or PLT group (causes of trachoma; psittacosis or "parrot fever"; lymphogranuloma venereum, a venereal disease; inclusion blennorrhea); the pleuropneumonia-like organisms[5] or PPLO (causes of respiratory and other diseases).

---

[1]A few microscopic, multicellular animals of medical importance, e.g., certain parasitic worms (microfilarias), are not listed here (Chapter 40).

[2]*Protos* is a Greek root meaning primitive; *zoa* is from the Greek *zoon*, for animal.

[3]A group of microorganisms named for their discoverer, James Howard Ricketts (Chapter 5).

[4]From the Greek *chlamys*, meaning a cloak or mantle. They were formerly thought of as "mantle viruses."

[5]Pleuropneumonia is a disease of cattle caused by one member of this group of microorganisms (Chapter 4).

16

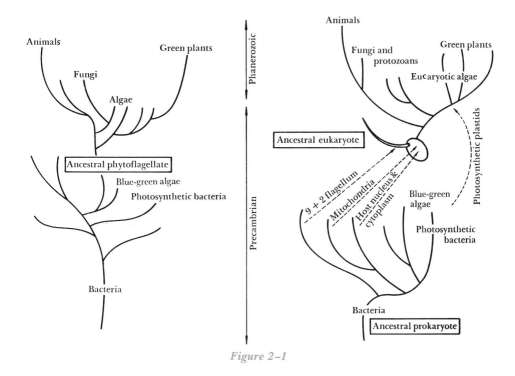

Figure 2-1

Comparison between the classic (*left*) and symbiotic (*right*) views of the evolution of plant and animal cells. The cell symbiosis theory holds that a primitive ameboflagellate, a heterotrophic cell, is ancestral to all eucaryotes: fungi, animals, nucleated algae, and higher plants. The photosynthetic blue-green algae symbionts became the plastids of algae and higher plants. Ancestral heterotrophs formed as a product of intracellular symbiosis; thus mitochondria-containing ameboflagellates developed in which mitosis and eventually meiosis evolved. Thus, according to this hypothesis, all organisms that contain mitochondria came from this organism. (Based on an article by Margulis, L.: The origin of plant and animal cells. *American Scientist*, 59:231, 1971.) See also alternate theory on page 6.

The chlamydias, rickettsias, and PPLO (*pleural pneumonia organisms*) were formerly listed as separate groups but are now regarded as modified forms of bacteria, having many structures and properties in common with typical bacteria.

    4. Viruses[6] — unclassified: neither cells in the general sense, nor alive as life is commonly defined (causes of poliomyelitis, influenza, measles, and other diseases).

Algae are green plants and *require sunlight* for growth. None is *pathogenic*[7] for man. Groups 2, 3, and 4, none of which requires sunlight for growth, contain pathogenic microorganisms and hence are of interest to the health profession. For convenience we shall give a brief general description of each main group and then turn especially to the bacteria for detailed discussion, not because they are most important but because they furnish convenient working material and are good illustrations of general

---

    [6]*Virus* is derived from a Latin root meaning "slimy substance" or poison (Chapter 6).

    [7]*Pathos* is Greek for sadness or pain; *genic* is from a Greek word meaning to produce or cause. Hence any agent, living or not, that produces pain or disease is said to be pathogenic.

Table 2–1. Characteristics of Major Groups of Microorganisms[1]

GREEN ALGAE	PROTOZOA	MOLDS AND YEASTS (EUMYCETES)	BACTERIA[7] (SCHIZOMYCETES)
Require sunlight; grow on lifeless media.	Grow in dark; some on lifeless media.	Grow in dark on lifeless media.	Grow in dark on lifeless media.
Multiply by fission and sexually.	Multiply by binary fission[2] and sexual means.	Multiply by budding,[4] conidia,[4] and sexually.	Multiply principally by binary fission.
Much larger than bacteria.	Much larger than bacteria; in volume usually hundreds to thousands of times greater.	Size much greater than bacteria—filaments and other structures often macroscopic.	Round forms do not exceed about 5 micrometers,[5] usually not over 2 to 3 μm in diameter; rod forms commonly 2 μm in diameter and 10 μm in length. Some curved species may exceed 500 μm in length but not over 1 to 2 μm in diameter.
Do not pass filters.	Do not pass filters.[3]	Do not pass filters.	Generally cannot pass filters.
Cell structure like higher plants.	Internal cell structures well developed; nucleus, vacuoles, "mouth" opening, etc.	Cell structure, especially nuclei, visible with ordinary microscopes.	No definite organs in the cell visible with ordinary microscopes. Granules, spores, capsules visible.[6]
Cannot ingest solid particles.	Can ingest solid particles (except a few parasitic forms).	Cannot ingest solid particles.	Cannot ingest solid particles.
Cellular.	Cellular.	Cellular.	Cellular.

[1] Not including helminths. Also not included: Slime molds, the symbiotic fungal-algal plant forms called lichens, rusts, smuts, mosses, perhaps even liverworts, and mushrooms.

[2] Multiplication by *binary fission* means that the cell divides into two new individuals (daughter cells), each sharing approximately equally genetic parts of the "parent" cell. Sex is not involved; hence multiplication by binary fission is asexual. In the process of budding, most yeasts divide into two or more unequal parts. This is not binary fission.

[3] *Filters* in this sense mean unglazed porcelain, clay, paper, or other fine-pored materials that permit the passage only of fluid and of microorganisms much smaller than algae, protozoa, yeasts, molds, or rickettsias. With a few exceptions (see PPLO), among microorganisms only viruses can pass through such filters.

[4] *Budding* and *conidia* formations are types of asexual multiplication in which daughter cells grow out from the parent cells like a bud or branch from a tree. Many buds may occur on a single parent cell. Each later becomes a complete, independent cell.

[5] Micrometer (μm) is a unit of length commonly used in microscopy. It is 1/25,400 (0.000,039) of an inch, 10^{-6} meter, or 0.0001 of a centimeter. The following line is 1 centimeter (cm.) in length: ——— (see page 22).

[6] For definitions of these structures see more detailed description of bacteria (Chapter 7).

[7] Not including blue-green algae, which are sometimes classed as blue-green bacteria (see Appendix A).

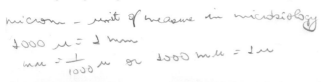

Table 2–2. Characteristics of Generally Smaller Forms of Microorganisms than Those Listed in Table 2–1

L FORMS OF BACTERIA	MYCOPLASMAS[1]	RICKETTSIAS AND CHLAMYDIAS	VIRUSES
Grow on lifeless media; their development from bacteria is promoted by high salt concentration or toxic agents, especially penicillin; they are pleomorphic forms of bacteria; some revert easily to the bacterial form while others do not.	Grow on lifeless media or on chick embryos or in tissue culture.	Grow only inside living cells.	Grow only inside living cells.
L forms are larger than mycoplasmas.	Multiply by modified form of bacteria-like fission and subdivision.	Method of multiplication probably binary fission.	Method of multiplication "biosynthetic."
L forms do not form a rigid mucopeptide cell wall, but they do contain DNA and carry on metabolism.	Highly pleomorphic; limp, fragile cell membrane; produce very minute forms that can pass bacteria-retaining filters. They are the smallest "free-living" cells.	Much smaller than bacteria. Rickettsias have rod, spherical, and spiral cells.	Extremely minute. Not visible with ordinary microscopes. By electron microscope some are seen to have a concentric, spherical, helical, cuboidal, or "tadpole" form.[2]
	Internal structure similar to bacteria; no cell wall.	One species of rickettsias can pass bacterial filters; chlamydias pass with difficulty, if at all.	Pass bacterial filters.
	Mode of nutrition includes serum (for plasma proteins) and often a steroid. They resemble bacteria without cell walls.	No definite internal structures visible with ordinary microscopes. Electron microscope reveals bacteria-like internal structure.	No internal structures visible with ordinary microscopes.
		Mode of nutrition like bacteria in some respects; dependent on certain enzymes of host cell.	Depend on genetically directed alterations of synthetic mechanisms, and use of genetic materials, of host cell.
Cellular.	Cellular.	Cellular.	Noncellular.

(handwritten annotation: an obligate parasite) grow only in living cells, don't grow on agar, etc

[1] Also called pleuropneumonia-like organisms (PPLO).
[2] Most of our first knowledge about viruses comes from studies with bacteriophage. special types of virus pathogenic in bacteria.

principles underlying the whole science of microbiology. Some general characteristics and relationships of microorganisms are seen in Table 2–1. This listing is continued in Table 2–2 for those organisms that are smaller than the bacteria (Schizomycetes). If all of the Protista are listed in order of relative size, the following approximation of a size relationship results:

protozoa > algae > yeasts and molds > bacteria > L forms > mycoplasmas > rickettsias > chlamydias > viruses.

However the student is warned not to regard this listing as an absolute fact. Many algae are much, much longer than some protozoa, while mycoplasmas may be as small as viruses or as large as bacteria.

UNICELLULAR ORGANISMS

With the exception of viruses, which have only a few of the fundamental properties of living matter, all living things, including ourselves, consist of living cells. Large animals and plants consist of billions of microscopic cells. These are differentiated into integrated systems of organs, such as liver and muscle in many-celled animals or *metazoa*, and into leaves, flowers, and stems in many-celled plants, or *metaphyta*. Each unicellular organism consists of a single microscopic cell. In a few species the cells form loose aggregates, but with a few possible exceptions among primitive animals, or *protozoa*, each cell is a complete organism and alone can reproduce the entire structure.

The Cell

The cell is the smallest and simplest unit of living matter capable of independent life and self-reproduction. Exceptions are seen in the modified smaller forms of bacteria now classified as chlamydias and rickettsias; these can reproduce only as intracellular parasites. Viruses are much smaller units, but they are not cells as currently defined, and so far as is known, they are incapable of independent life or reproduction. Cells vary in size, structure, and physiology according to their species (Fig. 2–2). The human body is made up of billions and billions of different tissue cells: liver cells differ from muscle cells, nerve cells differ from pancreatic cells and from bone cells, and so on. Basically, however, all cells are similar. Whether animal, vegetable, or protist, they *all* possess numerous structures and properties in common. The reader should not be misled and think of animal or plant cells when talking about bacteria. A drawing of a typical bacterial cell is shown in Figure 2–3.

PROTOPLASM.   The word is derived from the Greek *protos*, for first, original, or ancestral, and *plasma*, for substance. Before the advent of high-power microscopes protoplasm was thought to be the first and only known living substance, animal or vegetable. Thomas Huxley (1825–1895) called protoplasm "the physical basis of life." The term protoplasm, as the name of a single substance, is now obsolete. As seen with low-power lenses, "protoplasm," i.e., the contents of any living cell, appears to be watery, transparent, usually colorless, and very much like the raw white of an egg. When analyzed chemically, it is found to consist largely of carbon, oxygen,

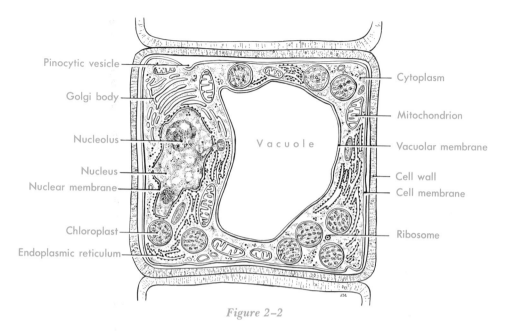

Figure 2–2

Diagram of a eucaryotic plant cell based on various cytological studies and use of the electron microscope. The *nucleus* controls hereditary properties and all other vital activities of the cell. Both nucleus and *nucleolus* have functions in the synthesis of cell material. The well-defined *nuclear membrane* appears to have pores or openings for communication with the cytoplasmic structures and direction of their synthetic and energy-yielding activities. The *cytoplasm* contains immense numbers of granules called *ribosomes*, concentrated especially along the periphery of a cell-wide labyrinth of connected, narrow sacs called the *endoplasmic reticulum*. These granules are involved in the continuous enzymic reactions which synthesize cell materials under direction from the nucleus. The *mitochondria* are involved in another set of enzymic reactions called *biological oxidation*, which yield the energy for all the cell activities. The *pinocytic vesicle* or invagination is a means of ingesting fluids or extremely minute food particles. *Golgi bodies* comprise an apparatus that may secrete the cellulose that in plants forms the thick, nonliving *cell wall*. This wall supports the plant body and is penetrated by many tiny holes that permit passage of materials between cells. Inside the cell wall is the *cell membrane*, or plasma membrane, a very thin structure that functions as a regulatory apparatus for the nutrients and waste products that must pass through it. *Chloroplasts* are the small bodies, typically disk-shaped, that contain the chlorophyll which imparts the color in green plants and participates in photosynthesis. *Vacuoles*, common in cells of plants and lower animals but rare in cells of higher animals, are bubble-like cavities filled with watery liquid and bordered by a thin vacuolar membrane. There are undoubtedly still other structures whose nature and function await elucidation by future cytological studies. Compare this complex cell with pictures of bacterial cells shown in this chapter and others. (From Villee, C. A.: Biology. 6th Ed. Philadelphia, W. B. Saunders Co., 1972.)

hydrogen, sulfur, phosphorus, and nitrogen. Many other elements, e.g., iron, sodium, chlorine, and magnesium, are usually present in smaller amounts.

Studies using the compound microscope, with ordinary (visible) light, and using the electron microscope, have revealed that, far from being a single "living distinct substance," protoplasm consists of many distinct submicroscopic bodies called *organelles* in a somewhat viscous matrix. In a typical animal or plant cell, organelles include: nucleus, mitochondria, chloroplasts, endoplasmic reticulum, ribosomes, and numerous other structures (Fig. 2–2).

The term protoplasm is sometimes used to mean "cell contents."

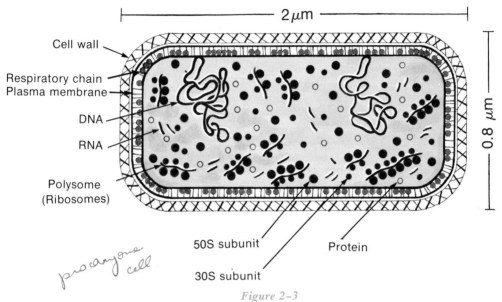

Cell wall

Respiratory chain
Plasma membrane

DNA

RNA

Polysome
(Ribosomes)

2 μm

0.8 μm

50S subunit   Protein

30S subunit

procaryone cell

Figure 2–3

Diagram of an *E. coli* cell containing two chromosomes 1 mm long (10^7 Å) attached to the cell membrane. 50S and 30S refer to ribosomal subunits of different molecular weights that can be separated on the basis of their sedimentation(s) coefficient. (From DeRobertis, Nowinski and Saez: Cell Biology. 5th Ed. Philadelphia, W. B. Saunders Company, 1970.)

Cell Structure

It might be imagined that since the contents of all living cells consist of a colloidal watery complex such as we have described, the cells, and tissues made of cells, would collapse, drain away, or dry up. How do living organisms maintain their shape and keep from being dissolved? It was discovered in 1838 by Schleiden and Schwann, German scientists, that the "watery" machinery of life ("protoplasm") is contained in tiny sacs or chambers called cells. The protoplasm of each cell forms its own self-containing cell membrane and, if a plant cell, a rigid cell wall. The entire structure, i.e., cell wall plus cell membrane and contents, and any external appendages such as flagella, pili, and capsules, are now generally included in the term cell.

Most cells are extremely minute (of the order of 1 to 20 μm in diameter[8]), and many millions of them are required to form so small an animal

[8] 1 μm = 0.001 millimeter or 1/25,400 or 3.937×10^{-5} inch.

A system of nomenclature for metric units now used by many microbiologists and the American Society for Microbiology follows:

m = *milli* = 0.001 = 10^{-3} meter or gram or ml (thousandth)
μ = *micro* = 0.000,001 = 10^{-6} meter or gram or ml (millionth)
n = *nano* = 0.000,000,001 = 10^{-9} meter or gram or ml (billionth)
p = *pico* = 0.000,000,000,001 = 10^{-12} meter or gram or ml (trillionth)
For example:
mm = millimeter = 10^{-3} meter (= 10^7 Å)
μm = micrometer = 10^{-6} meter (formerly, μ = micron)
nm = nanometer = 10^{-9} meter (formerly, millimicron = mμ)
Å = Angstrom = 10^{-10} meter (= 0.1 nm; 10 Å = 1 nm)
pm = picometer = 10^{-12} meter (formerly, micromicron = μμ)
pg = picogram = 10^{-12} g
ppm = μg/cc (ml); μg/g; 10^{-6} g/g or cc (ml)

as a flea. Cells vary greatly in size, however, and some are several inches in diameter. For example, all eggs are single cells. An ostrich egg is certainly far from microscopic, although it might be objected that much of the egg is reserve food substance and is not properly part of the actual microscopic reproductive cell itself. Some cells, such as nerve cells, may have portions several inches in length, although these filaments may be of microscopic fineness.

CELL MEMBRANE AND CELL WALL. The immediate covering of the "protoplasm" of each cell is a *cell* (or *cytoplasmic*) *membrane*, a thin, limp sac. The electron microscope shows it to consist of several layers and various minute granules and molecular aggregations that are absolutely essential to the life of the cell. This constitutes the external surface of most animal cells and also of PPLO.

In most "plant" cells, including algae, yeasts, molds, and bacteria (except PPLO), there is also a more or less rigid outer *cell wall*, which protects and supports the cell membrane and consists of a hard or tough substance formed by the cell. *Cellulose*, common in all familiar plants, is such a substance. A good example of cellulose structure is wood, which consists of a mass of microscopic cellulose chambers, each containing protoplasm. Another hard substance found in cell walls of many animals and a few eucaryotic plants (Eumycetes) is *chitin*. Examples of other structures made of chitin are the shells of insects, crabs, and lobsters. In bacteria the cell wall contains tough substances called *mucopolysaccharides* or oligosaccharides. Other constituents in bacterial cell walls, called *mucopeptides*, contain glucosamine and muramic acid. There are also teichoic acids, which are phosphate polymers of a rather complex nature. These are not entirely restricted to the cell wall but occur also between the cell wall and cell membrane.

NUCLEUS. A typical cell contains a definite organelle, usually situated near the center, which is called the *nucleus*. It is a very important part of the cell, since without it the cell soon dies. On the other hand, the nucleus may live by itself for some time. Indeed, there are some cells, e.g., spermatozoa, that appear to consist almost entirely of nuclear material. The nucleus is the center and controlling agency in all vital functions of the cell, and it takes a leading part in the processes of its reproduction and inheritance.

Eucaryon and Procaryon. On the basis of nuclear structure all cells, whether of animals or plants or protists, unicellular or multicellular, are divided into two great groups: eucaryons (Gr. *eu* = true; *karyon* = kernel) and procaryons (Gr. *pro* = primitive).

The nucleus of eucaryotic cells is enclosed within a true, morphologically distinct nuclear membrane that segregates the nuclear genetic material (DNA, see the following section) from the surrounding cytoplasm. During cell division or multiplication, sexual or asexual, the genetic material of the eucaryotic cell undergoes a series of striking morphologic changes involving the appearance of rodlike chromosomes and the phenomena of mitosis and, in sex cells, meiosis.[9]

---

[9]Actually, there are two other types of eucaryotic distinctions of cells, based on nuclear structure: the heterocaryons and the homocaryons. The heterocaryons are exemplified by a condition in fungi in which protoplasm and nuclei flow freely from cell to cell through the structure of the organism called the mycelium, and even occur in the spores. The result is that if more than one strain are growing in a flask, the different nuclei mix freely and express their genetic influence in all cells. In the homocaryon only one type of nucleus is present, although in the fungi one may still find four nuclei in one cell, two in another, and perhaps none in the third, at a specific moment.

The nucleus of typical procaryotic cells consists of a single, very long, circular, threadlike molecule of DNA that is not enclosed in a membrane, is not segregated from the surrounding cytoplasmic material and never manifests any mitotic or meiotic phenomena. The procaryotic nucleus is, therefore, commonly referred to as *nucleoid* (nucleus-like).

There are also numerous striking differences between eucaryotic and procaryotic cytoplasms. The cytoplasm of eucaryons contains numerous discrete, membranous and membrane-enclosed functional bodies (*organelles*) (Fig. 2-2). The cytoplasm of procaryons contains principally ribosomes; other functional portions, except certain curious membranes, are missing, obscure, or very primitive.

Knowledge of the differentiation between procaryons and eucaryons is important because these differences underlie many of the distinctive properties of the various microorganisms in relation to disease and its diagnosis, treatment, and prevention.

All animal cells and all "higher" plant cells are eucaryotic. The following are procaryotic:

1. Blue-green algae (Cyanophyceae).
2. Bacteria (Schizomycetes) including rickettsias, chlamydias, and mycoplasmas as described in following chapters.
3. Viruses, which are included here for convenience, though they are not truly alive or cells and therefore are neither eucaryotic or procaryotic.

The true molds and yeasts (Eumycetes) and protozoa described in this book are all eucaryotic organisms. Eucaryotic organisms, from protozoa to humans, are commonly referred to as more highly evolved organisms; the procaryons are less highly evolved organisms.

For years it has been thought by many microbiologists that certain eucaryotic organelles may have evolved from phagocytized, free-living, procaryotic organisms. Like these primitive cells, the mitochondria and the photosynthetic plastids of eucaryotic cells perform metabolic functions, have their own nucleic acids, and synthesize their own protein components. Certainly the influence of the nucleus may not be overlooked, but the Precambrian ancestors (primitive bacteria, perhaps) of these ingested cell organelles must have required at least a billion years to become true endosymbionts. A more recent and equally plausible theory is mentioned on pages 6 and 17.

Deoxyribonucleic Acid (DNA) and Ribonucleic Acid (RNA). These occur in all typical cells. The most important nuclear material is deoxyribonucleic acid (DNA). This determines the hereditable characters and the entire makeup and functioning of the cell. DNA is chemically very complex and is formed into long double-spiral strands or helices (Fig. 2-4). These strands are composed of regularly repeated molecular groupings called *nucleotides*, arranged in certain patterns. DNA contains D-2-deoxyribose (called simply deoxyribose), the purines adenine (A) and guanine (G), the pyrimidines cytosine (C) and thymine (T), and also phosphate. DNA extracted from cells by chemical means contains approximately 10,000 paired deoxynucleotide units on each strand. The nature and arrangement of these nucleotides determine hereditary characters. In some viruses the strands are single.

The chemical components of RNA nucleotides are D-ribose, the purines adenine (A) and guanine (G), the pyrimidines cytosine (C) and uracil

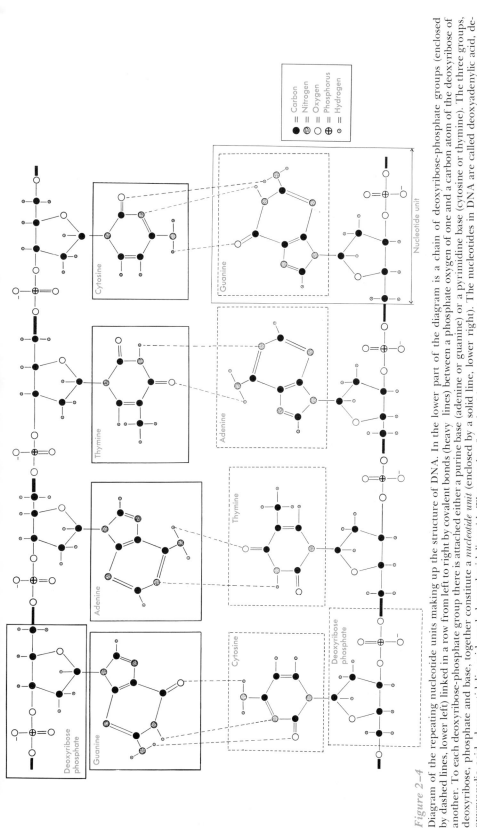

Figure 2–4

Diagram of the repeating nucleotide units making up the structure of DNA. In the lower part of the diagram is a chain of deoxyribose-phosphate groups (enclosed by dashed lines, lower left) linked in a row from left to right by covalent bonds (heavy lines) between a phosphate oxygen of one and a carbon atom of the deoxyribose of another. To each deoxyribose-phosphate group there is attached either a purine base (adenine or guanine) or a pyrimidine base (cytosine or thymine). The three groups, deoxyribose, phosphate and base, together constitute a *nucleotide unit* (enclosed by a solid line, lower right). The nucleotides in DNA are called deoxyadenylic acid, deoxyguanylic acid, deoxycytidylic acid, and deoxythmidylic acid. Thousands of nucleotide units are linked together, in varying sequences, in long twisted filaments of nucleic acid.

In the upper half of the diagram is a chain of nucleotide units corresponding to the lower half of the diagram but inverted. The upper chain is connected to the lower chain by hydrogen bonds (dashed lines) between the purine and pyrimidine bases as shown. Note that adenine always pairs with thymine, and guanine with cytosine. In DNA the two interconnected chains are commonly twisted together in a double helix. However, single-stranded DNA is known to occur in some viruses. In RNA there is commonly only a single strand. However, under some conditions of cell or virus reproduction double-stranded RNA has been observed.

25

(U), and phosphate, which links them together. In some viruses the sugar D-glucose may replace deoxyribose and 5-hydroxymethylcytosine may be present instead of cytosine. Cytosine may also be missing in some species that contain 5-methylcytosine. The genetic material of viruses may contain DNA or RNA, never (or very rarely) both.

Each hereditary character is associated with a particular segment of the long DNA (or RNA in some viruses) molecule. Such a segment may consist of (rarely) one to (commonly) hundreds of nucleotides. Each such segment constitutes a gene or genetic determinant. Any alteration in a gene produces a hereditary change in the organism of which the gene is a part. This change is called a *genetic mutation.* Such mutations are often produced by x-rays, ultraviolet light, atomic bomb radiations, various chemicals, and possibly by some viruses. The smallest unit of DNA subject to such mutation is spoken of as a *muton,* a nucleotide base pair.

In the nucleus of most cells, genes are arranged as long, microscopically visible threads called *chromosomes.* The supporting structure of a eucaryotic chromosome consists of basic nuclear proteins (usually protamine or histone) on which the DNA-containing genes are arranged. During asexual reproduction of cells the chromosomes replicate themselves and are divided between the daughter cells. In eucaryons this is accomplished by a process called *mitosis.* When eucaryotic sexual cells are formed, the maternal and paternal chromosomes in each cell combine, replicate, divide, and are redistributed to the sex cells in a complex process of cell division called *meiosis.* True sexual cells (gametes) do not occur in procaryons, though a primitive form of conjugation between certain cells of some species of bacteria is observed. Often genes are very closely linked on the same chromosome to neighbor genes, each of which produces almost identical phenotypic effects in the organism. For example, in a virus called T4 at least 40 such genes, also called *cistrons,* have been described. Although many microbiologists use the terms gene and cistron interchangeably, actually cistron should be used only to describe genetic material when applied to *complementation analysis,* a genetic method of studying hereditary DNA arrangement on the chromosome.

Nucleotides are adenine deoxyribose phosphate, guanine deoxyribose phosphate, cytosine deoxyribose phosphate, or thymine deoxyribose phosphate (see Fig. 2–4). The deoxyribonucleotide adenine deoxyribose phosphate also exists as deoxyadenosine-3'-monophosphate or as deoxyadenosine-5'-monophosphate, and so on. If any mutational structural change occurs in a single nucleotide pair, out of many thousands of polydeoxyribonucleotides within a single gene, the mutational unit may be referred to as a *muton.* When nucleotide pairs are involved in genetic recombination each single nucleotide acts as a recombination unit. This smallest unit, not divisible by recombination, is called a *recon.* As will be shown, a virus particle (called a *virion*) consists of a single molecule of NA coated with protein. Thus, a virus particle in many ways resembles an independently existing chromosome. In some viruses RNA is the genetic material, in place of DNA. The difference is that in DNA viruses one finds deoxyribose and thymine, whereas RNA viruses contain ribose and uridine. The other nitrogen bases are identical in both types of viruses.

The linear sequence of nucleotides in the double-helix DNA (Fig. 2–5) of the genes is exactly copied prior to cell division. The nucleotide DNA order template is also transmitted via the enzyme RNA polymerase

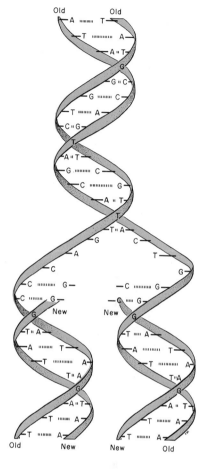

Figure 2–5

Diagram illustrating the semiconservative replication of DNA by a process involving the separation of the original base pairs and the unwinding of the two strands of the helix. Each strand then serves as a template for the synthesis of a new complementary strand. (From Villee, C. A.: Biology, 5th ed. W. B. Saunders Co., Philadelphia.)

to messenger RNA (mRNA). At least three other RNA types have been recognized to exist besides mRNA; they are nuclear RNA, also part of the chromosomes, soluble or transfer RNA (sRNA or tRNA), and ribosomal RNA (rRNA). By means of a complex mechanism RNA is then involved to transmit the message or *code* to ribosomes and to determine the order of amino acids that make up the enzymes of the cell. Thus the linear sequence of amino acids in the proteins (enzymes) synthesized in the cytoplasm is related directly to the linear sequences of nucleotides in the mRNA as copied from the DNA. The triplet code letters in messenger RNA have been determined with some certainty for all amino acids found in proteins. However, a specific amino acid may be linked to another specific amino acid not only by one set of code directions but perhaps by several. For example, Table 2–3 shows that alanine may be attached to a polypeptide under the direction of GCU, GCC, GCA, or GCG. The sequences of amino acids in the polypeptide repeating units (amino acids) of enzymes, arranged by mRNA according to the nucleotide sequence of the chromosomal DNA, determine whether a protein formed by a ribosome shall be a dehydrogenase, viral or other protein, or some other substance, or it may perhaps determine the quality of a beefsteak. We

Table 2–3.   Genetic Code*

[The nucleotide compositions of RNA codewords have been obtained by directing amino acids into protein in *Escherichia coli* extracts with randomly ordered polyribonucleotides synthesized with polynucleotide phosphorylase. Nucleotide sequence in codewords is not known; thus the order of bases is arbitrary. The tentative summary of RNA codewords shown in the table is considered to be *potential* codewords; that is, they code for amino acids in cell-free systems, but all codewords may not be applicable to cells in vivo. The genetic code may be regarded as quite universal in the sense that messenger RNA codons, when translated, are usually translated into the same amino acids in all organisms that have been examined. This applies to *E. coli*, human hemoglobin, bacteriophage T4, tobacco mosaic virus, yeast, *Neurospora*, and others.]

AMINO ACID		RNA CODEWORDS*				
1 Alanine	GCU	GCC	GCA	GCG		
2 Arginine	CGC	CGU	CGA	CGG	AGA	AGG
3 Asparagine	AAU	AAC				
4 Aspartic acid	GAU	GAC				
5 Cysteine	UGU	UGC				
6 Glutamic acid	GAA	GAG				
7 Glutamine	CAG	CAA				
8 Glycine	GGU	GGC	GGA	GGG		
9 Histidine	CAC	CAA				
10 Isoleucine	AUU	AUC	AUA			
11 Leucine	UUG	UUA	CUU	CUC	CUA	CUG
12 Lysine	AAA	AAG				
13 Methionine	AUG**					
14 Phenylalanine	UUU	UUC				
15 Proline	CCC	CCU	CCA	CCG		
16 Serine	UCU	UCC	UCG	UCA	AGU	AGC
17 Threonine	ACU	ACC	ACA	ACG		
18 Tryptophan	UGG					
19 Tyrosine	UAU	UAC				
20 Valine	GUU	GUC	GUA	GUG**		
CHAIN TERMINATION	UAA	UAG	UGA			

*The code triplets account for all 64 possible combinations (codons), as based on data presented by Jukes, T. H., and Gatlin, L.: Recent Studies Concerning the Coding Mechanism. Progress in Nucleic Acid Research and Molecular Biology, Vol. 11, 1971, Academic Press, New York.

This amino acid code was almost determined as shown here in Braun, W.: Bacterial Genetics, 2nd Ed. 1965, Philadelphia, W. B. Saunders Co.

**Starts the synthesis of a polypeptide chain ("initiator codons").

may think of some mutations as the result of one or more changes in the DNA structure such that a "nonsense" protein or enzyme is produced that has no biologic function. In some experiments certain nucleotide sequences, e.g., UAA, UGA, and UAG, have been shown to eliminate certain amino acids, create a gap rather than adding any known amino acid to a peptide chain. We may thus think of UAA, UGA, or UAG as determining the punctuation of the code rather than being part of the code itself.

Actually, there is no direct biochemical relationship between a codon[10] in mRNA and the amino acid that it specifies. The message is transmitted from mRNA to the anticodon of three consecutive nucleotides in a molecule of tRNA and then the specific amino acid is selected to be added to the peptide chain.

[10] A codon is the triplet code, like GCU, GCC, GCG, etc.

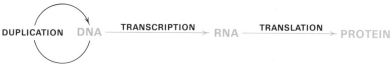

Figure 2–6

Flow of information from the genome. (From Ideas In Modern Biology. Proceedings Vol. 6, XVI International Congress of Zoology, The Natural History Press, 1965.)

A simplified version of how the genome of microorganisms duplicates itself is shown in Fig. 2–6. DNA sends the message by transcription via RNA, and translation of the code to protein which, as the enzyme, carries out the work the microorganism needs for its life processes.

THE NUCLEOLUS.   This is a spherical body inside the nucleus of eucaryotic cells. It consists only of nucleoprotein containing RNA. The nucleolus appears to play a role in protein synthesis within cells where it occurs.

Recently a new type of RNA has been discovered. It represents more than 75 per cent of the RNA synthesis of the cell and may be the precursor

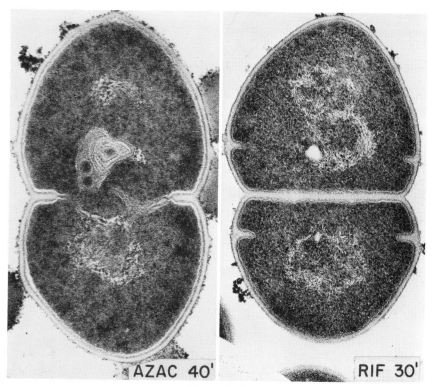

Figure 2–7

Electron micrographs of *Streptococcus faecalis* duplicating itself. *Left,* Nuclear material can be seen in the cell (treated with 5-azacytidine), before the septum has formed between the two daughter cells. *Right,* Nuclear material is also seen in the two cells (treated with the antibiotic rifampin) at the beginning of the four-cell stage. (Courtesy L. Daneo-Moore and M. L. Higgins: J. Bacteriol., 1972, *109*:1210.)

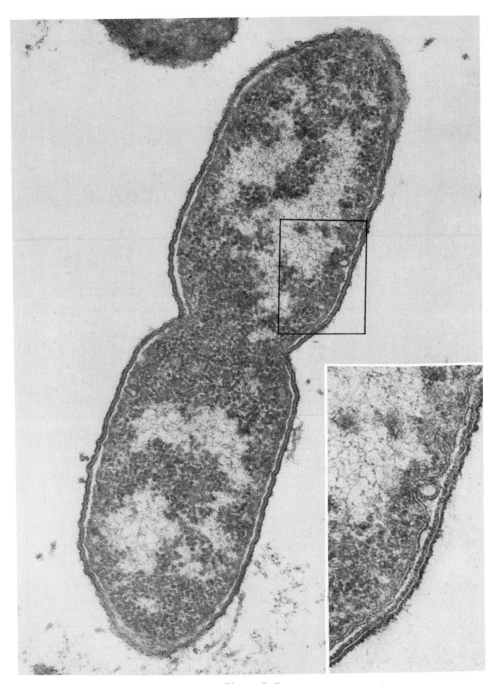

Figure 2–8

Electron micrograph of the bacillus *Erwinia amylovora*. The cell, fixed at room temperature, shows the double-track structure of the cell wall. The markers indicate 0.1 μm on the micrograph. (Courtesy of P. Huang and R. N. Goodman.: J. Bacteriol. 1971, *107*:361.)

of "true" messenger RNA; it has escaped detection because it is very unstable. Other RNA species with as much as 80 per cent adenine (the purine in DNA and RNA) have also been found. Their functions are at present unknown.[11]

CENTROSOME. This is a small condensed structure containing some DNA, usually located near the nucleus of eucaryotic cells and having a function that is associated with the process of cell division.

CYTOPLASM. The remainder of the protoplasm is called the *cytoplasm*. The cytoplasm of a living cell consists of all the portion enclosed within the cell membrane (cytoplasmic membrane) except the nucleus. The cytoplasm may contain many food particles (for example, fat, starch, and sulfur), pigment granules, and special protein and vitamin complexes (coenzymes) with various functions related to digestion and reproduction.

The cytoplasm of eucaryotic cells contains such structures as mitochondria, the sites of respiration; endoplasmic reticulum supporting millions of ribosomes, the sites of protein synthesis; Golgi bodies, the sites of secretion synthesis; lysosomes, sacs of digestive enzymes; chloroplasts, sites of photosynthesis; and other structures and organelles that may be seen and studied with special microscopic techniques, especially electron microscopes.

As previously mentioned, procaryotic (especially bacterial) cytoplasm contains chiefly ribosomes, possibly attached to membranous materials (Fig. 2–7). In photosynthetic species there are also *chromatophores* that contain the photosynthetic pigments bacteriochlorophyll and chlorobium chlorophyll. The procaryotic cytoplasm seems very sparsely furnished (Fig. 2–8).

HABITAT AND MODE OF LIFE

Unicellular, or single-celled, microorganisms of one type or another are found almost everywhere on the surface of the earth. Some live deep in the sea; others inhabit pools of stagnant water; and still others can exist only in the soil or in the blood or feces of various animals. The entire life work of unicellular organisms, whether plant or animal or bacterial, consists of feeding, excreting waste products, and multiplying. Their physiology is, therefore, relatively simple, although, strangely enough, the biochemistry[12] and mode of living and reproduction of all cells are remarkably alike and are obviously mere modifications of a single basic design, like different makes of automobiles.

---

[11] Bernhard, R.: Verdict of cancer meeting: information too sketchy. *Sci. Res.*, 1968, pp. 47–52, April 29.
[12] The chemistry of life.

Supplementary Reading

Braun, W.: Bacterial Genetics. 2nd Ed. 1965, Philadelphia, W. B. Saunders Co.
Cantarow, A., and Schepartz, B.: Biochemistry. 4th Ed. 1967, Philadelphia, W. B. Saunders Co.
Committee on Form and Style of the Council of Biology Editors: CBE Style Manual. 3rd Ed. 1972. Washington, D.C. American Institute of Biological Sciences.
Davidson, J. N., and Cohn, W. E. (Editors): Progress in Nucleic Acid Research and Molecular Biology II. 1971, New York, Academic Press.
DeRobertis, E. D. P., Nowinski, W. W., and Saez, F. A.: Cell Biology. 5th Ed. 1970, Philadelphia, W. B. Saunders Co.

Eck, R. V., and Dayhoff, M. O.: Atlas of Protein Sequence and Structure, 1967–1968. 1968, Maryland, National Biomedical Research Foundation.

Fawcett, D. W.: An Atlas of Fine Structure: The Cell. 1966, Philadelphia, W. B. Saunders Co.

Frobisher, M.: Fundamentals of Microbiology. 8th Ed. 1968, Philadelphia, W. B. Saunders Co.

Poindexter, J. S.: Microbiology. An Introduction to Protists. 1971, New York, The Macmillan Company.

Sharp, J. T.: The Role of Mycoplasmas and L Forms of Bacteria in Disease. 1970, Springfield, Ill., Charles C Thomas, Publishers.

Spencer, J. H.: The Physics and Chemistry of DNA and RNA. 1972, Philadelphia. W. B. Saunders Co.

Stanier, R. Y., Adelberg, E., and Douderoff, M.: The Microbial World. 3rd Ed. 1970, Englewood Cliffs, N.J., Prentice-Hall, Inc.

Villee, C. A.: Biology, 6th Ed. 1972, Philadelphia, W. B. Saunders Co.

Characteristics of Algae, Protozoa, Yeasts, Molds, and Helminths

ALGAE

Blue-green algae are of interest because of their procaryotic structure and other similarities to bacteria. Bacteria and blue-green algae are *the only known procaryotic organisms*. (See Appendix A.)

Although algae are of no known pathogenic significance to man, it is worth noting that some species of eucaryotic algae such as *Chlorella* are "cultivated" on the surface of sewage effluents in large artificial lagoons. They help decompose the organic matter in the sewage. They grow so luxuriantly that when harvested they furnish large amounts of vegetable matter that can be used as food for livestock and, in the Orient, for man (Fig. 3–1).

Eucaryotic algae will undoubtedly play an important role in the nuclear space age, as man travels to other planets, since, if cultivated under artificial sunlight (ultraviolet light) in submarines and space ships, they not only produce life-giving oxygen like other green plants but also take up poisonous carbon dioxide from the atmosphere, help purify human wastes, and provide at least some food. Although not commonly used as a food for man, eucaryotic algae synthesize several polysaccharide gums of commercial value. Agar, an important ingredient of microbiologic culture media (Chapter 9), is derived from a common seaweed alga, *Gelidium*. Similar gums are algin and carrageen.

PROTOZOA

Protozoans, relatively large in size but still mostly microscopic, are unicellular animals that are very complex in structure and activities. Many of these minute organisms grasp and take solid food particles into their single-celled bodies, swim or creep about, have a definite though simple sex life, and sometimes form quite complex communities. Most species of protozoa are harmless, living on dead organic matter or on bacteria (which are much smaller). They are found in the sea, lakes, rivers, sewage, and damp soil. A few protozoa are found only in animals and

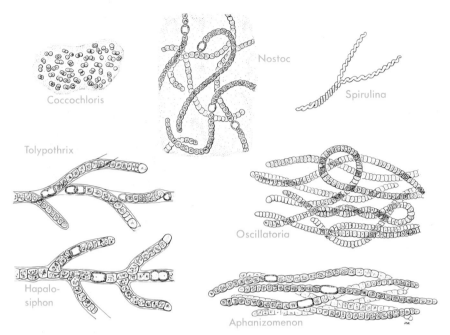

Figure 3–1

Some common species of blue-green algae. (From Villee, C. A.: Biology, 6th Ed. Philadelphia, W. B. Saunders Co., 1972.)

plants, where they cause disease. Good examples of pathogenic protozoa are those that cause malaria, those that cause amebic dysentery, and those that cause African "sleeping sickness" (trypanosomiasis). For purposes of study some can be propagated in test tubes or their reproduction can be watched under the microscope on glass depression slides.

STRUCTURE.   The protozoan cell is typically eucaryotic in structure and in general resembles other typical animal cells. Unlike typical plant cells, which have cell walls, animal cells, including protozoa, characteristically lack morphologically and chemically distinct cell walls. In many species of free-living protozoa, a much thickened and toughened outer membrane or plasmalemma serves most of the functions of a cell wall.

MULTIPLICATION.   Protozoa multiply by *binary fission,* that is, by dividing into two. First the nucleus divides by a process called *mitosis;* then the cytoplasm and cell membrane divide to surround the two nuclei; and the two *daughter cells* then separate as two new individuals. In addition to cell division, some species of protozoa exhibit definite differentiation of sexes, such as that seen in malaria parasites. The differentiation of sexes in dioecious species of protozoa is much more highly developed than in bacteria, yeasts, or molds.

NUTRITION.   The individual cells of most protozoa differ from all bacteria, and indeed from the individual cells of virtually all plants, in having the power to ingest solid food particles. Many also are nourished, as are yeasts, molds, bacteria and plant cells, by diffusion of dissolved food matter through the cell membrane. Ingestion of solid particles of

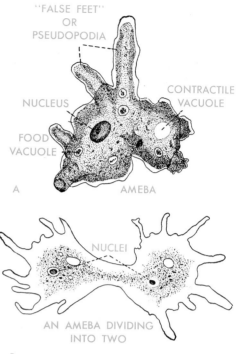

Figure 3–2

A species of harmless ameba from stagnant water; trophozoite stage. Others are not so harmless; for example, *Entamoeba histolytica*. Note the numerous pseudopodia, the nucleus, and the vacuoles inside the cell. This organism, itself microscopic in size, feeds upon bacteria and is thousands of times larger than bacteria. (MacDougall and Hegner: Biology. New York, McGraw-Hill Book Co., Inc.)

food is a distinctively animal characteristic and is often called a *phago-trophic* type of nutrition.

LIFE CYCLES. Many of the protozoa pass through a definite and readily demonstrable series of stages in their development and thus differ greatly from most bacteria. These *life cycles*, as they are called, differ for each species and often are relatively complicated. A good illustration of a protozoan life cycle is that of the malarial parasite (Chapter 40). Some protozoa, especially the malarial parasite, multiply sexually in one or more sanguivorous[1] arthropod[2] hosts (certain flies, mosquitoes, and other insects). The offspring then become mature inside the arthropod and are ready to infect man or other susceptible animals when the arthropod bites.

TROPHOZOITE AND CYST. The actively growing, feeding, and multiplying form of protozoa is called the *trophozoite*[3] stage (Fig. 3–2). Many protozoa also exhibit a thick-walled, inactive stage in which they are dormant and resist drying. This is the *cyst* stage (Fig. 3–3). The cyst stage is important in the transmission of the ameba (*Entamoeba histolytica*) that causes amebiasis (dysentery, liver abscess, and so forth).

CLASSIFICATION. All protozoa are motile in at least one stage of their life cycle. The means of motility differs among them and furnishes a basis for classification into four main groups, as shown in Table 3–1. At least one species of each group is a pathogen of man. Many others are pathogens of lower animals and plants. The important pathogens of man are discussed more fully in Chapters 26 and 40.

---

[1]Latin *sanguis*, blood; *vorare*, to eat; blood-eating, as a mosquito or flea.

[2]Greek *arthron*, joint; *podion*, foot; hence jointed-legged creatures such as mosquitoes, ticks, flies, and shrimp.

[3]Greek *trophe*, nutrition; *zoon*, animal; an actively feeding form of animal.

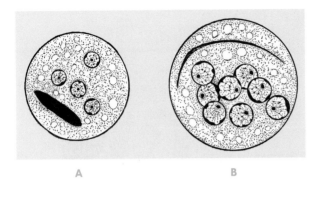

Figure 3-3

A, Cyst of *Entamoeba histolytica.*
B, Cyst of *Entamoeba coli,* generally considered harmless.
Compare as to size and number
of nuclei. The larger dark circular objects inside the cysts are
nuclei formed by nuclear fission
within the cell that produces the
cyst. The numbers and size of
the nuclei are characteristic of
species. The elongated bodies in
the cysts are food or other reserve material. Recognition of
the cysts in feces of patients is
an important means of diagnosis.
(Hegner, Root, and Augustine:
Animal Parasitology. New York,
Appleton-Century-Crofts, Inc.)

A   B

TRUE FUNGI (EUMYCETES)

Fungi are plants that lack chlorophyll, the green pigment responsible
for photosynthesis. The group of Eumycetes includes large, edible mushrooms, "puff-balls," and so on, as well as microscopic yeasts and molds.
Like the protozoa, the cells of Eumycetes are eucaryotic in structure.

Table 3-1.   Classification of Protozoa

Class I.	SARCODINA (move with pseudopodia*; reproduction asexual) *Entamoeba histolytica*—causes amebic dysentery (transmission like that of other enteric infections; Chapters 23, 25, 27).

Class II.	MASTIGOPHORA (move with long, whiplike lashes called *flagella;* reproduction asexual)
	Intestinal parasites
	    Giardia lamblia—possibly causes mild enteritis (transmission like that of other enteric infections)
	    Trichomonas hominis—pathogenicity and transmission same as *Giardia lamblia*
	Parasites in genitourinary tract
	    Trichomonas vaginalis—causes vulvovaginitis (transmission by sexual contact, also by fomites†)
	Blood parasites
	    Trypanosoma rhodesiense and *T. gambiense*—cause African sleeping sickness (transmission by insect vectors‡)
	    Trypanosoma cruzi—causes South American trypanosomiasis (Chagas' disease) (transmission by insect vectors)
	Blood and tissues
	    Leishmania donovani—causes kala-azar (transmission by insect vectors)
	    Leishmania tropica—causes oriental sore (transmission by insect vectors)
	    Leishmania braziliensis—causes espundia (transmission by insect vectors)

Class III.	CILIOPHORA (move with cilia; reproduction usually asexual; occasional conjugation) *Balantidium coli*—causes enteritis and ulcers of the colon (transmission like that of other enteric infections) *paramecium*
Class IV.	SPOROZOA (move with pseudopods in immature stages only; male form is flagellate; reproduction alternately sexual and asexual) *have to be carried like by mosquito* *Plasmodium* (*vivax, malariae, falciparum, ovale*)—causes different types of malaria (transmission by insect vectors)

*"False feet," or having the functions but not the structure of feet (Greek, *pseudo,* false or imitation;
podion, foot).
†Plural of fomes; any object that may transfer infectious microorganisms from one person to another,
e.g., eating utensils, toothbrushes, handkerchiefs, and so on.
‡A vector is any agent, living or inanimate, that transmits infectious agents.

More than 70,000 species of eucaryotic fungi have been described. Yeasts and molds were classed as plants and grouped (with algae and bacteria) as examples of the simplest forms of plant life. Except for some aquatic types (Saprolegniales), most true fungi are nonmotile. The cell walls of many true fungi resemble the outer cuticle of some animal cells in that they contain chitin, the tough, flexible substance (chemically resembling cellulose) in skeletal and shell tissues of insects and crustacea. True fungi and most bacteria are heterotrophic or chemo-organotrophic; i.e., they must have organic matter as part of their food. Mycology is the name given to the science concerned with the study of fungi (including molds and yeasts).

RELATION OF BACTERIA (SCHIZOMYCETES OR FISSION FUNGI) TO TRUE FUNGI (EUMYCETES).   Ideas concerning the classification of microorganisms vary considerably. Although there may be general agreement on the characteristics of a species, a genus, or even a family, as larger groupings are proposed differences of opinion held by specialists in *taxonomy*[4] may be very great. Table 3–2 illustrates the relative position of microorganisms in the plant kingdom, showing the relationship of true fungi (Eumycetes, eucaryotic) to the bacteria (Schizomycetes, procaryotic).

In a classification of bacteria now in preparation (eighth edition of *Bergey's Manual of Determinative Bacteriology*) the names and sequence of the groups of bacteria listed in Tables 3–2 and 3–3 are much altered; some are eliminated, others added. Since, at this writing, the new arrangement is not entirely complete, the time-honored system of the 1957 (seventh) edition of *Bergey's Manual* will be followed in this book except for a few newly adopted names in general use. For example, because of our use of a recent change of nomenclature for the Enterobacteriaceae (Chapter 23), the name *Salmonella typhi* is used instead of the older name *S. typhosa* given in the seventh edition of *Bergey's Manual*. An outline of the new arrangement is given in Appendix A.

CHARACTERISTICS OF EUCARYOTIC FUNGI.   Most true fungi grow as branching, filamentous tubes filled with protoplasm. When growing in this manner they are called *molds;* when growing in the form of ovoid, budding cells they are commonly referred to as yeasts. In many species, environmental conditions (e.g., temperature, oxygen supply, nutrition) may cause a "yeast" to grow in a filamentous form and a "mold" in a yeast-like form. The terms yeast and mold have no scientific status; they are used for convenience in discussing different forms of fungi.

YEASTS

Yeasts are typically unicellular organisms though several cells often cling together after fission (Fig. 3–4). Yeast cells are 20 to 100 times as large as most bacteria. Everyone is familiar with bakers' yeast, which is composed of countless numbers of these unicellular plants compressed together, dried, and granulated. Each granule contains millions of yeast cells. Stained smears of the moistened material on glass "slides" must be viewed with the microscope in order to see the yeast cells.

Yeasts are gram-positive (a type of staining process described later)

---

[4]Taxonomy is the science of the classification of organisms.

Table 3–2.   Classification of Fungi in the Plant Kingdom

Phylum I. Tracheophyta (vascular plants). Contain chlorophyll; require sunlight.
  Subphylum 1. Pteridopsida (ferns and seed-bearing plants such as lilies, grasses, roses, zinnias, oak trees).
  Subphylum 2. Sphenopsida (horsetails).
  Subphylum 3. Lycopsida (club mosses).
Phylum II. Bryophyta (liverworts and true mosses). Contain chlorophyll; require sunlight.
  Class 1. Musci (mosses: e.g., *Sphagnum*, *Polytrichum*).
  Class 2. Liverworts (e.g., *Marchantia*).
Phylum III. Thallophyta (nonvascular plants). May or may not contain chlorophyll. No differentiated
    leaves, stems, flowers, or roots. Relatively simple structure. Can generally grow in lifeless
    media.
  Subphylum 1. Red, brown, and green algae. Contain chlorophyll; require sunlight. (Represented
      by various seaweeds and green pond-scums.)
  Subphylum 2. Myxophyceae or Cyanophyceae (blue-green algae). Contain chlorophyll; require
      sunlight. (Some seaweeds, scums on stagnant water, etc.)
  Subphylum 3. Fungi. Do not contain chlorophyll. Do not require sunlight.* With exception of
      certain bacteria, can grow in lifeless media.
    Class 1. Myxomycetes. Slime molds. These have a motile ameboid stage and closely resemble
        protozoa. They reproduce by "spores," but are as far removed from the true fungi as
        are the bacteria. Some bacteriologists regard them as bacteria.
    Class 2. Basidiomycetes. Reproduce sexually by basidiospores, and also asexually. Represented by
        mushrooms, puffballs, and rust and smut diseases on plants.
    Class 3. Ascomycetes. Most yeasts and many molds. Reproduce sexually by ascospores, and also
        asexually. Some are parasitic on plants. Truffles are a type of ascomycete.
    Class 4. Phycomycetes. Molds with coenocytic hyphae. Multiply asexually by sporangiospores; also
        reproduce sexually. Represented by water molds, common bread mold, many saprophytes;
        some are parasites on plants and insects.
    Class 5. Fungi Imperfecti. Reproduce only by asexual spores. Many are very common molds. Most
        fungi that cause disease in man belong to the Fungi Imperfecti. In addition there are many
        that are parasitic on plants. Includes fungi that cannot be properly assigned to either
        class 3 or 4.
    Class 6. Schizomycetes or Fission Fungi (Bacteria).†   *procaryotic*
      Orders: 1. Pseudomonadales (gram-negative rods and rigid spirals).
            2. Chlamydobacteriales.
            3. Hyphomicrobiales.
            4. Eubacteriales (simple rods, cocci, and spirals).
            5. Actinomycetales (branching, moldlike bacteria).
            6. Caryophanales.
            7. Beggiatoales.
            8. Myxobacterales.
            9. Spirochaetales (flexible spirals).
           10. Mycoplasmatales (PPLO).
           11. Rickettsiales (cannot grow in lifeless media).

will be studied the most

  *A few species of harmless, photosynthetic bacteria are exceptions. Organisms in classes 1–5 are
eucaryons. Organisms in class 6 are procaryons.
  †Only the orders containing species of medical interest are described in detail in this book.
Table 3-3 further subdivides the class Schizomycetes.

Table 3–3. Class: Schizomycetes*

ORDER	FAMILY	GENUS	SPECIES†
Eubacteriales	Micrococcaceae	*Staphylococcus*	*S. aureus*
		Micrococcus	*M. epidermidis*
		Gaffkya	*G. tetragena*
		Sarcina	*S. lutea*
	Enterobacteriaceae	*Escherichia*	*E. coli*
		Salmonella	*S. typhi*
		Shigella	*S. dysenteriae, etc.*
		Proteus	*P. vulgaris*
		Aerobacter	*A. cloacae*
		Klebsiella	*K. pneumoniae*
		Serratia	*S. marcescens*
	Brucellaceae	*Pasteurella*	*P. pestis, etc.*
		Brucella	*B. abortus, etc.*
		Haemophilus	*H. influenzae, etc.*
		Moraxella	*M. lacunata*
		Bordetella	*B. pertussis*
		Actinobacillus	*A. lignieresii*
	Bacteroidaceae	*Bacteroides*	*B. fragilis, etc.*
		Fusobacterium	*F. fusiforme*
		Streptobacillus	*S. moniliformis*
	Achromobacteraceae	*Alcaligenes*	*A. faecalis*
	Neisseriaceae	*Neisseria*	⎰ *N. gonorrhoeae*
		Veillonella	⎱ *N. meningitidis*
	Lactobacillaceae	*Diplococcus*	*D. pneumoniae*
		Streptococcus	*S. pyogenes*
		Lactobacillus	*L. acidophilus*
	Corynebacteriaceae	*Corynebacterium*	*C. diphtheriae*
		Listeria	*L. monocytogenes*
		Erysipelothrix	*E. insidiosa*
	Bacillaceae	*Bacillus*	*B. anthracis* (aerobic)
		Clostridium	*C. tetani* (anaerobic)
Pseudomonadales	Spirillaceae	*Vibrio*	*V. cholerae*
		Spirillum	*S. minus*
	Pseudomonadaceae	*Pseudomonas*	*P. aeruginosa*
Actinomycetales	Mycobacteriaceae	*Mycobacterium*	*M. tuberculosis*
	Actinomycetaceae	*Actinomyces*	*A. bovis* (anaerobic)
		Nocardia	*N. asteroides* (aerobic)
	Streptomycetaceae	*Streptomyces*	*S. species* (soil)
Spirochaetales	Treponemataceae	*Treponema*	*T. pallidum*
		Borrelia	*B. recurrentis*
		Leptospira	*L. icterohaemorrhagiae*
Mycoplasmatales	Mycoplasmataceae	*Mycoplasma*	*M. hominis*
Rickettsiales	Rickettsiaceae	*Rickettsia*	*R. prowazekii*
		Coxiella	*C. burnetii*
	Chlamydiaceae	*Chlamydia*	*C. trachomatis*
		Miyagawanella	*M. psittacii*
			M. lymphogranulomatis
	Bartonellaceae	*Bartonella*	*B. bacilliformis*

*Adapted from Zinsser, H.: Microbiology, 13th ed. D. T. Smith, et al., Editors, Appleton-Century-Crofts.

†Only species of most significance in human disease are listed here.

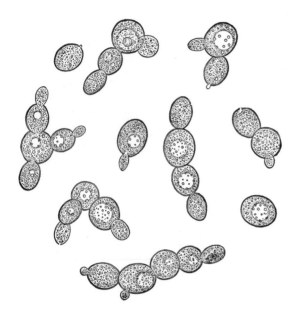

Figure 3–4

Yeast cells. Brewers' yeast actively multiplying by budding. This species is called *Saccharomyces cerevisiae*. The single large internal vacuoles and the numerous small fat drops are shown, as are also buds in various stages of development, and the cell wall. Nuclei not visible here. (Highly magnified.) (Sedgwick and Wilson.)

and may also be stained with simple dyes like methylene blue. Staining makes microscopic cells more readily visible. In general, yeasts are grown on simple media (nutrient materials) much as are bacteria, and their colonies [masses of growth visible to the naked eye (see discussion, Chap. 9)] resemble those of true bacteria. Sabouraud's agar is a favorite medium for the cultivation of yeasts and molds. It contains 1 per cent neopeptone (partly digested meat), 4 per cent maltose or glucose, 1.5 to 2.0 per cent agar (to solidify the medium unless broth is desired), and the pH is adjusted to 5.6 (acidic).

STRUCTURE OF YEAST CELLS.   Yeast cells are eucaryotic in structure. They are usually oval or egg-shaped, although in some species long filamentous cells, as well as filaments of cells, are formed resembling those of molds. There is a well-developed and rather large, globular nucleus and a thick cell wall, composed in part of a chitin-like substance. There are also vacuoles containing waste substances, and there are food granules of various kinds, some evidently of glycogen, and fat.

HABITAT OF YEASTS.   Yeasts are widely distributed in nature in much the same situations as are bacteria. They commonly occur on grapes and other fruits and plants, the spores passing the winter in the soil. The kind of wine made from grapes depends to some extent on the varieties of "wild" yeasts occurring upon them naturally. Yeasts are always found in dung, soil, and milk, and are not infrequently observed in throat cultures, river water, dust, and so on.

Multiplication of Yeasts

ASEXUAL.   Most species of yeasts reproduce asexually by a process called budding in which, instead of forming two equal cells as the bacteria do, the new cell is at first much smaller than the other and is referred to as a daughter cell. The daughter cells, or *buds*, often cling to the parent cell; clumps or chains of cells are thus formed (Fig. 3–4). A few species of yeasts reproduce by binary fission like bacteria and protozoa.

SEXUAL. Ascospores, i.e., spores in sacs, or *asci*, are formed during sexual reproduction by many species of Eumycetes, including yeasts. All sac-forming fungi are called *Ascomycetes*. In some yeasts (nonfilamentous Ascomycetes), the nucleus of a single cell undergoes meiotic division and the haploid daughter nuclei remain in the cell as ascospores. Later they fuse and form diploid cells that are released as budding diploid cells. Usually, four, six, or eight spores are formed by divisions of the nucleus within a sac, the number tending to be characteristic of the species. Ascospores are less resistant than bacterial spores, and they are killed by a temperature of 62 C. in a short time but they are dormant and resistant to drying. Bacteria commonly form only one spore per cell. Therefore spore formation in them is not an important means of increasing their numbers as it is in ascomycetes.

Often asci are formed following a process in which two adjacent haploid cells send out projections that meet and form a copulation canal, through which there is an intermingling of nuclear material. The fertilized diploid nucleus divides meiotically to form a number of haploid ascospores. These may reproduce indefinitely asexually as haploid cells. Some very interesting studies have been made of the heredity and breeding of yeasts (which are quite analogous to heredity and breeding in dogs, cattle, or men) and the development of progeny that have special value in fermentation processes and the like (Fig. 3–5).

ACTIVITIES OF NONPATHOGENIC YEASTS. Yeasts, especially yeasts of the genus *Saccharomyces*, which includes the bakers' and brewers' yeasts, very readily use various kinds of sugar as food. They give off enzymes that bring about the chemical changes in sugars, called fermentation, during which alcohol and carbon dioxide are formed. Both of these products are found in beer, new wine, and rising dough, all of which are yeast-fermented products. The holes in bread are due to CO_2 gas bubbles. The foam on beer and the effervescence of champagne also result from carbon dioxide formed by the yeast.

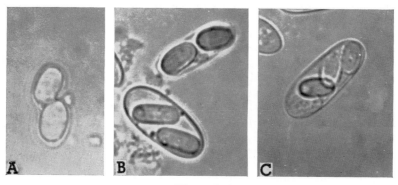

Figure 3–5

One form of sexual multiplication in a species of yeast (*Saccharomycopsis guttulata*). *A*, Two cells in sexual contact; the cell walls at point of contact have dissolved, and intermingling of intracellular (nuclear) materials is occurring. *B*, Fertilized cells (ascus; plural asci), which have formed two ascospores within each cell. *C*, Ascus with four ascospores. (Courtesy of Drs. M. Shifrine and H. J. Phaff. In *Antonie Leeuwenhoek*, Vol. 24.)

There are various species of "wild" yeasts and torulas,[5] which produce different by-products during their metabolic processes. Some of these give undesirable flavors and odors to beer and wines. The use of *pure cultures* of desirable yeasts is, therefore, of great importance in industry, where flavor and other qualities of the product depend on the particular species of yeast employed. Some species of *Torula* are cultivated for their nutritive value as stock feed.

MOLDS

The differentiation between yeasts and molds is not a sharp one, since, as previously mentioned, many yeastlike fungi have properties of growth like molds, and vice versa, depending on environmental circumstances. For purposes of this discussion only those forms that commonly grow in definitely woolly and filamentous colonies will be considered as molds. Molds are as widely distributed in nature as yeasts, most of them being saprophytes. Many live in the soil and take an active part in the decomposition of organic matter. Everyone is familiar with the green, brown, black, white, or yellow molds often seen on stale bread, fruits (especially over-ripe oranges), jars of jelly, or on rags, books, or old leather shoes that have lain in a damp place for a long time. If such growths are examined with a magnifying glass, they will be seen to consist of beautiful, almost fairy-like plants, all glistening and transparent. The "fruit" (spores) is usually deeply colored and grows in great profusion. Each little colored ball or frond is a mass of spores. Molds are cultivated and manipulated in the laboratory in much the same manner as are yeasts and bacteria.

Typical molds are made up of branching tubular filaments or *hyphae*, forming a woolly growth, the *mycelium*, from which the asexual reproductive cells (*spores or conidia*) develop. The mycelial filaments often penetrate into the medium on which the mold is growing, thus acting like roots.

In some molds (Phycomycetes[6] the filaments throughout the whole plant or mycelium are *coenocytic* (undivided by transverse walls), the nuclei being spaced more or less regularly in the filament. Only rarely are these species pathogenic for man. In other molds—Ascomycetes, Basidiomycetes (e. g., mushrooms), and Fungi Imperfecti—nuclei and cytoplasm seem to be segregated inside segments ("cells") of the hyphae by means of partitions called *septa*. Such molds are said to be *septate*. However, the septa in Ascomycetes are not restrictive of protoplasmic flow or the transfer of nuclei. For example, in *Neurospora crassa* (an ascomycete) the septa are perforated; protoplasm and nuclei pass freely through them (Fig. 3–6). Sometimes one may find several nuclei in one cell and in other cells none. The flow of protoplasm carries nuclei and cellular materials not only from cell to cell in the hyphae but also, at certain stages, from conidial spore to spore.

In molds we thus see the beginnings of *division of function* between *vegetative* cells, which provide for nutrition and anchorage, and *reproductive* cells. This is one step higher in organization than bacteria and the simpler species of protozoa, in which all the functions of the organism are carried on in the single cell.

---

[5]Torulas are yeastlike fungi that do not form sexual spores or cause alcoholic fermentation, e.g., *Fungi Imperfecti*.

[6]From the Greek *phykos*, seaweed; *mykes*, fungus; hence, marine and aquatic fungi. Some species are terrestrial.

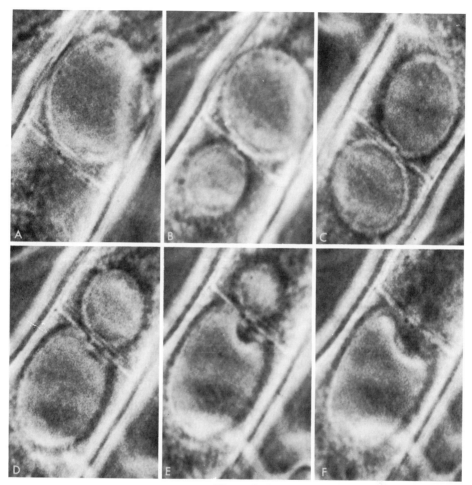

Figure 3–6

Protoplasmic flow through a septum of a hypha of *Neurospora crassa*. The result is complete mixing of nuclei and genetic determinants, thus enzymes and their metabolic products. If two strains are inoculated into one flask, the cultures grow like one organism.

Reproduction of Molds

ASEXUAL.   Molds reproduce *asexually* by one or more of five different methods, as follows:

Oidia*[7] *or Arthrospores.   These are short fragments of mycelium that become detached by *fragmentation*. This occurs only in septate molds.

Blastospores.   These are much like the buds of yeasts but they develop along mold hyphae.

Chlamydospores.   Along some hyphae certain cells develop thick protective walls and appear to go into a resistant, dormant stage. They separate and resume independent growth when conditions of warmth and moisture become favorable again, each forming a new mycelium.

---

[7]Oidium is from a Greek root meaning egg, i.e., an ovoid body.

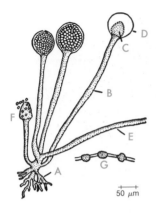

Figure 3–7

Characteristic structures of *Rhizopus*. The rootlike filaments (*rhizoids*) are seen at *A*, the stolon or spreading filament at *E* and a *conidiophore* or conidia-bearing hypha at *B*. Details of the sporangium are seen at *C* and *D* and conidia leaving the *columella* at *F*. Chlamydospores are seen at *G*. This is *asexual* reproduction. (From Conant, N. F., *et al.*: Manual of Clinical Mycology, 3rd Ed. Philadelphia, W. B. Saunders Co., 1971.)

Sporangiospores.   Sporangiospores are formed only by the Phycomycetes. In terrestrial species they are minute, rounded, thick-walled bodies resistant to climatic heat and drought. They are produced in large numbers in globular envelopes at the tips of special hyphae. The envelope is called a *sporangium*, hence the term sporangiospores (Figs. 3–7, 3–8). In most aquatic species they are liberated from the sporangium as flagellate, free-swimming zoospores.

Conidiospores.   Conidiospores are produced in long chains, free of an enclosing membrane, by certain Ascomycetes (Fig. 3–9). *Conidio* is from a Greek word meaning dust. The forms, arrangements, and colors of sporangiospores and conidiospores are very useful in the identification of molds. The green or blue powdery material on a spoiled orange is a mass of conidiospores. Since each conidiospore is able to grow into a new mycelium, it is easy to understand how quickly spoilage can spread.

SEXUAL.   Sexual reproduction occurs in Phycomycetes and also in

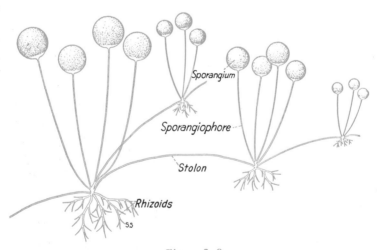

Figure 3–8

A species of *Rhizopus*, a coenocytic mold. Note the branches resembling roots (*rhizoids*), the long connecting filament by which the mycelium spreads (*stolon*), and the vertical branches (*sporangiophores*) holding the sacs (*sporangia*) full of *sporangiospores*. (Swingle, D. B.: Plant Life, 2nd Ed. D. Van Nostrand Co., Inc.)

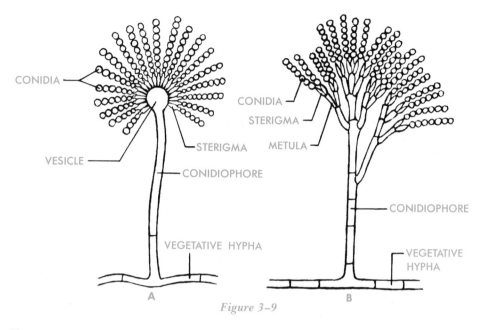

CONIDIA

VESICLE

STERIGMA

CONIDIOPHORE

VEGETATIVE HYPHA

A

CONIDIA

STERIGMA

METULA

CONIDIOPHORE

VEGETATIVE HYPHA

B

Figure 3-9

Two common species of molds, showing structures. *A, Aspergillus; B, Penicillium.* For discussion see text. (Carpenter, P. L.: Microbiology, 3rd Ed. Philadelphia, W. B. Saunders Co., 1972.)

the filamentous Ascomycetes. The process is very distinctive in each species or genus. For example, in two common genera of Phycomycetes called *Mucor* and *Rhizopus* two cells of the same culture grow into contact; the separating walls dissolve, and the cell contents mingle as one cell. This

Figure 3-10

Zygospore formation (sexual reproduction) by a species of *Rhizopus. A,* The tips of two coenocytic hyphae representing male and female gametes (sex cells) come together and a spore wall forms around them. *B,* The nuclei from each gamete then form pairs and fuse. *C,* A multinucleate spore in which all the nuclei are diploid results. *D,* Reduction division (meiosis) takes place just before the spore germinates to form a new coenocytic hypha tipped by a sporangium filled with asexual sporangiospores. (Swingle, D. B.: Plant Life, 2nd Ed. D. Van Nostrand Co., Inc.)

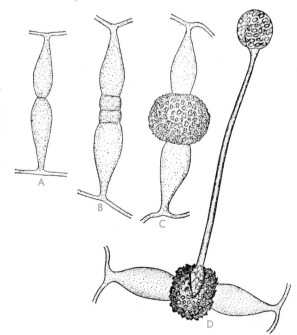

A

B

C

D

cell, called a *zygospore*, acquires a hard, thick outer shell and becomes dormant for a time, much as does a seed. Eventually, finding conditions of moisture, temperature, and nutrition favorable, it bursts or germinates, sending forth a filament (Fig. 3–10). During the resting stage the zygospores resist unfavorable conditions such as drought, food deprivation, and exposure to sunlight, in this respect resembling the spores of yeasts and bacteria. Although more heat-resistant than the spores of yeasts, they are very much less so than the endospores of bacteria (Chapter 12).

In the filamentous Ascomycetes, e.g., *Aspergillus* and *Penicillium*, the sexual spores are formed, as in *Mucor* and *Rhizopus*, by fusion of cells in the mycelium. However, instead of a single zygospore resulting, the fertile cell nucleus divides to form a number of spores that are held together for a time in a multiple sac or complex ascus. The structure holding these sexually produced spore-sacs is called an *ascocarp* and is usually found suspended in the mycelial network.

Fungi Imperfecti

This term is used for a large and rather miscellaneous collection of molds and yeasts that, although closely resembling well known species, have never been observed to produce sexual spores and are therefore designated imperfect. Many of the commonest molds are Fungi Imperfecti. They cease to be designated Fungi Imperfecti when we learn of their sex life.

Growth of Molds

Molds may be readily cultivated on ordinary bacterial media. Sabouraud's medium is often used (Fig. 3–11). They can grow on materials where

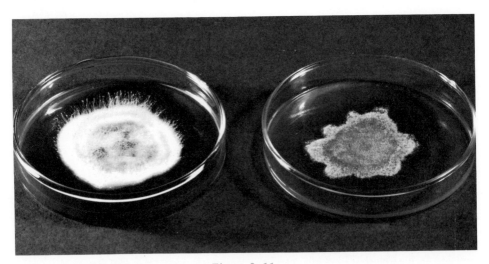

Figure 3–11

A giant colony of a species of *Aspergillus* (about one-half life size) which has grown for a week on nutrient agar in a Petri dish. Note the aerial conidiophores (left) and the mass of dark conidia in the central portion of an older colony (right). (Smith and Sasaki: *Appl. Microbiol.*, Vol. 6.)

there is relatively little moisture, and can get sufficient water from humid atmospheres. Because of their ability to obtain nutriment from solutions of high osmotic pressure such as syrups, jams, jellies, and pickling brines, they are often found on the surface of such materials on the housewife's preserve shelf. They are, in general, aerobic plants, but are injured by sunlight.

Common Species of Molds

There are several genera of molds that everyone commonly sees. We may mention *Aspergillus, Penicillium, Mucor,* and *Rhizopus.* The Ascomycetes *Neurospora crassa* and *Neurospora sitophila,* pink "bread molds," have been extensively studied in the laboratory by microbial geneticists because these species offer certain advantages for investigations of genetic fine structure and biochemical metabolic blocks and pathways. Some common species produce poisonous metabolic products (*aflatoxins, mycotoxins*) when growing in certain foods, especially in moldy livestock feeds.

ASPERGILLUS.   One of the commonest species of mold is *Aspergillus glaucus,* which forms gray-green conidiospores (Fig. 3–9A). It is seen on spoiled food and mildewed clothing, especially shoes, during the summer or in the tropics. A species causing infection in the lung is called *A. fumigatus. Aspergillus flavus,* common on spoiled stock feeds such as ground peanuts, produces *aflatoxin.* Just how common this poison may be in human foods is not yet clear.

PENICILLIUM.   Like aspergilli, the penicillia are very common in nature and contribute to the spoilage of food and other objects composed of organic matter. Various species of *Penicillium* form the familiar, dusty, blue-green growth seen on decaying oranges and other fruits. The conidiospores are borne at the ends of branched filaments in an arrangement suggestive of a tiny paint brush, from which the name *Penicillium* (from Latin *penicillus,* for paint brush or pencil) is derived (Fig. 3–9B).

Some species of *Penicillium* are known to give a characteristic flavor to cheese, such as *P. roquefortii* in Roquefort cheese and *P. camemberti* in Camembert cheese. The blue veins in the Roquefort cheese are made up of masses of conidiospores. The drug penicillin is named for *P. notatum,* the fungus from which it was first isolated.

MUCOR AND RHIZOPUS.   *Mucor* is the generic name for one of the many familiar white or grey molds that grow as cottony tufts on damp organic substances such as decaying manure. Some species of these molds occasionally cause infections of the lung called mucormycosis. The disease is often fatal.

The black mold seen on old bread is often a closely related genus called *Rhizopus.* These two genera belong in the group of Phycomycetes that reproduce by asexual *sporangiospores* and sexual *zygospores* (Fig. 3–10). They differ most distinctively in that *Rhizopus* has little rootlike attachments on the hyphae (Figs. 3–7 and 3–8).

HELMINTHS

The term helminth is used to designate worms that are parasitic in man or animals. Three major groups of helminths are the following: phylum Nemathelminthes, class Nematoda, *nematodes* or roundworms that are exemplified by hookworms, pinworms, and the trichina worms found in pork; phylum Platyhelminthes, class Cestoidea, *cestodes* or flatworms represented by various tapeworms; and class Trematoda, *trematodes* or flukes, large flattish worms, the most dangerous species of which are found in tropical areas, especially in the Orient.

None of the *adult* helminths found in the United States is a genuine microorganism, although some, e.g., the pork trichina worm (1.5 mm), are quite small. Diagnosis and study of helminthic diseases require the use of microscopes, however, to find and identify the microscopic eggs of the worms and to study the minute identifying structures of the adults. In the filarial worms, the nematodes that cause the tropical disease *filariasis*, one symptom of which is *elephantiasis*, the infective larvae of the worms are truly microscopic in size. They are transmitted by biting flies and mosquitoes and are found in the blood of patients.

Since adult helminths are highly complex animals and are not truly microorganisms, they are not discussed here in detail. The student who is interested in them will find numerous excellent textbooks devoted largely to them. In this book representative species are discussed among the organisms transmitted from the intestinal tract (Chapter 26) or from the blood (Chapter 40).

APPLICATION FOR THE HEALTH PROFESSIONS

As will be pointed out later in this book, the basic knowledge of the characteristics of protozoa, yeasts, molds, viruses, and helminths is frequently valuable in understanding symptoms, medical therapy, and the prevention of infectious diseases. It is not only interesting but it is also important to recognize and readily identify with some understanding the scientific names of microorganisms as they appear in professional literature and on medical records. Medical aspects of these organisms are discussed farther on in appropriate chapters.

Supplementary Reading

Barnett, H. L., and Hunter, B. B.: Illustrated Genera of Imperfect Fungi. 3rd Ed. 1972, Minneapolis, Burgess Publishing Co.

Bodily, H. L. (Editor), Updyke, E. L. (Coeditor), and Mason, J. O. (Assoc. Editor): Bacterial Mycotic and Parasitic Infections. 5th Ed. 1970, New York, American Public Health Association.

Burmeister, H. R., and Hesseltine, C. W.: Biological assays for two mycotoxins produced by *Fusarium tricinctum. Appl. Microbiol.,* 1970, *20:*437.

Christensen, C. M.: The Molds and Man. 3rd Ed. 1965, Minneapolis, University of Minnesota Press.

Colwell, R. R.: Genetic and Phenetic Classification of Bacteria, Annual Review of Ecology and Systematics 2. 1971, Palo Alto, California, Annual Reviews Inc.

Conant, N. F., Smith, D. T., Baker, R. D., and Callaway, J. L.: Manual of Clinical Mycology. 3rd Ed. 1971, Philadelphia, W. B. Saunders Company.

Conti, S. F., and Naylor, H. B.: Electron microscopy of ultrathin sections of *Schizosaccharomyces octosporus.* III. Ascosporogenesis, ascospore structure, and germination. *J. Bact.,* 1960, *79:*417.

Emmons, C. W., Binford, C. H., and Utz, J. P.: Medical Mycology, 2nd Ed. 1970, Philadelphia, Lea & Febiger.

Faust, E. C., Beaver, P. C., and Jung, R. C.: Animal Agents and Vectors of Human Disease, 3rd Ed. 1968, Philadelphia, Lea & Febiger.

Faust, E. C., Russell, P. F., and Jung, R. C.: Craig & Faust's Clinical Parasitology, 8th Ed. 1970, Philadelphia, Lea & Febiger.

Hayes, A. W., Wyatt, E. P., and King, P. A.: Environmental and nutritional factors affecting the production of rubratoxin B by *Penicillium rubrum* Stoll. *Appl. Microbiol.*, 1970, *20:*469.

Hegner, R. H.: Big Fleas Have Little Fleas, or Who's Who Among the Protozoa. 1938, Baltimore, The Williams & Wilkins Co.

Hsu, T. C., and Fuerst, R.: The Biology of *Neurospora crassa.* 16 mm. motion picture with sound. Released by the University of Texas, M. D. Anderson Hospital, January, 1958.

Lockhart, W. R., and Liston, J. (Editors): Methods for Numerical Taxonomy. 1970, Washington, D.C., American Society for Microbiology.

Rose, A. H.: Yeasts. *Sci. Amer.*, 1960, *202:*136.

Stanier, R. Y., Doudoroff, M., and Adelberg, E. A.: The Microbial World, 3rd Ed. 1970, Englewood Cliffs, N.J., Prentice-Hall.

Characteristics and Types of Bacteria

4

Bacteria are used in this book as convenient models to illustrate many basic phenomena of microbiology. Since many laboratory techniques and other health-related procedures are centered around bacteria, a general survey of bacteria is given in this chapter. Later chapters describe in detail the more important pathogenic species, the modes of their transmission, control, and so on.

CLASSIFICATION. Space prohibits a complete classification of all the microorganisms discussed in this book. Classifications of protozoa are to be found in textbooks on parasitology or on animal agents of disease; classifications of pathogenic yeasts and molds are found in books on clinical mycology and tropical medicine (see Supplementary Reading, Chapters 2, 3, and 37). As stated on page 37 under "Relation of Bacteria to True Fungi" a new classification of bacteria is in preparation (see Appendix A). For convenience, the classification and nomenclature of bacteria in this book follows the still widely used (though obsolescent) system given in the seventh (1957) edition of "Bergey's Manual of Determinative Bacteriology." Classifications of bacteria now include the mycoplasmas (PPLO), the L forms of bacteria, the rickettsias, and the chlamydias. Classifications of rickettsias, chlamydias (PLGT group), and viruses are discussed briefly elsewhere in this book. An overall classification of the bacteria as part of the plant kingdom is given in Tables 3–2 and 3–3 (pp. 38, 39).

THALLOPHYTES. Table 3–2 shows that the bacteria, although included by some in the kingdom Protista, are also traditionally included in the plant kingdom in one of its major subdivisions, the *thallophytes.* The thallophytes are distinguished from all other plants by having no specially differentiated organs such as roots, leaves, or flowers. A single cell may constitute the entire plant or, if the plant is multicellular like mold or seaweed, a single cell by continued cell fission may reproduce the entire plant asexually. Within this subdivision the bacteria, or class of Schizomycetes, are grouped with the fungi. All fungi[1] can grow without sunlight and are characterized by absence of the green coloring matter, chlorophyll, which is necessary for photosynthesis and is so familiar in trees and grass.

---

[1]Except a few alga-like bacteria of no medical significance.

THE SCHIZOMYCETES

The class Schizomycetes, the procaryotic fungi, according to the obsolescent system of classification as mentioned above (*Bergey's Manual of Determinative Bacteriology*[2]), comprises about 1700 known species, which are arranged in 216 genera and subgenera. The genera are arranged in tribes, which in turn are grouped into families. Finally, the families are grouped into ten orders and several suborders. The student in the health fields, however, need not feel discouraged by this vast array of bacteria, as only six of the ten orders contain species of medical importance, and only a dozen or so of these are of everyday concern in North America.

NOMENCLATURE OF BACTERIA.   The long and apparently meaningless names often borne by bacteria, as well as by higher plants and animals, need not be a source of confusion. They are based on a long-standing binomial (two-name) system; the first name is that of the genus, the second name that of the species.

NAMES OF GROUPS.   A *species* of microorganisms is a group of which all the individuals are essentially alike and identifiable as belonging to that group and not to some other group. (In actual practice, few bacterial species are so clearly distinguishable.) A *genus* is a group of similar species; a tribe, of similar genera, and so on.

A *strain* consists of the progeny of a particular group of individuals of the same species. For example, a species of protozoa (say, *Entamoeba histolytica*) derived from a patient named Albert Jones would be called the "Albert Jones" strain of *E. histolytica*.

A *clone*, in microbiology, consists of the progeny of a single cell.

Each species of organism, as has been said, has two names: The first name, that of the genus, is written with the initial letter *capitalized;* the second, the name of the species, is written with the initial letter *not capitalized.* When printed, genus and species names are properly italicized e.g., *Staphylococcus aureus.* When written by hand or typed, the genus and the species must be underlined; for example, Staphylococcus aureus. The names are usually of Latin or Greek derivation, and are often derived from the names of places or persons associated with the discovery of the organism. The names of the bacteria are also intended to be descriptive of the cardinal features of the organisms. This saves time and avoids confusion. For example, by having a general agreement as to just what characters are possessed by organisms classified in the genus *Bacillus*, it saves a great deal of time in writing and talking to use that word in place of the long list of properties to which it refers such as "strictly aerobic, sporeforming, rod-shaped bacterium." Similarly, by applying the name *anthracis* to the species of *Bacillus* causing anthrax, we save repetitions of long, detailed, pathologic and clinical descriptions. To give another example, the name *Salmonella typhi* indicates, by general agreement among microbiologists, a facultative, nonspore-forming, gram-negative, motile, rodshaped bacterium, not fermenting lactose, not liquefying gelatin, fermenting glucose without gas formation, and causing typhoid fever. Its generic name, *Salmonella*, is derived from an American microbiologist named Salmon. It is obviously efficient to use only two distinctive words to express all these facts.

---

[2]An eighth edition is in preparation at this writing.

Table 4-1. Some Useful Relationships of Measurements

1 inch = 2.54 cm
1 cm = 10 mm = 1/2.54 inch
1 mm = 1,000 μm (micrometer)
1 μm = 0.001 mm = 0.000,03937 or 1/25,400 inch = 1,000 nm (nanometer)
1 nm = 0.001 μm = 10.0 Angstroms (Å)
1Å = 0.000,1 μm = 0.000,000,1 mm = 1/254,000,000 inch

See also system of nomenclature of metric units on page 22.

Structure of Bacteria

SIZE OF BACTERIA. It is easy to understand why a microscope is necessary for the discovery and study of microorganisms when we realize that even very large bacteria are only about 100 μm long (Table 4-1). A common bacterium in the intestine, called *Escherichia coli*, is only about 5 to 10 μm in length. Nearly two billion (2,000,000,000) medium-size bacteria may easily be contained in a single drop of water, and about 30 billion would hardly weigh as much as a dime.

The highest power of an ordinary compound microscope (oil-immersion lens) magnifies about 1000 diameters. An object 0.5 μm in diameter when magnified 1000 times ($\times$ 1000) appears about the size of a period on this page. Most bacteria are of about this diameter, although their length may be greater. Most viruses cannot be seen at all with ordinary microscopes. Rickettsias are visible with ordinary microscopes and in general have forms like bacteria but are much smaller.

Another type of magnifying instrument called the *electron microscope* gives clear images of bacterial structures at enlargements up to one million and more diameters ($\times$). A human hair magnified to only about $\times$ 300,000 would have a diameter about twice that of a modern tunnel, like those leading into New York City below the river! Pictures made with an electron microscope are called electron micrographs. By means of the electron microscope, viruses can be made visible and their inconceivably minute anatomy studied. A complex microscope, an outgrowth in the development of the electron microscope, also uses electrons but gives a picture in as-

A   B

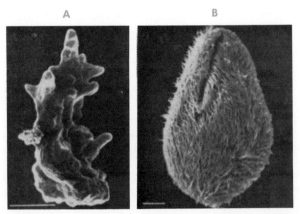

Figure 4-1

A, Amoeba proteus. Preservation of lobopods is shown (scale, 100 μm). *B, Nyctotherus ovalis.* Holotrichous ciliate from the hind gut of the roach *Blabarus discoidalis* (scale, 100 μm). (From Small, E. B., and Marszalek, D. S.: Scanning electron microscopy of fixed, frozen, and dried protozoa. *Science, 163*:1064, March 7, 1969. Copyright 1969 by the American Association for the Advancement of Science.)

tonishingly "3-D"-like perspective. The new instrument is called a scanning electron microscope. (See Fig. 4–1, also page 00.)

MORPHOLOGY OF BACTERIA.   Van Leeuwenhoek's drawings (Fig. 1–4) show that he observed spherical types of bacteria that today are called *cocci* (singular = coccus; from a Greek word meaning berry); elongated, cylindrical forms, some of which were cigarette-shaped, now classified under the general heading of *bacilli* (singular = bacillus; from a Greek word meaning rod); and others curved, wavy, or *helicoidal*, like a coiled wire spring, now known as *vibrios* and *spirilla*. Some of the helicoidally coiled bacteria are capable of flexing, twisting movements. These organisms are now grouped in a special order, Spirochaetales, commonly known as *spirochetes*. Figures 4–2 and 4–3 show four basic morphologic types of bacteria: cocci, rods, curved and helicoidal forms.

The *morphologic* **classification of bacteria** may be outlined as follows:

Spherical (cocci):
    Diplococcus (pairs)
    Streptococcus (chains)
    Staphylococcus (irregular clusters)
    Gaffkya (groups of 4)
    Sarcina (cubical packets)
Cylindrical:
    Bacilli (straight, commonly sausage or cigarette-shaped rods) many other
       elongated shapes and forms—outnumber all other bacterial forms
Helicoidal:
    Vibrio and *Spirillum* (from single curve of *Vibrio* to 5 and more corkscrew-like
       turns in *Spirillum; rigid*)
    Spirochetes (curved or spiral; *flexible;* Fig. 4–3)

Classification of Cocci.[3]   The division of the spherical and spheroidal bacteria into genera is based primarily on distinctive types of grouping

---

[3]According to a scheme of classification commonly used in the United States, found in *Bergey's Manual of Determinative Bacteriology,* 7th Ed. 1957, Baltimore, The Williams & Wilkins Co. This scheme will become obsolete on the publication of a new (8th) edition of *Bergey's Manual.* However, because of our use of a recent rearrangement and nomenclature for the enteric bacilli (Chapter 23), the newer name *Salmonella typhi* is used throughout instead of the older name *Salmonella typhosa* in the seventh edition of *Bergey's Manual.*

Figure 4–2

Some basic morphologic forms of bacteria, cocci, bacilli, and vibrios. Spiral forms are not shown here but are presented in Figure 4–3. Note that pleomorphic (abnormal, greatly distorted) forms of all these organisms are sometimes observed, as well as long filaments of very long rods that may then break up.

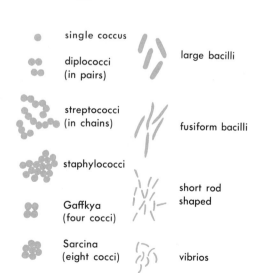

single coccus

diplococci
(in pairs)

streptococci
(in chains)

staphylococci

Gaffkya
(four cocci)

Sarcina
(eight cocci)

large bacilli

fusiform bacilli

short rod
shaped

vibrios

of the cells after fission. The cells of many species remain together in pairs after fission. In order to differentiate these pair-forming cocci they are called *diplococci*, the prefix *diplo* being derived from a word meaning *two* or *a pair*. There are two medically important genera of diplococci: *Diplococcus* and *Neisseria*. Other species of cocci cling together in long chains as they continue to divide, and this type is called *streptococci* (*strepto* = chain), e.g., genus *Streptococcus*. Still other cocci form neither regular pairs nor chains, but irregular groups and masses like clusters of grapes. These are often called micrococci or staphylococci (*staphylo* = cluster), e.g., genera *Micrococcus* and *Staphylococcus*. One type of coccus forms square groups of four cells and this organism is called *Gaffkya tetragena* ["producer of four"; Gaffky was a famous German bacteriologist (1850–1918)]. Another type of coccus, of little or no importance medically, produces cubical packets of organisms and is called *Sarcina*, from a Latin word meaning "packet."

Types of Bacilli.   Bacilli or rods are quite diverse in shape and size. Two groups that are of medical interest are spore-forming long rods that stain purple with Gram's stain; i.e., they are gram-positive. Others are slender and much smaller bacilli that do not form spores and are stained red by Gram's stain; i.e., they are gram-negative. Many gram-negative species belong to the genera *Escherichia*, *Salmonella*, *Shigella*, and *Proteus*. Many bacteria important in medicine belong to these genera.

To one group of the spore-forming rods just mentioned, which grow only in the presence of air, Cohn, their discover (1876), gave the name *Bacillus*. Strictly speaking, the term *Bacillus* is limited to the genus of spore-forming, rod-shaped, mostly gram-positive bacteria that grow only in the presence of air. When so used, the word *Bacillus* is italicized and begins with a capital B. The term bacillus, not italicized and with a small b, is widely used for *any* rod-shaped bacterium – gram-positive or gram-negative, spore-forming or not.

The other group of gram-positive, spore-forming rods is called the genus *Clostridium*. Members of the genus *Clostridium* grow only in the absence of air. This strange phenomenon, discovered by Pasteur and called *anaerobiosis*, will be discussed later. No bacteria other than the genera *Bacillus* and *Clostridium* (with possibly one or two exceptions) form highly heat-resistant spores.

Types of Helicoidal Bacteria.   There are two types of helicoidal bacteria: *rigid* and *flexible.* The *rigid* helicoidal species occur in several families of Schizomycetes. Some are coiled in several turns; others are merely comma-shaped. Of the former, only one species is pathogenic, *Spirillum minus*, the cause of rat-bite fever. Of the many comma-shaped species, only a few are important human pathogens, notably *Vibrio cholerae*, also called *Vibrio comma*, the cause of Asiatic cholera, and *Vibrio El Tor*, the cause of a cholera-like disease.

ORDER SPIROCHAETALES.   The *flexible* helicoidal bacteria are grouped in this order. Members of this order are commonly referred to as spirochetes. The pathogenic species are slender, spiral microorganisms about 0.2 to 2 μm in diameter and ranging from 5 to 50 μm in length. About half the known species of spirochetes are harmless saprophytes, living in the soil, in decaying organic matter, and in stagnant pools. Many have a rather complicated structure, like a plastic tube wrapped around a central fibrillar rod or axial filament composed of a kind of elastic protein, with properties suggestive of protozoa. Others have a crest or ridge of chitin-like substance along one side (Fig. 4–3).

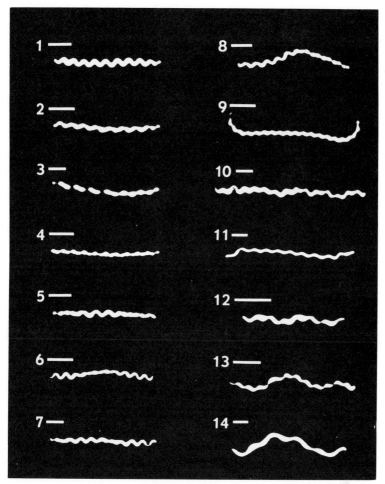

Figure 4–3

Dark-field micrographs of slowly rotating or stationary spirochaetes. Each bar equals 2 μm. (1–8), The Nichols virulent strain of *Treponema pallidum*. (9), *Leptospira* B-16 strain. (10), Reiter treponeme. (11), Kazan 8 treponeme. (12), *Spirochaeta zuelzerae*. (13), *Spirochaeta stenostrepta*. (14), *Spirochaeta aurantia*. Note that a single cell of *Treponema* is only 0.2 μm thick; thus, the illustration does not indicate how very delicate spirochetes really are. (From Cox, C. D.: *J. Bacteriol.*, 1972, *109*:943.)

The Anatomy of the Bacterial Cell

CAPSULES.   Capsules are a very important part of bacterial anatomy. Many, probably most, species of bacteria produce a gummy or slimy coating over their surface, which is spoken of as a capsule. It is sometimes a very thin film and invisible even when the bacteria are examined by special methods. At other times it is thick and may easily be demonstrated by simple methods (Fig. 4–4). Capsular material of many species of bacteria consists of starchlike or gummy substances called *polysaccharides*. The chemical composition of the capsule of any given type or species of bacteria is absolutely distinctive of that type or species and is said to be *type-* or *species-specific*. This distinctiveness is exceedingly valuable in medical

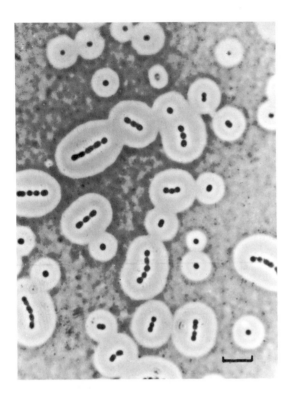

Figure 4–4

Photomicrograph of encapsulated streptococci suspended in India ink for
contrast. The small dark spheres are
cocci; the surrounding light areas,
capsules. These capsules are unusually
large. The straight line represents 10
micrometers at this magnification (about
× 1500). (Taylor and Juni: *J. Bact.*,
81:688, 1961.)

work, since it affords a reliable means of diagnosis in bacterial infections.
This is discussed in detail in Chapter 28. Capsules generally confer increased virulence on bacteria possessing them, probably because, like a
jacket or armor, they insulate the bacteria from the phagocytes, antibodies, and other defensive mechanisms of an infected body and from
many other deleterious influences.

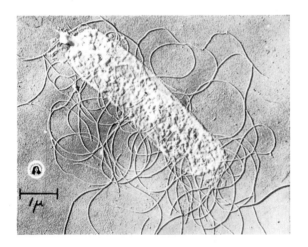

Figure 4–5

Electron micrograph of a common
bacterium (*Proteus vulgaris*) showing
peritrichous flagellation. (Line
shows size of 1 μm at this huge
magnification.) Note the fineness
of the flagella, their insertion
through the cell wall of the bacterium, and the apparent origin of
several flagella in a small granule,
suggestive of a blepharoplast. Note
also the diffuse, granular character
of the cell contents. (Courtesy of
Drs. A. L. Houwink, C. F. Robinow,
and W. van Iterson. From the collection of the American Society for
Microbiology. The small portrait
of Antony van Leeuwenhoek is in
the emblem of the American Society for Microbiology.)

In one order of filamentous aquatic bacteria numerous cells are arranged end-to-end inside a distinct and discrete tubular structure called a *sheath.* These organisms are not pathogenic. In some pathogenic species a thin, capsule-like surface layer on individual cells is often called a *sheath antigen.*

Capsules and Health. Easily identifiable capsules may not always be present on bacterial cells, and they constitute a variable factor in bacterial structure. Usually they are present on bacteria infecting the body. Hence, bacteria in pus, mucus, and feces from an infected person are particularly dangerous because of the increased virulence conferred on them by their capsule. This is a very important fact that should be remembered.

FLAGELLA. Flagella (flagellum, sing. = "whip") are long, extremely fine, hairlike appendages distributed on the outside of the cell in various ways. They enable flagellate organisms to swim about in fluids (Fig. 4–5). Many types of microorganisms have flagella, for example, protozoa and certain algae. Among bacteria, only certain species of rod-shaped bacteria (bacilli) and species of *Vibrio* and *Spirillum* have them. The spherical bacteria (cocci) generally do not have flagella.[4]

The means by which flagella move are not clear, since there are no known muscles in unicellular microorganisms. Recent evidence has shown that bacterial flagella consist of a protein called flagellin (mol. wt. 20,000) and are attached to protoplasmic material inside the cell and not to outside cellular slime, capsule, or cell wall. Unless prepared with certain stains, flagella are not readily visible with ordinary microscopes, but the motion produced by them is readily observed by mounting and examining a drop of fluid culture under a microscope, as described in Chapter 9.

Flagella located at one or both *ends* of rods are said to be *polar;* located indiscriminately on the surface of the rod, they are said to be *peritrichous.* The location of flagella is of use in identifying species.

PILI OR FIMBRIAE. Pili, like flagella, are very thin, hairlike, external appendages of a cell, protruding from the cytoplasm through the cell membrane, cell wall, and capsule if present. They are generally peritrichously arranged and around 150 in number. They consist of a specific protein called *pilin.* (See Fig. 4–9.)

Unlike flagella, pili are rigid, relatively short, straight, and not associated with motion. Their functions are not yet fully known but certain forms of pili (F pili) appear definitely to play a role in the primitive sexual conjugation processes in certain species of bacteria. They have so far been seen only on gram-negative bacteria.

SPORES. Of the 1700 or more species of bacteria only two genera (*Bacillus* and *Clostridium*) have the power of forming within each cell a small, round, or oval granule, glistening and apparently hard and thick-walled (Fig. 4–6). These are dormant *spores* and they contain the essential parts of the protoplasm of the cell in a condensed, probably dehydrated, form. Spores of these two groups of bacteria are far more resistant to drying and sunlight, heat, and disinfectants than the ascospores, conidiospores, and sporangiospores of yeasts and molds and the cysts of protozoa, though the term spore is sometimes used for all such bodies. Bacterial spores, more specifically called *endospores,* can resist drought, sunlight, heat (even boiling), disinfectants, and other unfavorable conditions for long periods (Fig. 4–7). Although the numerous spores produced by

---

[4]There may be one or two exceptions.

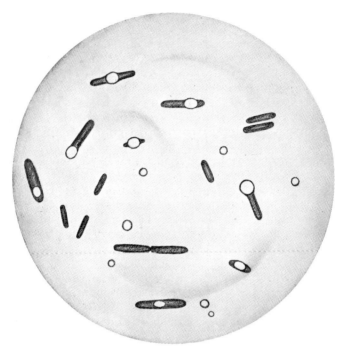

Figure 4–6

Various types of bacterial spores. Some of the spores have escaped from the sporangia. Stained with methylene blue, which does not penetrate inside the spore, only the outer surface of the spore is stained.

eucaryotic fungi are reproductive stages of normal life cycles, sexual or asexual, bacterial spores must be considered to be formed only as means of survival when conditions for growth and metabolism are unfavorable, since only one endospore (rarely two) is produced per cell.

Spores and Sterilization.   Spores are of tremendous significance in sterilization and surgery because they are so very resistant to chemical disinfectants, boiling, and so forth. It is of great importance that anyone working with (or against!) microorganisms learn what organisms produce spores and how to kill both the spores and the organisms. Detailed information on these points is given in Chapters 12 and 15 and Appendix C.

Spores and Dust.   A spore may leave a bacillus which then becomes nothing more than an empty shell, often called a *sporangium*. The spore may be blown about with dust, which contains the spores (also conidia, and so on) of many organisms and is always a potential source of contamination. When conditions are favorable for the active, vegetative, and reproductive life of the microorganisms, as in a surgical wound, in injured tissue, in unrefrigerated food (moisture, nutriment, and warmth are necessary), the spore "sprouts," or germinates, changes back to the ordinary vegetative form of the organism, and goes on growing. Only a few of the species of bacteria of importance in the health professions form spores, but the diseases they cause are often fatal. Among them are anthrax, tetanus (lockjaw), gas gangrene, and botulism (food poisoning).

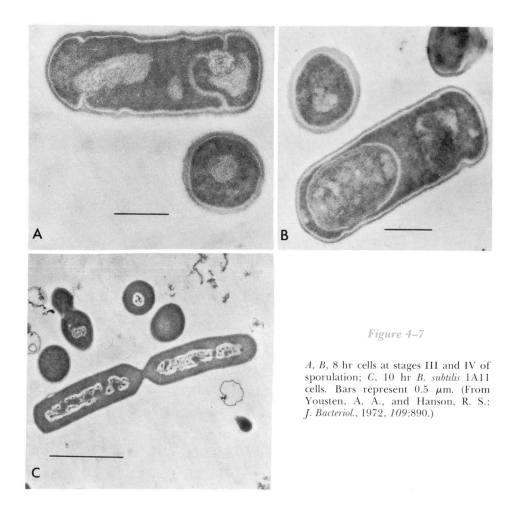

Figure 4-7

A, B, 8 hr cells at stages III and IV of sporulation; *C,* 10 hr *B. subtilis* 1A11 cells. Bars represent 0.5 μm. (From Yousten, A. A., and Hanson, R. S.: *J. Bacteriol.,* 1972, *109*:890.)

NUCLEI OF BACTERIA. The bacterial nucleus is unlike those of eucaryotic plants and animals because it has no nuclear membrane and no definite form. It is typical of procaryotic cells and is commonly referred to as a *nucleoid.* Because of the high RNA content in the cytoplasm of bacteria and the lack of a nuclear membrane it is difficult to demonstrate the nucleoid (also called chromatin body or nuclear body). However, special treatment shows the existence in most bacilli of two or more such bodies per cell. Nuclear division occurs first, and then cell division. Since the nuclear bodies (nucleoids) are attached to the cytoplasmic membrane by mesosomes during cell division, after septum formation the membrane pulls the nuclear bodies along into both of the daughter cells. No spindle fibers are needed. In experiments *Escherichia coli* was treated with an isotope-labeled nucleic acid constituent, tritiated thymidine. The isotope-containing chemical was taken up into the bacterial chromosome, which made it possible to trace the DNA after cell division with autoradiography (exposure of a photographic film to the isotope). The structure of the

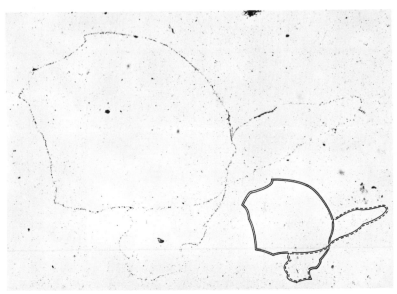

Figure 4–8

Autoradiograph of the chromosome of *Escherichia coli* Hfr K-12, labeled with tritiated thymidine for two generations and extracted with lysozyme in a dialysis chamber. Exposure time was two months. The inset is an interpretive diagram of the replication process. (From Cairns, J.: *J. Mol. Biol.*, Vol. 6: 208, 1963.)

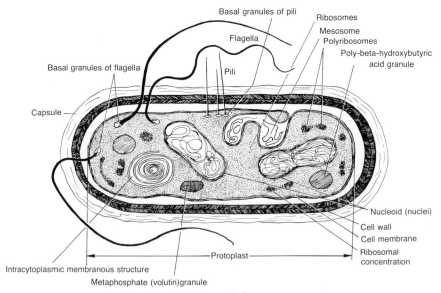

Figure 4–9

Diagram of a typical bacterial (procaryotic) cell showing all recognized structures. The space (theoretical) between cell membrane and cell wall is exaggerated to show the extent of the protoplast.

labeled chromosome strand was clearly shown (Fig. 4–8). The results indicated that the bacterium contained a circle of double-stranded DNA which when spread out would be about 1000 times as long as the bacterial cell itself. Important structural details of a common type of bacterial cell are shown diagrammatically in Figure 4–9. Lederberg's work on bacterial genetics will be discussed in detail in Chapter 7.

GRANULES OF BACTERIA. As noted in Chapter 2, cells of micro-organisms contain many granular structures; some have a role in repro-duction, some in the vital functions of food utilization (Fig. 4–10). In bac-teria some granules are obviously stored food material, such as fat or poly-beta-hydroxybutyric acid, and carbohydrates. These granules vary greatly in size and in number. Granules of complex groups (polymers) of inorganic phosphates are a stored form of phosphorus that is essential in the energy chemistry of the cell. Such granules have long been known as *"volutin."* In some species, such as the diphtheria bacillus or the bacillus of bubonic plague, they are so consistently present in characteristic numbers and lo-

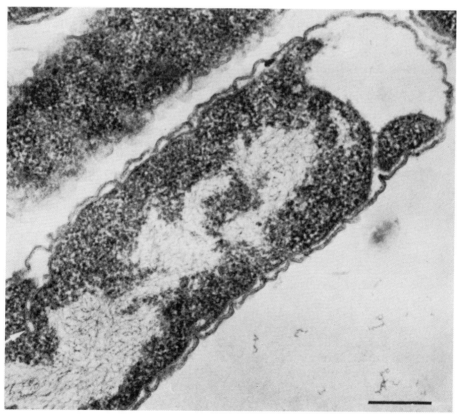

Figure 4–10

Electron micrograph of a cross section of a common non-sporing bacterium (*Escherichia coli*), showing nucleoplasm (light, centrally located amorphous masses) occupying a large portion in the cell. This cell shows the effects of experimentally induced plasmolyses, with the cytoplasm contracted at one pole. This photograph also shows the distribution of ribosomes throughout the cell and the laminated structures of the cytoplasmic membrane and the cell wall. (From Woldringh and van Iterson: *J. Bact.*, 111:801, 1972.)

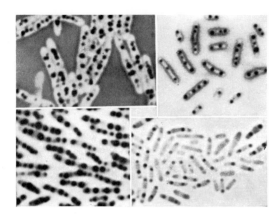

Figure 4–11

A common, harmless bacterium (*Entero-bacter aerogenes*) stained by the Albert-Laybourn method for demonstrating volutin granules. Volutin (inorganic phosphate—*polyphosphate* or "polyP") is a reserve food substance. Magnification originally × 3000. (Courtesy of Drs. J. P. Duguid, I. W. Smith and J. F. Wilkinson, Dept. of Bacteriology, University of Edinburgh, Scotland. In *J. Path. and Bact.*, Vol. 67, also *J. Bact.*, Vol. 68.)

cations in the cell that an experienced bacteriologist can diagnose these diseases merely by microscopic examination of pus and other substances containing the specific bacilli (Fig. 4–11). By certain staining procedures, some of these granules may be made to take on various colors different from the rest of the organism; therefore, they are sometimes called "metachromatic granules."

PIGMENTS. Many species of bacteria form pigments that range from white through the colors of the spectrum. Pigments may be hardly perceptible or very brilliant. The physiologic significance of most of these pigments is obscure, but they are of importance to the medical bacteriologist because they furnish an additional characteristic for the identification of species and the diagnosis of infections. They appear to have no relation to virulence. Pigments are easily observed in colonies of bacteria grown on solid medium in Petri plates. In some species of alga-like bacteria, the pigments are related to chlorophyll and carry on photosynthesis. They are of no medical importance.

THE MAJOR GROUPS (ORDERS) OF BACTERIA

ORDER EUBACTERIALES. The name of this order means "true bacteria." Most of the bacteria that are pathogens of man are included in this order. There are also many nonpathogens. The order includes only morphologically simple and undifferentiated forms: rods, spheres, and minor variations of these such as spheroidal, club-shaped, and fusiform (cigar-shaped). These bacteria exhibit no special anchoring or reproductive structures, as do molds or higher plants. They are not flexible, do not form branched structures, and do not grow upon stalks, as do bacteria in some other orders. Although various species of Eubacteriales differ widely from one another in form, motility, and enzymes produced, the Eubacteriales have in common an existence as unicellular fungi, each cell independent of the others (except when they may accidentally cling together in various ways after fission). When they are growing in colonies, there is nothing to suggest any functional specialization of certain cells such as occurs in molds and in the higher plants.

---

[5]According to the seventh (1957) edition of *Bergey's Manual of Determinative Bacteriology.*

The nearest approach of any of the Eubacteriales to the more complicated forms of plant life is the production of endospores (within the cells of only two genera, *Bacillus* and *Clostridium;* see Figure 4–7), and in the appearance of cells having irregular shapes, often suggestive of branching.

The Eubacteriales are probably close to the most primitive forms of living matter imaginable, having evolved, during hundreds of millions of years, little beyond single cells with special enzymatic powers. This order includes not only many bacteria important in medicine, such as the gonococcus (*Neisseria gonorrhoeae*) and the typhoid bacillus (*Salmonella typhi*), but also species of importance to the farmer, like the nitrogen-fixing bacteria (*Rhizobium* and *Azotobacter*) of the soil, and still others, such as the butyl alcohol bacteria (e.g., *Clostridium butylicum*), of importance in fermentation industries.

ORDER PSEUDOMONADALES.   This group is the largest in the entire class Schizomycetes. All but a few soil-living species are simple, unicellular forms, gram-negative, nonspore-forming, and either curved, spiral, or cigarette-shaped rods. A few are spheroidal. All motile Pseudomonadales differ from all motile Eubacteriales in that flagella of motile Pseudomonadales are located only at one or both ends of the cell (*polar* flagella), whereas flagella of motile species of Eubacteriales may appear at both ends as well as on all sides (*peritrichous* flagella).

Many species of Pseudomonadales are of great importance as soil builders, as scavengers, as nitrogen fixers, in photosynthesis, and so on. Many are important pathogens of valuable agricultural and horticultural plants and of lower animals. Fortunately, only four species are of importance in human disease. These are: *Pseudomonas aeruginosa*, a troublesome, nonspecific secondary invader of already injured tissues, often causing cystitis, otitis media, and infections of ulcers, in which it produces blue-green pus; *Spirillum minus*, previously named as the cause of one form of the rare (in North America) disease, rat-bite fever; *Vibrio cholerae*, cause of Asiatic cholera, which is common in the Orient but absent from the Western Hemisphere and Europe (unless accidentally introduced by personnel returning from Vietnam, etc.), and *Pseudomonas pseudomallei*, cause of a dangerous, glanders-like disease (melioidosis) in man, now being seen more and more frequently in our military personnel in Vietnam. These pathogenic Pseudomonadales will be discussed later on.

ORDER MYCOPLASMATALES.   This order comprises two (or three) groups of organisms that show differing degrees of relatedness to true bacteria, depending on stability of cell walls.

Mycoplasma.   The first of these curious organisms to be described was isolated in 1898 by Nocard and Roux, French scientists, from the pleural fluids (fluids collecting around the lungs) of cattle with an infectious disease called bovine pleuropneumonia. The organisms were (and still are) called pleuropneumonia organisms. The organism discovered by Nocard and Roux is now classified as the species *Mycoplasma mycoides* in the order of Mycoplasmatales.

These organisms are now considered to be modified bacteria. They are cultivable in the dark on lifeless media and like other bacteria are visible with ordinary microscopes. Unlike other bacteria, however, they have no cell wall and are enclosed only in a thin, limp, membranous sac. Consequently their shape and size are *extremely* variable; i.e., they are highly *pleomorphic* (Greek *pleon*, many, and *morphe*, form; appearing in many forms). Sometimes they produce elements that, like viruses, are small enough to pass through bacteria-retaining filters. The exact relationship of *Mycoplasma* to other bacteria is still under investigation by microbiologists. Although many different strains of *Mycoplasma* have been shown to cause diseases in cattle, goats, rats, chickens, cats, and so on, only two have been proved to be pathogenic in man, namely, *M. pneumoniae* (induces a type of pneumonia) and *M. hominis I* (genital tract abscesses).

PPLO.   After the discovery of pleuropneumonia organisms by Nocard and Roux numerous other organisms resembling them were found. These were not related to the disease pleuropneumonia but were found in other pathologic conditions and even in sewage, and were spoken of as *pleuropneumonia-like organisms*, or PPLO for short.

L Bodies.   During the last two decades, studies of certain bacteria have shown that under certain conditions of cultivation (e.g., in the presence of penicillin and some other substances that interfere with synthesis of, or destroy, cell walls) or as a result, apparently, of genetic mutations, many bacteria grow without a cell wall in a form called *protoplasts* (see Fig. 4–9) or *L bodies*. Continued studies have shown several supposed PPLO to be merely cell-wall-less forms of known species of bacteria. Many bacteria may readily be induced to assume either cellular or L body form. PPLO are frequently reported as being found in various pathologic conditions: arthritis, otitis media, pneumonia, urethritis, and so on. Some have been induced more or less readily to assume the parent bacterial form.

Whether the pleuropneumonia organisms (*Mycoplasma*) of Nocard and Roux are really a separate group of microorganisms, e.g., bacteria that have permanently lost (or never acquired ?) the ability to synthesize a cell wall, or are merely L forms of familiar bacteria that have not yet been observed to revert to a bacterial form, is still a matter of debate.

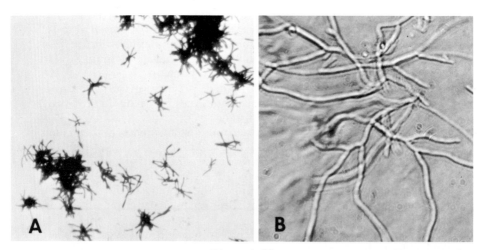

Figure 4–12

A pathogenic actinomycete, *Actinomyces israelii. A,* Smear from anaerobic (thioglycollate broth) culture (× 650). *B,* A very young colony on agar incubated anaerobically with 5 per cent carbon dioxide plus 95 per cent nitrogen at 37 C (× 1750). Note the true-branching mycelia. (Howell, Murphy, Paul, and Stephen: *J. Bact.,* Vol. 78.)

ORDER ACTINOMYCETALES.   These organisms represent a slightly more advanced stage in the evolution of the plant kingdom than do the Eubacteriales. They differ strikingly from the Eubacteriales in that the cells of Actinomycetales branch (Fig. 4–12), many as extensively as those of molds. In general, Actinomycetales may be cultivated in much the same manner and media as true bacteria, yeasts, and molds, and may be stained and studied in the same way. The name of the order is derived from the term *Actinomyces.* This was used by Harz in 1878 (*actino* = radially; *myces* = fungus) to describe the radially growing fungus-like organism (*Actinomyces bovis*) that causes "lumpy jaw" of cattle.

The diameter of the branching filaments, or *hyphae,* of the Actinomycetales is unlike that of molds, which are relatively enormous. The diameter of filaments of Actinomycetales, like that of all other bacteria, is around 2 μm. The length of the hyphae, however, may reach hundreds or thousands of microns (micrometers). The whole plant structure consisting of these branched, interlacing hyphae is spoken of as a *mycelium* and may form a colony ranging in size from less than one-fourth inch to an inch or more in diameter.

Those biologists who regard the primitive waters of the earth as the place in which life originated may find support for this view in the numbers of motile, aquatic, and marine forms of hundreds of species of bacteria. Many Eubacteriales, Pseudomonadales, and numerous others are essentially fluid-inhabiting, swimming organisms. The Actinomycetales, on the contrary, are mostly terrestrial, largely restricted to the soil, and, with one or two aquatic exceptions, nonmotile, i.e., not equiped for swimming. In keeping with a terrestrial or "dry-land" mode of existence, they can grow on solid surfaces exposed to the air, like old, damp shoes or wallpaper in damp houses, and require relatively little fluid moisture. They grow rather slowly and prefer damp atmospheres and comfortable room temperatures (20 to 30 C) to body temperature (37 C). They grow on a wide variety of nutrient substances.

In the seventh edition of *Bergey's Manual of Determinative Bacteriology,* the order is divided into four families, only three of which are of immediate interest to health personnel: the Mycobacteriaceae, the Actinomycetaceae, and the Streptomycetaceae.

The Family Mycobacteriaceae.   Cells of the Mycobacteriaceae occasionally branch to the extent of forming L, T, Y, V, and similar simple arrangements, but otherwise the Mycobacteriaceae resemble true bacteria (Eubacteriales) in size and form, being mainly slender, sometimes slightly curved, and often spindle-shaped, rods. This family contains only one genus of medical importance, called *Mycobacterium* (*Myco* = moldlike). This genus contains *M. tuberculosis* (the cause of tuberculosis) and *M. leprae* (the cause of leprosy, or Hansen's disease).

The Family Actinomycetaceae.   Actinomycetaceae contains two genera, *Actinomyces* and *Nocardia,* which branch somewhat more than mycobacteria. The genus *Actinomyces* includes *A. bovis* or *A. israelii,* or both, which are found in the mouths of man and cattle and sometimes cause ulcerative, invasive, and necrotic suppurative lesions in the jaws ("lumpy jaw" in cattle), tongue ("wooden tongue" in cattle), and adjacent parts by invading the tissues. The disease is called *actinomycosis* and is dangerous and often fatal.

Most species of *Nocardia* are harmless and live in fertile soil on rotting organic matter. They are numerous and widespread and help cause decay. A few species occasionally cause diseases of the lungs or other tissues, sometimes resembling actinomycosis and sometimes (in the lungs) tuberculosis. Such infections are called *nocardiosis.* Among the common pathogenic *Nocardia* are *N. madurae* (causing forms of Madura foot, an actinomycosis-like disease of the feet and legs); *N. asteroides* (causing an infection of the lungs, which may at times be mistaken for tuberculosis); *N. farcinicus* (causing lumpy lesions, or farcy, in tissues of cattle and horses). Actinomycosis and nocardiosis in man are relatively uncommon in North America and are not highly infectious to attendants, though often fatal to the patient.

The Family Streptomycetaceae.   This family of the order Actinomycetales is distinguished by the formation of extensive moldlike mycelia, the long hyphae branching freely. Coiled aerial hyphae are a striking feature. As in true molds, sporelike bodies called *conidia* appear on the ends of these, in long, brilliantly colored chains. These conidia (sometimes called spores) resist drying but do not have the high resistance to temperature that is characteristic of true bacterial spores and are readily killed by a few minutes of boiling and by vigorous disinfection. The forms of the coils of conidia serve as one basis of classification (Fig. 4–13).

To the health worker, only the genus *Streptomyces* is of importance, and only a few species need be mentioned here. One is *S. griseus,* the source of the antibiotic drug streptomycin; another is *S. aureofaciens,* the producer of the antibiotic chlortetracycline (Aureomycin); a third is *S. rimosus,* the source of oxytetracycline (Terramycin). These drugs will be mentioned later on. Numerous other species of *Streptomyces* valuable for the production of antibiotics have been discovered. None is an important pathogen of human beings.

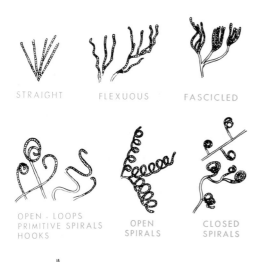

STRAIGHT   FLEXUOUS   FASCICLED

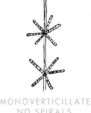

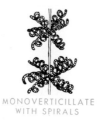

OPEN · LOOPS
PRIMITIVE SPIRALS   OPEN   CLOSED
HOOKS   SPIRALS   SPIRALS

Figure 4–13

Distinctive arrangements of conidial filaments of various types of *Streptomyces.* (Adapted from Pridham, Hesseltine and Benedict: *Appl. Microbiol.,* Vol. 6.)

MONOVERTICILLATE   MONOVERTICILLATE
NO SPIRALS   WITH SPIRALS

ORDER SPIROCHAETALES.   Some of the characteristics of this order have been mentioned previously in this chapter (also see Fig. 4–3). Spirochetes move in spiral or undulating fashion, or by rapid darting and wriggling motions. They progress because of their rotating spiral structure. Unlike most other bacteria, they can bend and twist themselves because of contractile elastic protein fibrils; true muscles are believed to be absent. Spirochetes resemble other bacteria in method of nutrition, multiplication, diameter, and procaryotic cell structure.

The order Spirochaetales contains some very dangerous pathogenic organisms, among them the organism causing syphilis (*Treponema pallidum*); that causing leptospirosis (including hemorrhagic jaundice), namely, *Leptospira icterohaemorrhagiae;* and that causing relapsing fever (*Borrelia*).

Except species of *Leptospira*, pathogenic spirochetes are difficult or impossible to cultivate, and require very special media. They also stain with difficulty and hence are usually observed alive with the darkfield apparatus, or with special phase-contrast techniques that will be described later.

APPLICATION TO HEALTH

The recognition of scientific names of bacteria and other microorganisms in laboratory reports will enable those who are sufficiently well educated to understand and bring important reports immediately to the attention of the physician. Recognition of the variability of bacteria should certainly be helpful in understanding some of the delays in laboratory studies. Knowledge of genetics and adaptability of microorganisms to chemotherapeutic agents is essential to intelligent administration of correct doses of sulfonamides and antibiotics at properly spaced intervals. This material on physiology, morphology, and structure of bacteria will also be referred to later under the discussion of pathogenic bacteria. The student will soon begin to associate names of organisms with morphology and with specific diseases.

As has been pointed out, the scientific names of microorganisms are clues to distinctive properties and characteristics of each organism. It would be tedious (but not impossible) to learn by rote the scientific names of all microorganisms important to the care of patients. Just to learn the names, however, would be pointless without learning the meaning and significance of these names. For example, the student will quickly learn that recovery of *Bacillus subtilis* from supposedly sterile packages in the operating room is a sign of danger, because *B. subtilis*, though usually regarded as harmless, is a spore-former, and its survival indicates that sterility has not been attained. Recovery of the same organism from the dust in the hospital wards, however, would not be a source of alarm, since the organism is generally nonpathogenic and ubiquitous.

Because of the widespread publicity about staphylococcal infections, the beginning student may view with deep concern reports of skin cultures that show the presence of *Staphylococcus epidermidis.* The more knowledgeable student, however, is able to discriminate and recognize that the species that is the culprit in serious infections attributable to this genus is *S. aureus*, and that the strains of this species that produce a golden-yellow (*aureus*) pigment and the enzyme coagulase are the primary causes of dangerous cases of staphylococcal infections. One of the best ways of learning microbial nomenclature is to look up the characteristics of each genus and species of organism that you encounter either in the classroom, in the laboratory, or in practice. If you continue this method of learning, each time you are not sure of the characteristics of a particular microorganism, a body of information will quickly become a part of your working knowledge, on which you can build the sound practice of your profession.

Supplementary Reading

Ainsworth, G. C., and Sneath, P. H. A. (Editors): Microbial Classification. 12th Symposium, Society for General Microbiology. 1962, New York, Cambridge University Press.

Breed, R. S., Murray, E. G. D., and Smith, N. R. (Editors): Bergey's Manual of Determinative Bacteriology, 7th Ed. 1957, Baltimore, The Williams & Wilkins Co.

Cairns, J.: Cold Spring Harbor Sympos. Quant. Biol., 1963, 28:43.

Frobisher, M.: Fundamentals of Microbiology. 8th Ed. 1968, Philadelphia, W. B. Saunders Co.

Hayflick, L.: The Mycoplasmatales and the L-Phase of Bacteria. 1969, New York, Appleton-Century-Crofts.

Hirota, Y., Jacob, F., Buttin, G., and Nakai, T.: On the Process of Cellular Division in *Escherichia coli*. I. Asymmetrical cell division and production of deoxyribonucleic acid-less bacteria. *Molec. Biol.*, 1968, 35:175–192.

Holmgren, N. B., and Campbell, W. E., Jr.: Tissue cell culture contamination in relation to bacterial pleuropneumonia-like organisms L-form conversion. *J. Bact.*, 1960, 79:869.

Klieneberger-Nobel, E.: Pleuropneumonia-like Organisms (PPLO): Mycoplasmataceae. 1962, New York, Academic Press, Inc.

Leifson, E.: Bacterial taxonomy: A critique. *Bact. Rev.*, 1966, 30:257.

Pease, P.: Evidence that *Streptobacillus moniliformis* is an intermediate stage between a *Corynebacterium* and its L-form or derived PPLO. *J. Gen. Microbiol.*, 1962, 29:91.

Purcell, R. H., Valdesuso, J. R., Cline, W. L., James, W. D., and Chanock, R. M.: Cultivation of Mycoplasmas on glass. *Appl. Microbiol.*, 1971, 21:288.

Sharp, J. T. (Editor): The Role of Mycoplasmas and L Forms of Bacteria in Disease. 1970, Springfield, Ill., Charles C Thomas.

Skerman, V. B. D.: A Guide to the Identification of the Genera of Bacteria. 2nd Ed. 1967. Baltimore, The Williams & Wilkins Co.

Theodore, T. S., Tully, J. G., and Cole, R. M.: Polyacrylamide gel identification of bacterial L-forms and *Mycoplasma* species of human origin. *Appl. Microbiol.*, 1971, 21:272.

Wittler, R. G., et al.: Isolation of a *Corynebacterium* and its transitional forms from a case of subacute bacterial endocarditis treated with antibiotics. *J. Gen. Microbiol.*, 1960, 23:315.

Characteristics of Rickettsias and Chlamydias

5

The rickettsias and chlamydias are both dealt with in this chapter because, although they possess structural and physiological properties that show their close relationship to other bacteria, they also have several other distinctive properties in common, notably, very minute size and inability to grow anywhere except *inside the living cells* of other organisms. In the seventh (1957) edition of *Bergey's Manual of Determinative Bacteriology*, they were classified together in the class Microtatobiotes (Greek *microtatus*, smallest; *biote*, life): order I, Rickettsiales; families Rickettsiaceae and Chlamydiaceae, respectively. These two groups of organisms are now considered to be modified bacteria. They have procaryotic structure and numerous bacteria-like enzyme systems. Because these enzyme systems are inadequate for independent, extracellular life, they can multiply only intracellularly; i.e., they are *obligate, intracellular parasites*. In this they resemble viruses.

THE RICKETTSIAS

The rickettsias are named for their discoverer, Howard Taylor Ricketts (1871–1910). In form, they are much like bacteria, but rickettsias are even smaller, averaging about one-tenth to one-half as large. Several species of rickettsias cause serious diseases in man such as typhus (not typhoid) fever and Rocky Mountain spotted fever.

CHARACTERISTICS. Rickettsias are larger than the largest viruses, yet smaller than the smallest bacteria. They range from around 0.2 to 0.5 μm in diameter and up to 0.8 to 2.0 μm in length, and they are variously shaped, like minute rods, spheres, or diplococcoid; they may be ellipsoidal or even filamentous. They can just be seen with ordinary microscopes and thus differ from all but a few large viruses. Typical viruses are far smaller and can be seen only with electron microscopes (Figs. 5–1 and 5–2). It is difficult to stain rickettsias with dyes like Gram's

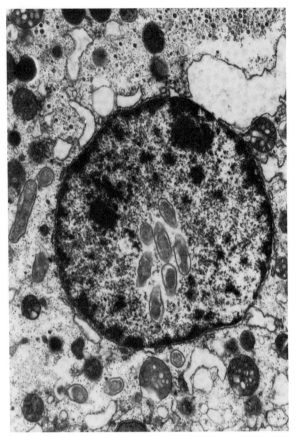

Figure 5–1

Ultrathin section of tick gut epithelium cell showing intranuclear growth of *R. canada.* × 14,500. Note bacterium-like size and form. (Burgdorfer, W., and Brinton, L. P.: Infection and Immunology, 2:112, 1970. Copyright American Society for Microbiology.)

stain (most are gram-negative; *Coxiella burneti* is gram-positive) and methylene blue, recommended for bacteria, but they are readily stained with complex mixtures of dyes, e.g., Macchiavello's, Giemsa's, and Wright's. The rickettsias are nonmotile and do not form spores. Only one strain, causing scrub typhus in man, has been shown to produce a toxin.

No true rickettsias have been cultivated in lifeless media. In this they resemble chlamydias and viruses. So far as is known, these organisms do not multiply outside the living cells of vertebrates or arthropods. Most rickettsias also resemble most bacteria in being nonfiltrable. Exceptions are the species of filtrable rickettsias that cause Q fever, *Coxiella burneti*, named for its discoverers H. L. Cox and F. M. Burnet. Like *all other cells*, and *unlike all viruses*, rickettsias contain both ribonucleic acid (RNA) and deoxyribonucleic acid (DNA), which occurs in strands. Viruses contain *either* RNA *or* DNA and are classified primarily on this basis. Rickettsias resemble bacteria in possessing muramic acid in their cell walls. Muramic acid is thought to occur only in bacteria, rickettsias, and chlamydias. In some species of rickettsias a capsule-like layer has been observed around the cell (Table 5–1).

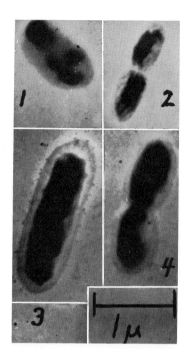

Figure 5–2

Electron micrographs of various representative rickettsias from yolk sac cultures. Note the bacterium-like form and structure, with cell wall, cytoplasm with intracellular granules, and what appears to be binary fission. Note also the small size as compared with bacteria. *1, R. mooseri; 2, Coxiella burneti; 3, R. rickettsii; 4, R. prowazekii.* (From the collection of the American Society for Microbiology, courtesy of Drs. H. Poltz, J. E. Smadel, T. F. Anderson, and L. A. Chambers. In *J. Exp. Med.*, Vol. 77.)

PROPAGATION.   Although rickettsias will not grow on lifeless media such as are used for yeasts, molds, and bacteria, they will multiply very well in the yolk sac of live embryonic chicks inside the egg. The yolk sacs are infected with a needle through a minute hole in the disinfected shell (Figs. 5–3 and 5–4). After inoculation of eggs with the appropriate rickettsias, and after several days of incubation, the yolk sacs, with their rickettsias, are removed from the eggs aseptically.[1] After various purifications and treatment with formaldehyde or some other means of killing the rickettsias, the material constitutes a vaccine that is used in immunizing persons likely to be exposed to the diseases caused by specific rickettsias. For example, persons traveling from the United States to certain areas where typhus fever (louse-borne) is prevalent are generally required to

[1]Completely avoiding contamination by any microorganisms from dust, eggshells, and so forth. Surgeons work as aseptically as possible.

Table 5–1.   Characteristics of Infectious Agents from Bacteria to Viruses*

MICRO-ORGANISMS	GROWTH ON ARTIFICIAL MEDIA	TWO NUCLEIC ACIDS	RESPONSE TO ANTIBIOTICS
Bacteria	+	+	+
Mycoplasma	+	+	+
Rickettsia	−	+	+
Chlamydia	−	+	+
Viruses	−	−	±

*From Debré and Celers: Clinical Virology, W. B. Saunders Co., 1970.

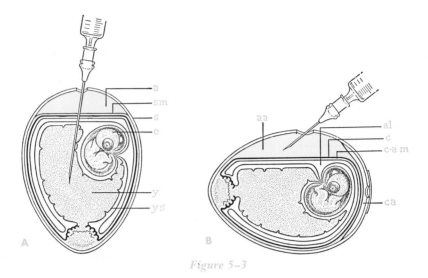

Figure 5–3

Methods of inoculating chick embryos. *A,* Injection into the yolk sac for cultivation of rickettsias. The normal air space is seen at a, the shell membrane at sm, and the shell at s. The living chick embryo is shown at e, while the yolk sac and yolk are seen at ys and y, respectively. *B,* Many microorganisms can infect the chorioallantoic membrane, seen at c-am. An artificial air space (aa) is created by allowing air from the normal air space to escape through the small opening seen at the right end of the egg as the opening for the needle is made. The collapsed air sac (ca) is then sealed up. Other important parts of the embryonic membranes and sacs are the allantoic sac (al) and the chorion (c). (Courtesy of E. R. Squibb & Sons. From Kelley and Hite.)

take "shots" (immunizing injections) of such a vaccine. Such antigens are also used in diagnostic serologic tests.

Habitat.   The rickettsias appear characteristically to inhabit the living cells lining the intestines of arthropods, both blood-sucking and nonblood-sucking. Several pathogenic species inhabit arthropods that bite human beings or animals, or both. Nonpathogenic (supposedly!)

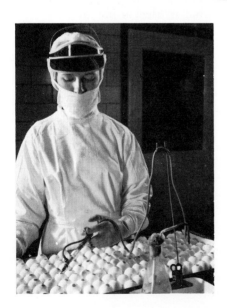

Figure 5–4

Carefully dressed technician using a pressure-fed syringe to inoculate fertile eggs with suspension of living rickettsias. The eggs, after suitable incubation, will be used in the preparation of vaccines or of antigens for diagnostic purposes. (Courtesy of E. R. Squibb & Sons.)

rickettsias, also, have been found in ticks, lice, bedbugs, spiders, and mosquitoes. The rickettsias, both pathogenic and nonpathogenic species, are found not only in the cells of the arthropod's intestines, but also frequently in the salivary glands, from which they may be transmitted to man by bites of the arthropod. Since they also occur in the intestinal contents, they appear in the feces. Thus transmission to animal hosts is often effected not only by bites, but by rubbing fecal material of arthropods into the skin. This is also true of certain arthropod-borne viral, bacterial, and protozoal diseases. The principal diseases of man caused by rickettsias are discussed in Chapter 39.

THE FAMILY CHLAMYDIACEAE

These organisms, formerly regarded as "large viruses," intermediates in size between "true" viruses and rickettsias, are now included, with rickettsias, as bacteria that have become adapted to *obligate* intracellular existence. Their cellular structure appears to be procaryotic though complete details are still lacking. Like all other cellular organisms and totally unlike viruses, they contain both RNA and DNA and they have synthetic enzyme systems; thus they are sensitive to most antibiotics. Remember that antibiotics act chiefly by inhibiting vital enzyme systems.

Chlamydias are larger than even the pox viruses (Fig. 6–2), but much smaller than any bacteria. Chlamydias characteristically occur in the form of very minute coccoid or roughly cuboidal bodies. These organisms are visible under ordinary microscopes, and they may be stained like bacteria. Like rickettsias (also many bacteria and viruses), they are cultivable in the chick embryo, especially in the yolk sac. They will not grow in the non-living media, and they are filtrable only with difficulty.

Chlamydias appear to parasitize their host cell for most of their energy and to lack most energy-yielding enzyme systems. Their method of multiplication is not binary fission like other bacterial cells, but it is totally unlike that of viruses. At times, very minute bodies called "elementary bodies" are formed, suggestive of the minute "minimal reproductive units" of PPLO. Like PPLO also, chlamydias have a thin, limp, grape-skin–like coating.

Members of this group include the agents of psittacosis and ornithosis; lymphogranuloma venereum[2] (sometimes called the PLGV group); others cause trachoma, a severe infection of the eye with corneal involvement often leading to blindness; and severe conjunctivitis, usually in the newborn (inclusion conjunctivitis) which is contracted from the genitourinary tract of the mother during birth. The inclusion conjunctivitis organism may also cause a urethritis in the adult. The trachoma and inclusion conjunctivitis organisms are often called TRIC agents.

ANTIBIOTICS AND CHLAMYDIAS. We have previously noted that viruses such as those of measles, polio, influenza, and most others are not significantly affected by most antibiotics. Indeed, microbiologists add certain antibiotics to tissue cultures of many viruses in order to suppress

---

[2]*Lymphogranuloma venereum* is a venereal disease causing destructive ulcerations, buboes, and obstruction of the lymph channels in the genitalia and adjacent parts. It is fairly widely distributed among sexually promiscuous persons. This is discussed further in a later section.

contaminating bacteria and molds and permit the viruses to grow. Viruses contain no enzyme mechanisms for the ordinary antibiotics to affect.

In contrast to the viruses, the chlamydias represented by the PLGV and TRIC groups generally resemble rickettsias and other bacteria in being quite susceptible to certain antibiotics. They have more advanced, more vulnerable enzyme systems than do the viruses. Rickettsias are generally susceptible to the same antibiotics as are the chlamydias, and for similar reasons.

Supplementary Reading

Burgdorfer, W., and Brinton, L. P.: Intranuclear growth of *Ricksettsia canada*, a member of the typhus group. *Infect. Immunol.*, 1970. *2:*112.

Carpenter, P. L.: Microbiology, 3rd Ed. 1972, Philadelphia, W. B. Saunders Co.

Davis, B. D., Dulbecco, R., Eisen, H. N., Ginsberg, H. S., and Wood, W. B.: Microbiology. 1967, New York, Hoeber Medical Division, Harper & Row.

Kramer, M. J., and Gordon, F. B.: Ultrastructural analysis of the effects of penicillin and chlortetracycline on the development of a genital tract *Chlamydia. Infect. Immunol.*, 1971, *3:* 333.

Lennette, E. H., and Schmidt, N. J. (Editors): Diagnostic Procedures for Viral and Rickettsial Infections. 4th Ed. 1969, New York, American Public Health Association, Inc.

Moulder, J. W.: The relation of the psittacosis group (chlamydiae) to bacteria and viruses. *Ann. Rev. Microbiol.*, 1966, *20:*107.

Ormsbee, R. A.: Rickettsiae (as Organisms). *Ann. Rev. Microbiol.*, 1969, *23:*275.

Tamura, A., and Manire, G. P.: Effect of penicillin on the multiplication of meningopneumonitis organisms (*Chlamydia psittaci*). *J. Bact.*, 1968, *96:*875.

Characteristics of Viruses

6

Viruses resemble chlamydias and rickettsias in that they cannot be cultivated outside of living cells. Viruses, chlamydias, and rickettsias are therefore said to be obligate intracellular parasites. There are viruses that infect either plants or animals or bacteria. Viral proliferation within cells results in injury ranging from death and dissolution to abnormal cellular multiplication, often accompanied by distinctive intracellular appearances (see later discussion of cytopathic effect).

Because of their small size, viruses cannot be seen with an ordinary microscope. However, with the electron microscope and special techniques, very high magnifications of viruses may be obtained. Clever use has been made of the fact that viruses can pass through clay or porcelain filters that can hold back yeasts, molds, most bacteria, rickettsias, and all larger organisms. Today more sophisticated devices (filters) for separating microorganisms by their cell sizes have been made available for the laboratory worker in microbiology. Figure 6–1 shows such a device; others will be discussed in Chapters 9 and 12. High-speed differential centrifugation is also commonly used.

For many years after the first discovery of a virus (tobacco mosaic virus-TMV) by Metchnikoff in 1882 viruses were known mainly by the diseases they caused. Common examples of human viral diseases are poliomyelitis, influenza, measles, mumps, warts, chickenpox, and the common cold. More than 300 viruses are known at present and new ones are constantly being discovered. In this book only a few of the common viruses will be discussed, and some general properties common to all of them will be described. The study of viruses is now a very large and complex field called *virology*. One of the most studied and best known types of virus is called *bacteriophage* (*bacterio* = bacteria; Greek *phagein*, to eat). The name is derived from an early and erroneous notion that the virus ate the bacteria from within. A single individual virus particle of any kind is called a *virion*; it is not a true cell, since it has no autonomous metabolism or life.

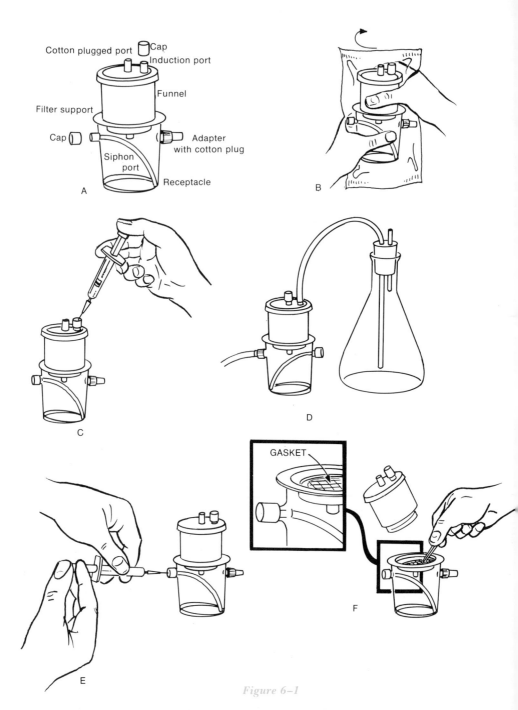

Figure 6–1

Filtration of viral suspensions under sterile conditions. *A*, The Falcon 150 ml filter units can be used free standing, clamped on ring stand, or connected in series to any vacuum source. I.D. tubing (3/8″ or 1/4″) may be used. *B*, Before removing filter unit from bag, grasp funnel portion with one hand while holding receptacle with other hand and apply firm pressure in a clockwise direction. Liquids to be filtered may be introduced by pouring directly into funnel, by syringe and needle through cap (*C*), or by tube from a source container (*D*). To remove filtrate, swab cap on siphon port with alcohol and insert needle and withdraw required volume (*E*). To remove membrane filter (*F*), grasp receptacle and unscrew funnel, then remove the rubber gasket by placing round nose forceps under the inner edge of the ring and lifting. (The gasket may be discarded or plated along with the filter.) Remove membrane filter by grasping the outer edge with flamed forceps. (Courtesy of Falcon Plastics, Division of BioQuest, Los Angeles, California.)

BACTERIOPHAGES

Bacteriophages, commonly called phages, are viruses that are pathogenic only for certain microorganisms, chiefly bacteria. Of importance in certain medical, diagnostic, and public health situations, they are commonly found in the intestinal tract. Because they are safe to handle, easily and cheaply cultivated in ordinary bacterial cultures, and relatively "hardy," phages have for years served as models for thousands of studies of viruses in general. It is essential to know what phages are, their properties and possible uses. They do not cause disease in man or lower animals. There are many kinds. Phages that attack a wide variety of protists have been discovered: coliphages, brucellaphages, actinophages, phages of yeasts (zymophages), lactic acid bacteria, and blue-green algae. They have long served as models of viruses in general.

MORPHOLOGY.   The electron microscope has enabled us to make pictures of many kinds of viruses, including phages (Fig. 6–2). The magnifications achieved in these electronic images (electron micrographs) are in the range of 10,000 to over 1,000,000 diameters, whereas ordinary optical microscopes give clear images up to only about 1200.

SIZE.   The diameters of some "large" viruses (e.g., smallpox) approach that of a small bacterium, *Escherichia coli* (about 1 μm = 1/25,400 inch); the diameter of some of the smallest viruses (e.g., yellow fever) is not much more than that of some protein molecules (e.g., egg albumin:

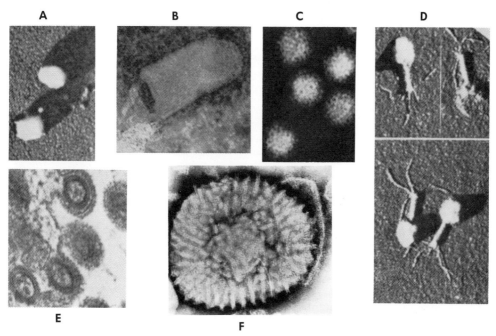

Figure 6–2

Various forms of virion. *A*, "Bun-" or brick-shaped Poxvirus (×24,000). (Courtesy Drs. F. P. O. Nalger and G. Rake: *J. Bact.*, Volume 55. *B*, Bullet-shaped rabies virus (×30,000). (From Murphy, Halonen, Gary and Reese: *J. Gen. Virol.*, 1968, *3*:289.) *C*, Icosahedral symmetry of reovirus (about ×10,000). (From Mayor and Jordan: *J. Gen. Virol.*, 1968, *3*:233.) *D*, Bacteriophage showing binal symmetry (×68,000). (Courtesy of Drs. R. C. Williams and D. Frazer: *Virology*, Vol. 2). *E*, Bittner (mouse mammary tumor) virus, showing cores and capsids and the manner in which viruses of this type acquire an envelope from the cell membrane on emerging from the infected cell (×60,000). (From Gay, Clarke and Dermott: *J. Virol.*, 1970, *5*:801.) *F*, A Poxvirus virion related to the virus in *A* but at ×150,000 magnification, showing details of irregular surface structure.

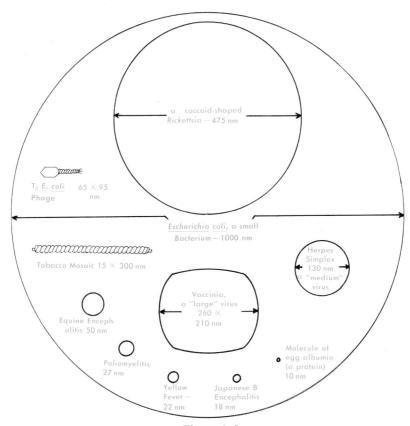

Figure 6-3

Diagrammatic comparison of sizes of viruses and related structures. The largest circle, enclosing the whole, represents the diameter of *Escherichia coli*, a small cylindrical bacterium about 1 μm (1000 nm) in diameter. The other objects are drawn to approximately the same scale. (Sketch and sizes based on Rivers and Horsfall: Viral and Rickettsial Infections of Man. Philadelphia, J. B. Lippincott Co.)

0.01 μm = 0.000,000,39 inch). It is easy to understand why viruses were formerly called ultramicroscopic (Fig. 6–3).

SHAPE.   The appearance of viruses in electron micrographs is quite striking and some of the viruses may be distinguished by their form. Some viruses that infect animals or man (zoopathogenic viruses) exhibit various types of polyhedral shapes such as icosahedral, cuboidal (various types of *cubic symmetry*), spherical, ovoid, bullet-shaped, or helical (*helical symmetry*). Bacteriophages commonly have tadpole-like shapes with polyhedral "heads" attached to slender "tails" (Figs. 6–4 and 6–5). Since they have two parts with different forms they are said to have *binal symmetry*.

In the electron micrographs of viruses shown in this book, the appearance of height or thickness is given by "shadowing." This is a technique of casting metallic vapors at an angle across the object to be pictured so that some parts are made opaque (shadowed), thus giving the illusion of perspective in the pictures.

STRUCTURE.   All viruses consist of an inner portion or *core* consisting entirely of RNA or DNA, never both. Note that the primary sub-

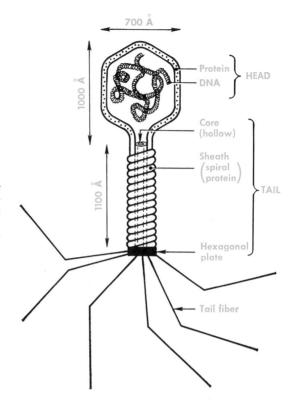

Figure 6–4

Diagrammatic representation of the structures observed in intact and triggered T-even phages of *E. coli.* (From Herskowitz, I. H.: Genetics. 2nd Ed. Boston, Little, Brown and Company, Inc., 1965.)

division of viruses is based on the kind of nucleic acid that they contain (see Table 6–1). For example, the first virus discovered, in 1892 by Iwanowski, causes a plant disease and is named after this disease, the tobacco mosaic virus (TMV). The TMV consists of a helical core of RNA (Fig. 6–6). The core is enclosed within an outer protective coating called a *capsid*. The capsid consists of protein units called *capsomeres*; their number, form, and arrangement around the core being symmetrical and distinctive

Figure 6–5

Bacteriophage T4r⁺ infecting *E. coli* (×210,000). The retracted tail sheath, base plate and fibers are evident. (From Margaretten, Morgan, Rosenkranz, and Rose: *J. Bact.*, 1966, *91*:823.)

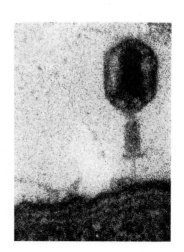

Table 6–1. Virus Classification on the Basis of Nucleic Acid and Lipid Content, Acid Sensitivity, and Size Estimate*

NUCLEIC ACID CONTENT	ETHER AND/OR CHLOROFORM SENSITIVITY	PH 3.0 SENSITIVITY	VIRUS FAMILY OR GROUP	NUMBER OF TYPES IN HUMANS	SIZE ESTIMATE (IN μM)	NUCLEIC ACID STRANDS†
DNA	Resistant	Resistant	Adenovirus (Respiratory infections)	31	70	Single
	Resistant	Resistant	Papovavirus (Warts, polyoma, papilloma)		40–50	Double
	Sensitive	Sensitive	Poxvirus (Cowpox, smallpox)	25	200–300	Double
	Sensitive	Sensitive	Herpesvirus (Herpes simplex, varicella-zoster, cytomegalovirus)		180	Single
RNA	Resistant	Resistant	Reovirus (previously ECHO type 10)		60–75	Double
	Resistant	Resistant	Enterovirus (subgroup of Picornavirus) (a) Poliovirus	64 3	15–30	Single

Table 6–1 *continued on opposite page.*

			Virus	Number of types	Size	Strand†
RNA	Resistant	Sensitive	(b) Coxsackie virus (c) Echovirus	{Group A=24 Group B= 6} 34		
	Sensitive	Sensitive	Rhinovirus (subgroup of Picornavirus)	over 70	15–30	Single
	Sensitive	Sensitive	Arbovirus (Dengue fever, yellow fever)	over 200	30–50	Single
		Sensitive	Myxovirus (a) Influenza	A,B,C, and subgroups 4	100–120	Single
			(b) Parainfluenza			
			(c) Mumps			
			(d) Newcastle disease			
			(e) Respiratory syncytial (RS virus)			
			(f) Rubeola	1		
	Sensitive	Sensitive	Rabies		60–175	
	Sensitive	Sensitive	Rubella	1	50–75	
	Sensitive	Sensitive	Avian infections (Bronchitis virus, IBV-like viruses)		80–160	

*After Diagnostic Procedures for Viral and Rickettsial Infections. American Public Health Association.
†Nucleic acid strands in RNA or DNA where experimental evidence exists.

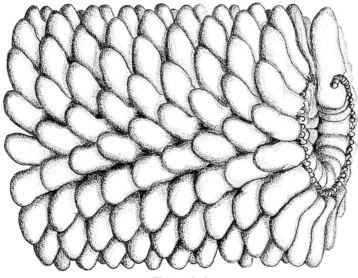

Figure 6–6

Diagram of the tobacco mosaic virus virion showing the outer protein subunits (capsomeres) and the inner helical coil of RNA. (Redrawn from Caspar, 1963, in Goodheart: An Introduction to Virology, W. B. Saunders Co., Philadelphia, 1969.

of each group of viruses. The core, plus capsid, is called a *nucleocapsid.* The nucleocapsid of many animal viruses (e.g., Arbovirus, Myxovirus, Poxvirus, Herpesvirus) is enclosed in a distinctively ether- or chloroform-soluble, sodium deoxycholate-sensitive, lipoprotein-containing *envelope* that is derived from host-cell membranes during emergence of the virus from the infected cell. Such viruses have a somewhat irregular morphology. Although the curious tadpole shape of phages is specially adapted for penetration of bacterial cell walls and is not commonly found in viruses that infect animal cells, which have no cell walls, nevertheless most of the properties and activities of animal viruses were originally discovered as a result of investigations of bacteriophage.

DEMONSTRATION OF BACTERIOPHAGE. If feces or sewage are emulsified in water and the fluid is then passed through a bacteria-retaining porcelain filter, the fluid that passes through, although entirely free of bacteria, contains an active agent (phage), invisible with ordinary microscopes and not cultivable in nonliving media, that will destroy young, actively growing bacteria (dysentery bacilli, for example) in broth cultures. This is often called the *Twort-d'Herelle phenomenon* after the British and French scientists who first described it in 1915 and 1922, respectively.

By transferring even a tiny quantity (e.g., one millionth of 1 ml) of the dissolved, filtered culture to a new culture of the same species of bacilli, the same process can be made to occur anew, and it will recur through an indefinite number of culture transfers and filtrations. Similar multiplications have been demonstrated with nearly all other known viruses, using cultures of animal cells (complicated and expensive) instead of bacteria (simple and inexpensive).

INFECTION BY BACTERIOPHAGE. The tail of a phage virion (never found in animal viruses) is of protein and has a rather complex structure.

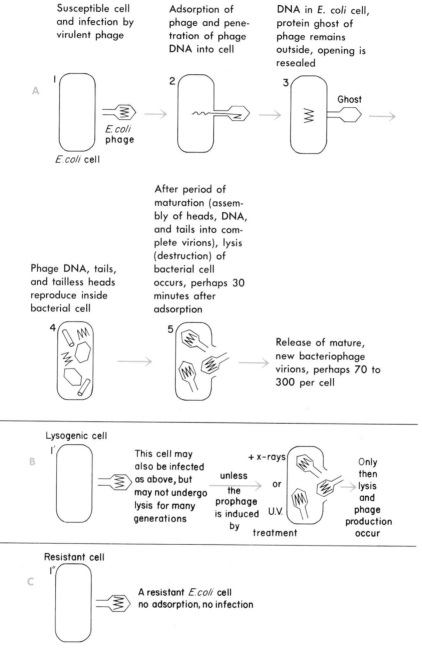

Susceptible cell
and infection by
virulent phage

Adsorption of
phage and pene-
tration of phage
DNA into cell

DNA in *E. coli* cell,
protein ghost of
phage remains
outside, opening is
resealed

A   1

E.coli
phage

E.coli cell

2

3

Ghost

After period of
maturation (assem-
bly of heads, DNA,
and tails into com-
plete virions), lysis
(destruction) of
bacterial cell
occurs, perhaps 30
minutes after
adsorption

Phage DNA, tails,
and tailless heads
reproduce inside
bacterial cell

4

5

Release of mature,
new bacteriophage
virions, perhaps 70 to
300 per cell

Lysogenic cell

B   1'

This cell may
also be infected
as above, but
may not undergo
lysis for many
generations

+ x-rays

unless
the
prophage
is induced
by

or

U.V.

treatment

Only
then
lysis
and
phage
production
occur

Resistant cell

C   1''

A resistant *E.coli* cell
no adsorption, no infection

Figure 6–7

A, Some bacterial cells are susceptible to phage and are destroyed (lysed). B, Lysogenic cells are infected but their progeny are lysed only when exposed to an inducing agent, e.g., radiation. C, Resistant cells are not infected.

At its tip is a *base plate* with *fibrils* that facilitate attachment of the virion to the bacterial cell that it parasitizes. Once attached (Fig. 6–7*A*) enzymes at the tip of the tail effect an opening through the bacterial cell wall and membrane. Through this opening the nucleic acid of the core passes into the infected bacterial cell. The protein head and tail remain outside, being now an inert "ghost." Most animal viruses, unlike the phage, appear to enter the cell by passage, intact, through the cell membrane; in many species this occurs by an ingestion or phagocytic process called *pinocytosis.*

By a complicated series of effects the nucleic acid core of any virus, once inside a susceptible cell and free of its capsid, dominates the synthetic mechanisms of the cell. New virions are quickly replicated. Phages and some other viruses, such as poliovirus, eventually occupy the entire interior of the cell and cause cell rupture or "lysis from within"; this is called *phage (or viral) lysis.* Not all viruses cause immediate death or lysis. Some infected animal cells continue to live for long periods, giving off new virions through the cell membrane. However, when liberated, the new virions attack new cells and continue the process unless inhibited by some extraneous agent: antibodies, drugs, interferon (see page 280).

When multiplying intracellularly the virions of many viruses tend to aggregate into regularly shaped translucent masses that resemble crystals (Fig. 6–8).

LYSOGENY.   The nucleic acid core of viruses is like a miniature chromosome. It contains the entire complement of genes (the genome) of the virus and is infective by itself. It has been shown that the genome of the bacteriophage can remain intact in an infected bacterium, apparently as a part of the bacterial chromosome. It is said to have been "reduced" to the *prophage* state. In this state it replicates with the bacterial chromosome through an indefinite series of cell fissions, sometimes contributing striking new genetic traits [e.g., virulence (toxigenicity) of diphtheria bacilli and of *Clostridium botulinum* or food-poisoning bacilli], a phenomenon called *viral conversion,* as though it were actually a part of the bacterium. Such a phage is said to be *temperate.* However, under certain circumstances (e.g., exposure to ultraviolet or x-rays or other *inducing agent*) it parts company with the bacterial genome, becomes actively *vegetative* and virulent, and causes phage lysis. A cell containing such a phage is said to be *lysogenic* (Fig. 6–7*B*). The same (or a similar) process appears

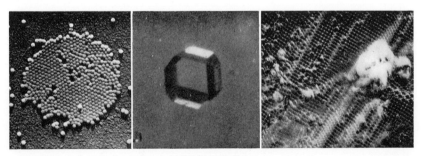

Figure 6–8

Poliovirus particles in a flat array (left) and in a three-dimensional crystal (center). A cut surface of a crystal (right) shows it to consist of virus particles in orderly arrays. (Burrows, after Schwerdt.)

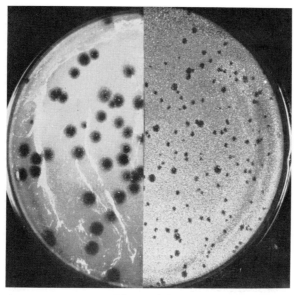

Figure 6–9

Bacteriophage plaques. On the surface of agar of appropriate composition was spread a culture of tubercle bacilli (*Mycobacterium tuberculosis*) mixed with bacteriophage specific for this organism. After incubation, the generalized growth of tubercle bacilli is seen as a whitish film. (Such growth of any bacteria on agar is often called a "lawn.") The plaques of phage are seen as dark, circular holes in the "lawn." Each plaque is, in effect, a colony of phage that has grown at the expense of the tubercle bacilli. Two different races or types of phage are shown here: a large-plaque and a small-plaque race. Different races of phages specific for other organisms show these and other colonial peculiarities. (Courtesy of S. Froman, D. W. Will, and E. Bogen, Olive View Sanatorium, Olive View, Calif. In *Amer. J. Pub. Health*. Vol. 44.)

to occur in some animal tumor virus infections (e.g., murine C-type viruses) and possibly also in herpes, though it has not been as clearly demonstrated as for phage.

VIRAL PLAQUES. If phage virions are mixed with a growing culture of susceptible bacteria in broth and then spread thinly on an agar surface and incubated, "colonies" of phage are seen as tiny holes (called *plaques*) in the ensuing growth (Fig. 6–9). Each plaque is in reality a colony of phage that has developed from a single phage virion which initially landed at that spot. Each plaque represents lysed bacteria and contains billions of phage virions.

Animal cells similarly cultivated in appropriate fluid media form thin films (*monolayers*) of cells in flasks or dishes. If such a sheet of cells is inoculated with an animal virus infective for those cells, readily visible and often very distinctive plaques are formed. The study of all kinds of viral plaques is widely used in diagnostic and other virological investigations.

PROPAGATION. In order to propagate viruses it is necessary to place them in contact with certain actively growing cells that they can *enter* (*infect*) and parasitize. They cannot grow independently outside living cells. Plant viruses require specific plant cells for growth; bacterial viruses are specific for certain bacteria; animal viruses are specific for certain animal cells. Three major techniques and types of living material are employed for the cultivation and study of animal viruses. In one, the developing chick embryo (Fig. 5–3), the yolk sac, chorioallantoic membrane, amniotic cavity, or other structures, depending upon the particular virus to be propagated, may be inoculated directly with virus-containing material (such as saliva, or an infected chick embryo that has been "homogenized" by being forced with the plunger through the opening in a syringe). In a second method, susceptible laboratory animals, such as mice, monkeys, and rabbits, are employed; the route of inoculation, age, and genetic background of the animal all affect the growth of the virus. A third method, widely used, is that of tissue cultures, i.e., mammalian cells in culture. Animal-tissue cells grow readily as a *monolayer* (a "sheet" of cells one cell in thickness) in glass vessels of any desired size or shape. The cultured cells are then inoculated with virus.

Tissue Cultures.   Extensive use has been made of living cells of various kinds, such as the HeLa (from human cervical cancer cells), L (mouse fibroblasts), and monkey-kidney cell lines for the propagation of animal viruses. Human tissues obtained as surgical by-products also provide a *medium* for the propagation of viruses. Although details are different, the essential components of all tissue cultures include a living cell system, a nutritional medium (nutrient solution) adequate for the maintenance and growth of cells, and antibiotics to control bacterial and fungal contaminants. Incubation is in a moist atmosphere rich in CO_2.

Some of the nutrient solutions for the tissue cells are very complex. Special methods of tissue culture (the work of Enders, Weller, Robbins, and others) have led to the preparation of polio (Sabin, Salk) and measles

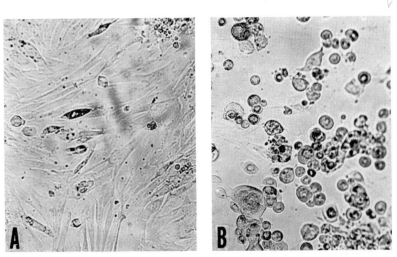

Figure 6–10

The cytopathic effect of a virus on human chorion cells in tissue culture. (The chorion is one of the membranes protecting the embryo in the uterus.) *A,* Normal cells: tissue culture five days old showing a fairly regular, organized network of uniformly elongated, spindle-shaped tissue cells of rather distinctive appearance. *B,* The same sort of cells 72 hours after being inoculated with the virus of herpes simplex ("fever blister"). The cells are largely destroyed. Those remaining have lost their distinctive form and arrangement, have undergone granular rounding, and will eventually become mere shapeless, disconnected, disorganized blobs (× 1500). (Courtesy of Drs. A. M. Lerner, K. E. Takemoto and A. Shelokov. In *Proc. Soc. Exp. Biol. & Med.,* Vol. 95. Copied by permission of The Society for Experimental Biology and Medicine.)

(Enders) vaccines. Numerous others (such as rabies and mumps) are now available. Several investigators are now trying again to develop a vaccine against gonorrhea. What a blessing for mankind (including women, of course) such a vaccine might be!

Animal and plant inoculations were formerly widely used in experimental and diagnostic virology. At present, except for special purposes, tissue cultures have replaced live animals to a considerable extent. Because viruses do not have any metabolic activities of their own that can be demonstrated in the laboratory, and multiply only in living cells, some authorities question whether viruses are living organisms. Outside the cell they seem to be totally inert. Inside the cell they use mostly cell materials and cause the cell synthetic mechanisms to synthesize the virus instead of the cell. Viruses are commonly spoken of as active or inactive instead of as alive or dead.

Cytophathic Effect.   When viruses grow in tissues, damage is produced in the cells; i.e., the viruses are *pathogenic* for the tissue cells. The effect of the viruses on the cells is said to be *cytopathic* (contraction of *cyto* = cell; *pathogenic* = producing disease in, or damage to). By the use of proper staining methods, the cytopathic changes produced by the viruses in individual cells may be seen and photographed (Fig. 6–10). The viruses themselves are visible only with the electron microscope.

INCLUSION BODIES.   A common response of the host cell to certain viral infections (such as smallpox, rabies, and measles) is the formation of rather prominent and distinct intracytoplasmic or intranuclear masses called *inclusion bodies*. These may be observed microscopically in infected tissues following fixation and staining. Some inclusions are aggregates or colonies of virus particles; others are probably sites of altered cellular metabolism. They may be intranuclear or cytoplasmic. Their morphology, location, and staining properties are often of great diagnostic value.

HEAT-RESISTANCE.   Nearly all viruses are readily inactivated by heat, most of them by boiling (100 C) within 20 minutes. There are two exceptions that should always be remembered: the virus of infectious (epidemic) hepatitis ("catarrhal jaundice"), and that of homologous serum jaundice (see page 369). Because of the heat-resistance of these two closely similar viruses, autoclaving[1] (20 minutes at 121 C) or oven sterilization (90 minutes at 165 C) is the only safe procedure for materials likely to be contaminated with them. These materials include, especially, infectious blood or bloody fluids, blood-contaminated instruments, hypodermic syringes and needles (most of these are now disposable), and in addition, for epidemic hepatitis, which is transmitted in feces, sewage-contaminated water, contaminated foods, dishes and clinical thermometers used by patients who have the disease, and other substances discussed in greater detail in Chapters 12, 14, and 15. Numerous viruses that cause diseases in animals or man are very fragile and do not remain active in body fluids, such as blood and sputum, for more than a few days at room temperature. Viruses that occur in the intestinal tract, e.g., poliomyelitis and epidemic viral hepatitis viruses, may survive for days in sewage. Curiously enough, if infected body fluids or tissues are rapidly dried, preserved with glycerin, or quickly frozen at extremely low temperatures, such as that of solid carbon dioxide ("dry ice," −76 C), even the most fragile viruses remain fully infective but in a static condition for many months, or even years.

---

[1]A method of heating in steam under pressure.

DISINFECTANT-RESISTANCE.   In general, viruses appear to be some-what more resistant to some chemical disinfectants, such as phenol, glycerol, and bichloride of mercury, than are most bacteria. In this, however, there are as many exceptions and variations as there are among bacteria. It is especially noteworthy that viruses in general are not affected by therapeutic treatment with sulfonamide drugs or antibiotics. This is because most antibiotics act by inhibiting cellular synthetic or energy-yielding enzymes; viruses do not have any such enzymes to be affected.

Diseases Caused by Viruses

Viruses may be studied by direct observation of infected cells with the electron microscope, or by observing viral growth and its effects in tissue cultures, as well as by chemical analyses, physical measurements, and so on. One of the most important methods of study of viruses is to observe their effects on cells and tissues of living hosts: bacterial, higher plant, invertebrate, or vertebrate. A virus is recognized primarily by its production of disease in a host or by its cytopathic effect (CPE) on living cells in tissue cultures (Fig. 6–9) as well as by the virus-specific *antibodies* that it evokes in the host animal (see next paragraph).

Viral infections often fail to produce any *recognizable* effect on cells or tissues. Such infections are often called "silent," "subclinical" or "inapparent." They may be detected by tests for certain specific proteins (gamma globulins; *antibodies*) that appear in the blood in response to infections. Such tests are called *serological* or *immunological* tests (see Chapters 9 and 19).

CLASSIFICATION.   Many diseases of plants, arthropods, other animals, and man are caused by viruses. Five general and not very sharply defined groups of *zoopathogenic* viruses may be mentioned as follows (see also Table 6–1).

Dermotropic viruses chiefly cause visible lesions of skin and mucous membranes (epithelial tissues) and include the viruses of:
    Smallpox
    Measles
    German measles (rubella)
    Chickenpox
    Herpes zoster (shingles)
Pneumotropic viruses cause respiratory diseases such as:
    Influenza
    Pneumonia or pneumonitis
Neurotropic viruses cause diseases of nervous tissues:
    Poliomyelitis (infantile paralysis)
    Rabies (hydrophobia)
    Encephalitis
Viscerotropic viruses cause diseases that chiefly damage internal organs:
    Yellow fever
    Hepatitis

The fifth group, the *enterotropic viruses*, are those that multiply primarily in the intestinal tract. Among these would be included poliomyelitis viruses, ECHO (Enteric Cytopathogenic Human Orphan), ECBO (Enteric Cytopathogenic Bovine Orphan), NITA (Nuclear Inclusion Type A) REO (Respiratory Enteric Orphan) viruses, and Coxsackie viruses. These are all discussed later (see Chapter 25).

This classification, although convenient for purposes of reference, is very imperfect and can be misleading, since several viruses cause more than one type of disease and may be localized in several kinds of tissue, besides changing quite unexpectedly. For example, the virus causing "shingles," or herpes zoster, which involves dorsal nerve roots, may be a neurotropic modification of one of the "dermotropic" viruses, that of chickenpox. Another example is the neurotropic poliomyelitis virus; it causes primarily an intestinal infection. A representative list of a number of widely known viral diseases of man is shown in Table 6–2. It includes the most common childhood diseases.

A binomial classification of viruses has been suggested and has been added as one appendix of this book (page 586) to satisfy the curious reader. It is not recommended that this particular system be used in any way other than as a ready reference at this time. A more commonly used system is based primarily on type of nucleic acid in the virus and secondarily on other chemical and physical properties (Table 6–1). The nucleic acids of viruses have been intensively studied. Some have single-stranded DNA or RNA, some double-stranded. The genetic strand (genome) of some viruses have approximately 400 genes or genetic units (vaccinia virus), while others have very few, e.g., a virus of mice has only 8 genes.

Modifications of Viruses

ZOOLOGIC MODIFICATION. An important property of viruses is their ability to adapt themselves to animal hosts other than those that they infect under natural conditions. This is sometimes called "zoologic modification." The virus of influenza, for example, which ordinarily appears to infect only human beings, may be induced to infect white mice under laboratory conditions so that it regularly produces a highly fatal pneumonia in them. The virus of rabies may, as shown by Pasteur, be passed artificially from rabbit brain to rabbit brain so that it becomes extremely pathogenic for these animals; yet, in becoming so adapted, it loses some of its virulence for human beings. The virus of fox distemper may be so modified by repeated transmission in ferrets that, although highly fatal for ferrets, it produces only a very mild disease in foxes and is successfully used in large silver-fox ranches, in immunizing the animals to the disease. These "adaptations" probably represent the *selective propagation* of mutants in the viral population best fitted to grow under the altered conditions.

As will be described, smallpox vaccination is probably based on zoologic modification.

HISTOLOGIC MODIFICATION. This occurs when a virus is continually induced to infect a tissue that it does not naturally invade. For example, yellow fever virus, normally infecting the blood, liver, and other viscera (viscerotropic), can be completely altered by injecting it into the brains of mice or other rodents. It becomes neurotropic and may not cause any visible infection if injected into the blood, and may be used for immunization purposes. An almost total loss of both viscerotropic and neurotropic properties will occur if it is cultivated in tissue cultures as described previously or passed through chick embryos, from egg to egg. The highly successful 17D yellow fever vaccine, now widely used to immunize persons traveling in yellow fever areas, is based on this fact. The Sabin oral vaccine is an infective, active-virus vaccine against poliomyelitis, of low virulence

Table 6-2. Representative Viral Diseases*

COMMON NAME OF DISEASE	TECHNICAL NAME OF DISEASE	BODY REGIONS INVOLVED	MODE OF TRANSMISSION	INCUBATION PERIOD	CHIEF SYMPTOMS OR CHARACTERISTICS
Smallpox	Variola	Chiefly skin	Usually dust, droplet or contact	7 to 18 days	High temperature, chills, headache, backache, and muscular pain; typical smallpox lesions on the body.
Measles	Rubeola	Chiefly skin	Dust, droplet or contact	10 to 14 days	Similar to an ordinary cold; high temperature; spots in the throat; typical skin rash.
German measles	Rubella	Chiefly skin	Dust, droplet or contact	14 to 21 days	Mild symptoms of a cold; rash; enlargement of lymph nodes back of ear.
Chickenpox**	Varicella	Chiefly skin	Dust, droplet or contact	14 to 16 days	Mild symptoms of a cold; the rash may appear as successive crops of vesicles.
Shingles**	Herpes zoster	Skin and sensory nerves	Dust, droplet	7 to 14 days	Small vesicles surrounded by redness; fever and aches; rash may follow the skin area supplied by the sensory nerve.
Fever blisters	Herpes simplex	Skin	Dust, droplet or contact		Sores on face or lips often follow colds, fevers, or severe diseases.
Warts	Verruca	Skin	Uncertain, probably contact	4 weeks to 6 months	Appearance of the characteristic wart-shaped bodies on the skin surface.
Mumps	Contagious parotitis	Salivary glands and often reproductive organs; occasionally central nervous system	Dust, droplet	17 to 21 days	Mild symptoms in children, more severe in adults; swelling of the salivary gland; may also involve the testes or ovaries.

Table 6-2 continued on opposite page.

Infantile paralysis	Poliomyelitis	Spinal cord and brain	Dust, droplet, food, feces.	7–21 days	Mild sore throat with respiratory coldlike symptoms followed by all degrees of paralysis from none to fatal.
Hydrophobia	Rabies	Brain and nerves	Usually bite of rabid animal	10 days to 6 months	Headache, difficulty in swallowing, convulsions, paralysis, violent spells; survival rare.
Sleeping sickness (North American)	Equine encephalo-myelitis	Nerves, brain, meninges, and blood	Bites of several types of mosquitoes	4–21 days	High fever, convulsions, vomiting, drowsiness, coma, and muscle twitchings.
Flu	Influenza	Respiratory tract including the lungs	Dust, droplet	1 to 3 days	Fever; aching in muscles of back, arms, and legs; headache; chest pains, which may be complicated by pneumonic type of disease.
Yellow fever	Yellow fever	Various internal organs	*Aedes aegypti* mosquito	3 to 6 days	Fever, abdominal pain, vomiting of blood; delirium and prostration; yellow coloration of the skin (jaundice).
Infectious hepatitis or catarrhal jaundice	Epidemic viral hepatitis	Liver, spleen, and lymph nodes	Food, milk, and water; perhaps direct contact; blood	10 to 40 days	Fever, weakness, nausea, vomiting, abdominal cramps; jaundice often is present; enlarged and tender liver.

*Adapted from Clark, R. L., Jr., and Cumley, R. W.: The Book of Health, 1st Ed. Elsevier Press Inc.

**The varicella-zoster virus (V-Z virus) is thought to cause chickenpox in non-immune individuals, but shingles in partially immune hosts.

for man, developed in tissue cultures of the poliovirus. Salk vaccine is inactivated (non-infective) poliovirus.

VIRAL VARIATION AND VACCINES.   As is true of the antigens (proteins, and so on) of different animals and plants (even antigens of closely related species of individuals), the antigens of viruses (even of those that cause the same types of disease) are often very different antigenically. If one vaccinates a group of people with influenza vaccine, one may be surprised and disappointed when many of the vaccinated people succumb to influenza during an epidemic. If it is shown, however, that the vaccine virus was type A and that the epidemic virus was type B, then one realizes the important fact that viral vaccines must include all the antigenic possibilities of the particular virus group involved. Influenza vaccine must contain influenza viruses of types A, B, C, and subgroups, and so on; polio vaccines must immunize against poliovirus I, II, III, and so on.

APPLICATION TO HEALTH

In addition to learning more about the principal characteristics of rickettsias, chlamydias, and viruses, you have acquired essential information concerning members of these groups of microorganisms that is useful in the health fields. Some outstanding examples of this type of information are: the highly parasitic nature of rickettsias, chlamydias, and viruses, which is an important clue to understanding the epidemiology of diseases caused by members of these three groups; the differences in susceptibility of varieties of viruses, chlamydias, and rickettsias to different methods of destruction, which we will use as part of the basis of discussions of sterilization and disinfection in Section Three; the methods of culturing rickettsias, chlamydias, and viruses, which are important in diagnosis and have made possible the development of vaccines, and which will be discussed more fully in Section Four; the effects of rickettsias, chlamydias, and viruses, which are important in understanding the symptoms of the diseases caused by members of these groups, and which will be discussed in greater detail in Section Five. Also, knowledge about rickettsias, chlamydias, and viruses is being sought very actively, so that students in all areas of health professions should be constantly on the alert for new information becoming available that they can utilize in their practice.

We hope that you are now beginning to see that the study of microbiology follows a very logical sequence and that one part builds directly on the preceding, that this science is fascinating and absorbing, and that the knowledge gained in this study is really vital to the health professions.

Supplementary Reading

Aaronson, S. A., Todaro, G. J., and Scolnick, E. M.: Induction of murine C-type viruses from clonal lines of virus-free BALB/3T3 cells. *Science,* 1971, *174:*157.

Akaro, R. J.: *Neisseria gonorrhoeae:* experimental infection of laboratory animals. Science, 1972, *177:*1200.

Braun, W.: Bacterial Genetics. 2nd Ed. 1965, Philadelphia, W. B. Saunders Co.

Debré, R., and Celers, J. (Editors): Clinical Virology: The Evaluation and Management of Human Viral Infections. 1970, Philadelphia, W. B. Saunders Co.

Eklund, M. W., Poysky, F. T., Reed, S. M., and Smith, C. A.: Bacteriophage and the toxigenicity of *Clostridium botulinum* type C. *Science,* 1971, *172:*480.

Fenner, F.: The Genetics of Animal Viruses. *Ann. Rev. Microbiol.,* 1970, *24:*297.

Goodheart, C. R.: An Introduction to Virology. 1969, Philadelphia, W. B. Saunders Co.

Hilleman, M. R.: Toward control of viral infections of man. *Science,* 1969, *164:*506–514.

Lennette, E. H., and Schmidt, N. J. (Editors): Diagnostic Procedures for Viral and Rickettsial Infections. 4th Ed. 1969, American Public Health Association, Inc., New York, N.Y.

Morgan, C., Rose, H. M., and Mednis, B.: Electron microscopy of herpes simplex virus. I. Entry. *J. Virology,* 1968, *2:*507.

Nii, S., Morgan, C., and Rose, H. M.: Electron microscopy of herpes simplex virus. II. Sequence of development. *J. Virology,* 1968, *2:*517.

Pollard, E. C., et al.: Inactivation of viruses. *Ann. N.Y. Acad. Sci.,* 1960, *83* (Art. 4):513.

Rapp, F.: Defective DNA Animal Viruses. Ann. Rev. Microbiol., 1969, *23:*293.

Schwartz, A. J. F., and Zirbel, L. W.: Propagation of measles virus in non-primate tissue culture, I. *Proc. Soc. Exp. Biol. & Med.,* 1959, *102:*711.

Sprunt, K., Redman, W. M., and Alexander, H. E.: Infectious ribonucleic acid derived from enteroviruses. *Proc. Soc. Exp. Biol. & Med.,* 1959, *101:*604.

Stent, G. S.: Molecular Biology of Bacterial Viruses. 1963, San Francisco, W. H. Freeman & Co.

Watanabe, K., Takesue, S., Jin-Nai, K., and Yoshikawa, T.: Bacteriophage active against the lactic acid beverage-producing bacterium *Lactobacillus casei. Appl. Microbiol.,* 1970, *20:*409.

Zinsser, H.: Rats, Lice and History. 1935, Boston, Little, Brown & Co. Also in paperback, Bantam edition: 1971, Bantam Books, Inc., New York.

Microorganisms and the World at Large

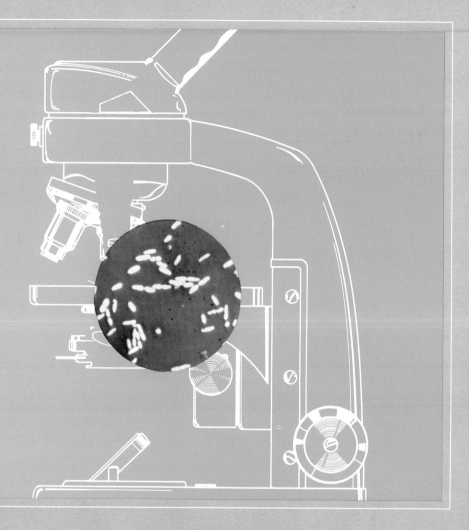

General
Bacterial
Physiology

7

THE BACTERIA

Bacteria are microscopic fungi of which most species can grow well in the dark. Like all other fungi they have no *chlorophyll*, as do ordinary plants. Also like all other fungi, including yeasts and molds, they can grow well on lifeless culture media. Viruses, chlamydias, and rickettsias require living cells for multiplication. Because bacteria characteristically multiply by binary fission, they are assigned to the class Schizomycetes (from Greek *schizein*, to divide; *mykes*, fungi), or *fission fungi*.

It is not easy for the beginner to realize the importance and complexity of bacteria; many typical species are only 1/25,400 (0.000039) inch (1 micrometer) in diameter (Fig. 6–3). It is also hard to understand how, being plants, they can live and multiply without leaves or flowers, stems or roots, in the absence of sunlight and often in the entire absence of air, and survive for years at temperatures hundreds of degrees below zero without water or food! Bacteria, moreover, through mutation and natural selection in different environments, have become adapted to life almost everywhere on the earth. Some can thrive in and at the bottoms of the seas, and in and on plants and animals, and can grow and multiply prodigiously, as they have done for millions of years. Not all species live everywhere, however, and some are rigidly restricted to certain environments such as marine depths or mucous membranes of the human body.

Physiology of Bacteria

"An unexpected knowledge of the secret life energies of bacteria has been revealed, through which they rule with demoniacal power over weal and woe, and even over the life and death of man."

Ferdinand Cohn
1828–1898

Metabolism

How Bacteria "Eat." Since even the most complex unicellular organisms (protozoa, eucaryotic algae) have only a cell membrane (and perhaps flagella, slime coating, and a cell wall), nuclear structures, and cytoplasm containing chloroplasts, mitochondria, enzyme granules, granules of stored food, fat, and so forth, it may seem strange that they are able to eat and breathe. In the case of bacteria, which are among the simplest of unicellular organisms, their eating involves no taste, chewing, swallowing, or other muscular or nerve activity. The food of bacteria (and all other plant cells) must be in solution, that is, dissolved in water. When bacteria are floating in solutions such as blood, beef broth, sewage, sea water, or water in the soil, the substances that they use as food permeate them through the cell wall and membrane. This passage of fluid and dissolved materials through a thin membrane is called *diffusion* or *osmosis*. Certain *permease enzymes* are often involved (page 99). Dissolved waste products in turn pass outward through the cell membrane and wall. Cell membranes seem to be permeable to just the right substances. Such a membrane is said to be *semipermeable* or *selectively permeable*. It allows only food substances to pass inward and waste products to pass outward. Except in animal cells, all substances passing through the cell wall and membrane are presumably in a soluble, not solid, form. Let us not forget, however, the possible exchange of gases; but this is another story, to be discussed later on.

If the volume of fluid in which the cells are suspended is small, as in a test tube or a tiny pool, the cells are soon surrounded by a mixture of food substances and waste products, all in solution. The food may then give out, or the accumulation of waste products may result in stopping the growth of the cells, or both factors may affect the cell population.

Nutrition solely by passage of foods dissolved in water through the cell membrane (and wall if present) is often called an *osmotrophic* mode of nutrition.

ENZYMES.   Although all plant and many animal cells are nourished only by soluble substances that are capable of passing through the cell wall, cell membrane, or both, from the surrounding fluids, many kinds of cells, including numerous species of bacteria, have considerable powers of making nutritive use of various solid substances that are neither in solution nor able to pass through the cell membrane. Thus, not only fats, starches, and proteins, but the shells of crabs, the trunks of trees, old rubber tires, petroleum, even (alas!) the paper on which this book is printed may ultimately serve as food for certain bacteria and other microorganisms of the soil or water that can "digest" or, more correctly, *hydrolyze*[1] (and thus solubilize) them. This hydrolysis or "extraneous digestion" is accomplished by means of *enzymes,* or digestive chemicals, that the bacteria (and other cells) secrete (see Fig. 7–1).

Enzymes are protein complexes that bring about chemical changes in a great variety of substances. Enzymes have the remarkable power of *catalysis,* that is, of bringing other substances together and greatly speeding up chemical reactions between them, much as a hostess brings a group of people together, introduces them, and causes them to play bridge—she catalyzes a party.

In general, enzymes are not destroyed in the catalytic processes. Thus

---

[1]From Greek *hydor,* water, and *lysis,* dissolution; a phase of enzymic digestion in which complex molecules such as starch, protein, or fat are split into simpler molecules such as glucose, amino acids, or fatty acids. Molecules of water are enzymically introduced into the molecules of starch, protein, or fat and then split, the result being the simpler molecules that are small enough to pass through the cell wall, membrane, or both and be used as food.

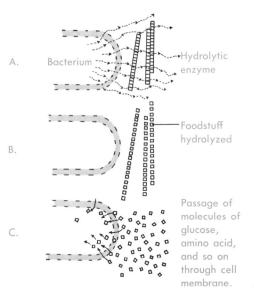

A.   Bacterium ········► ··► Hydrolytic
                                    enzyme

B.   Foodstuff
                               hydrolyzed

C.   Passage of
                               molecules of
                               glucose,
                               amino acid,
                               and so on
                               through cell
                               membrane.

Figure 7–1

Utilization of grossly large and insoluble food particles by extracellular digestion. Sketch *A* shows the bacterium secreting hydrolytic enzyme, which attacks the food particle (cellulose, chitin, starch, protein, fat). In *B* the foodstuff is hydrolyzed and its constituent molecules (glucose, amino acids, fatty acids, etc.) are separated from one another. In *C* the molecules derived by hydrolysis of the food pass (or are actively passed by permease enzymes) readily through the bacterial cell wall and cell membrane into the cytoplasm to be further metabolized.

very small quantities of enzymes will bring about extensive and continuous reactions. There are enzymes that can so change gelatin that it becomes permanently liquid and will no longer "set." Others cause sugar, water, and oxygen to react so that alcohol and carbon dioxide gas result and energy is yielded to the cell. Common bakers' yeast gives off an enzyme that does this, and the process is used in making beer, wine, and bread. Glandular cells in our stomach, the intestines, and in the pancreas produce hydrolytic enzymes such as pepsin, trypsin, amylase, lipase, and so on, which digest our foods to simple, soluble substances by catalyzing their combination with water (hydrolysis). The products of digestive hydrolysis in our stomachs are absorbed through the cells lining our intestines, eventually enter the circulating blood and lymph, and are used for energy or body substance. This natural analytical and synthetic chemistry is constantly going on in all living beings.

Exo-enzymes.   Enzymes that pass outward from the cell are called *exo-enzymes* (*exo* = outside of). These form physicochemical combinations with a great variety of substances, bringing about changes so that even the tough, hard, and chemically complex structures referred to previously are reduced to simple substances that dissolve rapidly and pass inward through the walls and membranes of living cells, there to be used as sources of energy and protoplasm (Fig. 7–1). Almost identical digestive processes go on in our own stomachs and enable us to assimilate tough old steaks, popcorn, and raw carrots. Actually, we can learn from embryology that the cells lining our mouth and digestive system are of the same lineage (ectoderm) as those that become our skin. Thus, technically we also digest on our outside (gastrointestinal tract). It is relatively easy to clean out the contents of our G.I. tract, but not so when we have absorbed toxins (poisons) or bacterial pathogens into our bloodstream.

Endo-enzymes.   Some enzymes are very closely attached to the cells themselves and are not released into the surrounding fluids. They are called *endo-enzymes* (*endo* = inside of), since they remain inside of or on the cell. They are mainly involved in cell synthesis and in liberating energy from foodstuffs and making it available for the cell's use in moving and

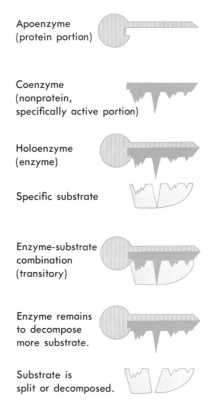

Apoenzyme
(protein portion)

Coenzyme
(nonprotein,
specifically active portion)

Holoenzyme
(enzyme)

Specific substrate

Enzyme-substrate
combination
(transitory)

Enzyme remains
to decompose
more substrate.

Substrate is
split or decomposed.

Figure 7–2

A typical enzyme consists of two complex molecular groups: a protein part called the *apoenzyme* (Greek, *apo*, part of), and a nonprotein part, the *coenzyme*. Most coenzymes are chemical derivatives of the so-called vitamins, which in microbiology are often called growth factors. The complete enzyme is called a *holoenzyme* (Greek, *holos*, whole). The coenzyme, because of its distinctive molecular structure, confers a high degree of specificity on the activity of the holoenzyme, and it is the coenzyme that carries on the specific activity of the enzyme. As seen in the drawing, the holoenzyme, by virtue of the peculiar structure of the coenzyme, is restricted to one kind of substrate having a corresponding molecular structure, as a complex key is capable of opening only correspondingly formed locks. In the drawing the enzyme has "split," or hydrolyzed, its specific substrate.

living. Probably most soluble proteins in a cell are active enzymes. *Permease enzymes* are involved in the permeation of food substances through cell wall and membrane by "active transport."

Specificity of Enzymes. There are probably thousands of different enzymes, each of which catalyzes a single, specific kind of chemical reaction with certain specific substances (called *substrates*) and not with others. Enzymes are therefore said to be *specific* in their action. Specificity may conveniently be thought of as resembling the relationship between a key and a lock. No other key will affect that lock (Fig. 7–2). For example, certain enzymes called peptidases hydrolyze proteins but not fats, carbohydrates, or any substance other than a protein. The enzyme β-galactosidase can hydrolyze lactose and related sugars, but not cane sugar or other carbohydrates; oxidases cause only oxidations and not hydrolysis. Enzymes can act only if *coenzymes* (nonprotein molecules that often are vitamin complexes) are also present. Coenzymes provide the needed specific physicochemical "fit" between substrate and enzyme (Fig. 7–2).

All cells have certain complex systems of enzymes that provide the energy and substance of life. In many cells these systems are virtually identical, just as the engines in automobiles are basically alike, differing only in minor details of arrangement. Not all cells produce *all* kinds of enzymes, however. Some of the enzymes or enzyme-like substances that certain bacteria produce are very poisonous (or *toxic*, from a Greek word meaning "poison"). These produce disease. Diphtheria toxin is a good example.

Later on we will also learn more about the effect of bacterial enzymes

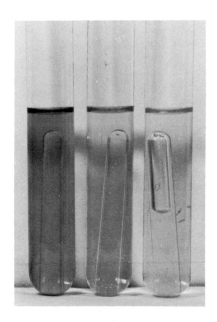

Figure 7–3

Carbohydrate fermentation reactions in glucose broth. The bacteria did not ferment the sugar in the left tube. Acid produced in the tube in the center changed the indicator color of the broth from red to yellow. The tube on the right shows acid (the broth also turned yellow) and gas production.

on a variety of substances, such as lactose (milk sugar), saccharose or sucrose (cane sugar), glucose (dextrose), gelatin, milk, coagulated serum and blood, and body tissues. Each species of microorganism has certain enzymic activities that are more or less characteristic of the species and that can therefore be utilized for diagnosis in the laboratory. Thus it is a relatively easy matter for the microbiologist to distinguish between the bacterium (*Salmonella typhi*) that causes typhoid fever and the common, usually harmless, intestinal bacteria (*Escherichia coli*). The latter ferments lactose and from it produces lactic acid and other substances, including a mixture of hydrogen and carbon dioxide gas, which is easily seen in special so-called "fermentation tubes" arranged to catch gas (Fig. 7–3). *S. typhi* does not attack lactose at all. It is easy, therefore, to realize the importance of bacterial enzymes in the identification of certain specific microorganisms in medical diagnosis.

Classification of Enzymes. Enzymes are classified according to the kind of chemical reaction they catalyze or the kind of specific substance (substrate) upon which they exert their influence. The names of most enzymes are derived from the chemical activity or the substrate plus the suffix "ase." For example, *oxygenases*, or oxygen transferases, and *oxidases*, catalyze oxidations which are important sources of energy in all living cells. *Hydrolases* bring about hydrolysis; *dehydrogenases* take hydrogen and electrons away from substrates. Dehydrogenation is an indirect and very common form of biologic oxidation. Like direct oxidation, it yields energy to living cells. Oxido-reductases catalyze the transfer of electrons in the energy metabolism of the cell; transferases catalyze the transfer of molecular groups from one molecule to another. Polymerases catalyze the syntheses of long-chain molecules like the combination of the nucleotide chains of DNA. Several enzymes discovered years ago bear unsystematic names, but because these names have become so widely known and have been generally used for such a long time, it would be very inconvenient to change them. *Ptyalin* (starch-digesting enzyme [amylase] of the saliva), *pepsin*, and *trypsin* (protein-digesting enzymes of the stomach and intestines, respectively) are examples of these. (See also Adaptive Enzymes, page 403.)

BIOLOGIC OXIDATION. According to Cheves Walling, "Oxygen which bathes all substances exposed to the atmosphere is the most ubiquitous of chemical reagents; through combustion and respiration it provides us with most of our available energy, and its ready availability makes it one of our cheapest raw materials."[2] With respect to animals with lungs or gills, the term "breathing" or respiration is quite applicable. Unicellular microorganisms, however, have no lungs or gills. The term *biologic oxidation* (biooxidation) is therefore used here, instead of respiration or breathing, to include all of the different energy-yielding (oxidation) mechanisms of all living cells. In some of these oxidative mechanisms the cells use the free oxygen of the air that is dissolved in the water around them.[3] In others the cells use an enzymic process called *dehydrogenation* by which hydrogen (with its electrons) is taken from the substrate, liberating the energy of the electrons. The hydrogen is then combined with free oxygen, or with oxygen from such substances as $NaNO_3$ or Na_2SO_4, forming H_2O as a waste product. Still others combine the hydrogen with *hydrogen acceptors* other than oxygen: with sulfur, for example, forming H_2S; with nitrogen, forming NH_3; or with carbon, forming CH_4. All the chemical reactions that yield energy to living things are forms of biologic oxidation, though oxygen may not be obviously involved. This may be demonstrated as:

$$AH_2 \quad + \quad B \quad \underset{}{\overset{Enzyme}{\rightleftharpoons}} \quad A \quad + \quad BH_2$$

| Hydrogen donor | Hydrogen acceptor | Oxidized product | Reduced product |

The substrate AH_2 is oxidized to A, while B, as the hydrogen acceptor, is changed to the reduced product BH_2. Energy is yielded to the cell.

The reader should remember that these reactions involve a transfer of hydrogen (and its electrons) that results not only in oxidation, whether or not oxygen itself is involved, but also in *reduction*. Oxidation is fundamentally a loss of electrons; reduction is the acquisition of electrons. Bacteria perform their electron-energy-transferring reactions by means of a series of carrier systems that involve numerous enzymes and coenzymes (cofactors) which act as carriers of hydrogen and/or its associated electrons. Important cofactors involved in numerous biochemical reactions that are part of the bacterial metabolism and often confuse the student because of their abbreviated nomenclature are listed in Table 7–1.

Sources of Energy

GREEN PLANTS AND PHOTOSYNTHESIS. The source of energy is one fundamental difference among living things. Green plants and a few species of bacteria and protozoa must have energy from the sun's rays. They utilize light energy by means of their photosynthetic pigments, the most familiar of which is the green pigment of leaves and grass called *chlorophyll*. In green plants (*not* bacteria) chlorophyll causes water and carbon dioxide of the atmosphere to combine so that starch, cellulose, and

---

[2]*Science*, 1966, *154*:640.
[3]By means of oxidases, oxygenases, and so on.

Table 7-1.   Some Coenzymes Used by Microorganisms*

COENZYME, OR GROWTH FACTOR	COENZYME COMMON SYMBOL	CHEMICAL STRUCTURE OF COENZYME
HYDROGEN CARRIER:		
Diphosphopyridine nucleotide	DPN+	Nicotinamide-ribose-phos-phos-ribose-adenine
= Nicotinamide adenine dinucleotide (Either name is used in the literature.)†	NAD'	
Triphosphopyridine nucleotide, also named	TPN+	Nicotinamide-ribose-phos-phos-phos-ribose-adenine
Nicotinamide adenine dinucleotide phosphate	NADP+	
Nicotinamide adenine dinucleotide phosphate reduced form	NADPH$_2$	
Flavin mononucleotide	FMN	Riboflavin-phosphate
Flavin adenine dinucleotide	FAD	Riboflavin-phos-phos-ribose-adenine
GROUP CARRIER:		
Adenosine triphosphate	ATP	Adenine-ribose-phos-phos-phos
Adenosine diphosphate	ADP	Adenine-ribose-phos-phos
Adenosine monophosphate	AMP	Adenine-phosphate
Coenzyme A	CoA	Adenine-phosphoribose-phos-phos-pantetheine (derived from pantothenic acid)
Folic acid or Pteroyl-L-glutamic acid	PGA	
Folinic acid = CF (Citrovorum factor)	CoF	N^5-formyltetrahydro-PGA (derived from folic acid)
Thiamine pyrophosphate	TPP	Thiamine-phos-phos
Uridine diphosphate glucose	UDPG	
Uridine diphosphate glucuronic acid	UDPGA	

*This list of coenzymes is not complete, but does contain most important coenzymes used by microorganisms.
   †See Figure 7-4.

other complex organic substances are formed in the plant. Free oxygen is released to the atmosphere. The chemical change involved in *green plants* may be symbolized as follows:

(1) $nCO_2 + 2nH_2O \xrightarrow{\text{Photosynthesis}} (CH_2O)n + nH_2O + nO_2 + \text{Energy absorbed}$

In the preceding reaction solar energy is absorbed and carbon dioxide is

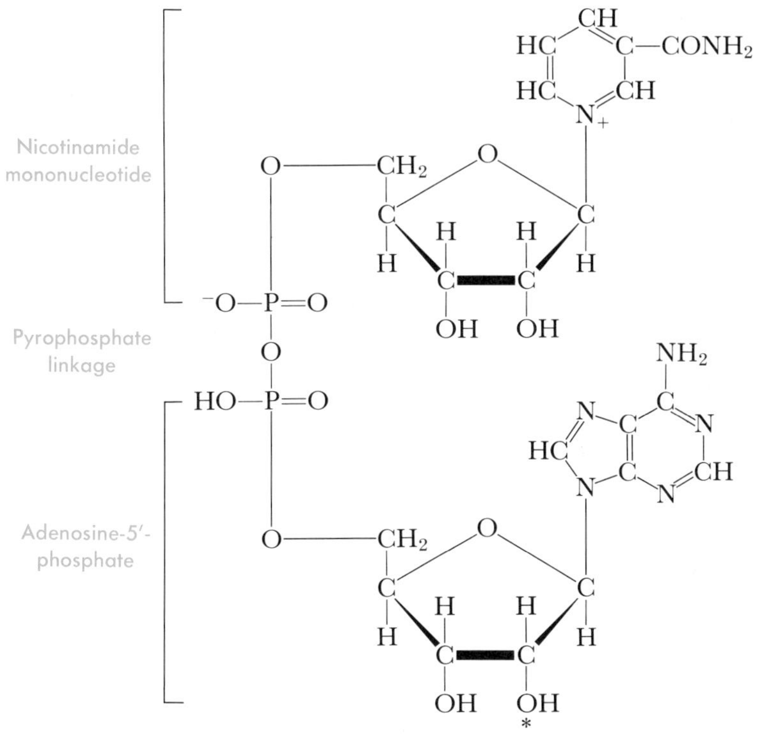

Figure 7-4

Nicotinamide adenine dinucleotide, also called NAD or, previously, DPN.
  *This indicates the attachment for H_3PO_4 in NADP, previously called TPN.

fixed from the air. $(CH_2O)n$ represents a carbohydrate like glucose where
$n = 6$. The reaction may thus also be written as

(2) $6CO_2 + 12H_2O \xrightarrow{\text{Photosynthesis}} (CH_2O)_6 + 6H_2O + 6O_2 +$ Energy absorbed

It is now known that 12 molecules of water are required in this reaction
for each molecule of glucose produced. $(CH_2O)_6 = 1$ molecule $C_6H_{12}O_6$.
    From the soil, the roots of terrestrial green plants draw up water con-
taining dissolved mineral compounds of nitrogen, sulfur, phosphorus,
potassium, and other elements. These, along with the energy furnished
by the sun and chlorophyll, are synthesized into the protoplasm and woody
and other structures of the plant. This synthesis, since it proceeds with the
aid of light, is called *photosynthesis*. That energy from the sun is actually
stored up in the plant is made evident when heat and light and motive
power are released, as in burning wood or coal in a steam engine or when
potatoes or sugar are transformed into human energy. The overall chemical change may be represented as the reverse of the photosynthetic reaction and this can be written in its simplest form, with O_2 being the hydrogen
acceptor and H_2O the reduced product.

(3) $(CH_2O) + O_2 \xrightarrow[\text{biological oxidation}]{\text{Combustion or}} CO_2 + H_2O$ (Energy is released)

This reaction as written is greatly oversimplified and actually consists of many individual chemical steps, yielding CO_2 and water as the carbohydrate is consumed. We shall show later how this process occurs in muscle tissue as well as in the fermentation process.

BACTERIA THAT ARE PHOTOSYNTHETIC. Only a relatively few species of bacteria are photosynthetic, and these are of no known medical interest. The photosynthetic process in bacteria is analogous to that in green plants but may be written as:

(4) $nCO_2 + 2nH_2A \xrightarrow{\text{Bacteriochlorophyll}} (CH_2O)n + nH_2O + 2nA$

Purple photosynthetic bacteria contain *bacteriochlorophylls* that permit a photochemical reaction to proceed from CO_2 to a carbohydrate but, unlike the reaction based on *chlorophyll*, oxygen is never produced in this process. H_2A may be any organic or inorganic useful chemical substrate instead of H_2O. Bacteriochlorophyll is also green, but may be masked by red or brown pigments present in the cell.

Some purple and some green bacteria can produce free sulfur by the following photosynthetic reaction:

(5) $nCO_2 + 2nH_2S \xrightarrow[\text{bacteria}]{\text{Purple sulfur}} (CH_2O)n + nH_2O + 2nS$

Even plain H_2 can serve as a specific hydrogen donor: Thus, H_2A can be any hydrogen donor.

(6) $nCO_2 + 2nH_2 \longrightarrow (CH_2O)n + nH_2O$

For example, species of *Rhodopseudomonas* produce acetone from isopropyl alcohol as shown in the following reaction:

(7) $CO_2 + 2$ isopropyl alcohol $\xrightarrow{\text{light}} (CH_2O) + H_2O + 2$ acetone

        (This could be any   (The product
        of many organic   depends on
        substances)   the precursor)

BACTERIA AND CHEMOSYNTHESIS. Unlike green plants, most bacteria, yeasts, and molds (fungi in general), as well as most protozoa, have no chlorophyll and many species are injured by prolonged exposure to sunlight. This is true especially of pathogenic species. The energy for the synthesis of bacterial protoplasm and that of yeasts, molds, and most animal cells comes not from the sun but from *chemical reactions* such as biooxidation of glucose (see reaction (3), page 103) or, in certain bacteria, some other substance such as hydrogen sulfide:

(8) $H_2S + 2O_2 \longrightarrow H_2SO_4 + $ energy

Such chemically energized self-synthesis is therefore called *chemosynthesis*. Virtually all microorganisms of medical importance are chemosynthetic. Sources of nitrogen, sulfur, phosphorus, and so forth, for chemosynthetic organisms are similar to those of green plants and may be organic, inorganic, or both, depending on species. Because microscopic plants like yeasts, molds, and bacteria, and most animal cells like protozoa, have no roots similar to large plants, they must actually be immersed in solutions of food (osmotrophic nutrition).

FERMENTATION. Although only a brief outline of fermentation can be given in this chapter, the topic is mentioned later in the book in connection with rising of bread, alcohol production, and spoilage of food. The

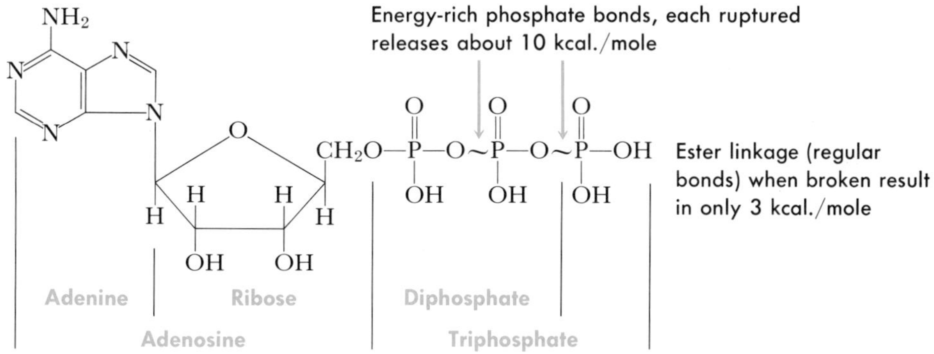

Figure 7–5

Adenosine triphosphate. Other nucleoside triphosphates may replace ATP in certain metabolic reactions. These are: GTP, guanine triphosphate; CTP, cytosine triphosphate; and UTP, uracil triphosphate. One kilocalorie (kcal) = 1,000 calories. The calorie is a unit of energy required to raise the temperature of 1 gram of water at atmospheric pressure 1 C.

chemistry of fermentation processes has been only partially outlined in Figure 7–6 (see page 106). The reader is referred to several references cited at the end of this chapter for a more informative treatment of the reactions involved.

Several fermentation pathways that are known are identified in the literature by a variety of names:

1. Hexose metabolism via the Embden-Meyerhof pathway is commonly called *glycolysis,* or also, yeast fermentation, anaerobic glycolysis, anaerobic carbohydrate metabolism of muscle, or dissimilation of glucose

2. The hexose monophosphate or *pentose phosphate pathway,* pentose cycle, pentose phosphate shunt, or even the Warburg-Dickens-Lipmann pathway also referred to as the monophosphate shunt

3. The glucuronic acid pathway or glucuronic acid cycle

4. The Entner-Doudoroff pathway

5. The glyoxylate cycle

Actually only glycolysis and the pentose phosphate pathway are well established routes of carbohydrate metabolism in microorganisms. Much research still needs to be done to ascertain the other cycles and pathways although they may be much more important in intermediary metabolism than current knowledge indicates.

In fermentation reactions microorganisms use energy-rich compounds like ATP (adenosine-triphosphate) for chemical loans of energy. This loan is then repaid with interest to the system (Fig. 7–5).

Without presenting the numerous enzymes and formulas involved, a fermentation scheme (glycolysis) from glucose to pyruvic acid is shown in Figure 7–6. In this process the hexose glucose, a 6-carbon compound, is broken down into two D-glyceraldehyde-3-phosphate molecules, triose, 3-carbon compounds, which are then transformed into 2 molecules of pyruvic acid per original mole of glucose. In this process 2 ATP energy-rich phosphate bonds, indicated by the symbol ~, are invested into the pathways and 4 ADP molecules are converted into 4 ATP molecules with a total gain of 2 ~ bonds.

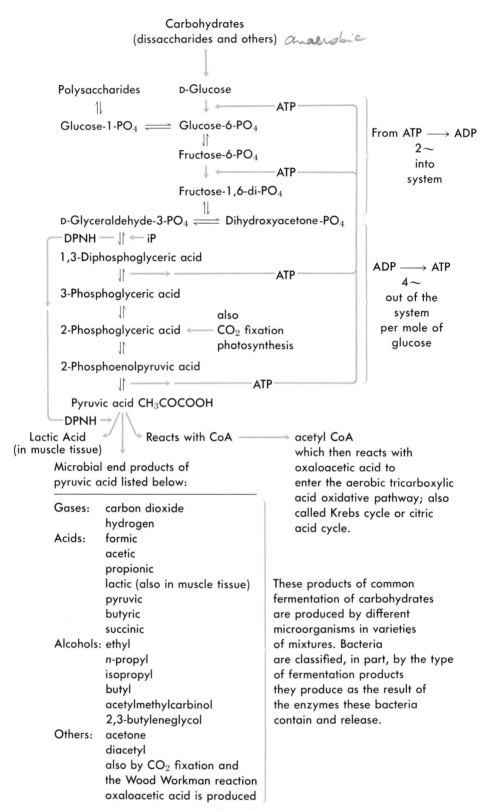

Carbohydrates
(dissaccharides and others) *anaerobic*

Polysaccharides   D-Glucose

Glucose-1-PO$_4$ ⇌ Glucose-6-PO$_4$ ← ATP

Fructose-6-PO$_4$

Fructose-1,6-di-PO$_4$ ← ATP

D-Glyceraldehyde-3-PO$_4$ ⇌ Dihydroxyacetone-PO$_4$

DPNH — iP

1,3-Diphosphoglyceric acid

3-Phosphoglyceric acid → ATP

2-Phosphoglyceric acid ← CO$_2$ fixation also photosynthesis

2-Phosphoenolpyruvic acid

Pyruvic acid CH$_3$COCOOH → ATP

DPNH

From ATP ⟶ ADP
2 ~
into
system

ADP ⟶ ATP
4 ~
out of the
system
per mole of
glucose

Lactic Acid
(in muscle tissue)   → Reacts with CoA ⟶ acetyl CoA
which then reacts with
oxaloacetic acid to
enter the aerobic tricarboxylic
acid oxidative pathway; also
called Krebs cycle or citric
acid cycle.

Microbial end products of
pyruvic acid listed below:

Gases:	carbon dioxide
	hydrogen
Acids:	formic
	acetic
	propionic
	lactic (also in muscle tissue)
	pyruvic
	butyric
	succinic
Alcohols:	ethyl
	n-propyl
	isopropyl
	butyl
	acetylmethylcarbinol
	2,3-butyleneglycol
Others:	acetone
	diacetyl
	also by CO$_2$ fixation and
	the Wood Workman reaction
	oxaloacetic acid is produced

These products of common
fermentation of carbohydrates
are produced by different
microorganisms in varieties
of mixtures. Bacteria
are classified, in part, by the type
of fermentation products
they produce as the result of
the enzymes these bacteria
contain and release.

Figure 7–6

Metabolism of carbohydrates. Anaerobic glycolysis – fermentation scheme.

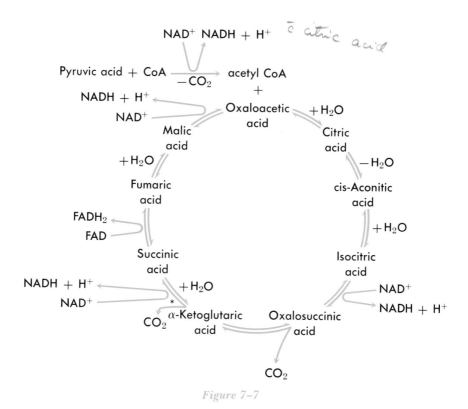

Figure 7-7

The Krebs cycle, tricarboxylic acid cycle, or citric acid cycle. The 2H⁺ produced in the citric acid cycle is carried by the respiratory chain through the cytochrome system to oxygen. (See Fig. 7–8.) The asterisk in the figure indicates that actually succinyl CoA is formed between α-ketoglutaric acid and succinic acid involving CoA, guanosine triphosphate, guanosine diphosphate, and an energy-rich phosphate bond. The coenzyme of thiamine has also been thought to be involved in this place in the cycle. For simplicity's sake, however, a simpler pattern is shown in the figure.

Glycolysis as an anaerobic system releases only a fraction of the potential energy of glucose. Without air many organisms use pyruvic acid to form some of the end products of the fermentation process as listed in Figure 7–6; others such as *Streptococcus* and *Lactobacillus* can reduce pyruvic acid to lactic acid; and some enter aerobic pathways such as the citric acid cycle (Fig. 7–7) and proceed to gain further energy through the electron transport system involving cytochrome pigments (Fig. 7–8).

Summaries of all these pathways are available in sources listed at the end of this chapter. The reader should realize that the estimated gain in energy depends on the enzymes a specific organism possesses and the reaction products it produces.

An approximation of energy released during glycolysis may be close to 35.0 kcal/mole, and the sum of energy released during the citric acid cycle, 57.6 kcal. The electron-transport-released energy is about 594.4 kcal. Thus 687.0 kcal/mole may be obtained from all the systems discussed in this chapter for the fermentation of glucose.

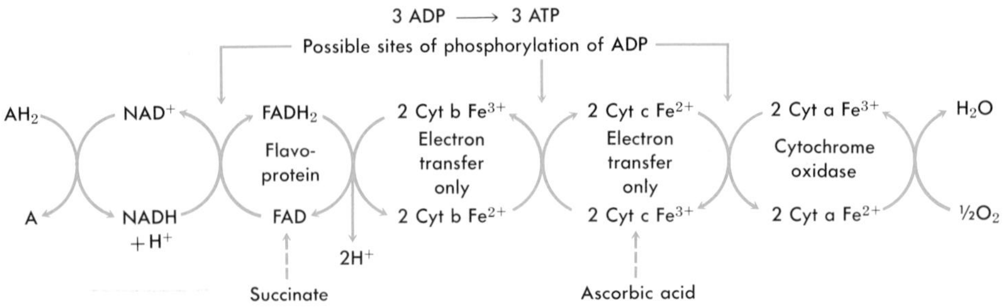

$$3 \text{ ADP} \longrightarrow 3 \text{ ATP}$$

Possible sites of phosphorylation of ADP

| AH$_2$ | NAD$^+$ | FADH$_2$ | 2 Cyt b Fe^{3+} | 2 Cyt c Fe^{2+} | 2 Cyt a Fe^{3+} | H$_2$O |

Flavo-protein | Electron transfer only | Electron transfer only | Cytochrome oxidase

A   NADH +H$^+$ FAD   2 Cyt b Fe^{2+} 2 Cyt c Fe^{3+} 2 Cyt a Fe^{2+} ½O$_2$

$2H^+$

Succinate   Ascorbic acid

Figure 7–8

Possible sites of coupling of phosphorylation with electron transport in cytochrome system (or liver mitochondria). Energy is gained in this "electron-transporting" mechanism. (Adapted from Fruton, J. S., and Simmonds, S.: General Biochemistry, 2nd Ed, 1958, New York, John Wiley and Sons, Inc.)

Some reference sources state that the conversion of glucose to carbon dioxide and water liberates energy as follows:[4]

$$C_6H_{12}O_6 + 6O_2 \longrightarrow 6CO_2 + 6H_2O; \; - \Delta F = 691 \text{ kcal/mole}$$

A total of 36 ATP are produced in the fermentation exchange of energy. By complete oxidation of glucose to CO_2 and H_2O by way of the Embden-Meyerhof scheme and the citric acid cycle, a total of 36 $\sim PO_4$ (36 energy-rich phosphates) are released.

The reader should never forget that some microorganisms may never employ the glycolysis scheme, but rather the pentose phosphate pathway; and fermentation products from pyruvic acid differ, depending on the enzymes produced. Furthermore, the "electron-transport" system may be entered at different sites of phosphorylation, if at all. Microorganisms differ in their genetic determinants and their enzymes produced and, consequently, in metabolic pathways and products of fermentation. All need energy, but how this energy is obtained determines many of their diagnostic characteristics and their success in the struggle for survival with other forms of life.

Viruses an Exception. The principal exception to these descriptions of how cells eat and oxidize their foods is the group of viruses. Their mechanisms of nutrition, energy derivation, and reproduction are not yet fully understood. In fact, viruses are not cells but, curiously enough, much like independently living chromosomes, or inheritance units of cells. They have no energy metabolism so far as is known at present.

Have no enzymes

Microbial Multiplication

We have seen that yeasts undergo a process of *unequal* fission called budding. When two *equal* cells are formed by the division of one cell, the process is called *binary fission*. Elongated forms of bacteria multiply by transverse binary fission; that is, the division occurs at right angles to the long axis. Flagellate protozoa divide lengthwise by *longitudinal* fission.

[4]See Mazur, A., and Harrow, B.: Biochemistry — A Brief Course. 1968, Philadelphia, W. B. Saunders Co.

Multiplication by fission is not confined to independently living micro-organisms. Fission occurs in cells that are part of large, complex, multi-cellular structures: dogs, trees, or humans.

REPRODUCTION AND FISSION. In trees, humans, or dogs, fission of body cells (not of sex cells) results only in increased size of the plant or animal, or in the replacement of some structural cells that have died (as in injury and the like). Reproduction (i.e., increase in numbers) of dogs, people, or trees is brought about only by the conjunction of sex cells. Among the unicellular microorganisms, only the eucaryons produce true gametocytes.

In bacteria, fission produces more than one cell and therefore more than one individual. This is their chief method of reproduction. A "pseu-dosexual" type of mating that results in genetic recombination, but not multiplication, and that will be discussed later in this chapter, has been demonstrated in certain species of bacteria.

GENETIC MECHANISMS IN MICROORGANISMS. In the eucaryons definite sexual phenomena are generally evident; there are contacts of more or less distinctive sex cells (gametes) and dissolution of separating cell walls, followed by intermingling of cell contents, especially of genes of genetic materials (DNA) that carry hereditary traits and characters (genetic recombination). In bacteria, which have only primitive nuclei (nucleoids), similar but more primitive conjugations have been described in several species (see later discussion of Conjugation).

In higher (eucaryotic) organisms such as zinnias or cats, sexual proc-esses are necessary for genetic recombinations and for reproduction.[5] Among unicellular eucaryons, sex, although present in most, is unneces-sary since most can multiply indefinitely by asexual fission. The bacteria not only indefinitely reproduce asexually, but, as is explained below, genetic recombination can occur by *transduction,* or by *transformation* in the entire absence of sex. Gene recombination also occurs in viruses, al-though sexual phenomena are entirely absent.

Transduction. In this process certain viruses (bacteriophages) that infect bacteria can invade one bacterial cell after another, carrying with them parts of the genetic material (genes; DNA) of the bacterial cells. This results in new genetic combinations. The DNA *of the phage itself* may also integrate temporarily with the bacterial DNA, giving the bacterium new traits, but only as long as the phage remains. This is often called viral conversion or "infective heredity." DNA from one *bacterial* cell, transferred by phage to another bacterial cell, imparts new hereditary traits to the second bacterium. The phenomenon is generally called *transduction.* Often the transduced DNA is rejected, resulting in *abortive transduction.*

Transformation. Various microorganisms may be made to "inherit" physiologic characters artificially by using DNA extracted in test tubes from live or dead microorganisms. Other, but closely related, microorgan-isms immersed in such extract acquire the DNA (with inheritable proper-ties) of the microorganisms from which the DNA was extracted. Thus the immersed microorganisms acquire new inheritable qualities by in vitro[6] inheritance without benefit of sex. This is called *transformation.* Studies

---

[5]*Propagation* by cuttings, grafts, and so on, does not involve genetic exchanges or sexual processes and is fundamentally merely continued growth of part of the same individual in a different place.

[6]From the Latin words for "in glass" (in the test tube).

with P^{32}-labeled DNA have shown just how the genetic material from the donor replaces DNA of the recipient bacterial strain in transformation. More than one genetic character can be transferred at one time in the transformation process. The DNA must be double-stranded, either native or renatured; it is not active in transformation if it is denatured or its two strands are separated after being heated for 10 minutes at 100 C. Recent evidence shows that transformation also occurs under natural conditions.

Conjugation.   Conjugation among bacteria is a primitive type of mating process discovered by Lederberg and Tatum in 1946 in *Escherichia coli.* In these organisms conjugation consists of a one-way transfer of genetic material from one cell, the donor, into another, the recipient. The donor cell is analogous to the male in higher biologic systems and the corresponding recipient is analogous to the female. Donor cells contain a cytoplasmic agent or episome called a *fertility* or "male" (F) factor and are designated F$^+$ cells. Recipient cells are designated F$^-$ cells. In mating, the F$^+$ cells readily transfer the F episome, but rarely genetic DNA, to F$^-$ cells which then become F$^+$ cells. DNA-containing elements (conjugons) other than the F factor have also been demonstrated. An episome of this type is the Cf conjugon, called "colicinogenic" factor (see Bacteriocins in Chapter 14), or the RTF (resistance transfer factors) that determine resistance or sensitivity to certain antibiotics. Thus, RTF$^+$ donor cells and RTF$^-$ recipient cells also exist. (See also Drug Resistance, later in this chapter).

Sometimes the F episome becomes integrated into the chromosome of the F$^+$ cell. This greatly increases frequency of genetic recombination (transfer of genetic DNA from donor cells to F$^-$ cells). Donor cells in which the F episome has become integrated into the donor chromosome are therefore called Hfr (high frequency of genetic recombination) cells. The mating process by these cells is often incomplete. The F factor in Hfr cells is the last part of the integrated chromosome to be transferred to the recipient cells. The chromosome usually breaks somewhere during the process. Therefore, in Hfr × F$^-$ matings, although F$^-$ cells frequently become genetic recombinants, they rarely become F$^+$ or Hfr. Note that Hfr denotes high frequency of *transfer of genes* but *not* high frequency of mating.

As can be seen in Figure 7–9 it is quite possible to interrupt the mating process by vigorous shaking at measured intervals and then to determine which "genes," genetic determinants, or markers have meanwhile been transferred from donor to recipient. It has been found that markers are always transferred in the same order and that the bacterial chromosome is a circular thread of DNA. This thread breaks at mating time and is transferred lengthwise from donor to recipient; the F factor is transferred last, if at all. In Figure 7–9 it is seen that the A gene passes into the recipient cell in 8 minutes, the C gene in 10 minutes, then the D, E, and F genes in that order. After 30 minutes the R gene (e.g., fermentation of galactose) is transferred. When, as is common, the chromosome is broken mechanically at the transfer bridge before completion of the mating, only a portion of the donor genes pass to the recipient. The time intervals may vary in different species.

We have learned much of the arrangement and sequence of markers ("genes") in the bacterial chromosome from interrupted mating experiments and the knowledge thus gained has enabled geneticists to form circular chromosome or genetic maps of bacteria. A typical genetic map of *E. coli* is shown in Figure 7–10.

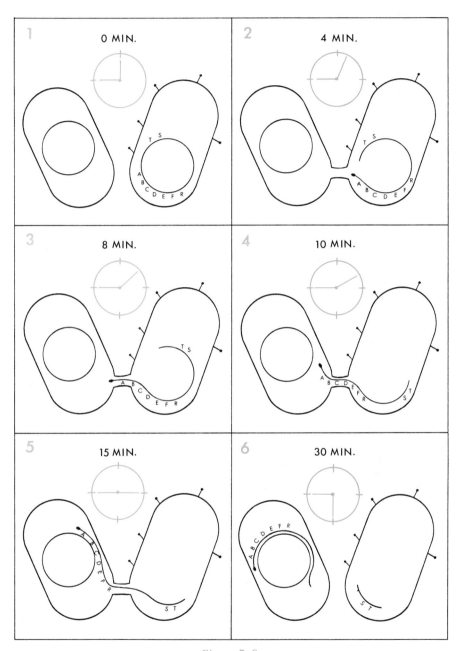

Figure 7–9

Bacterial genes are transferred from one bacterium to another in a linear order. Upon surface contact between a donor cell and a recipient cell, a conjugation tube is formed. The donor cell transmits a portion of its chromosome carrying genes A, B, C, D, E, F, R to the recipient cell. A recombinant cell is thus formed, containing genes from both parent types. The donor cell shows bacteriophage attached to the cell surface. Apparently the donor cell survives the loss of chromatin material because at this time the bacterial cell may be multinucleate. (Modified after Wollman, E. L., and Jacob, F.: "Sexuality in Bacteria." Copyright © 1956 by *Scientific American*, Inc. All rights reserved.)

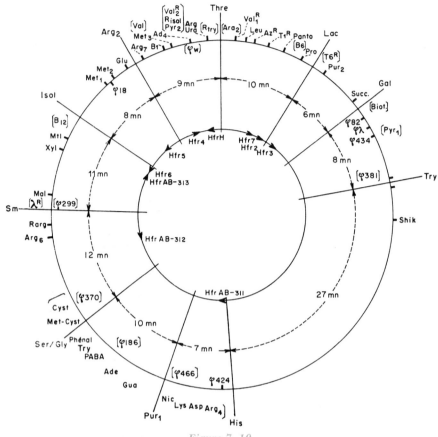

Figure 7–10

Schematic representation of the linkage group of *E. coli* K-12. The outer line represents the order of the characters (not their absolute distances). The dotted lines represent the time intervals of penetration between pairs of markers corresponding to the radial lines. The inner line represents the order of transfer of different *Hfr* types of donor high frequency genes. Each arrow corresponds to the origin of the corresponding *Hfr* strain.

Symbols correspond to synthesis of threonine (thre), leucine (leu), pantothenate (panto), proline (pro), purines (pur), biotin (biot), pyrimidines (pyr), tryptophan (try), shikimic acid (shik), histidine (his), arginine (arg), lysine (lys), nicotinamide (nic), guanine (gua), adenine (ade), para-aminobenzoic acid (PABA), tyrosine (tyr), phenylalanine (phenal), glycine (gly), serine (ser), cysteine (cyst), methionine (met), vitamin B_{12} (B_{12}), isoleucine (isol), thiamin (B_1), valine (val); to fermentation of arabinose (ara), lactose (lac), galactose (gal), maltose (mal), xylose (xyl), mannitol (mtl); requirement for succinate isoleucine (R_{isol}), tryptophan (R_{try}), location of inducible prophages 82, 434, 381, 21, 424, 466, and of noninducible prophages 186, 370, 299, 18, and W. Symbols in brackets indicate that the location of the marker with respect to neighboring markers has not been exactly determined.

The figures given for time intervals between two markers correspond to the average of several experiments of interrupted mating, using *Hfr* strains which inject early the region involved. (From Jacob, F., and Wollman, E. L.: Sexuality and the Genetics of Bacteria. 1961, New York, Academic Press.)

Recombination (Sex) in Bacteria.

Recombination (Sex) in Bacteria. Lederberg and numerous other microbial geneticists have crossed different strains of bacteria. Some genetic markers that have been used to test for recombination are shown in Table 7–2.

Table 7–2.   Symbols Used for Various Loci of *E. coli* K12*

NUTRITIONAL REQUIREMENTS

(Requirement of a substance is indicated by a superscript⁻; independence by a superscript⁺.)

STRAIN	SUBSTANCE	STRAIN
B^-	Biotin	B^+
B_1^-	Thiamine	B_1^+
C^-	Cystine	C^+
L^-	Leucine	L^+
M^-	Methionine	M^+
P^-	Proline	P^+
T^-	Threonine	T^+

SUGAR FERMENTATIONS

(Ability to ferment is indicated by a superscript⁺; inability by a superscript⁻.)

STRAIN	SUBSTANCE	STRAIN
Lac^+	Lactose	Lac^-
Gly^+	Glycerol	Gly^-

BACTERIOPHAGE RESISTANCE

(Resistance to phage is indicated by a superscriptʳ; sensitivity by a superscriptˢ.)

STRAIN	PHAGE	STRAIN
V_1^r	T_1 and T_5	V_1^s
V_6^r	T_6	V_6^s

RESISTANCE TO CHEMICAL AGENTS

(Resistance to chemical agents is indicated by a superscriptʳ; sensitivity by a superscriptˢ.)

STRAIN	SUBSTANCE	STRAIN
Cla^r	Sodium chloroacetate	Cla^s
A^r	Sodium azide	A^s

*Adapted from Lederberg, J.: *Genetics*, Vol. 32.

For example, a cross between two *E. coli* parental strains,

$$B^-M^-P^+T^+V_1^s \times B^+M^+P^-T^-V_1^r$$

may result in offspring of

79 per cent $B^+M^+P^+T^+V_1^s$ and 21 per cent $B^+M^+P^+T^+V_1^r$.

From this cross it is concluded that the gene for phage resistance V_1^r is about 21 chromosomal units away from the P and T genes on the *E. coli* chromosome, since V_1^s stays with P^+ and T^+ 79 per cent of the time, which means that the chromosome breaks occur only 21 per cent of the time, resulting in $P^+T^+V_1^r$ new combinations. By this system genes like B, M, P, and others may also be mapped on the chromosome.

Mutation.   Whatever alters the chemicophysical structure of molecules of genetic DNA (genes), whether the DNA is incorporated in a human sex cell or is floating free in a culture of bacteria, will alter the inherited characteristics of the organism which receives, sexually or asexually, that DNA. A *genetic mutation* may have occurred. This is manifested as a sudden change in inherited characters that will, in turn, be inherited by the progeny through indefinite generations. A *mutant* is an organism that has undergone mutation, be it man or bacterium. At this point, it is assumed that the student has not forgotten the definitions of the mutational unit, the *muton*; the recombination unit, the *recon*; or the complementation analysis unit, the *cistron*, all of which roughly refer to the *gene* (see Chapter 2). The term replicon has also been proposed as a common name for the bacterial chromosome and the conjugons (see page 110).

Mutagenic Agents and Cancer.   Some of the agents that can alter DNA or change the genetic structure and thus produce mutations in any type of cells are x-rays, ultraviolet light, and other irradiations; certain chemicals; possibly some viruses; and probably sex hormones. Such agents are said to be *mutagenic*, i.e., mutant-producing. "LSD" is said also to be a mutagen. It is interesting to note that many mutagenic agents are also carcinogenic, that is, cancer-producing or *oncogenic* (producing tumors, especially malignant tumors). A major concern of the human race is how much mutagenic effect is to be feared from radioactive fallout from thermonuclear bombs. Sometimes mutations occur for unknown reasons instead of as a result of exposure to a known mutagenic agent; then we hide our ignorance of the cause by calling the change a "spontaneous mutation." It seems that no living organism can escape *neutron* bombardment from outer space. Thus, even without any willful exposure to mutagenic agents, genetic material is always exposed to chance irradiation.

In 1962–1963 genetic material (DNA) was synthesized artificially in vitro. The man-made DNA, when applied to certain bacteria, altered their genetic characters just as effectively as though genetic mutation, transformation, or transduction had taken place. May we anticipate that by the use of various forms of predesigned, manufactured DNA, we may direct and control heredity in human beings, with purposeful production of supermen (or of frightful monsters)? Stranger things have happened.

Genotype and Phenotype.   The final, apparent or visible organism, be it fly, mouse, bacteria, or man, resulting from any given genetic makeup (*genotype*) is called the *phenotype* (*pheno-* is from a Greek word meaning that which shows) or the *phenotypic expression* of the genotype. An organism is generally modified to some extent by its environment. Response to environment, however, is controlled by its genotype. A phenotype, therefore, is generally the result of combined hereditary and environmental factors. For example, some hydrangeas have red flowers if growing in acid soil, but blue ones if growing in soil containing iron or alum. Such noninheritable, environmentally produced, temporary changes are sometimes called *fluctuations* or *modifications*.

Variable Bacterial Characters.   Among the phenotypic characters of bacteria that commonly vary because of mutation or fluctuation are size, shape, virulence (if pathogenic), color (if pigmented), capsule formation, motility, spore formation (if spore-forming), production of certain enzymes, or colony characteristics. Many other less readily observable changes occur, such as in chemical (antigenic) composition and nutritional requirements, i.e., the active enzymes. These and other, still obscure alterations underlie alterations in virulence of pathogens.

DRUG RESISTANCE.   A variation of particular importance to the members of the health group is the appearance of bacterial mutants resistant to sulfonamide drugs and antibiotics. This is a problem of major importance in hospitals, especially in communicable disease control, surgical and maternity wards, and nurseries. This aspect of microbial variation directly affects everyone working or living in any hospital. Drug resistance in microorganisms has already been mentioned as resulting from transmission of the RTF (page 110) and will be discussed in greater detail later.

Variation and Diagnosis.   While the offspring of a single bacterial cell may vary widely from its parent, there are certain limits beyond which variation does not go under ordinary conditions of laboratory study. Once the common fluctuants or mutants of a species are known, the diagnostic microbiologist should have no difficulty in recognizing that species. Unless a given species of microorganism is subjected to some unusual environmental condition producing a marked fluctuation or mutation of its properties, it tends to retain its well known characters. Any change in culture medium, pH,[7] and so on, may cause properties of all the cells in a culture to fluctuate. Certain kinds of variation, due either to mutation or fluctuation, are especially common or important in diagnosis and may be briefly described here.

Colony Variant Types.   Four commonly observed types of colony resulting from variation of the constituent cells when cultivated upon solid media like nutrient agar, are the rough or "R" type, the smooth "S" type, the mucoid "M" type, and the minute or dwarf colony type. The surface of rough colonies is rather dry and dull, often wrinkled and crumbly or granular looking, while the edges are irregular (Fig. 7–11A). They are often brittle in consistency. Smooth colonies are pasty or butyrous (buttery) in consistency and have perfectly regular margins, with smooth, glistening surfaces (Fig. 7–11B). Mucoid colonies tend to be smooth and glistening and rather voluminous and watery; they may "run" if the surface on which they grow is tilted. If touched with a wire they spin out long, mucoid threads like saliva or thin taffy. A fourth type of colony variant is the dwarf or small form. These colonies are extremely minute. S, R, M, and minute

---

[7]The symbol pH, with a number (e.g., pH 6.5), is a measure of acidity. (See next chapter.)

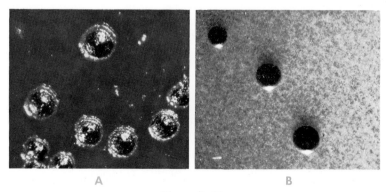

A   B

Figure 7–11

A, Rough (R) colonies of the diphtheria bacillus. *B*, Smooth (S) colonies of the diphtheria bacillus. (About three times actual size.)

colony forms have been observed in many species of bacteria. There are several other less commonly seen varieties of colony form.

Variations in Virulence.[8]   Extensive studies of bacterial variation have revealed that virulence (when present) is usually associated with the S type. The substances and conditions that promote the S and, consequently, virulent, type of bacteria are present in human and other animal bodies. Therefore, microorganisms in—or freshly isolated from—blood, serum, feces, and other materials from the diseased body are especially dangerous to persons who come into contact with this infectious material. S type variants are frequently encapsulated, and this is usually related to virulence. As will be seen later, capsules are protective mucoid coatings on the surface of bacteria; capsules help bacteria evade the defensive mechanisms of the body.

This point is emphasized to the student because health workers usually come into contact with bacteria just as they leave the infected patient and at the time they are most virulent and most capable of causing infection. The pathologist doing an autopsy, the laboratory technician handling infectious tissues, blood, or other body fluid specimens, and the nurse, the surgeon, and the physician dealing with an infectious patient must constantly bear this fact in mind.

After bacteria have been cultivated outside the body on artificial media such as meat broth for a few days or weeks, they tend to "degenerate" and to lose their truculent, invasive character (virulence) and become the pampered and softened pet of the bacteriologist.[9] They also tend to lose their capsule and form R colonies.

---

[8]Virulence is the degree of ability to produce disease. It is discussed more in detail later in this book.

[9]This is not always the case, and no one should assume that a living pathogenic microorganism has lost its virulence at any time except under certain carefully controlled conditions of attenuation of virulence (Chapter 20). Fatal accidents have resulted from such assumptions!

Supplementary Reading

Baker, J. J. W., and Allen, G. E.: Matter, Energy and Life, 2nd Ed. 1970, Reading, Massachusetts, Addison-Wesley Publishing Co.

Baum, S. J.: Introduction to Organic and Biological Chemistry. 1970, London, The Macmillan Company.

Braun, W.: Bacterial Genetics, 2nd Ed. 1965, Philadelphia, W. B. Saunders Co.

Cantarow, A., and Schepartz, B.: Biochemistry, 4th Ed. 1967, Philadelphia, W. B. Saunders Co.

Hassid, W. Z.: Biosynthesis of oligosaccharides and polysaccharides in plants. *Science*, 1969, *165*:137.

Herskowitz, I. H.: Genetics, 2nd Ed. 1965, Boston, Little, Brown & Co.

Kornberg, A.: The synthesis of DNA. *Sci. Amer.*, 1968, *219*:64.

Lengyel, P., and Soll, D.: Mechanism of protein biosynthesis. *Bact Rev.*, 1969, *33*:264.

Mahler, H. R., and Cordes, E. H.: Biological Chemistry. 1966, New York, Harper & Row.

Mazur, A., and Harrow, B.: Biochemistry—A Brief Course. 1968, Philadelphia, W. B. Saunders Co.

McGilvery, R. W.: Biochemistry: A Functional Approach. 1970, Philadelphia, W. B. Saunders Co.

Miller, J. H.: Experiments in Molecular Genetics. 1972, Cold Spring Harbor Laboratory, Cold Spring Harbor, N.Y.

Pardee, A. B.: Membrane transport systems. *Science*, 1968, *162*:632.

Spencer, J. H.: The Physics and Chemistry of DNA and RNA. 1972, Philadelphia, W. B. Saunders Co.

Stent, G. S.: Molecular Biology of Bacterial Viruses. 1963, San Francisco, W. H. Freeman.

Physiology of
Microorganisms
in Their Environment

Several physical and chemical factors are of absolutely critical importance to the growth and reproduction of living cells, be they bacteria or cells of our own body. Among the most important factors are moisture, nutrients, absence of toxic (poisonous) substances, specific temperature and pH ranges, the presence or absence of oxygen, the proper osmotic pressure, and others discussed later in this chapter. These factors not only control microorganisms but are the basis of several extremely important aspects of health care procedures as will be discussed in this book.

MOISTURE

Abundant moisture is essential for life and multiplication of all *vegetative*[1] cells, including those of our own bodies, but not for spores, cysts, and other *dormant* cells.

In the absence of water, microorganisms may survive but cannot grow; hence, many industrial commodities and foodstuffs, such as hay, meats, fruits, vegetables, and soups, are preserved by drying. These substances putrefy and spoil through growth of saprophytic[2] microorganisms only if they are kept in moist conditions. Although drying prevents growth of microorganisms, it does not necessarily kill them and, in fact, preserves many saprophytic and saprozoic microorganisms in foodstuffs. One method used by microbiologists to keep certain microorganisms alive for long periods (20 years or more!) is to dry them and store them in a refrigerated vacuum. In one process, which is effective in preserving even the most fragile and sensitive microorganisms, the microorganisms are

---

[1] Actively growing and multiplying; not dormant.
[2] From Greek *sapros*, rotten, and *phyton*, plant; hence a plant living on inanimate organic matter. Animals similarly nourished, especially protozoa, are said to be *saprozoic*.

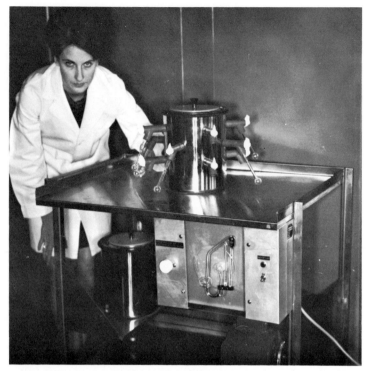

Figure 8–1

Lyophilization (quick-freeze drying) of bacterial cultures at the Microbiology Research Laboratory at the Texas Woman's University. Shown is a Virtis Co. lyophilizer.

first rapidly frozen and then subjected to a high vacuum to draw off the moisture. This is the basis of the procedure called *lyophilization*. The American Type Culture Collection (ATCC) uses this method to store for years many bacterial strains, which are supplied to laboratories when requested. A lyophilization apparatus is shown in Figure 8–1.

Certain fragile pathogenic microorganisms, such as the gonococcus (*Neisseria gonorrhoeae*, cause of gonorrhea), the spirochete that causes syphilis (*Treponema pallidum*), and vegetative trophozoite forms of the cause of amebic dysentery, *Entamoeba histolytica*, which can be dried while frozen, are extremely sensitive to drying at temperatures near those of the body. Certain other pathogenic bacteria (tubercle and diphtheria bacilli) and cyst forms of protozoa may survive at room temperatures, whether frozen or not, for long periods in dried mucus, pus, sputum, or feces.

NUTRIENTS

METABOLISM. By metabolism is meant the digestion and utilization of food to synthesize the proteins, fats, carbohydrates, and other substances of which living cells are made and to furnish the energy necessary for life and reproduction. Among bacteria the biochemical processes constituting metabolism are remarkably like those of all other cells: from your own brain cells down to the most primitive cellular microorganism (not viruses) imaginable. This is probably because all the higher forms of life are derived by evolution from the same, or similar, earlier forms on earth. The cell substance of all living things is therefore almost identical chemically; all living cells utilize the same general sorts of foods, metabolizing these foods by means of the same general chemical activities. As in designs of automobile carburetors, fuel pumps, and transmissions, differences in form exist, but the basic functions are the same.

Foods of Microorganisms

Since all cells consist mainly of carbon (C), hydrogen (H), oxygen (O), nitrogen (N), phosphorus (P), and sulfur (S), with smaller amounts of magnesium (Mg), iron (Fe), copper (Cu), sodium (Na), potassium (K), and a few other elements, nutrients of all cells must contain these elements. The form in which these nutritional elements can be used, however, varies widely with different kinds of cells. The elements may be utilized in one or both of two general forms:

Organic:[3] proteins, carbohydrates, fats, and related or derived substances, all of which are fairly complex compounds of carbon, oxygen, hydrogen, sometimes with phosphorus, nitrogen and sulfur, and so on. In addition, many species require organic complexes such as vitamins, e.g., nicotinic acid ("niacin"), thiamin, and riboflavin, and use them in much the same manner that human beings do. Indeed, in most fundamental respects, as mentioned before, the composition and metabolism of human cells are much like those of many microorganisms.

Inorganic:[4] simple salts such as sodium chloride, water, carbon dioxide, sulfur, iron, hydrogen. Some of the inorganic nutrients are required in such minute quantities that they are referred to as "trace elements." Trace elements will be mentioned later when microbiologic media for different bacteria are discussed. Some of the trace elements are: Zn, Mn, Co, Ca, and sometimes even substances that would be highly toxic in higher concentrations.

Nutritional Types

All living organisms may be subdivided on the basis of their sources of life energy. Thus, all green plants, including the eucaryotic green algae (seaweeds, and so forth) and the procaryotic blue-green algae (Cyanophyceae) and a small group of medically negligible bacteria, typically obtain all their energy for self-synthesis from sunlight, or equivalent radiant energy from an artificial source. Such organisms are said to be *photosynthetic* or *phototrophs*.

All typical animal cells and all fungi, including bacteria and related

---

[3]Since 1828 chemists have defined organic compounds as those that contain the element carbon.

[4]Inorganic compounds are those that do not contain carbon. However, CO, CO_2 and H_2CO_3 are on the borderline; they are ordinarily dealt with in inorganic chemistry.

forms (except the few species of photosynthetic harmless bacteria just mentioned), can live entirely without radiant energy and may even be injured by it. They obtain all their vital energy for self-synthesis from chemical reactions called *biooxidations*, or respirations, that are independent of light. They are said to be *chemosynthetic* or *chemotrophs*.

Each of these groups may be subdivided into two groups on the basis of the kinds of materials (not sources of energy) on which their growth depends. Some phototrophs may use only inorganic donors of hydrogen (e.g., H_2O for green plants, H_2S for certain bacteria) for the reduction of CO_2 in photosynthesis; these are called *photolithotrophs*. If they require organic donors of hydrogen for reduction of CO_2 in photosynthesis they are called *photoorganotrophs*. Chemotrophs whose energy-yielding chemical reactions (biooxidations) are restricted to oxidation of inorganic substances are said to be *chemolithotrophic*. Chemotrophs whose oxidation substrates must be organic substances are called *chemoorganotrophs*.

Organisms were formerly classed as *autotrophic*[5] if they could use CO_2 as a sole source of carbon, and *heterotrophic*[6] if they required carbon in organic combination. Because of numerous inconsistencies and overlappings, these groupings have been replaced by the previously mentioned terminology: *photolithotrophic, photoorganotrophic, chemolithotrophic,* and *chemoorganotrophic*.

Viruses, which receive both their energy and (most of) their substance from their hosts (i.e., from infected cells), are neither chemotrophic nor phototrophic; they are said to be *paratrophic*.

Some chemolithotrophic bacteria, common in the soil, rivers, and sea, live entirely on inorganic matter. They are restricted to carbon dioxide from the air as a source of carbon, i.e., they are examples of *autotrophs*. For the other requisite elements they may (and some must) use only the salts in soil or sea water. They obtain their nitrogen in the form of atmospheric nitrogen or ammonia or other simple nitrogenous compounds. From these simple substances they synthesize their own complex vitamins, carbohydrates, proteins, and fats. These bacteria gain their energy by oxidizing sulfur, iron, nitrogen, and a few other elements. Such bacteria are independent of all other forms of life and may be descendants of some of the earliest living things on this planet.

Some species of chemoorganotrophic microorganisms of the soil, sewage, and so forth can digest solid organic substances like wood, crab shells, and old rubber tires. Certain pathogenic species can digest the living tissues of your body. This is because the cells of these various species secrete the appropriate enzymes to liquefy (digest) these solid organic substances and then absorb them. Could you dine on old tires or sawdust? Theoretically you could, easily, if the cells of your alimentary tract secreted the same enzymes as the microorganisms. It is evident that all of the apparently enormous and spectacular metabolic differences between men and different species of microorganisms represent mainly differences in the enzyme equipment of the different species. "One bacterium's meat is another man's poison." Cats do not enjoy raw carrots, whereas some human beings (and rabbits) relish them. It should be noted that all microorganisms of medical importance are chemoorganotrophs.

SAPROPHYTES AND SAPROZOA. From the most primitive chemo-

---

[5] From Greek *autos*, self, and *trophe*, feed; self-feeding.
[6] *Hetero* is a Greek word meaning others.

organotrophic (or photoorganotrophic?) species of microorganisms there (probably) evolved species that could utilize more and more complex organic foods, i.e., "higher" forms. Presumably these "more advanced" species of plants and animals depended on the "lower" or more primitive forms for complex, organic foods. Such foods resulted from the waste products and dead cells of the lower species. The higher forms metabolized the dead organic matter and, thus, began the process of decay so necessary for the disposing of dead bodies, plants, excreta, and other refuse. Such microorganisms are the modern chemoorganotrophs and they are of many varieties. They occur in every drop of ocean or pond water, ditch mud, soil, and feces, in short, wherever dead organic matter may be found.

PARASITES AND PATHOGENS. Presumably through the ages the chemoorganotrophic microorganisms "progressed"; i.e., they finally became adapted to prey upon other living organisms. They became able to live in and on the bodies of other plants and animals; they became *parasites*. Because many of them are poisonous, giving off poisonous products, or actually invade healthy tissue and utilize valuable food substances, they seriously injure the host in which they live. The result is disease in the infected host. These parasites are *pathogenic*.

It must not be thought that the lines of division between saprophytic, parasitic, and pathogenic species are entirely clear and distinct. Some saprophytes, such as tetanus and botulism bacilli, are highly pathogenic. They do not invade healthy tissues but give off deadly toxins into dead tissues or into foods in which they grow. These toxins produce disease when (and if) they are absorbed by the body. Some parasites are not usually pathogenic. Examples are the numerous species of usually harmless bacteria and fungi of the respiratory and alimentary tracts and on external mucosa and skin. There are many intergradations, inconsistencies, and overlappings. The great groups named, however, are sharply enough defined for purposes of the present discussion.

PRESENCE OF TOXIC SUBSTANCES

When living cells metabolize foods, either for cell synthesis or as energy sources, or both, by means of their enzyme systems, they give off as waste products various substances such as hydrogen, toxic hydrogen sulfide, carbon dioxide, and many other compounds. These may range from fairly strong sulfuric acid, as in certain sulfur-oxidizing harmless chemolithotrophic bacteria of the soil, to complex organic compounds like toxic alcohols and organic acids, indole and acetylmethylcarbinol, as in the reactions discussed in Chapter 7.

DISTINCTIVE WASTES. Each species of microorganism is recognized by its food peculiarities, its particular waste products, its motility, form, pigment, and other properties.

In addition to their own deleterious waste products, substances from many other sources may be toxic to microorganisms: for example, dyes, acids, and metallic residues of industrial chemical plants dumped into rivers. Many common substances are so toxic that they serve well as disinfectants; phenol and its derivatives such as cresols and hexachlorophene, chlorine compounds like laundry bleach (5 per cent NaOCl, or Clorox) and so on.

Table 8–1. Table of Equivalents of Celsius (Centigrade, C) and Fahrenheit (F) Thermometer Temperature Scales*

C	F	C	F	C	F
−40	−40.0	9	48.2	57	134.6
−39	−38.2	10	50.0	58	136.4
−38	−36.4	11	51.8	59	138.2
−37	−34.6	12	53.6	60	140.0
−36	−32.8	13	55.4	61	141.8
−35	−31.0	14	57.2	62	143.6
−34	−29.2	15	59.0	63	145.4
−33	−27.4	16	60.8	64	147.2
−32	−25.6	17	62.6	65	149.0
−31	−23.8	18	64.4	66	150.8
−30	−22.0	19	66.2	67	152.6
−29	−20.2	20	68.0	68	154.4
−28	−18.4	21	69.8	69	156.2
−27	−16.6	22	71.6	70	158.0
−26	−14.8	23	73.4	71	159.8
−25	−13.0	24	75.2	72	161.6
−24	−11.2	25	77.0	73	163.4
−23	−9.4	26	78.8	74	165.2
−22	−7.6	27	80.6	75	167.0
−21	−5.8	28	82.4	76	168.8
−20	−4.0	29	84.2	77	170.6
−19	−2.2	30	86.0	78	172.4
−18	−0.4	31	87.8	79	174.2
−17	+1.4	32	89.6	80	176.0
−16	3.2	33	91.4	81	177.8
−15	5.0	34	93.2	82	179.6
−14	6.8	35	95.0	83	181.4
−13	8.6	36	96.8	84	183.2
−12	10.4	37	98.6	85	185.0
−11	12.2	38	100.4	86	186.8
−10	14.0	39	102.2	87	188.6
−9	15.8	40	104.0	88	190.4
−8	17.6	41	105.8	89	192.2
−7	19.4	42	107.6	90	194.0
−6	21.2	43	109.4	91	195.8
−5	23.0	44	111.2	92	197.6
−4	24.8	45	113.0	93	199.4
−3	26.6	46	114.8	94	201.2
−2	28.4	47	116.6	95	203.0
−1	30.2	48	118.4	96	204.8
0	32.0	49	120.2	97	206.6
+1	33.8	50	122.0	98	208.4
2	35.6	51	123.8	99	210.2
3	37.4	52	125.6	100	212.0
4	39.2	53	127.4	101	213.8
5	41.0	54	129.2	102	215.6
6	42.8	55	131.0	103	217.4
7	44.6	56	132.8	104	219.2
8	46.4				

*Degrees Celsius (Centigrade, C) may be converted to degrees Fahrenheit (F), and vice versa by the following formulas:

C to F: 1.8 C + 32

To change +54 C to F: $(1.8 \times 54) + 32 = 129.2$ F

−38 C to F: $(1.8 \times -38) + 32 = -36.4$ F

F to C: 0.556(F−32)

To change +54 F to C: $0.556(54-32) = 12.2$ C

−38 F to C: $0.556(-38 + -32) = -38.9$ C

TEMPERATURE

MESOPHILS.[7]   Just as is true for roses or cabbages, if microorganisms are to grow, not only must food and water be present but the temperature must be favorable. For example, microorganisms that live in the soil and shallow streams grow best at summer temperature, or about 20 to 30 C (Table 8-1). Bacteria that have become highly adapted to growth in the human body will flourish only at or near body temperature (37 C). These temperatures (from 20 to 37 C) represent the medium or middle range, and microorganisms growing best in such a temperature range are said to be *mesophilic* in respect to temperature (Fig. 8-2).

PSYCHROPHILS.[8]   Some microorganisms, such as those that live at the bottom of the sea, grow best at temperatures (4 to 10 C) near freezing and are said to be *psychrophilic*. Since relatively few species of microorganisms in the environment of man are extremely psychrophilic, low temperatures are widely used to prevent or greatly retard the growth of many kinds of bacteria, and other organisms that cause "souring," "spoiling,"

[7]From Greek *mesos*, moderate, and *philos*, loving.
[8]From Greek *psychros*, cold.

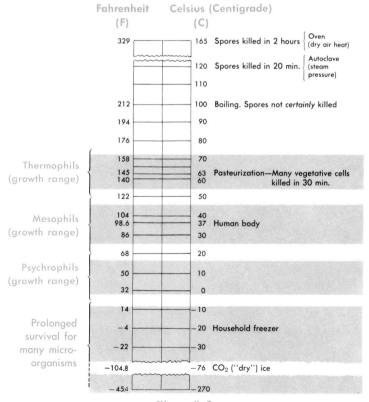

Figure 8-2

Some temperatures of significance in microbiology. Note the slow killing action of dry air heat and the relatively rapid killing action of steam (moist heat) at lower temperature. Boiling kills some but not all spores. Note overlapping growth ranges of thermophilic, mesophilic, and other forms.

and rancidity. Furs, confectionery, milk, vegetables, wood pulp, and many other products (serums, vaccines, antibiotics, drugs, and so on) may be preserved by efficient refrigeration.

Low temperatures, however, are seldom fatal to most microorganisms. Many species will survive in a dormant state, frozen for years, and can grow vigorously when thawed out. Some can survive the temperature of liquid air (−312 F.). A method of preserving microorganisms for future study, and bovine and other spermatozoa for artificial insemination, is rapid freezing with "dry ice" (solid CO_2) at −76 C (−159 F). The method is also used to preserve certain diagnostic specimens, sera, viruses, and so forth, during long distance transportation. Human tissue cells cultivated in artificial media are routinely kept with liquid nitrogen at −195 C (−319 F) for long periods. Some microorganisms will stand temperatures as low as −269 C (more than 450 below zero F).

THERMOPHILS.[9]   Still other species of microorganisms (certain algae and bacteria) will grow only at high temperatures. Any organisms that grow only at temperatures above about 50 C are called *thermophils*. For many species there is an inverse relationship between temperature and pH. In neutral or alkaline (pH 8.0) natural springs, some bacteria can grow at boiling temperatures (100 C). Increases in acidity to pH below about 3.0 are increasingly inhibitory as temperatures rise above about 70 C. Some thermophils are found in hot sulfurous springs such as those in Yellowstone National Park, in Iceland, and elsewhere. Thermophils are not infectious to man, since they cannot grow at 37 C.

Exposure to temperatures of 75 C or above for more than about 20 minutes is fatal to the actively growing (vegetative) forms of all pathogenic bacteria, higher fungi, and protozoa. This fact is used in various methods of sterilization and disinfection to be described. Bacterial *endospores*, however, as previously pointed out, are much more resistant and may survive boiling and even higher temperatures (350 F) for several hours. These will be discussed in detail later. Certain viruses also are exceptions.

OXYGEN

STRICT AEROBES.   Many microorganisms require, for the purpose of biooxidation, free access to the oxygen supply of the atmosphere; they are limited to the use solely of uncombined oxygen as hydrogen (electron) acceptor because of their enzyme production. They cannot grow without free oxygen. Such microorganisms are said to be *strict aerobes.* Examples among bacteria are *Pseudomonas fluorescens*, a common saprophyte of river waters, and *Bacillus cereus*, a common saprophyte of soil and dust.

FACULTATIVE AEROBES.   Some microorganisms that can use free oxygen as an electron (hydrogen) acceptor can also use oxygen obtained under anaerobic conditions from easily reducible compounds that contain it, e.g., $NaNO_3$:

$$NaNO_3 + H_2 \longrightarrow NaNO_2 + H_2O$$

Because they can use as hydrogen acceptor either free or combined oxygen, such organisms are said to be *facultative aerobes* (or facultative ana-

---

[9]From the Greek *therme,* heat.

erobes). Examples among bacteria are *Salmonella typhi* (cause of typhoid fever) and *Staphylococcus aureus* (cause of boils, etc.).

STRICT ANAEROBES.   However, there are also numerous species of bacteria that are extremely sensitive to the presence of free oxygen and are soon killed by it. These grow in the depths of the soil, in swamp muck, the animal intestine, and other places where the air cannot penetrate or where a very low oxidation-reduction (O-R) potential is maintained. Such bacteria are called *strict anaerobes*. Examples are *Clostridium tetani* (cause of lockjaw — tetanus) and *Bacteroides fragilis;* both are inhabitants of the human and animal intestinal tract.

Strict anaerobes typically do not obtain energy from biooxidation by the use of oxygen, free or combined, but by enzyme controlled dehydrogenation. The release of hydrogen from an organic substrate also releases electrons (energy). These organisms use, as hydrogen acceptors, organic substances such as pyruvic acid:

$$\underset{\text{pyruvic acid}}{\begin{matrix} \text{CH}_3 \\ | \\ \text{C}=\text{O} \\ | \\ \text{COOH} \end{matrix}} \; + \; \text{H}_2 \; \longrightarrow \; \underset{\text{lactic acid}}{\begin{matrix} \text{CH}_3 \\ | \\ \text{H}-\text{C}-\text{OH} \\ | \\ \text{COOH} \end{matrix}}$$

Cultivation of Anaerobes.   When studying strict anaerobes special means must be used to exclude the atmospheric oxygen or to maintain a low O-R potential. This may be accomplished in several ways. A simple method is to melt the contents of a tube of beef-extract agar[10] and introduce the desired bacteria into the depths, allowing the agar to harden. Oxygen is thus excluded, and the bacteria will grow in the depths of the tube (Fig. 8–3). Other methods require that the cultures be placed in jars

---

[10]Agar (a clear, jelly-like substance derived from certain seaweeds) is added to many nutrient solutions for microorganisms (culture media) to cause the nutrient solutions to solidify. The solidified medium has the consistency of stiff jelly. It liquefies on being heated to boiling and "sets" at about 38 C. In some respects agar resembles pectins such as "Certo" used to make jelly.

Figure 8–3

Deep tubes of agar inoculated with bacteria of various oxygen relationships. *A*, Fairly strict anaerobe, like *Clostridium botulinum*. *B*, Less strict anaerobe, like *Cl. perfringens*. *C*, Facultative aerobe-anaerobe, like *Escherichia coli*. *D*, Microaerophilic organism like *Brucella abortus*. *E*, Strict aerobe, like *Pseudomonas fluorescens*.

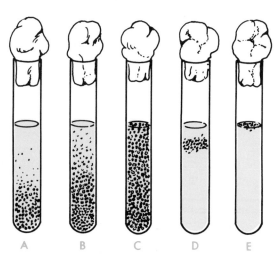

A   B   C   D   E

Figure 8–4

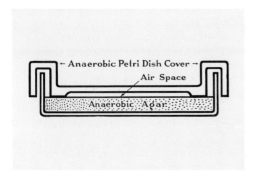

The Brewer anaerobic culture dish. The cover fits over a Petri dish so that the flat rim of the cover rests on the agar surface, trapping a very thin layer of air over the surface of most of the agar. (Petri was one of the early students of bacteriology under Robert Koch, about 1876.) Sodium thioglycollate in the agar then absorbs the oxygen from this thin layer of air so that growth on the agar surface is entirely anaerobic. (Courtesy of Baltimore Biological Laboratories, Baltimore, Md.)

or flasks from which all oxygen is removed by means of vacuum pumps, by chemical combination, or by replacing the oxygen with some inert gas such as hydrogen or nitrogen. Doubtless some of the methods will be demonstrated in the laboratory.

One of the simplest and most effective methods is to add to ordinary culture media a harmless chemical that absorbs oxygen as fast as it diffuses into the medium from the air. Cysteine and sodium thioglycollate are two chemicals commonly used for this purpose. Thioglycollate broth and agar media are commonly used in medical microbiology (Fig. 8–4).

MICROAEROPHILS. Some microorganisms appear to grow best in a situation where the amount of oxygen is somewhat reduced. These are called *microaerophilic* organisms. See Figure 8–3D. An example of this type of microorganism is *Brucella abortus*.

OSMOTIC PRESSURE

Many substances attract water. They are said to be *hygroscopic* or *deliquescent*. For example, observe grains of table salt or certain candies exposed on a plate during very humid weather. Let such a deliquescent substance be dissolved in water. Let the solution then be enclosed in a tightly sealed sac of material like cellophane or the outer membrane of an egg or a living cell. If the sac or cell is then immersed in distilled water, the deliquescent *solute* (substance in solution) attracts water, which passes inward through the membrane by a process called *osmosis*. The passage of water inward builds up pressure (*osmotic pressure*) inside the sac or cell, the amount of pressure depending on the nature and concentration of the solute. The cell may burst, a phenomenon called *plasmoptysis;* for example, *hemolysis* (laking) of red blood cells by water. Conversely, if a living cell is immersed in a concentrated solution of a deliquescent substance (e.g., strong brine or sugar syrup), water is drawn out of the cell, which then collapses (*plasmolysis*) and may or may not die. Cells vary greatly in their resistance to unfavorable osmotic conditions, but it is clear that osmotic pressure is of fundamental importance in all cell life. Some, but not all, pathogenic bacteria and most actively growing (nondormant) animal cells are relatively sensitive to continuous exposure to osmotic extremes.

Many saprophytic microorganisms that cause spoilage of food and other products are dehydrated by immersion in strong brines or syrups, and although not necessarily killed, cannot grow and produce spoilage.

They are held in a dormant state. This principle is used in the preparation of many sorts of pickles, corned beef, salt fish, jams, and jellies. Soaking in brine was a first step used by the ancient Egyptians in the preservation of mummies. The extremely dry climate helped maintain the mummified state afterward.

Halophilic[11] organisms are those that can thrive in strong brines such as are used in "corning" beef and making certain pickles (20 to 30 per cent salt). Others have become adapted to the high salinity of the Dead Sea and Great Salt Lake. These cannot thrive in ordinary fresh water or even in sea water. None is pathogenic.

ACIDITY AND ALKALINITY

Many microorganisms, especially those that cause disease, are adversely affected by even moderate degrees of acidity or alkalinity. So sensitive are they that it is necessary to adjust the reaction of the fluids used for their cultivation by adding acid or alkali, as may be required, so that the fluid becomes neutral or faintly alkaline like blood.

HYDROGEN ION CONCENTRATION. Hydrogen atoms, when dissolved in water, immediately assume a positive electrical charge. They are then called hydrogen *ions,* and the acidity of the solution is determined by them. Acids, such as hydrochloric or acetic acid, possess the property of acidity because they give off hydrogen ions (i.e., they *ionize*) in aqueous solutions. If a solution contains a large number of these ions it is very acid,

[11]Salt-loving.

Figure 8–5

A modern electronic instrument (pH meter) for determining the concentration of hydrogen ions in fluids. The fluid to be tested is placed in the beaker at the right. The two electrodes are then inserted in the fluid. Between the two electrodes an electrical potential develops that is dependent on the pH of the fluid. The instrument measures this potential and expresses it on the dial as pH. The instrument is therefore a sort of calculating voltmeter. (Courtesy of Photovolt Corp., New York City.)

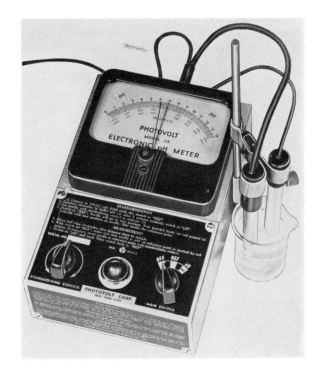

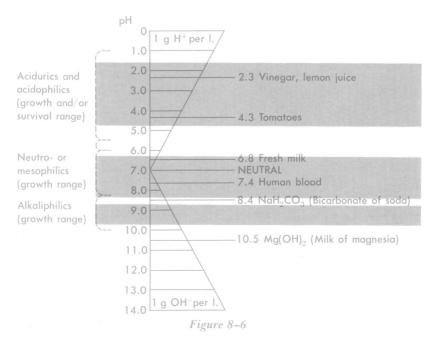

Figure 8–6

Some pH units of significance in microbiology. The slanting lines starting at pH 7.0 indicate increasing concentration of H⁺ or OH⁻ to the maximum of 1 gram of ions per liter.

and is said to have a high *hydrogen ion concentration*. If it is only slightly acid, or is alkaline, it is said to have a low hydrogen ion concentration.

PH. Hydrogen ion concentration is usually expressed by numbers used with the symbol pH, which stands for the negative logarithm of the hydrogen ion concentration. The hydrogen ion concentration (pH) of most solutions used in microbiology and medical work is easily measured by means of dyes that assume a distinctive color at a certain pH. Dyes are also used in pH paper which is employed for simple but relatively rough measurements. More commonly, exact pH determinations are now made by using pH meters, electrical instruments of many different types, some of which are accurate to two decimal places (Fig. 8–5). A pH of 14 is the lowest acidity[12] and pH 7 is neutral. pH 0 is the highest acidity in this system and represents 1 g of hydrogen *ions* per liter of solution. Any pH between 0 and 7 is acidic, any pH between 7 and 14 is alkaline. The pH of human blood is about 7.4; that of freshly drawn milk is around 6.8 (Fig. 8–6). Most pathogenic bacteria are inhibited by acidities of near pH 5 and alkalinities around pH 8.5 and prefer a pH close to 7.4[13] Some free-living chemolithotrophs of the soil thrive at an acidity of pH 1.5.

The preservation of fish, meat, vegetables, and other foods by pickling in vinegar is based, in part, on the sensitivity of spoilage-causing microorganisms to the acidity of the vinegar. Salt, sugar, and spices are added for flavor and for osmotic effects. Some spices are said to have a preserva-

---

[12]Actually, it is equal to strong alkali.

[13]The numbers used with pH are logarithms of fractions, i.e., negative logarithms. They are therefore inversely related to actual degree of acidity (concentrations of hydrogen ions). Note carefully in reading, therefore, that a low pH means a high concentration of hydrogen ions or acidity, and vice versa.

tive action, but the main reason vinegar-pickled foods "keep" is that the acid prevents bacterial growth. The un-ionized acetic acid of vinegar also is toxic per se.

RADIATIONS

SUNLIGHT AND ULTRAVIOLET (UV) WAVES. It has already been pointed out that all bacteria of medical significance, all higher fungi and all typical animal cells (including protozoa) differ from all green plants in not possessing the photosynthetic pigment chlorophyll. The chlorophyll-deficient organisms therefore cannot utilize sunlight as a source of energy; in fact, many species, especially unpigmented varieties of bacteria (which includes most, *but not all*, pathogens) are killed within a few minutes or hours by direct sunlight. The ultraviolet rays of sunlight in the range of about 3000 Å wavelength are its most bactericidal components. Their greatest lethal effect is exerted on the DNA and enzyme proteins of the cell.

Ultraviolet rays in sunlight are absorbed to a great extent by carotenoid and other pigments. Thus many pigmented species of bacteria, including many harmless environmental species that are adapted to life in sunlight and air, are protected from UV by their own pigments. Some very dangerous pigmented pathogens, e.g., *Staphylococcus aureus*, are also protected and can resist sunlight. In general, UV rays have very little power to penetrate anything except certain substances like quartz or certain plastic or special-glass window materials. Sunlight passing through ordinary window glass loses most of its UV rays and therefore its disinfecting power.

Excessive exposure to UV radiation, solar or artificial, is to be avoided because UV rays can severely damage the eyes and are also definitely mutagenic and carcinogenic or oncogenic. Sublethal exposures to UV radiation are commonly used in research to induce mutations in many species of microorganisms.

Part of the "purifying" action of sunlight on decaying organic matter is due to the fact that it warms and dries and, in addition to its UV contents, certain of the visible rays, in the presence of oxygen, induce microbicidally destructive photooxidation of enzymes and other vital cell components, thus helping to suppress odorous decomposition of organic matter.

Various kinds of equipment that produce ultraviolet rays are available and are used in the treatment of skin infections and disinfection of blood plasma, swimming pool water, and so forth. Special lamps producing large amounts of ultraviolet rays are now used to prevent the growth of surface molds and bacteria in meat-storage warehouses, in many research laboratories, even in some commercial kitchens and to disinfect the air in operating rooms (Fig. 8–7).

X-RAYS AND OTHER RADIATIONS. These are called ionizing radiations because, being of much shorter wavelength than UV (less than about 1000 Å), they have much greater powers of penetration. They can cause disruptive ionizations of various components of the cell, especially DNA and proteins. These effects are commonly lethal; some cells have enzyme controlled mechanisms for the repair of the damage induced, if it is not too extensive. If exposures are not too intense or prolonged they may, like UV, produce mutations or carcinogenic alterations.

Among the ionizing radiations fatal to microorganisms are x-rays and radium emanations. Radium gives off three kinds of particles or radia-

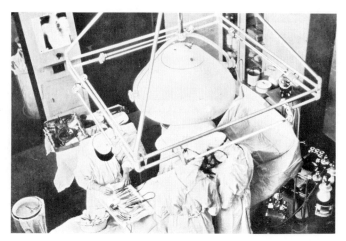

Figure 8–7

Maintenance of asepsis in surgery by means of bactericidal radiation from above. The large dome is for ordinary illumination. The ultraviolet radiations are given off by the special tubular lamps attached to the rectangular framework. Note the eyeshades on the surgeons. Direct exposure of the eyes to ultraviolet light is very deleterious. (Courtesy of Westinghouse Electric & Manufacturing Co.)

tions: *alpha rays* (actually helium ions traveling at very high velocities), *beta rays* (negatively charged particles at high velocities), and *gamma rays* (somewhat like "hard" x-rays). Hard x-rays differ from soft x-rays in being of shorter wavelengths and having greater powers of penetration.

Unicellular organisms vary greatly in resistance to radiation. A protozoan may require 300,000 R (roentgens) to be killed, but 0.01 R is sufficient to affect the growth of *Phycomyces blackesleeanus*, a fungus. The median lethal dose within 30 days ($LD_{50}/30$) of x-ray irradiation for man is about 450 rem (roentgen equivalent, man), for yeast 30,000 rem, for some bacilli 150,000 rem, but for *Paramecium* (a protozoan) as high as 350,000 rem. Although theories exist to explain this range of responses on the basis of nuclear volume, oxygen tension, and so on, it is still not certain why some organisms may be highly radiosensitive, and others resistant.

It is probable that within a few years various radiations, especially Co^{60} gamma rays and cathode rays (streams of moving electrons), will be used for sterilizing a variety of things, such as canned foods, ready-cooked foods now available only as frozen foods, and surgical materials. The ionizing rays penetrate the closed packages and kill the microorganisms in them, without any unwholesome change in the product. The flavors and textures of some foods suffer.

OTHER PHYSICAL INFLUENCES

ELECTRICITY AND MAGNETISM.   These appear to have little or no direct effect on bacteria, although detrimental effects of extremely high magnetic fields on bacteria have been reported. A powerful electric current passed for a long time through a broth culture generates heat and certain chemical compounds that may kill the bacteria.

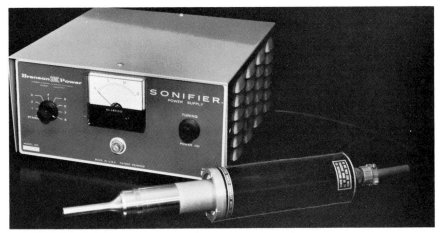

Figure 8–8

Sonic disintegrator. (Branson Sonifier courtesy of Scientific Systems Corp.)

SOUND WAVES.   Most sound waves audible to the human ear appear to be without effect on bacteria. Waves of certain rapidities, however, can disintegrate microorganisms of some species under proper experimental conditions.

SUPERSONIC VIBRATIONS.   If cultures are subjected to certain very rapid vibrations, higher in pitch than the highest capable of being heard by man (*supersonic* or *ultrasonic vibrations*), many microorganisms are entirely disrupted and literally shaken to pieces. This fact is utilized in research when it is desired to investigate intracellular substances without using chemicals to rupture the cells. Figure 8–8 shows a sonic disintegrator, which is frequently used to rupture cells and to free enzymes for biochemical studies.

APPLICATION TO HEALTH

In many ways, the relation of microorganisms to their environment directly determines the methods that may be used for their control, as will be discussed in Section Three. Altering certain environmental factors may be all that is needed to slow down the growth of microorganisms or to kill them. For example, high temperatures alter the characteristics of the cells so that life is no longer possible. The presence or absence of oxygen may determine whether a pathogenic organism is capable of producing an infection or a toxin which is detrimental to the host. It must be remembered, however, that what seem to us to be extremely minute or almost nonexistent quantities of nutrients, moisture, and oxygen may be sufficient to support the life of millions of microorganisms. It is seldom reliable to trust in the removal of food, water, and oxygen for inhibition or destruction of microorganisms. The primary means of reducing or destroying microbial growth are altering temperatures and subjecting the microorganisms to poisonous substances, i.e., disinfectants (see Section Three). Ultraviolet rays are sometimes used to destroy microorganisms in hospitals (operating rooms, nurseries, communicable disease units) but are truly effective only when all other methods of control have been adequately carried out.

Supplementary Reading

Benedict, R. G., et al.: Preservation of microorganisms by freeze-drying. II. The destructive action of oxygen. Additional stabilizers for *Serratia marcescens.* Experiments with other microorganisms. *Appl. Microbiol.,* 1961, *9:*256.

Bernstein, I. A., (Editor): Biochemical Responses to Environmental Stress. 1971, New York, Plenum Press.

Brock, T. D., and Darland, G. K.: Limits of microbial existence: Temperature and pH. *Science,* 1970, *169:*1316.

Farrell, J., and Rose, A. H.: Temperature effects on microorganisms. *Ann. Rev. Microbiol.,* 1967, *21:*101.

Flannery, W. L.: Current status of knowledge of halophilic bacteria. *Bact. Rev.,* 1956, *20:*49.

Foote, C. S.: Mechanisms of photosensitized oxidation. *Science* 1968, *162:*963.

Frazier, W. C.: Food Microbiology, 2nd Ed. 1967, New York, McGraw-Hill Book Co., Inc.

Harrison, A. P., Jr.: Survival of bacteria. *Ann. Rev. Microbiol.,* 1967, *21:*143.

Haynes, R. H., Wolff, S., and Till, J. (Co-editors): Structural Defects in DNA and Their Repair in Microorganisms. Radiation Research, Supplement 6. 1966, New York, Academic Press.

Josephson, E. S., Brynjolfsson, A., and Wierlicki, E.: Engineering and economics of food irradiation. *Tr. N.Y. Acad. Sci.,* 1968, Ser. II, *30:*600.

Ladanyi, P. A., and Morrison, S. M.: Ultraviolet bactericidal irradiation of ice. *Appl. Microbiol.,* 1968, *16:*463.

Mazur, P.: Cryobiology: The freezing of biological systems. *Science,* 1970, *168:*939.

Morgan, K. Z., and Turner, J. E.: Principles of Radiation Protection. 1967, New York, John Wiley & Sons, Inc.

Nagington, J., and Lawrence, M. F.: Notes on the storage of tissue culture cells with liquid nitrogen. *Monthly Bull. Minist. Health,* 1962, *21:*162.

Rose, A. H. (Editor): Thermobiology. 1967, New York, Academic Press, Inc.

Shaw, M. K.: Formation of filaments and synthesis of macromolecules at temperatures below the minimum for growth of *Escherichia coli. J. Bact.,* 1968, *95:*221.

Shilling, C. W. (Editor): Atomic Energy Encyclopedia in the Life Sciences. 1964, Philadelphia, W. B. Saunders Co.

Laboratory Study of Microorganisms

9

PURE CULTURES

ISOLATION. The microbiologist must work with pure cultures of microorganisms. In order to determine accurately the identity of a specific microorganism obtained from a patient, he must first isolate the organism from all others with which it is mixed. Mixtures of microorganisms are common in clinical material such as feces, sputum, and the like. The activities of extraneous organisms (contaminants) in the tests to be made with the organism that is being studied inevitably completely mask and confuse the results. What is needed is a *pure culture.* The extraneous organisms may greatly change the pH; they may produce antibiotics; they may influence, injure, modify, or kill the desired microorganisms in a hundred subtle ways.

PURE, MIXED, AND CONTAMINATED CULTURES. A pure culture is one containing only one kind of microorganism. A *mixed culture* contains two or more kinds of microorganisms. A pure culture may be likened to a bed of roses. In such a bed there is nothing but roses and we might say that the gardener had made a *pure culture* of roses. If some geraniums or other kinds of plants were also put in the bed, we might say that the gardener had prepared a *mixed culture*. If weeds got in accidentally, we would say that the culture of roses was *contaminated*. Likewise, when some undesirable microorganisms get into our pure culture by accident, we say that it is contaminated. Sometimes a contaminated culture is called a mixed culture.

PURE-CULTURE METHODS. In preparing a pure culture of bacteria, or of yeasts or molds, it is very convenient to have a solid surface on which to spread out the mixture of microorganisms (like spreading coins on a table to sort the different kinds) and then to pick out the kinds we want and put each separately into its own test tube of medium to multiply and grow as a pure culture.

Agar. A very useful substance for this purpose is the pectin-like, polysaccharide vegetable gum called agar. Dried agar is added to a nutrient fluid such as beef broth and the broth is boiled at 100 C to melt the agar. It remains a liquid until the temperature falls below 45 C. About 2 g of agar per 100 ml of broth are used. If some of this beef-broth agar is

133

sterilized and then poured into a sterile and flat, round, covered dish (generally called a Petri dish) and allowed to cool, it solidifies. We can then spread, on its moist, jelly-like surface, a droplet of the microorganism-containing sample to be analyzed (saliva, for instance). If we are working with yeasts, molds, or bacteria, and we keep the dish at body temperature for 24 hours (this process is called *incubation*), it is very easy to select a pure culture of the microorganisms we wish from among many others that may be present.

COLONIES.   The question at once arises: if microorganisms are so small that they are invisible, how can we select one from a mixture of perhaps hundreds on a jelly surface? It is simplicity itself. If the agar contains beef broth (or another appropriate nutrient substance), it will nourish the microorganisms. When the dish is put in a warm place, each viable[1] cell multiplies at the site on the agar surface where it initially landed. In 24 or 48 hours, or longer, depending on the species of microorganisms, small, separate masses, called *colonies,* of the microorganisms are visible to the unaided eye on the surface of the agar. Each colony consists of all the descendants of the single microorganism that landed previously on that particular spot (Fig. 9–1). All of the cells in a single colony, being descendants of a single cell, are of one kind. All that is now necessary to obtain a pure culture from any colony is to touch it with the end of a sterile needle (Fig. 9–2) and transfer the microorganisms adhering to the needle to

[1]Capable of living and multiplying.

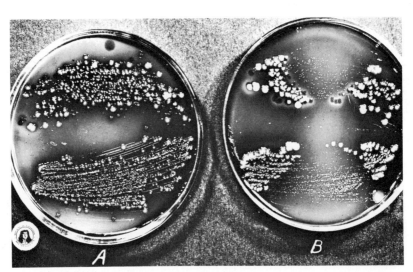

Figure 9–1

Bacterial colonies on blood-agar in Petri plates (about one-half actual size). This picture also illustrates a method of *selective cultivation* of a particular species of bacteria; in this case the organisms of whooping cough, or pertussis. A nasopharyngeal swab with mucus from the patient was passed over both plates, and the mucus was spread over the agar with a sterile loop. At the same time a drop of penicillin solution was placed on two sides of plate *B*. The plates were then incubated at 37 C for three days. Plate *A* shows the customary heavy growth of common bacteria usually found in the nasopharynx. The pertussis organisms (*Bordetella pertussis*) are completely overgrown and obscured. Plate *B* shows two areas where the common organisms have been completely inhibited by the penicillin, permitting *B. pertussis* (tiny white colonies) to grow unhampered by competition of the other organisms. (Courtesy of Dr. William L. Bradford. From the collection of the American Society for Microbiology.)

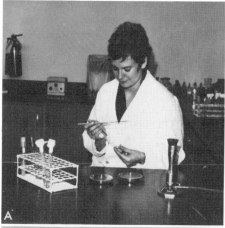

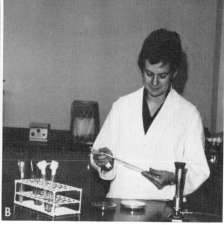

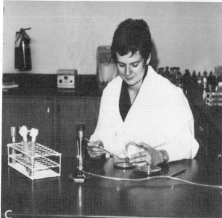

Figure 9–2

Subculturing bacteria. Transfer of bacterial colonies from Petri dish to tubes containing sterile culture media. By this method the desired strains of bacteria are isolated in pure culture. Note the holding of the cotton plug and the needle used, also the Bunsen burner for flaming (sterilizing) the entire wire of the needle. For details of the technique shown here (which may vary in different laboratories), the reader is referred to Fuerst: *Laboratory Manual and Workbook for Microbiology in Health and Disease*. 5th Ed. 1973, Philadelphia, W. B. Saunders Co. (Photographs through the courtesy of Mr. Stephen E. Fisch.)

Figure 9–3

Pure culture preparation on a commercial scale. Incubation of pure cultures in special bouillon for preparation of toxins, vaccines, and so on. This photograph shows a portion of a large incubator used for various types of culture growth. This room is kept at exactly 37 C, human body temperature. (Courtesy of Parke, Davis & Co.)

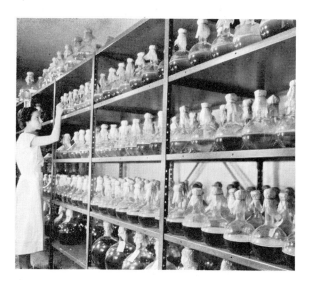

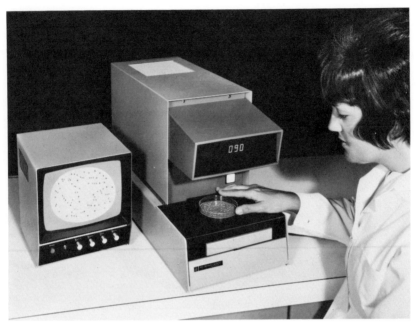

Figure 9-4

With automatic bacterial colony counters such as this, the technician can determine at a glance the number of colonies growing in a Petri dish. The colonies are scanned, the count is registered digitally, and the colonies are marked and shown on a vidicon screen. Courtesy New Brunswick Scientific Co., Inc., New Brunswick, N.J.

whatever kind of medium is desired. The medium in turn is *incubated* (Fig. 9-3) for as long as is necessary to result in visible growth of the pure culture of organisms.

Automatic bacterial colony counters are now available. Such a model produced by Aminco called Petri-Scan is shown in Figure 9-4. The technician places the Petri dish on the stage of the counter, presses a button, and takes the reading for the number of colonies per plate from the visual display.

Prevention of Contamination.   To prevent contamination of the pure culture by extraneous bacteria, yeasts, or molds, which are always present in the air, on dust, on the hands of the bacteriologist and, in fact, everywhere open to the general surroundings, all glassware and media used in microbiology are sterilized before use. Precautions used routinely to prevent contamination of pure cultures consist of cotton plugs, or plastic or metal caps on all tubes; glass, plastic, or metal covers on Petri plates; sterilization of needles or pipettes used to inoculate; minimal exposure to air and dust; the use of special, so-called "bacteriological hoods," with controlled air flow away from the technician; and rapid work by a skilled microbiologist.

APPEARANCE OF COLONIES.   Microbial colonies vary greatly in appearance. Some look like dewdrops; others are white and glistening like the head of a white pin; still others have various colors. These peculiarities are used in identification. Some of the ways in which the form of the colonies arising from a pure culture may vary have been described in the discussion of microbial variation.

When bacteria grow in broth, they sometimes cause a cloudiness, or *turbidity;* sometimes they form a surface film called a *pellicle,* and sometimes a *sediment.*

GROWTH OF BACTERIA.   Under the most favorable circumstances a single bacterium of certain species may divide in 10 to 30 minutes. Calculation will show that in 12 hours a single organism could give rise to over 68 billion. If conditions were always suitable, the earth would be overrun with bacteria. Like all other living things, however, they have to struggle for existence, and when conditions are unfavorable they multiply slowly or not at all. Food gives out and noxious waste products accumulate, the acidity increases, and other changes occur so that rapid growth soon ceases. The same principles apply equally to yeasts, molds, and most other *cellular* microorganisms (viruses are not cellular). If the numbers of cells in a pure culture are counted at regular intervals, starting with the inoculum (the cells that are transferred), and the logarithms of the numbers are plotted against time, a curve is obtained showing the changes in numbers with time and altered growth conditions. This is called a "growth curve," but is actually a population curve since it is generally equally applicable to most populations, which includes pure cultures of living bacteria such as *E. coli* (Fig. 9–5).

CULTURE MEDIA.   In the laboratory certain substances are used to induce microorganisms to multiply so that the student will be able to work with readily visible masses of them instead of with single invisible cells. The substances used are of many kinds, depending on the species of microorganisms. They are combined in various suitable mixtures called culture media.

The most commonly used medium for the growth of heterotrophic species of bacteria is *nutrient broth,* easily converted into *nutrient agar* by the addition of 1.5 to 2.0 per cent agar agar.[2] *Nutrient broth* is essentially meat extract, or weak "beef tea." Several modifications of this medium exist, all based on the following formula:

Nutrient Broth
Meat extract................................... 3 g
Peptone... 5 g

These ingredients, in dry form, are dissolved in 1000 ml of distilled water. The final pH as adjusted for dehydrated medium is 6.8, although a slightly alkaline pH is desirable in a freshly prepared medium (not commercial).

It is now not necessary to prepare beef extract by boiling fat-free beef, weighing out *peptone* (partially digested meat), filtering both, and thus making an *infusion broth.* In the modern laboratory, one reads the label on a bottle of dehydrated commercially prepared culture medium, adds water to a weighed amount of dried powder, as directed, and fills test tubes not more than half full with the medium. The tubes are plugged with cotton or closed with plastic or metal caps and sterilized in the autoclave.

Various substances are added to broth or agar media to help the desired microorganisms to grow. This is also helpful in determining what

---

[2] Agar agar is often used to designate the agar material used to add to liquid medium in order to make it solid. By the term agar (above) the microbiologist often means "nutrient agar" a special medium made from nutrient broth with agar agar added.

Table 9–1.   An Example of a Bacterial Assay Medium as Available Commercially in Dehydrated Form for the Quantitative Assay of the Amino Acid *l*-Leucine*†

Bacto-Dextrose (Glucose) .... 50 g	Adenine Sulfate .... 0.02 g
Sodium Acetate .... 40 g	Guanine Hydrochloride .... 0.02 g
Ammonium Chloride .... 6 g	Uracil .... 0.02 g
dl-Alanine .... 0.4 g	Xanthine .... 0.02 g
l-Arginine Hydrochloride .... 0.484 g	Thiamine Hydrochloride .... 0.001 g
Bacto-Asparagine .... 0.8 g	Pyridoxine Hydrochloride .... 0.002 g
l-Aspartic Acid .... 0.2 g	Pyridoxamine Hydrochloride .... 0.0006 g
l-Cystine, Difco .... 0.1 g	Pyridoxal Hydrochloride .... 0.0006 g
l-Glutamic Acid .... 0.6 g	Calcium Pantothenate .... 0.001 g
Glycine .... 0.2 g	Riboflavin .... 0.001 g
l-Histidine Hydrochloride .... 0.124 g	Nicotinic Acid .... 0.002 g
dl-Isoleucine .... 0.5 g	*p*-Aminobenzoic Acid, Difco ...... 0.0002 g
l-Lysine hydrochloride .... 0.5 g	Biotin .... 0.000002 g
dl-Methionine .... 0.2 g	Folic Acid .... 0.00002 g
dl-Phenylalanine .... 0.2 g	Monopotassium Phosphate .... 1.2 g
l-Proline .... 0.2 g	Dipotassium Phosphate .... 1.2 g
dl-Serine .... 0.1 g	Magnesium Sulfate .... 0.4 g
dl-Threonine .... 0.4 g	Ferrous Sulfate .... 0.02 g
dl-Tryptophane .... 0.08 g	Manganese Sulfate .... 0.04 g
l-Tyrosine .... 0.2 g	Sodium Chloride .... 0.02 g
dl-Valine .... 0.5 g	in H$_2$O to .... 1 liter

*The growth of *Leuconostoc mesenteroides* (a special bacterial strain) is measured acidimetrically or turbidimetrically on this medium with small measured amounts of l-leucine added. From the results in these "control samples" a standard curve is constructed for comparison with the "unknown." An unknown amount of leucine in a sample of material is also added to the above medium and the quantity of *l*-leucine present is determined by comparison with the known amounts of leucine in the control samples as indicated on the standard curve.

†From Difco Manual of Dehydrated Culture Media and Reagents for Microbiological and Clinical Laboratory Procedures. 9th Ed. 1965, Detroit, Difco Laboratories.

changes are produced in the food substances by the microorganisms. In medical microbiology blood (which is free of microorganisms when carefully obtained from a healthy animal) is frequently added. The broth is then spoken of as "blood broth." With agar added, it becomes "blood agar," a very useful medium for the growth and identification of many human pathogenic bacteria. Various kinds of carbohydrates, such as sucrose, melibiose, *d*-mannitol, glucose, starch, or lactose, may be added along with the blood or instead of it, and the broth then takes its name from the substance added. Examples are: lactose broth, maltose broth, etc.

Other varieties of media are prepared from eggs, various vegetables, broth of beef, pork or veal, milk, and other substances.

Synthetic Media.   For many purposes, such as research and the making of vaccines, it is desirable to use media made up of chemically pure compounds in absolutely exact, reproducible proportions. Such media are called *synthetic* or *defined media.* They range in complexity from simple, weak, aqueous solutions, such as: 1 g KH$_2$PO$_4$; 1.5 g NaNH$_4$HPO$_4$; 0.2 g MgSO$_4$; 3 g Na citrate (or glucose); 1 liter water, to very complex solutions containing a score or more of amino acids, various vitamins, one or more carbohydrates, purines, pyrimidines, salts, and so on. The formula used depends on the nutritional requirements of the species of organism being cultivated (Table 9–1).

CULTIVATION AND STUDY OF VIRUSES

CELL CULTURES.   As has been previously mentioned (in Chapter 6), viruses can be cultivated only in susceptible, actively metabolizing cells. Consequently, any culture of viruses really involves a twofold system: first, the virus itself, and second, the living host cell that will support the growth of the virus. The host cell may be a susceptible plant, animal, or bacterium, depending on the particular virus under consideration, or it may be a developing chick embryo, which has already been described in detail as a laboratory host for microorganisms. Tissue culture techniques provide an indispensable laboratory or "test tube" (in vitro) device for the investigation of viruses.

Tissue cell cultures may be grown as a single (mono-) layer or sheet of cells on glass surfaces (e.g., flasks, Petri dishes, test tubes) and maintained in a complex fluid culture medium. Following the inoculation of such cultures, viral multiplication in the growing cells may be detected by microscopic observation of the cytopathic effects (CPE) due to virus in the cells.

Following inoculation of the sheet of cells with a suspension of virions, the cell culture may be overlaid with a thin film of agar gel to immobilize both cells and virions. After an appropriate incubation period, multiplication of virions may be detected by the presence of a readily observable clear, cell-free zone around each original virion. This zone is caused by destruction of the cells by the virus growth. The clear area is called a *plaque.* The rest of the plate, without plaques, is covered with unaffected cells.

OBSERVATION AND STUDY OF VIRUSES.   Obviously, one of the simplest methods of studying viruses would be to observe them directly. Unfortunately, because of their small size as well as other properties, only some of the larger viruses may be investigated in this way. Most viruses are studied by use of the *electron microscope,* which will be explained later in this chapter.

Ultracentrifugation.   Viruses and many types of molecules, such as DNA or proteins, may be separated, purified, and studied by a number of physical and chemical procedures, which because of their variety and complexity need not be considered in detail here. One such procedure, however, is differential or density gradient *ultracentrifugation,* or centrifugation at extremely high speeds in layered fluids stratified as to specific gravities. This results in particulate matter forming a sediment at different levels, the strata depending on the weights, shapes, and sizes of the particles. Thus a virus suspension may be purified by this physical process of differential sedimentation.

Ultrafiltration.   Another method of isolating viruses and studying their particle size and form is by *ultrafiltration.* Here, suspensions of virus-containing materials (following coarse filtration to remove bacteria and other large particles) are passed through membrane filters. These filters are made of material with pores of a size that will retain particles of a given dimension, for example, a "large" virus, at the same time permitting others, such as "small" viruses, to pass through and, thus, provide a means of separating viruses according to their particle size.

Immunology.   The use of various antigen-antibody reactions (e.g., agglutination and complement fixation reactions, fluorescent antibody staining, and immunoelectrophoresis) as means of detecting the presence of viruses will be considered under the general topic of immunity (Chapter 19).

MICROSCOPY

OBSERVATION OF MORPHOLOGY.[3]   In order to work with any kind of object it is obviously important, although not absolutely essential, to see it. In identifying an unknown microorganism, important first steps are determination of its form, motion, staining reactions, and other visible characteristics, all of which require a clear view of the individual cells. Although Leeuwenhoek could see bacteria at magnifications of ×200 to 300, modern analytical and differential microbiology necessitates the use of the "ordinary" or *optical* compound microscope that uses ordinary, visible light (Fig. 9–6), and also the electron microscope that uses no light at all but streams of invisible electrons (Fig. 9–8).

THE OPTICAL MICROSCOPE.   Simple magnifying glasses were in use in very ancient times, but the use of combinations of two or more lenses arranged in a tube so that one lens magnifies the image produced by another (the compound microscope) originated, probably, with a Jesuit scholar, Athanasius Kircher (1602–1680). Because the magnified image is seen directly with the eye, microscopes using visible light are often called *optical microscopes* in contrast to microscopes that use invisible x-rays, ultraviolet rays, and electrons (see page 143).

The lens nearest the object being observed is called the *objective*. In optical microscopes used in microbiology the objective lens is small, it has a very short focal distance, like a nearsighted eye, and it must be very close to the object. The second lens, which magnifies the image made by the objective, is some inches above the latter. Since the eye is nearer to the second lens, this lens is called an *eyepiece* or *ocular*. To make the image clear and free from distortion, modern microscope manufacturers have added various accessory lenses to both objective and ocular, but the basic principle still holds. The highest magnification given by the ordinary objective is about ×90. This image is magnified usually by a ×10 ocular, giving a total enlargement of the image ×900. Several combinations of other objectives and oculars, giving total magnifications of from around ×50 to somewhat above 1000 are usually available with a good microscope. Direct magnifications of ×2000 yield "fuzzy" outlines. Clear pictures at ×2000 are obtained only by photographic enlargements of pictures taken at lower magnifications under ideal light conditions. They actually do not show much more detailed structure than the original direct image.

Because of the small lenses used in high-power objectives a strong source of light is focused upward through the object. All high power compound microscopes also have a system of lenses between the light source and the object, which collects the light rays and brings them to a focus on the object so that it is well illuminated. This is called a *substage condenser*. An *iris diaphragm* is included with the condenser so that for the more open, lower-powered objectives, the light may be somewhat diminished in order not to dazzle the observer.

In using a compound microscope the object to be examined, mounted on a glass slide, is placed on the flat metal plate, or *stage*, immediately over the condenser and beneath the objective. The latter is then focused by

---

[3]From Greek *morphe*, form; morphology is the study of form and structure.

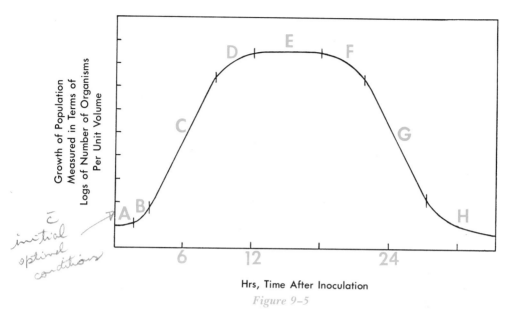

Hrs, Time After Inoculation

Figure 9–5

Growth curve of cellular organisms under initially optimal conditions of growth. This is a typical population curve whether it applies to bacteria, yeast cells, animal or human populations. The curve shows changes in numbers of cells or organisms expressed as logarithms (logs) of the actual numbers. For rapidly growing organisms such as *Escherichia coli* the units of time shown could be five hours each. For slow-growing organisms such as tubercle bacilli (*Mycobacterium tuberculosis*) they could be five days each. For humans in the United States, though not unicellular, the time units could be 30 or 40 years each. (Who knows in what part of the growth curve the population of the United States is today?)

At inoculation into a new culture tube at time 0 a certain number of organisms constitute the start of the new population. During phase *A* these organisms get adjusted to the new medium and environment; there may even be a slight decrease in total cell number. This part or phase of the curve (*A*) is referred to as the lag phase. Other succeeding parts are *B*, the phase of accelerated growth; *C*, logarithmic growth phase, during which numbers increase at a steady rate, such as doubling in each unit of time. The curve in this phase is a straight line. As living conditions become unfavorable, because of exhaustion of food or oxygen and the accumulation of poisonous waste products, growth slows down (*D*, phase of negative growth acceleration), remains briefly at a *steady maximum* (*E*) begins to decline (*F*, accelerated death phase; *G*, logarithmic death phase), finally levels off at a slowly declining minimum, and the culture finally dies out altogether (*H*, phases of readjustment and death). If both living and dead organisms in the culture are counted, the curve for total organisms does not decline. Will a nuclear war make phase *F* of the growth curve of the United States assume a perpendicular position and eliminate phases *G* and *H*?

If a few cells in the culture are transferred to a new tube with medium, the individuals taken from phase *C* will adapt to the new environment quickly, phase *E* less quickly, and cells from phase *H* perhaps not at all. How will the human population adapt itself to new planets when this test tube called "earth" has become contaminated beyond redemption with radioactive waste and industrial pollution products of our civilization?

means of a knob, which raises or lowers it to the correct focal distance. There is usually a large knob for coarse adjustment and a small knob for fine, final adjustments. A *mechanical stage* is often provided to hold the slide and move it in various directions smoothly and accurately. It is a convenience but not a necessity. The modern laboratory microscope is quite complicated, and a few directions for its use and care may not be out of place.

Oil Immersion Lens. The object lens commonly used in medical microscopy is called an *oil immersion* objective (×90). The procedure for focusing and adjusting it must be learned. First, put a small drop of special optical immersion oil on the object or material to be examined. The oil eliminates reflections and loss of light from surfaces of the lens and from the upper and lower surfaces of the slide. The object (e.g., bacteria) is usually contained in a "smear" (page 147) of fluid (say blood, saliva, or water), which has been spread, dried, and stained on the glass slide.

Place the slide upon the stage of the microscope with the stained area directed upward and above the condenser lens. Adjust the illumination and diaphragm so that maximum light passes up through the smear. Now, with the large knob (coarse adjustment) lower the barrel of the microscope, *watching the lowest point of the objective,* until the latter just touches the oil. Next, very carefully, lower the barrel still more until it almost touches the smear. Place your eye near the ocular and raise the barrel with the large knob very slowly until the smear comes into view. Make any subsequent adjustment of focus with the small knob (fine adjustment).

Never lower the barrel with the large knob unless you are watching the tip of the objective from the side of the microscope; otherwise, you may break the slide and ruin the lens.

Keep the instrument in its case when not in use to exclude dust.

Do not attempt to clean or repair the inside lenses or mechanism of your microscope yourself. Consult the instructor or someone familiar with such work.

If you have trouble with focusing, it may be due to a poorly adjusted or dirty mirror (in older microscopes), a poor source of light, dirty lenses, a closed diaphragm, a poor stain, or the fact that the smear is not under the lens, the slide is upside down, or the lens is pressed down on the slide.

Many new, modern microscopes have:

1. Substage direct light
2. Stops so that slides cannot be broken
3. Green and other color filters
4. Adjustments knobs — synchronized for fine and coarse, for continuous turning
5. Binoculars, cameras attached, and so on.

THE PHASE CONTRAST MICROSCOPE. The phase contrast microscope is an improvement of the optical microscope. It does not provide greater magnification, but it does give a more "three-dimensional" view of the material examined. It may be used to look at living, unstained material. Some phase contrast condensers permit a viewing of a certain part of a cell. This is done by simply turning the condenser and increasing or decreasing contrast with respect to other cell components.

FLUORESCENCE MICROSCOPY. Fluorescence is a property of a substance, organic or inorganic, by virtue of which it reflects light rays of a color (wavelength) different from that of the incident rays. Many fluorescent substances give off a bright reddish (wavelength about 800 nm), yellowish (wavelength around 680 nm), or greenish radiance (wavelength around 600 nm) when illuminated with invisible ultraviolet ("black") light (wavelength around 250 nm). Nonfluorescent objects are invisible in ultraviolet light.

If microorganisms are illuminated with ultraviolet light and then observed with the optical microscope through filters that permit only the fluorescent (visible) colors to reach the eye and withhold the eye-damaging ultraviolet rays, fluorescent (e.g., green, yellow) parts of the organisms are readily seen. If nonfluorescent objects such as bacteria are stained

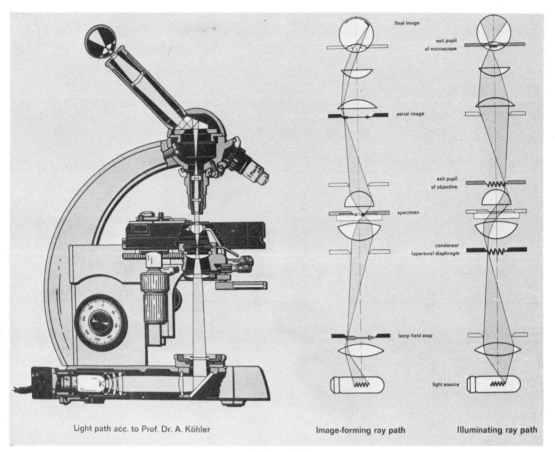

final image

exit pupil
of microscope

aerial image

exit pupil
of objective

specimen

condenser
(aperture) diaphragm

lamp field stop

light source

| Light path acc. to Prof. Dr. A. Köhler | Image-forming ray path | Illuminating ray path |

Figure 9–6

Vertical section of a widely used type of compound optical microscope. At the foot is an adjustable built-in light source; above it a *lamp field stop* and an *aperture diaphragm* for light control. Immediately above the diaphragm is a multilens condenser on a vertical-motion rack-and-pinion mount. Above the condenser is the stage with a specimen on a slide. Immediately above the stage, one of several objectives (available on the revolving nosepiece) is in place beneath the barrel of the microscope, the barrel being mounted on a vertical rack-and-pinion arrangement for focusing. At the top is the eyepiece of ocular lens combination, which magnifies the image produced by the objective lens combination. Final image is formed on the retina by the image-forming rays. (Courtesy of Carl Zeiss, Oberkochen, Württemberg.)

on a microscope slide with a fluorescent dye such as auramine and all excess "background" dye is washed away, then each bacterial cell, when illuminated with ultraviolet light, is visible as a glowing object in the otherwise dark field. This method is used especially in the diagnosis of tuberculosis.

Fluorescent dyes may also be used to stain selectively certain cell components of interest to the microbiologist. With delicate, sensitive detection devices, cell components may even be determined quantitatively in cells stained by this method.

THE ELECTRON MICROSCOPE. Scientists who are curious about extremely minute objects, such as molecules, soot particles, tiny crystals, and the minute, inner structural details of bacteria, protozoa, and viruses (Figs. 9–7 and 9–8), have been aided greatly by the *electron microscope* (Fig.

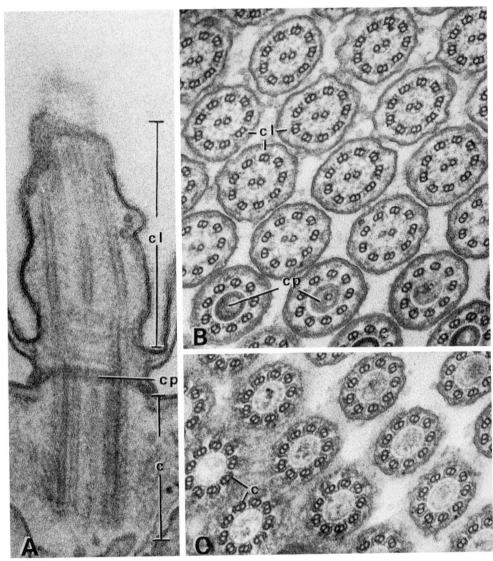

Figure 9–7

Electron micrographs of cilia in longitudinal and cross sections. *A*, cilium of *Paramecium aurelia* showing the centriole or basal body (*c*), the ciliary plate (*cp*) and the cilium (*cl*) proper. *B* and *C*, cross sections through cilia of *Euplotes eurystomes*. *B*, the section passes through the cilium proper showing the typical structure and the ciliary plate (*cp*). *C*, the section passes through the centriole or basal body (*c*). Notice the absence of central tubules and triple number of peripheral tubules. *A*, × 110,000; *B* and *C*, × 72,000. (Courtesy of J. André and E. Fauret-Fremiet.) (De Robertis, Nowinski, and Saez: Cell Biology, 5th Ed. Philadelphia, W. B. Saunders Co., 1970.)

9–8A), which makes possible direct magnifications up to 250,000 diameters. The direct image may be photographed and the photograph enlarged up to ×8, giving final magnifications of up to two million, revealing particles never before seen. This magnification is so enormous that a human hair, magnified to this degree, would take on a diameter of about 1000 feet,

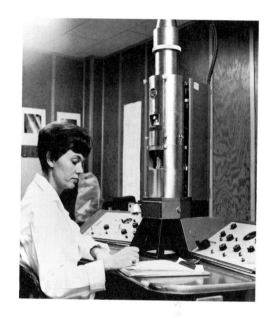

Figure 9–8

Dr. Burke Brown at the Texas Woman's University preparing the RCA electron microscope for examination of bacterial cells magnified 30,000 times.

several times the diameter of a vehicular tunnel such as one under the Hudson River. Visible light consists of a spectrum of electromagnetic waves with wavelengths that range from about 4000 Ångström units[4] (violet) to about 7700 Å (red). Objects smaller than bacteria do not reflect such long waves to the eye in a clear pattern (i.e., are not *resolved*), and are therefore not clearly visible.

Electrons create electromagnetic waves of very much shorter length (about 0.05 Å), and when focused magnetically, as is done in electron microscopes, are capable of *resolving* objects much smaller than even the smallest bacteria or rickettsias, notably viruses and their internal structures, enzyme granules, and even some large molecules. Electron waves are not visible to the human eye, however, just as ultraviolet or x-rays (other types of short, electromagnetic waves) are not. The magnified image produced by electron beams in an electron microscope must therefore be viewed on a fluorescent screen much like that used in clinical x-ray fluoroscopy. Photographs of these images, as mentioned previously, are usually greatly enlarged. These enlargments are called electron micrographs. Several are shown in this book. There are numerous other types of microscopes, such as x-ray, phase contrast, interference, and dissecting scope. Most of these are used mainly for research purposes.

HANGING DROP. An excellent method for observing cellular microorganisms in their natural, living state is by means of the *hanging drop* (Fig. 9–9), which will probably be demonstrated in the laboratory. Briefly, it consists in focusing the highest non-oil immersion lens (about ×45) of the microscope (the so-called high-dry lens) on a droplet of fluid containing the microorganisms, and observing them there. To prevent drying and accidental spilling, the drop of fluid is placed on a thin square of glass (a coverslip) and this is inverted over a concave depression in a special slide called a hollow ground or depression slide. The diaphragm of the

---

[4]Å = 1/1,000,000 mm or 0.1 nm. Ångström was a famous Swedish physicist.

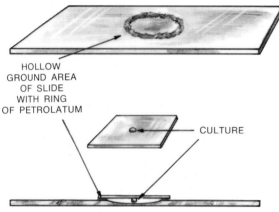

HOLLOW
GROUND AREA
OF SLIDE
WITH RING
OF PETROLATUM

CULTURE

DROP HANGS FROM COVERSLIP

Figure 9–9

Hanging drop preparation.

microscope must be partly closed. In a simpler procedure called a "wet mount," the drop may be placed on a plain slide and allowed to spread under a coverslip.

Much can be learned about microorganisms by the use of the hanging drop. Some bacteria, for example, have the power of motion (when in the early part of their growth curve), and in a hanging drop they may be seen darting, rolling and squirming about, bumping into one another, and so on (Table 9–2). The power of progressive movement of most motile bacteria is due to flagella. These propel the bacteria through the liquid. Highly motile bacteria can move at rates approaching 100 μm per second; that is, they can travel a distance equal to their length hundreds of times in a second. An automobile would have to travel nearly a thousand miles an hour to accomplish the same thing. Bacteria and other microorganisms, however, can move only in fluid—not through the air or on dry solid surfaces. In order to travel over any considerable distance, such as several feet or thousands of miles, microorganisms must be transported by human beings, birds, dust, airplanes, winds, rivers, and so on.

BROWNIAN MOVEMENT.   Minute particles of any sort, suspended in water, whether motile or not, acquire a rapid, irregular *nonprogressive*, vibratory motion because they are constantly being pushed about by moving molecules of water. Their motion is like that of a person in a dense

Table 9–2.   Motility or Nonmotility of Some Common Bacteria as Ordinarily Observed*

MOTILE		NONMOTILE
Genus *Clostridium* except	→	*Clostridium perfringens.*
Genus *Bacillus* except	→	*Bacillus anthracis.*
Genus *Salmonella.*		Genus *Shigella.*
Genus *Escherichia.*		*Mycobacterium tuberculosis* and related species.
Genus *Vibrio.*		*Corynebacterium diphtheriae* and related diphtheroids.
Genus *Spirillum.*		All cocci, including staphylococci, streptococci,
Genus *Treponema*, genus *Borrelia*, and genus		gonococci, meningococci, and pneumococci.
Leptospira.		

*Only young cultures show motility even in the organisms listed here as motile.

crowd of milling people; one is constantly pushed from side to side. Bacteria often show brownian movement, which may be confused with true progressive motility.

STAINING

In their natural state unicellular microorganisms such as bacteria (not viruses; why?) appear under the microscope as tiny, colorless, translucent spheres, rods, or spirals, which are difficult to see clearly. In order to see them distinctly and study them closely, they are stained with aniline dyes. To do this, a droplet of the fluid containing them (pus, broth, or blood) is spread in a thin film on a slide. The smear is allowed to air dry and is then warmed by passing it through the Bunsen flame. *Do not scorch the film.* It should never be hot enough to burn the hand. The heating dries the microorganisms and fixes the film to the slide so that it will not easily wash off. The film is now ready to stain. (*Note:* Neither the heat nor the staining can be depended upon to kill pathogenic microorganisms!)

There are several methods of staining microorganisms. A widely used, simple method is by means of a dye called *methylene blue*. A few drops of a solution of the dye are put on the film (prepared as just described), allowed to remain about 30 seconds, and then washed off with a *gentle* stream of water. The slide is blotted dry (not rubbed), and is then ready to be examined with the microscope.

THE GRAM STAIN. A simple stain such as methylene blue shows very well the shape and size of the organisms, but there are other methods that give more information. The most generally used stain for identifying bacteria was devised by a Danish scientist named Gram and bears his name. It is called a *differential stain* because it divides bacteria into two groups, the *gram-negative* and the *gram-positive* (Table 9–3). Many modifications of this method exist, but in general they are all based on the same principle of identifying two types of bacteria, although many morphological differences are also observed with the same stain.

The *Gram stain* is applied as follows:

Stain the fixed film for about 3 minutes with a gentian violet (also called crystal violet) solution made alkaline by adding a drop or two of bicarbonate solution. Rinse with "Gram's iodine" or "Lugol's iodine" solution and allow to stand for

Table 9–3. Some Common Bacteria Listed According to Their Reaction to the Gram Stain

GRAM-POSITIVE	GRAM-NEGATIVE
All common members of the genus *Bacillus,* including *Bacillus subtilis, Bacillus anthracis, Bacillus cereus,* and *Bacillus polymyxa.*	All intestinal bacilli of the typhoid-dysentery-paratyphoid group, i.e., the Enterobacteriaceae, including *Salmonella typhi, Shigella dysenteriae, Escherichia coli,* and others.
All members of the genus *Clostridium.*	*Vibrio comma,* also called *Vibrio cholerae.*
All streptococci (especially in blood, serum, or media containing these).	All in the genus *Neisseria.*
All micrococci and staphylococci.	All brucellas, including *Brucella abortus.*
Pneumococcus.	All in the genus *Haemophilus.*
Corynebacterium diphtheriae and related diphtheroids.	All in the genus *Pasteurella* and *Yersinia.*
Mycobacterium tuberculosis and related species.	
Yeasts.	

about 2 minutes. Wash gently with water from a washbottle and de-stain with ace-
tone-alcohol by allowing the mixture to flow over the film, drop by drop, until
the drippings show no tint of color (usually less than 10 seconds). Wash again
with water.

At this point it is necessary to explain the difference between gram-positive
and gram-negative bacteria. Gram-positive bacteria retain the gentian violet and
iodine in spite of the alcohol. When viewed under the microscope they appear
dark purple. Gram-negative bacteria do not hold the stain and iodine when the
acetone alcohol is applied, and under the microscope appear almost colorless and
as nearly invisible as when first put on the slide. Therefore, in order to make these
bacteria visible the organisms are *counter stained* for about 30 seconds with a red
dye called safranine, or some other dye having a color that contrasts well with the
bacteria already stained purple. Or, one may use Bismarck brown (especially
recommended for color-blind persons who may not see the contrasts with the other
dyes), brilliant green, basic fuchsin (carbol fuchsin), or eosin (red). Wash, blot,
or drain dry and examine under the oil immersion lens of the microscope.

The purple bacteria are gram-positive; the pink, brown, or green, as
the case may be, are gram-negative. Sometimes, in material such as feces,
both kinds can be seen in the same smear and differentiated. The differentiation is not absolute, and it is sometimes very difficult to be sure
whether a bacterium is gram-positive or gram-negative. The Gram stain
may only be considered reliable when the bacteria stained were obtained
from a "young" culture, perhaps best 18 hours after inoculation and
proper incubation, not made acid by fermentation, and so on.

NEGATIVE STAINING. Not all microorganisms readily take up
ordinary stains. Among those that do not are some protozoa and spirochetes such as *Treponema pallidum*, the cause of syphilis. A very convenient
method of demonstrating the outward form and size of such microorganisms is by means of the so-called *negative staining* process.

The suspension of microorganisms to be examined is mixed with a
little black dye called nigrosin, or with India ink. The mixture is then
smeared on a slide and allowed to dry. On examination with the microscope the microorganisms are seen to be unstained and to appear colorless
on a black background. The dye does not actually stain them at all (Fig.
9–10).

Other methods of staining, like the "acid-fast" stain and others, will

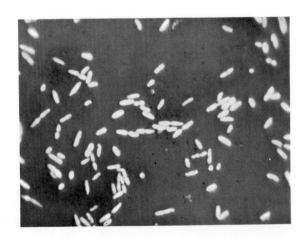

Figure 9–10

Negative staining or relief demonstration. The background is darkened by nigrosin. The bacilli (agriculturally   important   *Azotobacter
chroococcum*) are unstained and transparent (×978). (Starkey.)

be discussed later in connection with certain bacteria for which they are especially appropriate.

Spirochetes and similar microorganisms are also beautifully demonstrated in their living, motile state, by a special means of illumination called the darkfield. This is described in the section dealing with spirochetes.

DIFFERENTIAL DIAGNOSTIC METHODS

In addition to microscopic examination, preparation of pure cultures, staining and examination of smears, determination of motility, arrangement (chains, clumps, pairs), and other features, the diagnostic microbiologist also observes the way in which an organism grows on different food substances, the appearance of colonies, their size, shape, color, and other characteristics. Usually the microbiologist must also study the enzymes each organism forms that are peculiar to its species and that differentiate it from other organisms. These data, combined with its appearance under the microscope and its staining reaction, usually give the diagnostician definite clues as to the species of microorganism with which he is dealing and a possible diagnosis of a patient's illness.

STUDY OF ENZYMES.   In order to observe the activity of enzymes, the microbiologist induces the organisms under investigation to grow in various kinds of specially prepared media in which they can multiply rapidly and exhibit their enzymic activity to the best advantage. Many distinctive enzyme activities are readily studied by testing for the by-products of the action of the enzymes in pure cultures. As has been mentioned, bacteria, yeasts, and molds, by means of their enzymes, can cause a great variety of chemical changes very quickly under favorable conditions. Species differ greatly and may be identified by the chemical reactions their enzymes catalize and the end products that are formed. For example, in suitable culture media certain species such as paratyphoid bacilli can form acids and gases by fermenting glucose. Others (which cause gas gangrene) clot milk, liquefy gelatin, and bring about the changes that we call putrefaction, fermentation, and disease. Not all microorganisms can do all these things, but the ability of each kind of organism to produce certain chemical changes is known. The microbiologist therefore studies what the "unknown" organism can do, as well as what it and its colonies look like.

RAPID METHODS FOR CULTURAL IDENTIFICATION.   At least two types of rapid procedures for such studies are often used. In the first, instead of awaiting the relatively slow growth of large numbers of microorganisms in the test cultures, one prepares a very heavy suspension of the desired cells by collecting the billions that grow overnight on an agar slant. Two drops of such a suspension contain an enormous number of enzymically active, young bacterial cells. These are added to tubes containing a test substance, such as lactose, in a suitable medium such as agar or broth. The billions of young, active cells bring about the desired changes in the test media within two to six hours. The tubes with the carbohydrate fermentation broth medium may be arranged to catch gas produced by the microorganism as was shown in Chapter 7 (Figure 7–3). If an agar medium is used in test tubes, gas becomes evident as bubbles and cracks in the agar.

A second type of rapid procedure consists in placing previously prepared dried tablets or disks of filter paper, saturated with the test substance such as lactose, on the surface of agar medium previously inoculated with a heavy suspension of bacteria. On incubation, lactose in the paper disk is attacked by the growing organisms. Acid is formed and produces a color change in an indicator, such as phenol red, in the paper disk or in the agar around the disk.

Various ingenious improvements of both of these procedures are constantly being devised, especially in industrial microbiology where rapid and massive microbial action is also essential. One of these methods permits nine tests in one simple procedure. It is called the "Enterotube."

MEMBRANE FILTER METHODS.   When microbiologists want to detect and identify bacteria in fluids such as milk, drinking water, or a patient's blood, they ordinarily take a sample of 1 to 50 ml of the fluid. This is put into tubes and flasks of culture media and incubated. Growth and identification of the bacteria that may be in the specimen may take one to ten days or more.

It often happens that no bacteria are found in small samples, but that if larger samples had been examined, bacteria certainly would have been found. "The wider the net, the more the fish."

The use of very large volumes (for example, quarts of milk or gallons of water) in test tubes and flasks might yield better results but are awkward and expensive to handle. It is easier to pass large fluid samples through small, fine sieves or filter disks about 5 cm in diameter, thus collecting all the bacteria in the sample on one small area and discarding the bulky fluid. When the filter disk is removed from its holder, with the microorganisms on it from the fluid that passed through it, it is laid on a pad already saturated with an appropriate medium. The pad is placed in a Petri dish in an incubator, and each live bacterium on the filter disk will grow into a colony where it can be counted, isolated, and studied. If we include test substances in the medium in the pad, we can make some tentative inferences as to the identity and numbers of the bacteria on the disk according to the visible changes they produce (such as changes in color) in the test substances in the medium (Fig. 9–11).

These advantages are obtained by the use of the *membrane filter.* These filters are paper-thin disks of specially prepared plastic with pores so fine that they trap bacteria and even virus particles, and yet large enough to permit the ready passage of any watery solution. Placed in special metal,

Figure 9–11

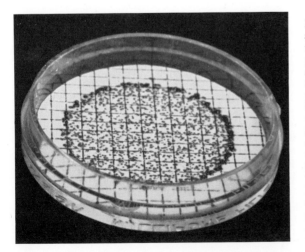

Disposable plastic dish containing a membrane filter disk through which a sample of river water was passed. After filtration of the water sample, the filter disk with the bacteria from the sample on it was placed in the dish on a pad saturated with culture medium. The whole was then incubated overnight at 35 C. Each bacterium on the filter disk, supplied with nutrient from the pad wet with culture medium, has multiplied into a visible colony. The colonies thus formed are seen here as dark spots. The grid-marks on the filter are to locate and identify specific colonies. (Actual size.) (Courtesy of Millipore Filter Corporation, Bedford, Mass.)

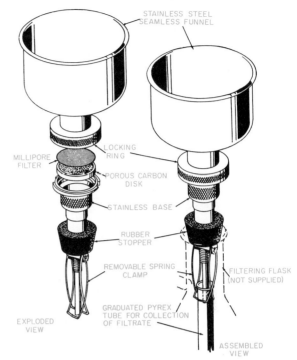

Figure 9–12

Use of a membrane filter to sterilize a fluid. The "exploded view" on the left shows the various parts separately. The porous carbon disk serves merely to support the fragile membrane (Millipore) filter. It plays no role in the filtering process. The whole assembly, mounted in a receiving flask (dashed lines, right), is sterilized before use. (Courtesy of Millipore Filter Corporation, Bedford, Mass.)

funnel-like holders, they are sterilized and used as just described (Fig. 9–12). Fluids to be passed through them are first clarified of coarse particles (silt, erythrocytes, and so on), which would clog the fine pores of the filters. This is done by sedimentation, centrifugation, or other means.

Membrane filters are also available that may be inserted into a syringe; fluid is then pushed through the filter under pressure. The advantages of this rapid method of filtration are obvious. It should also be noted that this method permits the injection of filter-sterilized, but previously nonsterile, solutions in animal experiments.

ANIMAL INOCULATION. In studying microorganisms suspected of being pathogenic, it is frequently necessary to inject or inoculate them into animals (Fig. 9–13). This is the only way in which their action on the living body can be studied directly and exactly, since we cannot ordinarily experiment on human beings. Animals react to many kinds of microorganisms in much the same way as man reacts, and the organisms often cause the same kinds of changes in their bodies. Diagnosis of disease may often be made only by this means. (It should be pointed out, however, that some microorganisms that cause fatal infections in man will not infect animals and vice versa, and that different animals may react differently to a given bacterium.) Microbiology and medicine could never have developed without the study of the action of microorganisms on animals and the experiments that can be performed on them. Animals commonly used for this purpose are guinea pigs, white mice, and rabbits.

Furthermore, the inoculation of animals may be useful in making a more rapid diagnosis because some microorganisms grow better and more quickly in the bodies of animals than in test tubes. For instance, the bacilli

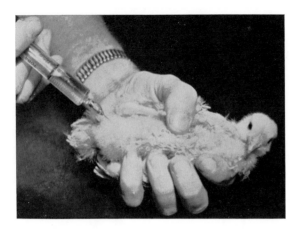

Figure 9–13

Inoculation of a chick to determine the pathogenicity or nonpathogenicity of bacteria isolated from a child with a sore throat. The material (broth culture of diphtheria bacilli) is being injected into the peritoneal cavity of the chick. If the bacilli are virulent, the chick will be dead in 24 hours. If they are not virulent the chick will live, perhaps to become a broiler! (Courtesy of U.S. Public Health Service, Communicable Disease Center, Atlanta, Ga.)

of "rabbit fever" (tularemia) and of tuberculosis grow slowly and not always with certainty on culture media in the laboratory, but by inoculating a guinea pig with the suspected material a positive diagnosis may often be obtained more surely. The animal will develop tularemia (or tuberculosis) and an autopsy will demonstrate the condition. It is of the greatest advantage to a patient who is suffering from an infection to determine as soon as possible what microorganisms are causing his trouble, and the inoculation of animals often helps toward this end.

SEROLOGIC TESTS.   Occasionally an infection in human beings or in experimental animals is so mild that it is imperceptible by ordinary means. It is said to be "subclinical" or "silent." The only way of demonstrating that an infection has occurred is to test the blood (or the fluid part of it after clotting, called *serum*) for distinctive protein substances (types of globulins, especially gamma globulins or immunoglobulins) called *antibodies*. Antibodies (immunoglobulins) are produced by the body tissues in response to the infection. Antibodies are discussed more fully in the section on immunology. Each type of infection usually evokes antibodies that react with the *specific* infectious agents (antigens) that stimulated their production by the tissues. Thus, the detection of specific antibodies can have great diagnostic value. Many of these serologic tests for antibodies are used daily in every diagnostic laboratory. The names of some are the *agglutination*, the *precipitin*, and the *complement fixation* tests. They are used in the diagnosis of bacterial, viral, and rickettsial diseases, syphilis, enteric diseases, fungal and protozoal infections, and so on. Many of these tests are named for the individuals who devised them: (e.g., the Widal, Krauss, Kahn, Eagle, Hinton, Wassermann, and Bordet-Gengou tests), although lately it has become more fashionable and efficient to use abbreviations for the names of some tests, e.g., VDRL (Venereal Disease Research Laboratories of the National Communicable Disease Center).

A ROUTINE LABORATORY PROCEDURE.   To illustrate the practical application of some of the procedures outlined in this chapter, let us suppose the microbiologist in your hospital laboratory receives a specimen of feces from an adult patient with gastroenteritis and fever of four days' duration. One immediately suspects infection by one of the organisms that (in the geographical location of your hospital) commonly cause enteric disease in adults: possibly the ameba (*Entamoeba histolytica*) that causes

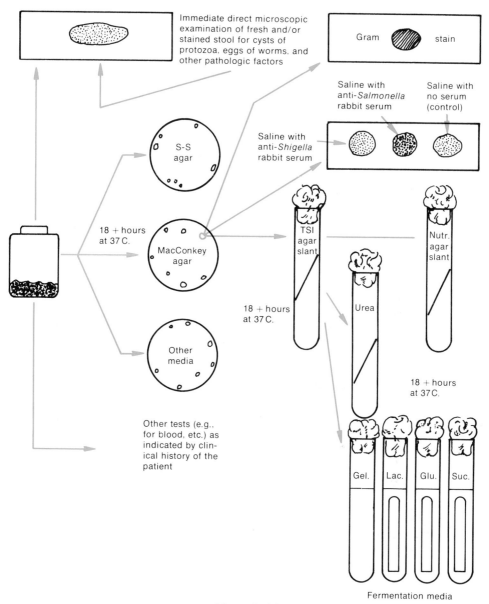

Immediate direct microscopic examination of fresh and/or stained stool for cysts of protozoa, eggs of worms, and other pathologic factors

Gram   stain

Saline with anti-*Salmonella* rabbit serum

Saline with no serum (control)

Saline with anti-*Shigella* rabbit serum

S-S agar

18 + hours at 37 C.

MacConkey agar

TSI agar slant

Nutr. agar slant

18 + hours at 37 C.

Urea

Other media

18 + hours at 37 C.

Other tests (e.g., for blood, etc.) as indicated by clinical history of the patient

Gel.   Lac.   Glu.   Suc.

Fermentation media

Figure 9–14

Steps in a typical examination of stool for pathogenic microorganisms (not including viruses). The specimen is examined immediately for protozoa and helminths by direct microscopic observation. It may also be subjected to tests for blood. Inoculated onto one or more plates of selective media, such as S-S agar (*Salmonella-Shigella* agar), it is incubated for 18 or more hours at 37 C. Colonies thought to be those of pathogenic enterobacteria are examined microscopically in a gram-stained smear. If gram-negative rods, they are tested for agglutination with group- or genus-specific (poly-valent) agglutinating sera. They are also transferred to a triple-sugar-iron (TSI) agar slant and incubated for 18 hours at 37 C. This medium gives distinctive reactions suggestive of *Shigella*, *Salmonella*, and other groups of *Enterobacteriaceae* (Chapter 23). Growth from this slant is transferred to tubes containing urea media, nutrient gelatin, and broth with lactose, glucose, sucrose, and many other substances to determine the species of bacterium being dealt with. These cultures are incu-bated for about 18 hours at 37 C. A plain agar slant is also inoculated to be used for further sero-logic and cultural tests if desired.

dysentery, possibly one of the dysentery bacilli (one species of *Shigella*[5]),
or a species of the genus of typhoid-like *Salmonella*[6] bacilli. There are other
possibilities that can be considered: a viral infection, a fungal infection,
no infection at all but accidental poisoning, or a condition requiring surgery (appendicitis) and so on. We will observe the microbiologist at his
work on only the three most likely of the various possibilities. (See Fig.
9–14.)

After the patient's name, the room or ward, physician, date, and other
identifying data are recorded, a minute portion of the stool specimen is
streaked on a Petri plate containing a medium that is selective for *Shigella*,
Salmonella, or both; i.e., it contains nutrients for *Shigella* and *Salmonella*
and also substances that inhibit virtually all the millions of other intestinal
bacteria. These are discussed more fully later on. Often plates of several
media designed for this purpose, but of different formulas, are used to
increase the chances of isolating a pathogenic bacterium. After overnight
incubation of the plates at 35 C the microbiologist searches for certain
colorless, grey, or black colonies, which are recognized (from training and
experience) to be those of *Shigella* or *Salmonella*.

With a sterile needle portions of some of the suspected colonies are
transferred, in pure culture, to slants of agar medium, each colony to
a different slant in a separate tube. A bit of one colony may also be mixed
in two drops of water (or saline solution) on two separate microscope
slides. From one drop a smear is made, dried and gram stained. If one
finds on microscopic observation that gram-negative, nonspore-forming
rods, and no other types, are present, presumably one has a pure culture.
These could be *Shigella* or *Salmonella*, since both are gram-negative, non-

---

[5] Genus of bacteria named for their discoverer, the Japanese microbiologist Shiga.
[6] Genus of bacteria named for an American bacteriologist, Salmon.

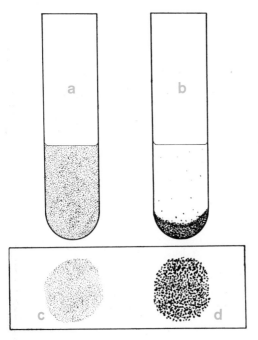

Figure 9–15

Agglutination in a tube and on a slide.
In tube *a* bacteria were smoothly suspended in sterile saline solution containing nonspecific serum (in this example, *Shigella* serum). The bacilli
remained evenly suspended throughout
the fluid even after incubation for two
hours at 35 C and 18 hours at 4 C.
In *b* the saline solution was mixed with
serum containing agglutinins specific
for the bacteria (in this example, anti-
Salmonella rabbit serum). After incubation as noted above, the bacteria in tube
b had settled to the bottom of the tube
in flocs. On the slide at *c* the bacteria
were smoothly mixed in a few drops of
serum-saline as in *a*. The saline at *d*
contained *Salmonella*-agglutinating
serum. The *microscopic* appearance of
agglutinated bacteria is seen in Figure
9–16.

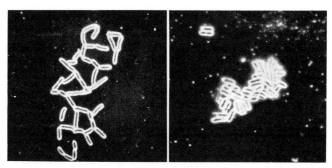

Figure 9–16

Agglutinated bacteria as seen with the microscope by dark-field illumination. Two different types of agglutination are seen here: left, *flagellar, flocculent* or *H*; right, *somatic, granular* or *O*. (After Adrianus Pijper.)

spore-forming bacilli and look exactly alike. This hypothesis is not conclusive, however, because dozens of harmless species look exactly like the pathogens. Further data are necessary.

Of the other drop of bacterial suspension, one portion (A) is mixed with a small amount of diluted serum from a rabbit that has received many injections of dead *Shigella* bacilli. A second portion (B) of the same drop is mixed with a small amount of diluted serum from a *Salmonella*-injected rabbit. This may be done on a glass slide or in test tubes (Fig. 9–15). Now, let us say that the serum of the *Salmonella* rabbit causes the bacilli in portion B to clump (or agglutinate) together like minute curds of sour milk. This clumping is due to antibodies called *agglutinins* in the animal serum. These tiny masses of agglutinated bacilli may be visible to the naked eye (Fig. 9–15). They can also be readily seen with the microscope (Fig. 9–16). The bacilli in portion A remain unaffected. The microbiologist may also observe the still wet saline suspension of the bacilli with the microscope and see that the bacilli are actively swimming about.

It is now known that one can practically eliminate the possibility of *Shigella* because the bacilli were not agglutinated by *Shigella* serum; they were agglutinated by *Salmonella* serum, and *Shigella* are *very rarely* motile, whereas *Salmonella* are, as a rule, actively motile. A tentative diagnosis may now be made—*Salmonella* infection or salmonellosis. One cannot say, however, what species of *Salmonella* is present. Hence, it is best to proceed to determine this, and, since a single test may be misleading, to confirm his preliminary diagnosis by additional examinations.

The species of *Salmonella* can be determined by further agglutination tests using successive lots of rabbit serum, each especially prepared to agglutinate a single, different species of *Salmonella*.

After some hours of incubation of the pure culture, one can confirm and extend the tentative diagnosis of salmonellosis by transferring a bit of the growth from one of the previously inoculated agar-slant pure cultures, to tubes of sterile broth containing test substances such as lactose, gelatin, glucose or other carbohydrate fermentation media, and the like. After incubating these test cultures 24 hours or longer, the reactions obtained are noted and either compared with those on a table of known test reactions in a book on diagnostic bacteriology[7] or, being an adept and expert diagnostician (such as we hope our reader will become!), these reactions are known by heart and we can arrive at a final diagnosis immediately by inspection of the test cultures (see Table 23–2, page 330). This description of a diagnostic procedure is a simplified one, but it gives an idea of a routine, relatively easy laboratory diagnosis.

We might add that the stool specimen of this patient, on direct microscopic examination, also revealed the cysts of the ameba of dysentery (Fig. 3–3), and thus the patient suffered from a double infection and had a very bad time. Expert medical treatment and skillful care, however, cured the patient of both infections and restored him to health and prevented the spread of the infection to personnel in the hospital and to visitors.[8]

---

[7]Such as Breed et al.: Bergey's Manual of Determinative Bacteriology. (See Supplementary Reading.)

[8]The patient afterward married his nurse, a most attractive young woman, and they now live in Tanganyika.

Supplementary Reading

B. B. L. Manual of Products and Laboratory Procedures. 5th Ed. 1968, Baltimore, Baltimore Biological Laboratory, Inc.

Blair, J. E., Lennette, E. H., and Truant, J. P. (Editors): Manual of Clinical Microbiology. 1970, Bethesda, Md., American Society for Microbiology.

Bodily, H. L., Updyke, E. L., and Mason, J. O. (Editors): Diagnostic Procedures for Bacterial, Mycotic and Parasitic Infections. 5th Ed. 1970, New York, American Public Health Association.

Breed, R. S., Murray, E. G. D., and Smith, N. R. (Editors): Bergey's Manual of Determinative Bacteriology. 7th Ed. 1957, Baltimore, The Williams & Wilkins Co.

Collins, C. H.: Microbiological Methods. 1964, London, Butterworths.

Difco Manual of Dehydrated Culture Media and Reagents for Microbiological and Clinical Laboratory Procedures. 9th Ed. 1965, Detroit, Difco Laboratories.

Frobisher, M.: Fundamentals of Microbiology, 8th Ed. 1968, Philadelphia, W. B. Saunders Co.

Lennette, E. H., and Schmidt, N. J. (Editors): Diagnostic Procedures for Viral and Rickettsial Infections. 4th Ed. 1969, New York, American Public Health Association.

Lillie, R. D., et al.: H. J. Conn's Biological Stains. 8th Ed. 1969, Baltimore, The Williams & Wilkins Co.

Lynch, M. J., Raphael, S. S., Mellor, L. D., Spare, P. D., and Inwood, M. J. H.: Medical Laboratory Technology and Clinical Pathology. 2nd Ed. 1969, Philadelphia, W. B. Saunders Co.

Microorganisms in Our Ecological System

10

BACTERIAL ECOLOGY

The study of the relationship between living organisms and their environment is called *ecology*, a term introduced by Haeckel in 1869. A "biotic community" includes *all* the organisms living in any given environment; an *ecosystem* includes the biotic community and the inanimate (or physically limiting) parts and factors that make up the total environment. For a microbiological example we may cite the human colon, with its enclosed biotic community of billions of microorganisms of hundreds of different species: bacteria, protozoa, yeasts, and so on. The colon is not an inanimate environment but it contains and supports the whole living system within it and is the physically limiting boundary of this entire, very complex universe or ecosystem. Numerous other types of microbial ecosystems are found in various kinds of soil, in the sea, and so on.

Microorganisms are almost ubiquitous on the surface of the earth and are therefore important factors in the human ecosystem. Their ecological relationships with man and all other forms of life are extremely complex and important. Some microorganisms may rapidly kill humans by thousands or millions (e.g., the 1971 cholera epidemics in East Pakistan, now Bangla Desh); others are of tremendous value to man in his industries and of vital importance in agriculture and related human activities.

MICROORGANISMS AS BENEFACTORS

Health personnel—doctors, nurses, medical technologists, dieticians, attendants, and so forth—are perhaps inclined to think of all microorganisms as causes of disease and as enemies of human life, whereas comparatively few species are known to be pathogenic to man. Microorganisms may be divided into two great groups according to their activities: the harmful and the useful ones. The first kind, the *pathogenic* microorganisms (viruses, bacteria, protozoa, yeasts, molds) cause disease merely because they are able to live on or in the bodies of human beings, animals, or plants and, unfortunately, damage the *host* (infected plant or animal) in greatly varying degrees.

The second kind live in the outside world and are harmless to man. These are *saprophytic* or *saprozoic*, unless they are pathogenic for plants or some animals. Many of them, especially yeasts, molds, and bacteria, are used to manufacture alcohol, lactic acid, butter, cheese, solvents for paints and oils, antibiotics such as penicillin, and other products, and to increase soil fertility. Of more than 1700 known kinds of bacteria, only about 70 cause disease in human beings, and of these only a dozen or so are, as a rule, really dangerous.

Many of the pathogenic microorganisms can thrive only in the body, finding the outside world cold, dry, and unfriendly, and they soon die if they are cast forth into it. Conversely, microorganisms adapted only to life in the outside world find conditions in the human body unsuitable to their growth so that they cannot multiply there. There are, however, numerous exceptions in each group.

Before studying the disease-producing microorganisms, with which medicine and public health are chiefly concerned, we should get a wider view of the activities of useful microorganisms and their place and importance in the world.

DECAY, PUTREFACTION, AND FERMENTATION. *Decay* (or rot) is a general term denoting gradual decomposition of organic matter such as dead animals and plants and their wastes, on and in the soil. Strictly speaking, *putrefaction* and *fermentation* are, respectively, decomposition under anaerobic conditions of proteins and of carbohydrates. The terms decay and putrefaction are often loosely used interchangeably. Under natural conditions a great variety of saprophytic microorganisms, including yeasts, molds, bacteria, algae, and the like, may be involved in all three processes. These processes transform organic refuse into useful plant foods, but if they are disturbed our ecological system suffers. Industrial waste may not only kill animals and plants directly, but also indirectly by preventing their (and our!) food production by microorganisms in the soil.

When tissues of dead animals or plants are buried in the ground, microorganisms from the soil and those already in the animal's intestine (or on the plant) enter the tissues. There, by means of their various enzymes, microorganisms cause the fats, proteins, carbohydrates, and so forth, of the tissues to disintegrate. The gases (carbon dioxide, ammonia, hydrogen sulfide, and so on) and water that are formed pass off into the earth or air. Other substances that the microorganisms produce by decomposition of the animal's or plant's body contain nitrogen, phosphorus, sulfur, and other necessary elements combined in water-soluble molecular forms. In this way the dead matter disappears; the complex organic molecules of which it was made up during life are broken apart by enzyme action, and are used over again to nourish plants. Animals and men then use the plants for food. After their death they, in turn, are changed into food for plants. It is through this decomposing work of microorganisms that undue accumulation of dead animal and vegetable matter is prevented and the earth kept fit for living beings. Without microbial activity, higher life would be impossible. The alternating cycle of the elements between animate matter and inanimate matter is carried on largely by the saprophytic yeasts, molds, bacteria, and related microorganisms.

The conditions most favorable for putrefaction, fermentation, and decay in the outside world are those that are most suitable for the growth of microorganisms living in soil, rivers, lakes, and oceans. A temperature about that of hot summer weather is generally best.

PURIFICATION OF SEWAGE AND WATER

Until quite recently every well designed sewage disposal plant was merely a man-made device to control and exploit the decomposing activities of certain groups of saprophytic microorganisms. Only now industrial processes of a different nature begin to replace this type of installation. People can live in large communities under sanitary and healthful conditions only when there is some way of taking care of their wastes. Great epidemics have been caused in the past by the accumulation of human excreta in cities, with resultant contamination of water supplies by pathogens of the intestinal tract: typhoid, cholera, and so on. In ancient times, and even more recently in some underdeveloped communities, it has been the custom to throw the contents of household "slop pails" out the window to lie in the streets. The community water supplies may then become contaminated with feces. Some of the plagues and pestilences that we read of in historic writings were undoubtedly spread in this way. Today the activities of soil and water microorganisms are used in "purifying" sewage. The microorganisms utilize the organic substances of the sewage as food and convert them into harmless, inoffensive materials that are food for plants. A common type of septic tank for suburban or rural use is shown in Figure 10–1A. A more modern, actively aerating home disposal system is shown in Figure 10–1B.

MUNICIPAL SEWAGE. A much used method for purifying municipal sewage is first straining out extraneous objects by passing the "raw" (untreated) sewage through metal screens or racks, then allowing it to flow very slowly through large tanks. In Figure 10–2A these are of a type known as *Imhoff tanks*. In such tanks the solid matter in suspension settles to the bottom. This solid material is slowly decomposed through the hydrolytic action of microbial enzymes (mostly by anaerobic and facultative bacteria). It eventually forms a sort of mud or sludge, rich in plant food, which is pumped out, dried, and frequently used for garden fertilizer. *Milorganite* is a familiar example. It is sterilized before packaging.

The fluid part of the sewage is sprayed on the surface of large beds (*trickling filters* in Figure 10–2A, B) of coarse gravel, during which process it becomes fully aerated. On the surfaces of the pieces of gravel or sand a slimy film develops. This film consists of the growth of aerobic microorganisms, which get their nourishment by decomposing and oxidizing offensive materials in the sewage as the sewage trickles slowly through the gravel. Any solid matter (*humus* in Fig. 10–2A, B) is collected in a final sludge-digestion tank (e.g., Dortmund in Fig. 10–2A) and pumped onto sludge-drying beds. The fluid part, now largely deodorized and much cleansed, is collected in drains and led away to a convenient water course or run into fields for irrigation with fertilization.

Many sewage disposal plants combine these operations in efficiently designed "package plants," consisting of a single, compact unit. A large

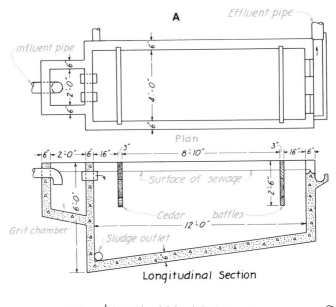

A

Plan

Longitudinal Section

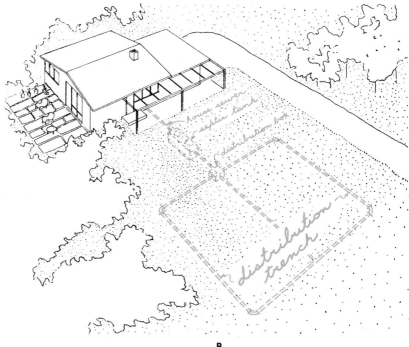

B

Figure 10–1

A, Septic tank arrangement for home or other small group. The sewage is brought first to the *grit chamber.* Insoluble grit and heavy extraneous objects are caught here. The bulk of the sewage flows into the larger chamber. Here solid organic matter settles; grease forms a scum on top and may eventually have to be removed. The settled solids undergo anaerobic microbic digestions in the sump at the bottom of the tank. They are finally reduced to largely inorganic *sludge,* which is pumped out from the sludge outlet. Sometimes several such tanks are connected in tandem. In such a tank sewage fluid is cleared of odor and solid material before it flows onto the filter beds or, if available, into a stream. (Bulletin No. 16, Engineering Experiment Station, University of Washington.)

    B, A common form of sewerage layout for rural or suburban home, showing location of septic tank and drain-tile system for disposal of the fluid effluent from the septic tank. (U.S. Housing and Home Financing Agency, Division of Housing Research, Construction Aid # 5, Superintendent of Documents, Washington D.C. 20402)

(*Figure 10–1 continued on opposite page.*)

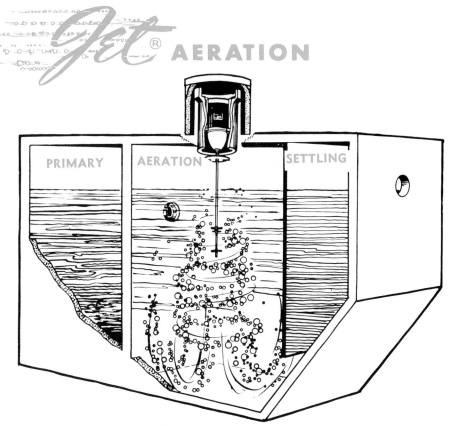

Figure 10–1 (Continued)

C, A compact, aerating sewage disposal unit. This is designed to provide a clear, colorless, and odorless effluent within 24 hours under normal conditions of use. (Courtesy of Jet Aeration Company, Cleveland, Ohio.)

number of rapidly growing communities have discovered that their present methods of sewage disposal are hazardous. These communities spend millions of dollars to protect their inhabitants from potential infectious microorganisms that enter and exit from the human gastrointestinal tract. Yet the construction process of newer and better disposal plants is never finished. As one plant is completed it is being redesigned to take care of a greater load *ad infinitum.*

Activated Sludge. In *activated sludge* processes, aeration of the sludge and the sewage is accomplished by violently agitating the sewage with large volumes of air (Fig. 10–2C). Solid matter is torn into small granules or particles. The particles of sludge contain millions of active aerobic microorganisms that use the air to oxidize and decompose rapidly the offensive matter in the sludge. Aeration is the key objective in the form of sewage disposal shown in Figure 10–2A, B, C.

Some other modern facilities make use of a process that is entirely different, yet also familiar to the microbiologist. It consists of a "giant"

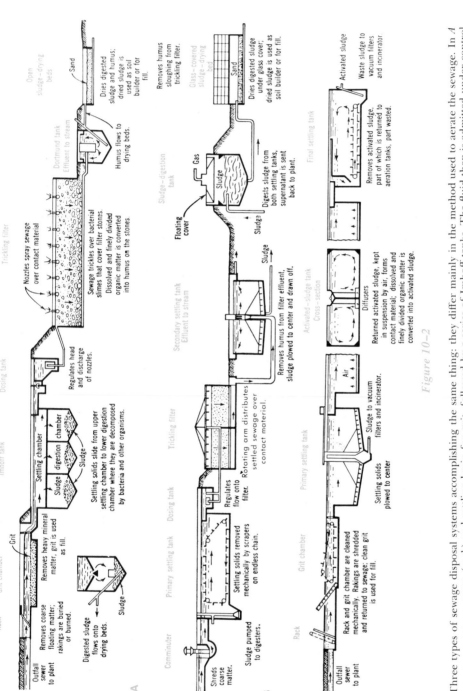

Figure 10–2

Three types of sewage disposal systems accomplishing the same thing; they differ mainly in the method used to aerate the sewage. In *A* are seen a coarse screen (rack) and settling basin for grit, followed by a series of Imhoff tanks. The fluid then is admitted under control (dosing tank) to a trickling aerating filter. The aerated fluid then passes through a secondary tank (Dortmund tank) from which residual solids (humus) are removed to sludge-drying beds. In *B* the solids are comminuted mechanically and collected mechanically from a primary settling tank. The aerating filter is of the sparger type. A secondary settling tank removes residual sludge or humus to a digestion tank which has a "floating" cover to trap sewer gas for use as fuel. The sludge is finally removed to a covered sludge drier. In *C* the partly clarified fluid is aerated and treated by the activated sludge process instead of by trickling filters. (Fair and Geyer in Water Supply and Wastewater Disposal, New York, John Wiley & Sons, Inc.)

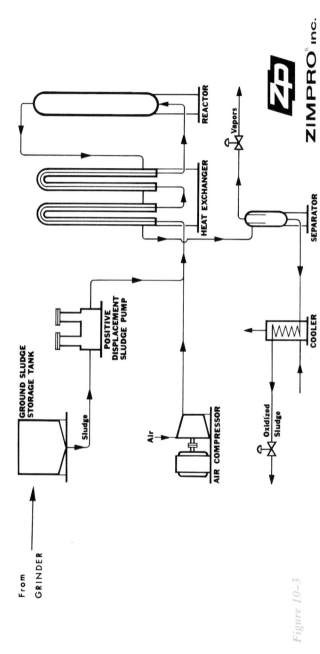

WET AIR OXIDATION PROCESS

ZIMPRO® inc.

Figure 10–3

A simple schematic of the sludge oxidation and dewatering system. Sewage sludge is pumped through the grinder to the ground sludge storage tank (existing digester) and from there it is pumped by the centrifugal sludge feed pump to the high pressure pump where the sludge pressure is raised to the system pressure, approximately 350 psig. Compressed air is introduced at this point and the sludge and air mixture is passed through a series of heat exchangers where the mixture temperature is raised to 280 to 310 F. Steam from the boiler is injected near the bottom of the reactor, into the heated sludge and air mixture, increasing its temperature to the required reaction temperature of about 350 F. The resultant mixture passes through the reactor, which provides sufficient retention time to allow the oxidation and *sterilization* to be accomplished. The reactor products (gas, steam, and oxidized sludge) then pass back through the heat exchangers to preheat the incoming sludge and air. The reactor products leave the heat exchangers at 110 to 150 F. In the separator, the gas and steam portions of the reactor products are separated from the liquid and solid portions. The gas and steam are depressurized through the pressure control valve and pass through the vapor diffuser located in the bottom of the primary clarifier feed manhole. The oxidized sludge (liquid and solid reactor products) passes through the oxidized sludge cooler, where it is cooled by effluent water. It is them depressurized through the level control valve and discharged into the drying beds. The liquid or effluent, which is drained from the oxidized sludge, is recycled through the treatment plant. (From Operating Manual, Zimpro Wet Air Oxidation Unit, Denton, Texas.)

pressure cooker, related to the principle of the autoclave. Once exposed to this much heat, all organisms are killed in the sewage. Usually this step follows the aerobic digestion process.

The purpose of the Wet Air Oxidation Unit (Fig. 10–3) is to partially decompose the organic material in sewage sludge, and to render the remaining sludge sterile and readily drainable on the sludge drying beds, producing a sludge cake which is nonputrescible and unrecognizable as being of sewage origin. The filtrate is nontoxic and highly biodegradeable, and is recycled to the treatment plant. When sewage sludge and air are mixed and retained in a reaction vessel at proper temperature and pressure conditions for a sufficient period of time, oxidation and degradation of organic compounds in the sludge takes place, and the residue is sterilized. This process operates continuously, providing that air, water, and combustible material in proper quantities are furnished, and products of combustion are removed. Steam is injected into the mixture after entering the reactor to bring the sludge and air up to required oxidation temperature.

DRINKING WATER.   Many saprophytic microorganisms are indigenous to the waters of rivers, lakes, springs, and oceans. They are often present in drinking water and are harmless to the human body. We take considerable numbers of them into the body with food, water, and milk every day. Water polluted with "raw" (untreated) sewage, however, usually contains pathogenic microorganisms, among which may be the typhoid or dysentery bacilli, cholera vibrios, polio and hepatitis viruses, the amebas that cause dysentery, and others. The water of streams, rivers, and lakes is so likely to be contaminated with sewage or fresh feces that it is always unsafe to drink it without disinfection. Dug or open wells are also dangerous, as they frequently receive drainage from cesspools, barnyards, and sink drains. Water from drilled wells is usually, but not always, safe, since polluted water may reach them through crevices in the rocks or be drawn into them by continuous pumping. There are no simple tests that tell whether or not water is bacteriologically safe to drink. Positive tests for synthetic detergents in drinking water reveal pollution of the water with household or other wastes, provided detergent is used and the pollution is recent.

Except for water from approved supplies, the only safe way is to boil all water or to treat it with chlorine a few hours before use. Tablets of hypochlorite or other chlorine compounds for this purpose are available from campers' outfitters or chemists. Ordinary laundry bleach (5 per cent sodium hypochlorite, *Clorox* for example), purchasable in any grocery store, makes an excellent disinfectant for water as well as for many other things such as dishes, laundry, urine, and feces. The manufacturers usually provide ample instructions for use as disinfectant on the label of the bottle. The individual who is faced with the problem of disinfection in the home will do well to remember this. There are also excellent iodine disinfectants, *Wescodyne*, for example.

Municipal Water Reclamation.   In many large cities, water is usually first allowed to clarify by the process of *sedimentation*, or settling out while the water is stored for weeks or months in reservoirs or lakes. It is then usually subjected to some sort of screening process, in order to remove dead fish, leaves, and other solid matter. The water is pumped (from different intakes) into the "water works," "filtration plant," or "water purifi-

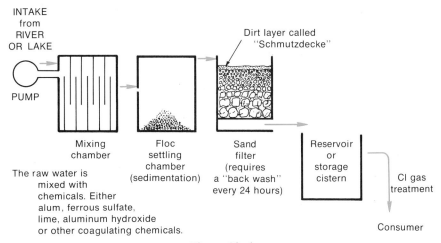

INTAKE
from
RIVER
OR LAKE

PUMP

Dirt layer called
"Schmutzdecke"

Mixing
chamber

The raw water is
mixed with
chemicals. Either
alum, ferrous sulfate,
lime, aluminum hydroxide
or other coagulating chemicals.

Floc
settling
chamber
(sedimentation)

Sand
filter
(requires
a "back wash"
every 24 hours)

Reservoir
or
storage
cistern

Cl gas
treatment

Consumer

Figure 10–4

Shown here is a schematic diagram of one of the simplest and oldest established water purification systems, as used in many towns in the United States. It was first introduced in St. Louis to
purify water from the Mississippi River. All other "water reclamation" systems are variations and/or
improvements of the one shown here.

cation plant," now often called *"water reclamation plant"* (Fig. 10–4).
Previous chemical experimental testing determines what chemicals are
required to be mixed with the raw water to bring about a *"floc."* This means
that the organic substances in the water flocculate with the mixture of
added chemicals, e.g., alum, ferrous sulfate, lime, aluminum hydroxide,
and others in the mixing chamber. Different waters require different treatments. This floc settles in the "floc settling chamber," also called the *sedimentation basin.* These may have a capacity of a million gallons or more to
permit the mud, silt, and floc to collect on the bottom. The water then
flows onto a *filter bed* consisting of layers of sand built up over layers of
gravel. This may be many feet thick and cover an area of many thousands
of square feet. Any remaining microorganisms, floc and other solid particles are removed by the sand, and the filtered water then resembles
spring water purified by filtration through the earth. Under the gravel are
drains that carry the filtered water to storage cisterns. Before release for
consumption, the water is chlorinated to retain 0.1 to 0.2 ppm of chlorine
at the last outlet in the supply system. Fluorine is also often added. All
these processes are developments in engineering based on principles of
microbiology. In our modern civilization about 125 gallons of fresh water
are used per person per day. Obviously this is not all for drinking or even
bathing, but in large part for industrial needs associated with our way of
life.

Bacteriologic Examination of Drinking Water.   Certain bacteriologic
tests, prescribed for legal purposes by the American Public Health Association, are carried out daily in every public health department laboratory.
They are used to keep watch on the probable safety of public water supplies. These tests are designed to reveal the presence of certain well known
and generally harmless intestinal bacteria of the group known as "coliforms," one species of which, *Escherichia coli,* is especially significant in
determining pollution with feces or sewage. When cultivated in lactose

E. coli — is nonpathogenic but can pollut H₂O

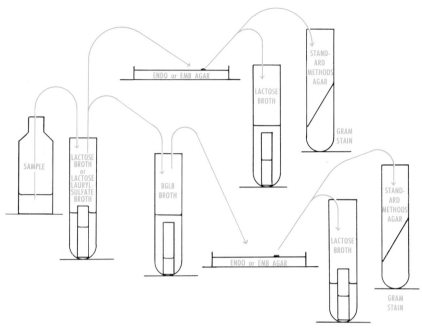

Representative steps in determination of coliform organisms in water, milk, and so forth. The media and procedures are standardized according to criteria set by the American Public Health Association and affiliated organizations. For explanation see text. (Adapted from Standard Methods for the Examination of Water and Wastewater, 13th ed., 1971, American Public Health Association.)

broth these bacteria produce gas (CO_2 and H_2). The gas bubble is easily seen. Some bacteria unrelated to feces or sewage also produce gas under the same conditions. It is necessary, therefore, when gas occurs in the cultures, to determine whether it is due to coliforms or to nonintestinal microorganisms. Ingenious selective[1] media are used.

For this purpose samples of water [or other fluid to be tested for intestinal (coliform) bacteria] in amounts of from 0.01 to 50 ml, depending on suspected intensity of pollution, are placed in fermentation tubes containing lactose broth, or lactose broth with sodium lauryl sulfate which inhibits virtually all noncoliform organisms (Fig. 10–5). After 24 hours (or 48 hours, if necessary for gas to appear) at 35 C, a drop is transferred from one or more cultures showing any amount of gas to tubes of brilliant green-lactose bile broth (BGLB) which inhibits nearly all noncoliform organisms. If gas appears within 48 hours at 35 C, the test for coliform organisms is said to be "Confirmed." To complete the test, however, transfers are made from tubes of BGLB showing gas to plates of Endo or EMB agar, which are selective[1] for coliform organisms. If, after 24 hours at 35 C, colonies that have the distinctive coloration of coliform colonies appear on these media, such colonies are transferred to fresh fermentation

[1]Media containing substances such as antibiotics, certain dyes, and salts that inhibit unwanted microorganisms but permit the desired species to grow freely; also, media containing all nutrients essential to the desired species, but lacking in one or more essential growth factors (e.g., vitamins) necessary to unwanted species.

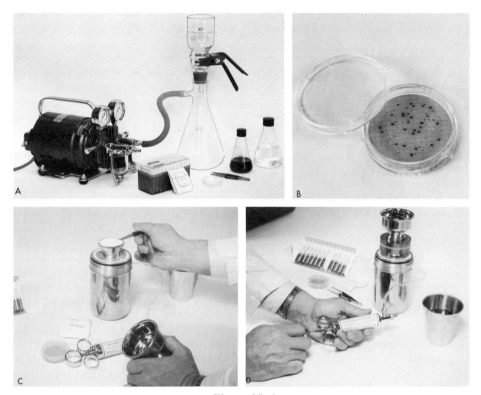

Figure 10–6

Rapid portable water laboratory procedures. *A,* Basic equipment and materials required for routine coliform water analysis in the laboratory. *B,* Pink or red coliform colonies exhibit green metallic sheen after incubation on MF-Endo medium. Colonies may be picked for subculturing. *C,* After sterilizing the apparatus, a sterile type HA Millipore filter is placed aseptically on the filter holder base. *D,* Several short strokes of the syringe are used to pull the water sample through the filter. (From Millipore Corporation: Microbiological Analysis of Water, 1969.)

tubes of lactose broth and to slants of plain nutrient agar. If gas appears in any fermentation tube within 48 hours at 35 C and *only* gram-negative, nonspore-forming rods appear on the corresponding agar slant, then coliform organisms have been isolated in pure culture from the sample. The test is "Completed." By arrangement of the tests in multiple series, and by calculating from the numbers of highest dilutions yielding coliforms, the results can be made roughly quantitative ("most probable numbers").

In the preceding procedure the transfer from the initial lactose or lactose-lauryl sulfate broth tubes to confirmatory BGLB tubes may be bypassed as shown and the initial broth culture spread directly on Endo or EMB agar plates. This short-cut is not the preferred method for the confirmed test.

MEMBRANE FILTER METHOD.   In still another approved procedure the samples of fluid are passed through a membrane filter, which is then incubated in contact with special media (e.g., M-Endo) selective for the coliform group. Typical coliform organisms produce colonies of characteristic pink or red color with green metallic sheen (Fig. 10–6). This method is more rapid than the fermentation methods previously outlined and has the advantage of simplicity, which is valuable in field work. The membrane filter method, using media specially adapted to the organisms sought for, is widely applicable in microbiology. If *E. coli* is found in water, it is probable that the water contained feces. It therefore may contain typhoid, dysentery, or cholera organisms, as well as poliomyelitis and hepatitis viruses and other intestinal pathogens, since these are discharged with the feces from patients, convalescents, and *carriers.*[2]

MICROORGANISMS IN THE AIR

Under ordinary conditions numerous microorganisms may be found in the air all about us. Many of these are the spores of molds and yeasts, conidia of *Streptomyces,* and spores of bacteria of the genera *Bacillus* and *Clostridium.* Spores and conidia are admirably adapted to survive floating about on dust in the air for weeks or years.

In considering microorganisms in the air one must remember that microorganisms cannot fly and have no power to leave any surface of their own volition. They are, however, great "hitchhikers." Indeed, the number of microorganisms in the air usually depends on the amount of dust, since most of the microorganisms are riding around on dust particles. They are usually of the harmless kinds found in soil and soon die in the dry air and sunlight. The air of dark, badly ventilated rooms, especially if they are not kept clean, however, may contain many pathogenic bacteria, especially when occupied by persons who have such organisms in their noses and mouths. These may easily gain access to the air as will be described.

With the recent increase in air pollution, smog problems and industrial growths of cities, car exhausts, and even smoking exhalations by people who should know better, bacteria find it easier to be carried over great distances from host to host. This is one price we have to pay for civilization.

In recent years much attention has been given to air as a means of disease transmission, especially in hospitals. It is known that every drop of saliva and nasal exudate, even from healthy persons (even health personnel and friendly hospital visitors!) contains microorganisms capable of causing disease. Among these are staphylococci, pneumococci, streptococci of scarlet fever, puerperal sepsis and septic sore throat, as well, sometimes as diphtheria bacilli, tubercle bacilli, and numerous viruses (polio, influenza, adenoviruses, and so on). By means of bacteriologic examination of air, the presence of all of the bacteria just listed has been demonstrated in sick rooms, hospital wards, and even such carefully guarded places as operating rooms.

DROPLET INFECTION. The air of classrooms, theaters, schools, and public buses must swarm with microorganisms, especially in winter when sneezing and coughing add to the general pollution of the atmosphere by bacteria- and virus-laden sprays of saliva and mucus. Transmission of disease by droplets of saliva or mucus is often called "droplet infection." These sprays contaminate dust, and when dry, this dust carries the bacteria about (Fig. 10–7).

---

[2]Persons, lower animals, or plants that harbor pathogenic microorganisms without showing any perceptible evidences of disease but that can transmit the infection to others; the condition may be transitory, intermittent, or continuous.

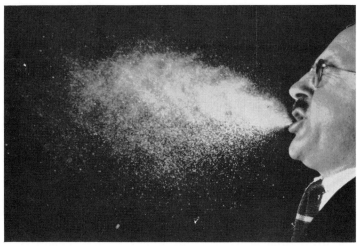

Figure 10–7

The atomization of droplets into the air during sneezing. A violent, unstifled sneeze, not quite completed. Photo taken in a strong light. (Courtesy Dr. M. W. Jennison, Syracuse University, Department of Plant Sciences, Syracuse, N.Y.)

DROPLET NUCLEI. The droplets of saliva and the bacteria contained in the dried particles of mucus float about in the air and are inhaled like dust. Such dried particles are spoken of as *droplet nuclei*. These land on floors, furniture, lips, hands, surgical wounds, foods, and so on. The possibilities are obvious.

MICROORGANISMS IN FOOD

Many saprophytic microorganisms, and some dangerous pathogenic bacteria, grow well in foods that are moist, at warm room temperature, and not too acid. Such foods include milk, cooked cereals, macaroni dishes, custards, and soups. The bacteria come from dust, dishes and hands, ingredients in the foods, water, and utensils. We eat large numbers of saprophytic microorganisms in foods every day with no bad results. Many microorganisms flourish so well in some foods, such as soups, stews, or broth, gelatin, potatoes and milk, that these substances are often used for cultivating such microorganisms in the laboratory. The growth of certain microorganisms in some kinds of food is advantageous. The good flavors of butter and cottage cheese are produced by the action of certain harmless streptococci purposefully added to them. Varieties of cheese are largely determined by the kinds of microorganisms (bacteria and molds) present in them. For this reason it is customary to add "starters" (materials containing the desired bacteria) to cream before it is churned into butter, and to milk that is to be made into cheese. Pickles and sauerkraut are fermented by certain flavor-producing bacteria (*Lactobacillus, Leuconostoc*).

PROTEIN DECOMPOSITION. Excessive growth of saprophytic microorganisms in food, or in any other product for that matter, results in spoilage. The anaerobic decomposition of proteins (muscle, egg white, fish, and similar foods) by microorganisms (*putrefaction*) is usually accompanied by very bad odors due to the formation of ammonia, hydrogen sulfide, mercaptans, and other volatile substances. Ordinarily, putrefied materials are disagreeable, but we sometimes eat "putrefied" milk in the form of Limburger and Liederkranz cheeses! Putrefied materials are not necessarily dangerous unless they contain pathogenic microorganisms.

CARBOHYDRATE DECOMPOSITION.   The series of changes that microorganisms bring about in carbohydrates under anaerobic conditions is called *fermentation*. The chief substances formed as a result of fermentation are acids of different kinds, such as lactic acid, and also alcohol and gases, especially carbon dioxide. Many bacteria, as well as yeasts and molds, can cause fermentation.

There are different kinds of fermentation. One of the most familiar is the production of alcohol by yeast from the sugar of fruit juices, as in the making of wine and hard cider. A familiar microbial action (which, being strictly aerobic, is not true fermentation) is the change of cider or wine into *vinegar* when bacteria called *Acetobacter* form acetic acid from the alcohol of the cider or wine. These aerobic bacteria collect on the surface as scum called "mother of vinegar."

The souring of milk is due to the formation of lactic acid by certain streptococci (*Streptococcus lactis*), which ferment the sugar of milk (lactose). These harmless streptococci, along with many ordinary saprophytic bacteria, gain entrance to the milk from dust in the barns, the cow's skin, milker's hands, and unsterilized buckets. Fresh market milk commonly contains thousands or millions of harmless saprophytic bacteria per cubic centimeter, which cause it to spoil if it is not refrigerated. In many modern dairies much contamination is avoided by drawing milk from the udder directly into sterilized milking machines and, thence, via a closed system of sterile pipes, directly into refrigerated tanks, "untouched by human hands." Also, some milk that reaches the market today is actually made from dried powder; thus all nonspore-forming microorganisms in this milk have been killed by heat.

The raising of bread, also, is due to fermentation. The yeast cells multiply in the dough and decompose sugar derived from the flour starch, forming alcohol and carbon dioxide gas. The bubbles of gas, imprisoned in the dough, raise ("leaven") the bread. Baking dries and firms the bread and drives off the alcohol.

A few microorganisms are sometimes present in eggs even before they are laid. Microorganisms can also pass through the shell after the egg is laid. Many people have, in ignorance, washed dirt from the outside of an egg into the egg.

The spoiling or decay of foods is caused by the growth of various saprophytic microorganisms in them. Tainted meat, rancid butter, rotten eggs, and decaying fruit and vegetables are all the result of the growth of microorganisms. Spoiled foods, while unpleasant, are not necessarily harmful or infectious.

FAT DECOMPOSITION.   Chemically, fats are organic salts or esters, being commonly composed of glycerin (one type of alcohol or organic base) and one or more fatty acids, such as butyric, oleic, or stearic. One form of decomposition of fats by microorganisms is hydrolysis, which liberates the glycerol and butyric acid and similar volatile fatty acids. These acids are the principal factors in the odor and taste of rancidity.

CONTAMINATION OF FOODS.   Sometimes pathogenic bacteria get into various foods such as milk, meat, sandwich fillings, salads, and puddings. The bacteria come from the unclean hands and respiratory droplets and secretions of cooks, or from flies, roaches, rats, or mice that come to exact their tribute from, and to pollute, the kitchen. If food, unknowingly polluted, is held at room temperature and is not promptly and sufficiently cooked after being contaminated, the pathogenic bacteria may multiply in the food and cause disease in the people who eat it. The food, far from appearing spoiled, may seem to the eye, nose, and taste to be perfectly wholesome. The bacteria may, under certain circumstances (especially lack of refrigeration or insufficient cooking), give off potent poisons into the food, which, when swallowed, cause distress and sometimes death. These matters will be discussed more fully later.

Moist food should never be allowed to stand unrefrigerated unless it has been thoroughly cooked and remains in a closed vessel. No moist food should be allowed to remain uncovered and unrefrigerated for more than a short time before cooking or eating. It is important to remember this, for protection not only of others but also of yourself and your family.

MICROORGANISMS IN INDUSTRY

Besides the alcohol and lactic and acetic acids produced by microorganisms during fermentation of carbohydrates, many other substances of equal or greater value are formed and are widely used in industry. It has been said that microorganisms have gone into business.

Industrial fermentations are often carried on in great vats or tanks holding thousands of gallons. Here the skill and knowledge of the microbiologist, engineer, and chemist are pooled for the common good. In addition to products already mentioned, butyl alcohol, glycerin, antibiotics, vitamins, and many other substances of great value and importance are produced in the culture vats, depending on the species of microorganisms present, the culture medium, and so on. The fermentative, putrefactive, synthetic, and other enzyme controlled powers of microorganisms are also utilized in the manufacture of products such as rubber, coffee, cocoa, tobacco, linen, spices, leather, stock feed, pickles, and drugs. Purified and concentrated, the microbial enzymes themselves are widely used in industry. Added to laundry detergents they are very undesirable since, being proteins, they can induce allergic states and reactions.

BACTERIA AND SOIL NITROGEN

We have already dealt in some detail with the work of bacteria in decomposing complicated organic substances into simple, soluble substances that can be used as food by plants. Here we shall point out how bacteria operate in the opposite direction and synthesize complex materials from simpler ones.

MICROORGANISMS, NITROGEN, AND LIFE

NITROGEN FIXATION.   Although we are surrounded by an atmosphere 80 per cent of which is nitrogen, and although nitrogen is absolutely essential to life since it is a part of all living substance, man has always been totally unable to utilize atmospheric nitrogen (until relatively recent advances were made in chemical engineering). We have been wholly dependent on "lower" forms of life to prepare it for us by combining it with other elements, mainly oxygen, hydrogen, and carbon. The process of combining nitrogen of the atmosphere with other elements is called *nitrogen fixation.*

Nonsymbiotic Nitrogen Fixation. It is worth noting that the evolution of our entire grand and glorious nuclear and space age has depended in good part on certain humble bacteria of the soil that "fix" nitrogen of the air by at least two distinct methods: nonsymbiotic and symbiotic. By nonsymbiotic nitrogen fixation we mean the direct combination of atmospheric nitrogen as part of the substance of a living cell without the cooperation of any other organism. For example, atmospheric nitrogen can be built up directly into complex enzymes, DNA, and so on, by the bacteria of the genus *Azotobacter* (*Azo* = nitrogen) and by several other microorganisms, including some algae, certain eucaryotic fungi, and bacteria of the genus *Clostridium*. These useful species abound in all fertile soils. A farmer, allowing a field to lie fallow or unplanted, permits the *Azotobacter, Clostridium,* and some other microorganisms to accumulate nitrogen from the air as a gift of nature. Nitrogen in the form of commercial fertilizers is very expensive.

Symbiotic Nitrogen Fixation. The little nodules on the roots of *legu-*

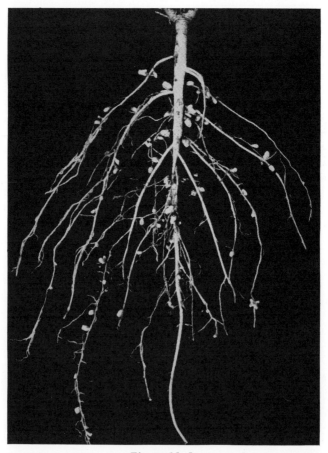

Figure 10–8

Nodules on the roots of Alsike clover. These contain symbiotic nitrogen-fixing bacteria of the genus *Rhizobium.* (Swingle, D. B.: Plant Life. New York, D. Van Nostrand Company, Inc.)

minous plants such as clover, beans, peas, and alfalfa contain multitudes of bacteria belonging to the genus *Rhizobium*. These, growing together with the plant, have the power of taking nitrogen out of the air and combining it into substances essential for the growth of both the bacteria and the plants. This fixed nitrogen is released into the soil on the death of the plants. The process is *symbiotic* (living together for mutual benefit), since neither the *Rhizobium* (root-living) nor the plants could effectively accomplish the nitrogen fixation alone, whereas together they act for mutual advantage (Fig. 10–8). Crops of beans, peas, alfalfa, clover, and so on do not grow well without the indispensable *Rhizobium*. It would be good for human beings, as individuals and as nations, to be more symbiotic!

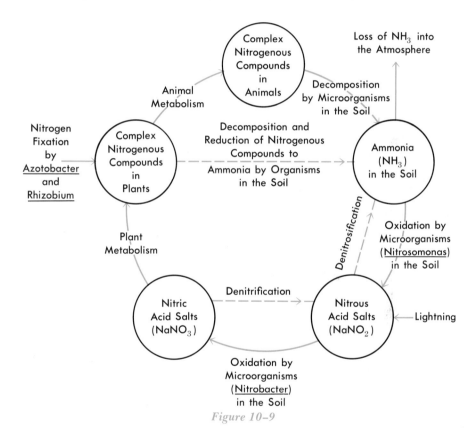

Figure 10–9

The nitrogen cycle. At the right, ammonia (NH_3) and oxides of nitrogen are brought into the cycle. Ammonia is nitrogen in its most reduced form. Oxides of nitrogen are carried to the soil in rain. Ammonia is derived principally from decomposing organic matter (center of diagram). Some escapes to the atmosphere.

Proceeding in a clockwise manner, the process of nitrosification, carried on by soil bacteria (e.g., *Nitrosomonas*) oxidizes the NH_3 to nitrites. Other soil bacteria (e.g., *Nitrobacter*) oxidize the nitrites to nitrates, in which form the nitrogen is available to plants (left of diagram). Facultative and anaerobic bacteria of the soil are constantly acting to reverse these processes, as indicated by the lines marked "denitrification" and "denitrosification." After nitrogen is at last incorporated in plants as proteins, and so forth, it is converted into animal tissues (top of diagram). When plants and animals die, and their wastes decay, the saprophytic microorganisms in the soil convert the nitrogen back into the form of ammonia, and the cycle recommences.

At the left of the cycle are shown the means by which atmospheric nitrogen is converted directly into living matter by the processes of nonsymbiotic and symbiotic nitrogen fixation carried on by soil bacteria: *Clostridium, Azotobacter, Rhizobium*, and so forth. Once it is in this form, it follows the same course in the cycle as do other vegetable proteins, and so on.

NITRIFICATION.   Nitrogenous compounds released into the soil by leguminous plants may be in part taken up by other plants and partly decomposed by putrefaction, yielding ammonia (NH_3). As ammonia, nitrogen is generally useless, or almost so, to most green plants. To be most readily available to plants the nitrogen of ammonia must first be oxidized to nitric acid (HNO_3). Ammonia is first oxidized to nitrous acid; this is oxidized by other species to nitric acid. These important functions are carried on by soil bacteria of the family Nitrobacteriaceae. The nitric acid they form immediately combines with various substances to form nitrates, which can be used by plants. Many commercial fertilizers contain some nitrates. Oxides of nitrogen are also produced in small amounts by lightning flashes and are washed into the soil by rain. The process of changing nitrous acid into nitric acid is called *nitrification.* The nitrifying bacteria, as well as the nitrogen-fixing microorganisms, are clearly of immense importance to agriculture. The great store of nitrogen in the air would be useless for the needs of many living things if it were not for the nitrifying and nitrogen-fixing microorganisms (Fig. 10–9).

Below a soil depth of four feet, microorganisms become less numerous, and at a depth of ten to 12 feet there are usually none.

MICROORGANISMS IN AND ON HUMAN BEINGS

Numerous microorganisms find their optimum (and for several pathogenic species their only) habitat in or on the bodies of man or of animals. The healthy human body harbors millions of microorganisms on the skin, in the mouth, eyes, ears, genitourinary tract, and in the intestine, in short, on every surface that comes in contact with the outside world, with respired air, or with food (Table 10–1). The human body is a complete ecosystem. Most of these microorganisms rarely or never cause disease under normal conditions, but some may, under certain circumstances (e.g., in wounds or after surgery), gain entrance to the deeper parts of the body, where bacteria are not usually present and produce what we call an infection. Each region of the body in contact with the exterior normally has its characteristic microorganisms.

The skin carries large numbers of bacteria, picked up from the various things with which it comes in contact. In addition, *Staphylococcus aureus,* the common cause of boils, carbuncles, breast abscess, infantile impetigo or pemphigus, and other conditions, is found at times in the hair follicles and sweat ducts. The skin cannot be made absolutely sterile even with the most thorough scrubbing and the application of antiseptics because although the bacteria in the outer layers of the skin can be removed, it is impossible to get rid of those in the deeper layers and in the sweat and sebaceous glands, hair follicles, and so on. Therefore gloves, which can be made sterile, are worn in the operating room and in other situations where sterile conditions are essential.

Inhaled air contains particles of dust, some of which have microorganisms attached. The air around persons who have been coughing or sneezing contains a bacteria-carrying mist of nasal secretion and saliva droplets. To demonstrate this for yourself, watch someone sneeze who is sitting near the window of a darkened room where the sun is shining brightly against one windowpane (Fig. 10–8). Hold a Petri plate with nu-

Table 10–1.   Microorganisms That May be Found More or Less Regularly in or on Apparently Normal Persons

Scalp:
  Staphylococcus epidermidis (S. albus)†
  Corynebacterium acnes†

Conjunctivae:
  Corynebacterium xerosis
  Staphylococcus epidermidis
  Haemophilus sp.*

Ears:
  Mycobacterium phlei
  Corynebacterium sp.
  Staphylococcus epidermidis†

Perianal folds and area:
  Mycobacterium smegmatis
  *Escherichia coli** and coliforms
  Enterococci
  Clostridium sp.†
  Lactobacillus sp.
  Corynebacterium sp.
  Staphylococcus epidermidis†
  Spores of fungi and yeasts

Nose, mouth, and pharynx:
  *Streptococcus pyogenes**
  Streptococcus salivarius
  Streptococcus mitis
  Streptococcus faecalis†
  *Diplococcus pneumoniae**
  Corynebacterium pseudodiphtheriticum
  Corynebacterium xerosis
  *Corynebacterium diphtheriae**
  *Haemophilus influenzae**
  Borrelia vincentii†?
  Borrelia buccalis
  Fusobacterium fusiforme†?
  Trichomonas sp. (*tenax*?)

  *Staphylococcus aureus**
  Staphylococcus epidermidis
  Neisseria catarrhalis
  *Neisseria meningitidis**
  Mycobacterium phlei
  Lactobacillus casei
  Lactobacillus fermenti
  *Candida albicans**
  Spores of *Bacillus,* yeasts, and molds
  Any microorganisms of food or air
  Filamentous actinomyces-like organisms
    around teeth (*Leptotrichia buccalis*?)
  Influenza and adenoviruses*

Axillae:
  Mycobacterium smegmatis
  Mycobacterium phlei
  Staphylococcus epidermidis†
  Corynebacterium sp.

Genitalia:
  Mycobacterium smegmatis
  Treponema refringens (esp. male)
  Corynebacterium sp.
  Lactobacillus acidophilus (vagina)
  *Trichomonas vaginalis**

Glabrous skin:
  Staphylococcus epidermidis†
  *Staphylococcus aureus**
  Corynebacterium acnes,† etc.
  Any organisms of surrounding air, clothing, etc.
  Spores of *Bacillus,* molds, etc.

Hands:
  Variable, depending on materials being handled;
    commonly microorganisms of skin, respiratory
    tract, feces, and perianal region

Colon:
  *Escherichia coli** and coliform group
  Shigella sp.*
  Salmonella sp.*
  *Bacteroides fragilis**
  *Bacteroides serpens**
  Clostridium perfringens†
  Clostridium tetani†
  Streptococcus faecalis and enterococci†
  Alcaligenes faecalis
  Lactobacillus bifidus (esp. infants)
  Lactobacillus acidophilus

  Pseudomonas aeruginosa†
  Proteus vulgaris†
  *Candida albicans**
  Giardia lamblia
  Trichomonas hominis
  Entamoeba coli
  *Entamoeba histolytica**
  Enteroviruses*
  Poliovirus*
  Virus of epidemic hepatitis*

*Primary invaders. †Secondary invaders, opportunists or lesser pathogens. *Note:* Fungi that cause dermatomycoses (skin infections) are not included in the table, although, in an unsuspectedly high percentage of our population, apparently normal persons have these organisms on their scalp, skin, ears and feet.

trient agar in front of the mouth of someone coughing or sneezing, or even talking, and then incubate it. It will then be plain that we both inhale and exhale considerable numbers of microorganisms daily.

The inside of the nose is especially adapted for dealing with these microorganisms. It contains a complicated, scroll-like arrangement of bones (the turbinates), covered with mucous membrane. As the air passes over these surfaces it is not only warmed and moistened (nature's air-conditioning apparatus), but the microorganism-laden dust sticks to the moist surface and is finally carried to the outside in the nasal secretion. In a healthy nose few microorganisms can gain a permanent foothold. If the nasal passage is stopped up by adenoids or by other obstructions, or if the normal defense mechanisms are held in abeyance by diseases such as influenza, measles, or whooping cough, microorganisms may find suitable conditions for growth and cause such diseases as sinusitis, rhinitis, or pneumonia.

The mouth and throat constantly contain numerous kinds of microorganisms. These live and multiply in the secretions of the nose, oral cavity, and among the teeth; hence, good oral and dental hygiene are desirable. Commonly found are streptococci (*Streptococcus pyogenes*) of several pathogenic varieties, staphylococci, pneumococci (*Diplococcus pneumoniae*), and certain spirochetes (*Borrelia vincentii*). Also occasionally present are diphtheria bacilli (*Corynebacterium diphtheriae*), *Haemophilus influenzae*, the influenza virus, adenoviruses, tubercle bacilli, as well as saprophytes from food, dust, and fingers. Microorganisms of many types grow readily in a neglected mouth because conditions of warmth and moisture are favorable, and bits of food and desquamated epithelium around the teeth provide nourishment.

In patients with febrile and various other diseases, the mechanisms ordinarily holding oral microorganisms in check are weakened and decompositions occur, giving rise to the oral fetor or halitosis common in such patients. Bacteria may aid in decay of the teeth. The tartar that collects around the gums is composed partly of microorganisms, and the white coating on the tongue is a mixture of microorganisms, bits of foods, and castoff cells from the tongue. The mouth would contain more microorganisms than it does if it were not for the saliva, which acts as a continuous mouthwash. The microorganisms are swallowed with the saliva, and many are killed by the acid gastric juice. Persons who have been in contact with meningitis, scarlet fever, pneumonia, or diphtheria patients may carry the bacteria causing these diseases in their mouths and throats, although they may not develop any symptoms.

The normal conjunctivae usually contain bacteria of a harmless kind, which are related to the diphtheria bacillus and are called "diphtheroids." One common species is known as *Corynebacterium xerosis*. Similar bacteria are found in the nose and throat (*Corynebacterium pseudodiphtheriticum*), in the wax of the ears, on the skin, and around the genitalia.

Harmless bacteria called *Mycobacterium smegmatis*, closely related to tubercle bacilli (*Mycobacterium tuberculosis*), are common on and around the genitalia. They are important because they sometimes get into urine specimens and may be confused with tubercle bacilli in attempting bacteriological diagnoses. This explains the necessity of taking urine specimens intended for bacteriologic examination by means of a sterile catheter into a sterile tube.

The stomach normally contains few live microorganisms because of the disinfectant action of the strongly acid gastric juice. After meals the acidity has been reduced by the food and many bacteria may grow and pass through the stomach unharmed.

The neonatal intestinal contents are sterile, but microorganisms enter with the first feeding. The intestine of the adult contains enormous numbers of microorganisms, and billions are thrown off every day in the feces. In connection with these immense numbers of organisms it should be remembered that the intestine is about 26 feet long, and conditions of food, warmth, and moisture in it are ideal for microorganisms, especially the anaerobic and facultative types. They are more abundant in the large than in the small intestine.

Prominent among the intestinal bacteria is the relatively harmless *Escherichia coli*, which as already mentioned is viewed as an index of fecal pollution when found in drinking water. Other important species are the organisms that cause gas gangrene (*Clostridium perfringens* and numerous related species) and *Clostridium tetani*, the cause of lockjaw. In some backward places where ignorance and filth are everywhere, fecal material (containing *Cl. tetani*) gets into the stump of the umbilical cord of infants at birth and causes tetanus neonatorum (tetanus of the newborn). In some sections of aboriginal Africa, the land of witch doctors, it is said that over 50 per cent of the infants die of this disease. Many harmless bacteria are also present in the intestine, including *Streptococcus faecalis*, one species of the group called enterococci. Always present in feces and fresh sewage, it is sometimes used by microbiologists instead of *E. coli* as an indicator organism of fecal pollution.

The vagina normally contains certain distinctive nonpathogenic bacteria, including *Streptococcus faecalis* and *Lactobacillus* species. The uterus is normally free of bacteria. Immediately after childbirth, however, it is an excellent place for the growth of pathogenic bacteria, especially *Streptococcus pyogenes*, which may be carried in during parturition, or afterward on dirty hands, instruments, or dressings, and cause puerperal fever. This is one of the reasons why sterile precautions are so necessary at childbirth.

MICROORGANISMS IN THE BLOOD.   In certain diseases the causative microorganisms circulate in the blood for periods ranging from hours to days, sometimes intermittently. This is true in typhoid fever, brucellosis (undulant fever), syphilis, malaria, yellow fever, typhus fever, and numerous others. When the microorganisms are bacteria, the patient is said to have a *bacteremia* (presence of bacteria in the blood). Similarly, when the microorganisms are viruses, the patient is said to have a *viremia*. Microorganisms may also sometimes be present in the blood of perfectly healthy persons. The vessels that drain the blood from the lower intestines into the liver (portal veins) often contain a few intestinal microorganisms. These are quickly removed from the blood by certain cells in the blood vessels, especially in the liver and spleen.

RETICULOENDOTHELIAL SYSTEM.   These cells constitute part of the lining of the blood vessels. They have the power of engulfing minute foreign particles in the blood (bacteria, cell fragments). They are said to be *phagocytic.*[3] The entire group of these phagocytic tissue cells throughout the body, as distinguished from the freely wandering phagocytic cells called leucocytes, is called the *reticuloendothelial system* (Chapter 18). Some-

---

[3] From the Greek *phagein*, to eat, and *cyte*, cell; phagocytes are therefore "cells that eat."

times after the extraction of a tooth, a local injury, or some unnoticed trauma, a few dangerous pathogenic bacteria may circulate in the blood for a few minutes before being taken up and killed by the phagocytic cells.

MICROORGANISMS IN BLOOD BANKS.   These temporary bacteremias would be of little or no significance were it not for the danger that the bacteria might get into blood being drawn for blood banks or transfusion. Some of the organisms normally on the skin can also get into blood bank blood when the *venipuncture* (placing the needle in the vein) is made. With properly sterilized equipment and clean, expert technique, this very rarely happens. If the bacteria are numerous in blood bank blood, however, they can cause reactions that are always serious and sometimes fatal.

Precautions with Blood Bank Blood.   The blood in a blood bank container must not be exposed to contamination from any source whatever. The blood must be kept refrigerated. It must not be allowed to stand at room temperature for more than a few minutes before being stored or after removal from the refrigerator for use in a patient. Some of the most troublesome bacteria in blood can grow well even at the low temperature at which blood is stored. Nearly all of them can grow rapidly at room temperature. Bacteria sometimes found in blood bank blood and blood products include species of *Pseudomonas, Salmonella, Escherichia, Staphylococcus, Bacillus,* and *Corynebacterium.* Syphilis organisms do not survive in blood bank blood for more than two days. Malaria organisms die in about five days. A constant danger is the virus of homologous serum jaundice (infectious hepatitis B) against which special safeguards must be constantly maintained. Blood bank blood must be used within the date limit. It must *never* be used if there is evidence of hemolysis (i.e., if the clear, fluid part looks red), discoloration, or other abnormality. If there is any doubt in your mind about the blood, notify your superior at once.

APPLICATION TO HEALTH FIELDS

The beginning student of microbiology frequently views with alarm the fact that microorganisms are around us constantly. As has been pointed out, however, relatively few of these are harmful. A knowledge of where *pathogenic* microorganisms are likely to be found is extremely helpful so that you can be constantly on the alert to protect yourself and others from infection.

Supplementary Reading

Aaronson, S.: Experimental Microbial Ecology. 1970, AIBS Books, New York, Academic Press.

Alexander, M.: Introduction to Soil Microbiology. 1961, New York, John Wiley & Sons, Inc.

Barth, E. F. (Editor): Advanced Waste Treatment and Water Reuse Symposium, Dallas, Texas, Jan. 12–14, 1971, Session Two, Sponsored by Environmental Protection Agency.

Bernstein, I. A. (Editor): Biochemical Responses to Environmental Stress. 1971, New York-London, Plenum Press.

Brody, A. L.: Flexible Packaging of Foods. Cat. No. 0103/106, The Chemical Rubber Co.

Current List of Water Publications 1965–1970, Robert A. Taft Sanitary Engineering Center, Office of Information, Ohio Basin Region, Federal Water Quality Administration, U.S. Department of the Interior, Cincinnati, Ohio.

Fair, G. M., Geyer, J. C., and Okun, D. A.: Water and Waste-Water Engineering. Vol. I, 1966; Vol. II, 1968; New York, John Wiley & Sons, Inc.

Foster, E. M., Nelson, F. E., Speck, M. L., Doetsch, R. N., and Olson, J. C., Jr.: Dairy Microbiology. 1957, Englewood Cliffs, N.J., Prentice-Hall, Inc.

Frazier, W. C.: Food Microbiology. 2nd Ed. 1967, New York, McGraw-Hill Book Co., Inc.

Frobisher, M.: Fundamentals of Microbiology. 8th Ed. 1968, Philadélphia, W. B. Saunders Co.

Furia, T. E. (Editor): CRC Handbook of Food Additives. 1968, The Chemical Rubber Co.

Furia, T. E., and Bellanca, N. (Editors): CRC Fenaroli's Handbook of Flavor Ingredients. 1971, The Chemical Rubber Co.

Gafford, R. D., and Richardson, D. E.: Mass algal culture in space operations. *J. Biochem. & Microbiol. Tech. & Engin.*, 1960, *2:*299.

Geldreich, E. E., et al.: Fecal-Coliform-Organisms Medium for the Membrane Filter Technique. J. American Water Works Association 57, No. 2, Feb. 1965.

Geldreich, E. E., et al.: Technical Considerations in Applying the Membrane Filter Procedure. Health Laboratory Science 4, No. 2, April, 1967.

Gray, W. D.: The Relation of Fungi to Human Affairs. 1960, New York, Henry Holt & Co.

Gray, W. D.: The Use of Fungi As Food and In Food Processing. Cat. No. 0104/106, The Chemical Rubber Co.

Gregory, P. H.: Microbiology of the Atmosphere. 1962, New York, Interscience Publishers, Inc.

Hassall, K. A.: World Crop Protection. Vol. 2, Pesticides, 1969, The Chemical Rubber Co.

International Standards for Drinking Water. 2nd Ed. 1963, Geneva, World Health Organization.

James, G. V.: Water Treatment. 4th Ed. 1971, The Chemical Rubber Co.

King, C. J.: Freeze-Drying of Foods. Cat. No. 0105/106, The Chemical Rubber Co.

New Technology for Treatment of Wastewater by Reverse Osmosis, Environmental Protection Agency, Water Quality Office, Cincinnati, Ohio. Superintendent of Documents, U.S. Government Printing office, Washington, D.C.

Odum, E. P.: Fundamentals of Ecology. 3rd Ed. 1971, Philadelphia, W. B. Saunders Co.

Richards, T.: Spoilage of industrial materials by microorganisms. *Nature,* 1954, *173:*102.

Rook, J. J.: Microbiological deterioration of vulcanized rubber. *Appl. Microbiol.,* 1955, *3:*302.

Rose, R. E.: Effective Use of Millipore Membrane Filters for Water Analysis. Water and Sewage Works, 1966.

Rosebury, T.: Microorganisms Indigenous to Man. 1962, New York, McGraw-Hill Book Co., Inc.

Rushing, N. B., et al.: Growth rates of *Lactobacillus* and *Leuconostoc* species in orange juice as affected by pH and juice concentration. *Appl. Microbiol.,* 1956, *4:*97.

Slade, F. H.: Food Processing Plant. 2 Vols. 1967, The Chemical Rubber Co.

Standard Methods for the Examination of Water and Wastewater. 13th Ed. 1971, New York, American Public Health Association.

Stapley, J. H., and Gayner, F. C. H.: World Crop Protection. Vol. 1., Pests, Diseases and Controls, 1969.

Teitell, L., et al.: The effect of fungi on the direct current surface conductance of electrical insulating materials. *Appl. Microbiol.,* 1955, *3:*75.

Underkofler, L. A., Barton, R. R., and Rennert, S. S.: Production of microbial enzymes and their applications. *Appl. Microbiol.,* 1958, *6:*212.

Wallis, C., and Melnick, J. L.: Concentration of viruses from sewage by adsorption on millipore membranes, Bull. WHO, 1967, *36:*219–225.

Water Pollution Control, Report of a WHO Expert Committee. 1966, Geneva, World Health Organization, WHO Tech. Rept. Ser. No. 318.

References on Filtration

Manual for Swimming Pool Operators. Texas Beach and Pool Association, 1100 West 49th Street, Austin, Texas.

Manual for Waterworks Operators. Texas Water and Sewage Works Association, 2202 Indian Trail, Austin 3, Texas.

Minimum Standards for Public Bathing Places. American Public Health Association, 1790 Broadway, New York, New York.

Municipal and Rural Sanitation. New York, McGraw-Hill Book Company.

Oklahoma Public Bathing Place Act Interpretive Code. Bureau of Sanitary Engineering, Oklahoma State Department of Health, Oklahoma City, Oklahoma.

A Short Course in Swimming Pool Operation. Texas State Department of Health, Division of Sanitary Engineering.

Swimming Pools (*PHS publication No. 665*), U.S. Government Printing Office, Washington, D.C.

Swimming Pool Age. 425 Fourth Avenue, New York, New York.

Swimming Pool Operation. Circular No. 125. State of Illinois, Department of Health, Springfield, Illinois.

Destruction, Removal and Inhibition of Microorganisms

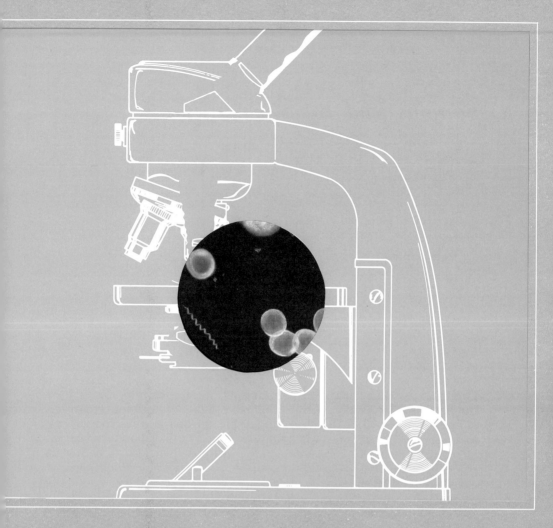

Definitions and Basic Principles 11

Until it was known that microorganisms cause communicable disease, the need for sterilization, disinfection, and sanitation was not recognized. Instruments had to be developed to see microorganisms; microorganisms had to be cultivated and studied in pure culture in the laboratory; and the effect of various substances and conditions upon them had to be investigated. Someone has said, "If we know more about science today, it is because we stand on the shoulders of geniuses who preceded us." Thousands of years ago the Egyptians and Hebrews used certain aromatic oils for preservation of perishable materials and followed certain laws of sanitation that we can understand today because of our comparatively recent information in the field of microbiology. Alexander the Great was advised by Aristotle to have his armies boil all drinking water and bury their excreta and the dung from the beasts of burden. The ancient Romans built aqueducts to bring pure water to the city. What amazingly practical wisdom in a world that was completely unaware of microorganisms!

In the seventeenth century Molière said, "Presque tous les hommes meurent de leurs remèdes et non de leurs maladies."* But even in the early nineteenth century, hospitals were dingy, dirty buildings, not the gleaming structures of the twentieth century. Patients were often placed on mats on the floor or at best on low beds close together; the dead and dying were often crowded together in the same beds. These same conditions exist in some parts of the world today. The poor went to these "pest houses." Nearly as many patients died in hospitals as recovered (Fig. 11–1).

Picture a surgeon making "rounds" in a first-rate hospital even as recently as 1870! Typically, he wears a black frock coat. Linen thread is wound around one of his buttons so that it will be available as suture material. His scalpel is sticking out of his breast pocket to be used periodically for lancing infections. If the scalpel is not sharp enough, it can be sharpened conveniently on the heel of his boot. The only reason the doctor

*Nearly all men die as a result of their remedies and not of their maladies.

182

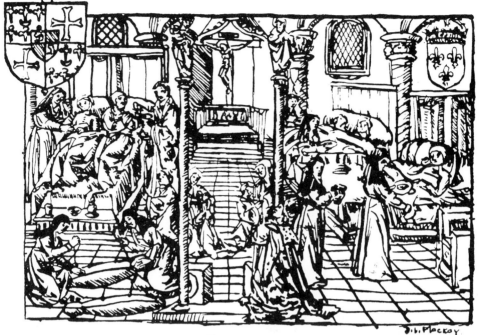

Figure 11–1

A ward in the Hôtel Dieu of Paris. Facsimile of a wood engraving at the head of a sixteenth century manuscript. Note the attendants sewing a corpse into its shroud (lower left), patient and corpse in the same bed (upper left), more than one patient in a bed (upper right), and the generally unsanitary surroundings. Reproduced from Hoffbauer: Paris, A Travers les Ages, I. (Courtesy of Modern Hospital Publishing Co.)

might wash his hands would be that they get obviously soiled with pus and blood. The only reason for turning back the cuff of the coat is to keep it from getting dirty. In those days, hospitals were truly pest houses.

During this period Pasteur proved (ca. 1863) that infections were caused by microorganisms; Koch discovered (ca. 1865) many microbial causes of disease and improved the criteria for determining the cause of disease; Lister first used dilute carbolic acid (phenol) (ca. 1867) to prevent and treat infections in surgery; Semmelweis (ca. 1848) insisted that doctors wash their hands before delivering babies; and Oliver Wendell Holmes (ca. 1843) also insisted on handwashing in maternity practice. From these men, the modern practice of asepsis, antisepsis, and disinfection began. The early attempts at disinfection relied largely on aromatic substances and on chemicals that are deodorants. Even today, the odor of antiseptics is associated (sometimes erroneously) with cleanliness.

One of the earliest systematic and purposeful uses of heat to destroy microorganisms in foods (although the microorganisms themselves were still unknown) was in response to a demand by Napoleon Bonaparte for better foods for his armies. A process of preserving canned foods by heat was developed by a French scientist, Nicholas Appert, about 1805. The process, then called "Appert-izing," involved steam, heat, and pressure; essentially, it was autoclaving, a method of sterilization used today in the canning industry, public health clinics, and every hospital.

Another early use of heat for destruction of microorganisms was devised by Pasteur. In 1863 he found that spoilage of beer and wine could be prevented by subjecting them to temperatures of 50 to 60 C for a few minutes. In 1898 this procedure was adopted in Denmark for disinfection of milk. The process later became known as *pasteurization*.

Koch used a method of intermittent heat at 100 C to make culture media sterile. Tyndall, a British scientist, perfected the method of fractional sterilization in order to destroy spore-forming bacteria and it has since become known as tyndallization. About 1880 Pasteur constructed an apparatus, similar to the modern pressure cooker, that was a miniature, early autoclave.

More than only a working knowledge of various modern methods of destroying or eliminating microorganisms is required in the control of our water supply and in sewage disposal; in industrial preparations; in storage and shipping of foods; in the pharmaceutical industry; in the prevention, control, and cure of diseases; and in other areas of applied microbiology.

In the health profession it is necessary to become conscious of the invisible. One must constantly bear in mind that microorganisms are always present unless special precautions have been taken to kill or eliminate them. It is also necessary to realize that, although most microorganisms in our environment are harmless and we take millions of them into the body every day, pathogenic species are often mixed with them. In many circumstances it is essential to destroy or eliminate these pathogenic microorganisms, and to this end certain modern features of surgical, public health, hospital, and laboratory techniques have been devised.

As in many technical procedures, the results obtained depend largely on the intelligence and skill of the person doing the work and only secondarily on the apparatus. Elaborate and expensive equipment is available in hospitals, but the ingenious person realizes that simple equipment available in the home, such as a bottle of grocery store hypochlorite solution (Clorox, or Purex), a household refrigerator, a pan of boiling water, a "double-boiler," an antiquated oven, or a pressure cooker, if intelligently used, can achieve the killing or inhibition of microorganisms as effectively as the gleaming and expensive equipment available in the most streamlined hospital.

DEFINITIONS

The following terms are often used erroneously and sometimes interchangeably. The student must learn to use them correctly.

DISINFECTION.   This is any process that kills pathogenic organisms. The term is easily understood by simply separating the word into "dis" and "infect." It is sometimes used incorrectly as a synonym for sterilization. An example of disinfection without sterilization is the pasteurization of milk. This destroys the pathogenic organisms present in milk. The milk is disinfected; however, it is not sterile since it still contains many living, though harmless, microorganisms, as is evidenced by the putrefaction of pasteurized milk. Another example of disinfection without sterilization is the use of iodine or other disinfectant on the skin in preparation for surgery. The application of a suitable chemical on the skin destroys most harmful bacteria present on the surface, but because of the layered and pitted structure of the skin and the bacteria as well as spores, under the layers and in the hair follicles, such disinfectants never achieve absolute freedom from microorganisms. In careful surgical procedures the surgeon discards the scalpel he has used to cut through the outer skin and then uses a second, sterile scalpel for cutting underlying tissues.

Disinfectant. A disinfectant is any agent, usually a chemical like iodine or phenol (carbolic acid), that kills pathogenic microorganisms, organisms that infect. The term generally applies to preparations intended for use on inanimate objects, as distinguished from living tissues (see *antisepsis*). Liquid[1] chemical disinfectants are not expected to kill bacterial spores and rarely do so. This is an important fact and should never be forgotten or overlooked. A *germicide*[2] is essentially the same as a disinfectant. A *bactericide* is similar to a germicide, but it is restricted to bacteria and does not affect their spores. A *fungicide* kills fungi and a *virucide* inactivates viruses.

STERILIZATION. This is achieved by any process that completely removes or *destroys all living organisms* in or on an object. Any process designed to sterilize must be adequate to destroy bacterial spores. Few chemical methods of inhibiting and killing microorganisms are true sterilization procedures, since spores resist ordinary (mostly liquid) chemical disinfectants. Various methods of heating are therefore commonly employed for sterilization. The use of *ethylene oxide* and *beta-propiolactone*, which are germicidal gases or vapors capable of killing bacterial spores, is replacing heat in some selected applications, however. *One should never talk of sterilizing one's hands because as long as any tissue or body part is living it cannot, by definition, be called sterile.*

BACTERIOSTASIS. Bacteriostasis is the process of inhibiting (stopping or greatly slowing) the growth of bacteria. Freezing and drying are two common methods. Some of the sulfonamides, and antibiotics like chlortetracycline, are bacteriostatic (inhibitory) rather than bactericidal (killing) in their action. Usually a substance is said to be bacteriostatic if the bacteria are alive after an hour or so of contact with it, although they have been made dormant.

Selective Bacteriostasis. In diagnostic work substances are often used that inhibit one type of microorganism but permit another type to grow. A selective bacteriostatic agent would act against some types of microorganisms but not affect others. For example, in cultivating viruses (Chapters 6, 9) antibiotics are used to prevent the growth of bacteria. The antibiotics selected for this purpose have no effect on viruses or on the tissue cells in the culture.

A good example of bacteriostasis in bacteriology is the use of the dyes *eosin, methylene blue,* and *basic fuchsin. Sodium desoxycholate,* a salt derived from bile, is used for the same purpose. These bacteriostatic agents are mixed with nutrient agar designed for the isolation of certain species of intestinal bacteria, such as *Salmonella typhi* (cause of typhoid fever) and *Escherichia coli.* These organisms grow readily in the presence of the bacteriostatic substances used, although nearly all the other organisms in feces are more or less inhibited.

---

[1]Some gaseous disinfectants can kill spores and are, in fact, sterilizing agents (see page 206).

[2]The suffix "cide" indicates "killer." Thus a germicide is a germ killer; bactericide, a bacteria killer; and so on.

ANTISEPSIS. This is any process that prevents or combats infection or sepsis (the growth of pathogenic bacteria in living tissues) by killing or inhibiting the bacteria. This term is not as widely used as the related word "antiseptic." Because the word *antiseptic* has been much exploited for commercial purposes, the term has been defined in the Federal Food, Drug and Cosmetic Act, which states that "The representation of a drug in its labeling, as an antiseptic, shall be considered to be a representation that it is a germicide (i.e., kills bacteria), except in the case of a drug purporting to be, or represented as, an antiseptic for inhibitory use as a wet dressing, ointment, dusting powder, or such other use as involves prolonged contact with the body."[3] It is seen in this definition that an antiseptic must kill or inhibit bacteria. This definition prevents unscrupulous manufacturers from flooding the drug stores of the country with worthless (or nearly so!) "antiseptic" lotions, toothpastes, salves, mouthwashes, and other products. In practice *antiseptics are diluted disinfectants*, but the reverse is *not* necessarily true.

SANITIZATION. Sanitization is a useful term for the process of making objects free from pathogenic organisms, and esthetically clean as far as organic material (saliva, mucus, and feces) is concerned. This term has been applied to the process used in restaurants and other eating establishments for cleaning dishes. In hospitals, nurses and others have for years talked about "sterilizing bedpans," although this is really not true. Most of the procedures in use *sanitize* bedpans. It would be the rare medical or surgical patient, indeed, who needed a sterile bedpan, but certainly all patients should be given sanitized bedpans. Bedpans from patients with enteric infections, such as typhoid fever, poliomyelitis, or amebic dysentery, must be thoroughly disinfected.

GENERAL INFORMATION

Before inhibition and destruction of microorganisms are discussed in specific detail, it is important to relate to these problems some data presented in Chapter 2. These are: all microorganisms are composed chiefly of complex organic materials that are largely protein in nature; some vegetative cells have a protective substance such as wax closely associated with the cells, e.g., the tubercle bacillus; some cells are capable of producing resistant forms, e.g., all species of genera *Bacillus* and *Clostridium* produce extremely thermostable spores, and certain protozoa produce cysts; and microorganisms differ in susceptibility to adverse changes in their environment.

In addition, students must remember that, in practice, they are attempting to utilize information about disinfection and sterilization in a variety of situations unlike the laboratory situations in which they learned about sterilization and disinfection. In the testing laboratories the effectiveness of a particular process is frequently studied with pure cultures of the microorganisms, to which protein material may or may not be added. The organisms selected for study are usually not the more resistant types or forms. In practice, however, disinfection and sterilization are required in situations in which mixtures of various types of microorganisms are almost inevitable, resistant forms of microorganisms are common, living

---

[3]Federal Food, Drug and Cosmetic Act and General Regulations for Its Enforcement. U.S. Department of Health, Education, and Welfare, Food and Drug Administration, Revision of June, 1958. Government Printing Office, Washington, D.C.

human tissue as well as feces, mucus, pus, or blood may be involved, and delicate materials or instruments may be present. The health worker must, therefore, evaluate each situation and decide on the best possible procedure. Only a thorough knowledge of principles of microbial destruction, removal, or inhibition will enable the individual to do this.

The following are several means of accomplishing each of these three objectives:

I. *Destruction* by
   A. Fire (burning of used dressings, etc.)
   B. Heat (autoclaves, pressure cookers, ovens, etc.)
   C. Chemicals (liquid disinfectants or gaseous agents)
   D. Radiations (such as x-rays, gamma radiation, ultraviolet light)
   E. Mechanical methods (crushing, shattering, ultrasonic vibrations, etc.)

II. *Removal* (especially of bacteria) by
   A. Passing fluids containing them through very fine filters
   B. High-speed centrifugation ("slinging" the bacteria to the bottom of tubes held in a rapidly rotating rotor of a centrifuge)

III. *Inhibition* by
   A. Low temperatures (refrigeration, "dry ice," etc.)
   B. Desiccation (drying processes)
   C. Combinations of desiccation and freezing ("freeze-drying")
   D. High osmotic pressures (syrups, brines, etc.)
   E. Bacteriostatic chemicals and drugs
      1. Certain dyes such as eosin and methylene blue, crystal violet, and desoxycholate
      2. Chemotherapeutic drugs such as sulfonamides and antibiotics

It is certain that in time other means will also be used routinely to destroy specific microorganisms selectively. This may be accomplished through the use of bacteriophage (see Chapter 25), bacteriocins (such as colicins; see Chapter 14), immunologic methods or others.

Destruction by Heat and Chemical Agents

The rate and effectiveness of heat and chemicals in destroying microorganisms are determined by the following major factors: characteristics of the microorganisms, characteristics of the agent used, and factors influencing the interaction between the agent and the microorganisms.

CHARACTERISTICS OF THE MICROORGANISMS. Important in this connection are the degree of resistance of various types of vegetative organisms to agents used for their destruction, spore formation, and numbers of organisms present.

Resistance of Nonspore-Forming Bacteria. The tubercle bacillus is an example of a nonspore-forming organism relatively resistant to certain common forms of destruction, especially chemical disinfectants. This is partly the result of the existence of a waxy substance, present either as a part of the cell wall or closely associated with the cell in some other way. The gonococcus and the meningococcus, conversely, are examples of organisms that are very fragile and very susceptible to all common methods of destruction. *All of the nonspore-forming pathogenic bacteria are readily destroyed by boiling at 100 C for 5 to 10 minutes.*

Resistance of Bacterial Spores.   Spore-forming bacteria, on the contrary, are highly resistant to destruction by heat and chemicals because of their spores. Many bacterial endospores can resist boiling and baking temperatures for an hour or more, and only two or three chemicals suitable for general use as disinfectants can kill bacterial spores within a reasonable period of time, at reasonable cost, or with certainty. Such spores can be killed most efficiently (for most purposes) only by adequate exposure to steam under pressure (autoclaving: 121 C for 20 to 30 minutes) or by two hours of exposure to relatively high temperatures (165 C) in an oven.

In many hospital and industrial applications and for certain materials ruined by heat, two effective chemical sterilizing agents have been adopted. These are *ethylene oxide* gas and *beta-propiolactone* vapor. Both will be discussed later. Certain microbicidal radiations, such as ultraviolet or cathode rays, have been employed experimentally for sterilization but are not yet in general use.

The ascospores of yeasts and the conidia of molds and of *Streptomyces* (mold-like bacteria) are much less resistant to heat and as a rule are killed after about 15 to 30 minutes of boiling at 100 C, although possibly not in 10 minutes.

Numbers of Microorganisms.   When large numbers of microorganisms are present in material such as feces, sputum, and some other body discharges, more than minimal amounts of disinfectant or a longer duration of application of heat or disinfectant must be allowed. This resistance of large numbers in such situations may be due to the clumping together of organisms in masses of mucus, feces, and so on, which interferes with the penetration of the disinfecting agent to all of the organisms present. Also, in any large group of organisms, some of the individuals are more resistant than the majority. Furthermore, the inert organic material in feces, mucus, and similar substances exerts a protective action by coating the microorganisms with a tough layer of coagulum and also by combining with the disinfectants, and thus diverting them from the bacteria.

CHARACTERISTICS OF THE AGENT USED FOR DESTRUCTION.   If heat is used for sterilization it may be either "dry heat," as applied in an oven, or "moist heat," as applied by boiling in water, or the use of steam.

With regard to chemical disinfectants, important properties from the practical standpoint include the chemical nature of the substance, the concentration necessary for best effect, its solubility, the ability of the agent to affect the vital parts of microorganisms, its effect on surface tension, its destructive, toxic (poisonous), irritating, and other undesirable properties and its cost and availability.

"Chemical Nature."   This refers to the constituents in a disinfectant that may be inhibitory or lethal to microorganisms. For example, chlorine is of no value as a disinfectant in the form in which it occurs in table salt (sodium chloride), but it is one of the most effective disinfectant substances in a free form either as moist gas, an alkaline aqueous solution, or in the state in which it is present in bleaching solution (NaOCl). Certain organic acids, such as benzoic and acetic, are mild disinfectants because they are especially poisonous to certain microorganisms. They are often used to preserve foods. Phenol, or "carbolic acid," has acidic and other properties (e.g., surfactant) that render it especially efficacious for some uses. In concentrations above about 1 per cent it exerts a coagulative action and can be very destructive to human tissues.

Substances strongly acidic or basic are likely to be highly bactericidal, but may be too corrosive for general use as disinfectants. Salts of some heavy metals, such as silver, copper, and mercury, are effective disinfectants because they coagulate protoplasm (protein), or are poisonous to certain enzymes in living cells, or both. Some agents oxidize vital portions of organisms (potassium permanganate, hydrogen peroxide). Some active disinfectants react especially with certain molecular groups in the cell structure; e.g., amino, hydroxyl, sulfhydryl, DNA, RNA, etc. The mode of action depends on the chemical nature of the disinfectant. In many instances the mode of action is multiple, or it may still be obscure.

Necessary Concentration. In selecting or dealing with chemical disinfectants, it is desirable to know the most effective concentration of each on a specific microorganism. The use of an unnecessarily high concentration is wasteful and often irritating or destructive to human tissues. The use of very low concentrations fails to disinfect or requires prohibitively long exposures for adequate results. For example, a 2 per cent solution of saponated cresol is effective against most vegetative nonspore-forming forms of bacteria within 30 minutes. A 20 per cent solution of this disinfectant is no more effective, is very irritating and poisonous to tissues, and very expensive and wasteful. Solutions under 0.1 per cent are of some value, but ample time must be allowed for their action.

Intensity of heat. The susceptibility of different organisms to heat varies greatly. Some thermophilic, or "heat-loving," bacteria inhabit hot springs with temperatures approaching boiling. So far as is known, with the exception of the viruses of hepatitis (infectious or epidemic hepatitis, and serum hepatitis), no organisms of significance in medicine resist more than 5 to 10 minutes of actual boiling (212 F or 100 C at sea level) unless they form spores. Bacterial spores may resist boiling for hours. Only temperature like that of saturated steam under 15 pounds pressure (autoclaving: 121 C for 15 to 20 minutes) is effective against the spore-forming organisms. If oven baking (dry heat) is used instead of steam, a much higher temperature must be applied for a longer time (165 C for two hours). The viruses of hepatitis also survive this treatment for 30 minutes and possibly longer (see Chapters 25 and 38).

Conversely, some nonspore-forming (vegetative) pathogenic organisms, e.g., diphtheria bacilli, are susceptible to temperatures as low as 55 C applied for 10 minutes. The pasteurization procedure (62.8 C [145 F] for 30 minutes or 71.7 C [161 F] for 15 seconds) is based on the fact that most organisms that cause epidemic disease and that occur in milk are nonspore-forming and are destroyed by such exposure.

Moisture and coagulation. It is clear from the earlier discussion that dry heat sterilizes less efficiently than moist heat. This is because, when moisture is present, the proteins, protein complexes, and other unstable constituents of living cells are more readily coagulated, hydrolyzed, or both, than when dehydrated. Egg albumen, or "white," if nearly dehydrated, coagulates only at temperatures of a "moderate to hot" baking oven (about 170 C, or 340 F). In a fully hydrated condition it is readily coagulated at much lower temperatures (about 75 C). The same is true of the proteins in microorganisms.

Water-Solubility. Since some disinfectants depend on ionization, which occurs only on solution in water, the water-solubility of chemical agents used to inhibit or kill microorganisms is of obvious importance.

The resistance of bacterial spores to heat and chemicals may be partially explained by the dehydrated form, for the most part, of the proteins and other organic complexes of the spores. Thus neither heat nor chemicals can readily affect them.

Effect on Vital Parts of Microorganisms.   The ability of a noncoagulative agent to affect vital parts of microorganisms is of obvious importance in inhibiting and killing them. This is, in part, the basis of the action of antibiotics and sulfonamide drugs. Among the most vital parts of microorganisms are the enzymes and related structures in the cell, by means of which they obtain energy or synthesize cell substances. Enzymes are readily affected by heat and by most chemical and physical agents that affect proteins. If these vital enzyme systems are interfered with, the organisms die or are held inert by bacteriostasis. Suboptimal but nonlethal temperatures, osmotic pressures, or pH may prevent the functioning of certain enzymes, but these do not necessarily kill the organisms. Thus, unfavorable physical factors in cell environments may inhibit without destroying; such factors are microbistatic.

For example, a temperature of 37 C (body temperature) is advantageous to the growth of pathogenic microorganisms because their oxidative enzymes and other biochemical functions proceed well at this temperature. Temperatures above 50 C are usually harmful to them because many enzymes do not function at this higher temperature. Freezing temperature decreases or stops enzyme activity and slows down chemical reactions and, in the case of some susceptible organisms, destroys them. Many pathogenic organisms, however, particularly the *Salmonella* and *Shigella* groups (causes of typhoid fever, food infection, and dysentery), may survive for months frozen in ice.

Surface Tension.   An exceedingly important property of disinfectants is the surface tension of their solutions. So vital is this property that millions of dollars are spent annually by large manufacturing companies in producing disinfectants with solutions of low surface tension.

Without going into a detailed explanation of the physics of surface tension, we may gain some understanding of it from illustrations of its effect. Surface tension is responsible for the property of "wetness" of a fluid. Mercury is a fluid (at ordinary temperatures) with very high surface tension (466 dynes per cm). Because of its high surface tension it refuses to come into intimate contact with (or wet) most objects and draws itself away into tiny spheres; therefore, it would refuse to spread and contact bacterial or other surfaces if one tried to use it as a disinfectant. Alcohol, on the other hand, has very low surface tension (about 28 dynes per cm). An alcoholic solution of iodine (tincture of iodine) spreads very well, comes into intimate contact with rough, dry surfaces, and gets into narrow spaces where bacteria may escape aqueous solutions with surface tensions of 77 dynes per cm. An aqueous solution of iodine (e.g., Lugol's solution) wets much less efficiently than the alcoholic tincture of iodine unless a surface-tension reducer is added to the aqueous solution. This is done in aqueous iodine disinfectants of low surface tension, such as *Wescodyne* and *Ioclide*.[4] Thus, if a substance has the power to lower surface tension of aqueous solutions, it is of great value in disinfection because it allows the solutions to *wet* and therefore brings the disinfectant into intimate contact with the microorganisms.

Many substances, although not disinfectants per se, have the power

---

[4]These and similar disinfectants are often called *iodophors* because the iodine is in loose chemical combination with an organic substance, which thus "carries" the iodine (phor is from the Greek word *phoros*, carrying).

to lower the surface tension of aqueous solutions, i.e., to make them wetter. Among these surface-tension reducers are many household detergents[5] and soaps.

Some surface-tension reducers are also disinfectants, e.g., alcohols and substances like cresol. Saponated cresol solution is aqueous cresol, with soap added as a surface-tension reducer. The whole group of quaternary ammonium compounds, of which *Zephiran* is a well-known representative, are surface-tension reducers and disinfectants at the same time. They are discussed in more detail farther on. Surface-tension reducers are often called "surface-active" substances or, more briefly, "surfactants." They are characteristically effective in producing foaming or "suds," the housewife's delight (and the sanitarian's dilemma!). Foaming suds are one of the most annoying and difficult chemical contaminants to control in our public waters. The use of "biodegradable" detergents readily decomposed by microorganisms in sewage has eliminated much of this difficulty.

Adsorption.[6] An important property of water-soluble surface-tension reducers in general, including disinfectants that reduce surface tension, is that they accumulate at surfaces and tend to adhere there. This accumulation of surface-tension reducers at surfaces is called *adsorption.* Water-soluble surface-tension reducing disinfectants such as cresol and its many derivatives (among them hexachlorophene) and quaternary ammonium compounds (among them Zephiran, Ceepryn) tend to be adsorbed and to remain in very thin films on the surfaces of hands and objects and to maintain disinfectant action there. Special precautions are necessary in the use of disinfectants based on phenolic compounds (see page 218.)

Surface disinfection.   Floors, surgeons' and nurses' hands, and other surfaces, therefore, if washed with appropriate and properly prepared solutions of surface-tension reducing disinfectants, tend to remain disinfected for some time, perhaps hours, afterward. Some other applications of surface-tension reducing disinfectants will be mentioned later in the book.

Surface-tension reducers in media.   A derivative of a long-chain fatty acid, sold under the name Tween 80, permits the growth of many microorganisms if present in liquid media. This is due to the action of Tween 80 as a non-disinfectant surface-tension reducer. Thus, for example, the tubercle bacillus grows and multiplies quite profusely when Tween 80 is present in Dubos' medium, an aqueous solution that would not otherwise come into effective contact with (i.e., wet) the waxy tubercle bacilli.

Toxicity.   The living substance of all cells is chemically very similar whether in plant cells or in animal cells of any kind. Chemical agents that are toxic for the cells of microorganisms may therefore also be toxic for human cells. Violently poisonous or corrosive chemicals may be used for the disinfection ("sanitization") of inanimate objects like bedpans, pails, or other containers. Disinfection processes to be carried out on or in living human tissues, however, must be selected with due and careful consideration for their toxicity. If disinfectants (for example, phenol at high con-

---

[5]From the Latin *detergere,* to wash away. The basis of the cleansing action of most commercial detergents is lowered surface tension. These act mainly by *emulsifying* lipids (fats, grease, and so on). Lipid *solvents* such as alcohol and gasoline act as detergents because they *dissolve* lipids.

[6]Do not confuse with *absorption,* which means the taking up, by capillary action, of fluids by finely divided, powdery, or fibrous materials such as absorbent cotton or dry plaster.

centration, strong lye, or sulfuric acid) are used, not only is damage done to the patient but the dead tissues become an excellent medium for the growth of pathogenic microorganisms. An example of the misuse of poisonous disinfectants is the once common practice of pouring strong (7 per cent) tincture of iodine into open cuts. This is highly irritating and toxic to the exposed tissues and does more harm than good. The ideal disinfectant for use in contact with living animal tissue is nontoxic to animal cells and tissues, nonirritating, not destructive to materials, odorless, inexpensive, highly water soluble, chemically stable, easily available, and lethal to all microorganisms. Such an ideal substance is not known at present, but several available disinfectants and drugs approach this ideal in some respects. Some will be discussed later.

FACTORS INFLUENCING THE INTERACTION BETWEEN AGENT AND MICROORGANISM.   Important in this connection are temperature, absence of organic material, contact, time, surface tension and pH.

Temperature.   In sterilizing by means of autoclaving or oven baking, the temperature is important. It is also of some importance in improving the efficiency of some chemicals such as disinfectants. For example, a warm solution is likely to be more effective than an ice-cold one, because warming lowers surface tension and heat increases the speed of the chemical reactions involved in disinfection.

Organic Material.   Organic materials such as blood, serum, mucus, pus, feces, and foods are important obstacles to the inhibition and killing of microorganisms for two main reasons:

(1) Agents such as bichloride of mercury, which coagulate protein, will coagulate the organic material of pus, mucus, or feces to form a coating surrounding the microorganisms. This leaves live microorganisms inside the coagulated mass, protected from the disinfectant. It is thus clear that whenever large masses of organic material are to be disinfected, the disinfection process will be more efficient if it is possible to break up the masses mechanically. For example, when feces from a patient who has typhoid fever or other intestinal communicable disease are disinfected, large masses should be broken into the smallest possible particles before the disinfectant is added unless they are to be deposited directly into a sewer. Chlorinated lime, phenol, or saponated solution of cresol would be chosen rather than bichloride of mercury because each has less strong coagulative powers.

(2) Many chemical disinfectants combine as readily with extraneous organic materials such as blood, mucus, and similar substances as with vital organic complexes in the cell. If large amounts of organic material are present, these may take up or inactivate all or most of the disinfectant so that insufficient disinfectant is left free to kill the microorganisms. For this reason, in addition to breaking apart solid masses of mucus and feces, it is necessary to add extra large amounts of disinfectant in order to be sufficient to combine with both the organic matter and the microorganisms.

Contact.   It is obvious that for any sterilizing or disinfecting agent to be effective it must come into contact with the microorganisms to be killed. This is true of both chemicals and heat. As has been indicated previously, contact of chemical disinfectants with microorganisms is directly related to the presence of organic material and surface tension. In addition, in the practical application of any method of killing microorganisms, all parts of the article or substance to be sterilized or disinfected must be in contact with the agent. This means complete immersion of the object

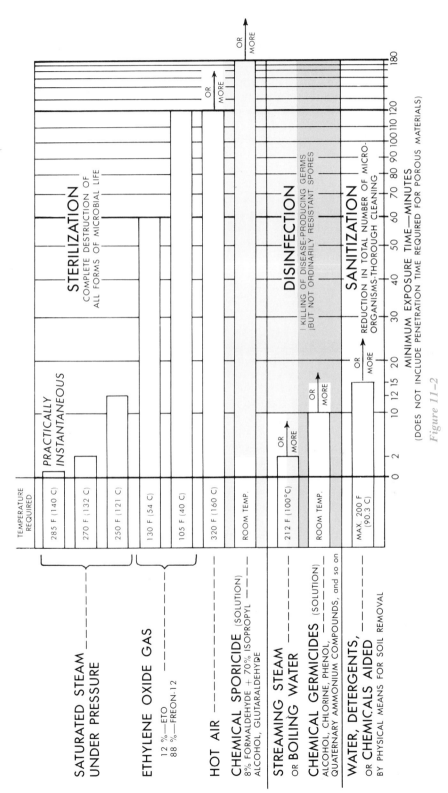

Figure 11-2

Methods for controlling microbial life. *Note:* Chemical sporicide is recommended in practice for high-level disinfection, not routine sterilization. (Courtesy of Research and Development Section, American Sterilizer Co.)

in the chemical or in boiling water with no air bubbles that might prevent contact of the agent with the object. This also means correct packing of materials in an autoclave or oven so that all parts can be contacted by the steam or hot air.

Some substances, e.g., alcohol, dimethyl sulfoxide (DMSO),[7] that dissolve lipids can penetrate through lipid-rich cell walls and membranes of microorganisms and thus make good "carriers" for disinfectants that are soluble in them.

Clean, smooth instruments can be sterilized or disinfected in a shorter period of time than soiled, contaminated objects that have crevices which may be difficult to penetrate. Instruments that have been oiled recently cannot be disinfected by an aqueous solution of disinfectant. This applies also to rectal thermometers lubricated with petrolatum or petroleum jelly because aqueous solutions do not penetrate films or droplets of oil or grease. Cleaned clinical thermometers can be sterilized by sporicidal gases that do not require too high a temperature (e.g., beta propiolactone), but this is not used for individual thermometers. Electronic thermometers with disposable covers are now used extensively.

Time.   Time of contact or application is extremely important in disinfection and sterilization and this should be constantly in the mind of the individual when he is carrying out these procedures. The time necessary to disinfect various substances is dependent on contact, concentration, penetration, and the other factors just listed. For this reason no chemical can be expected to act instantaneously, and only moist heat at 100 C or above acts very rapidly. Some organisms (not spores) are killed in a few seconds by temperatures around 80 C; others may resist 100 C for many minutes. Chemicals require time to make contact with the organisms and to react with them.

As a general rule, at least 10 minutes of boiling (at sea level) or one hour of contact with disinfectant may be used. Many circumstances will change these recommendations. Neither boiling nor ordinary chemical disinfectants may be depended on to sterilize or to kill spores.

Figure 11–2 shows a comparison of methods that are commonly used to destroy microbial life. The reader should note that sterilization by steam under pressure takes less time than sterilization by ethylene oxide or hot air. Also, in Figure 11–2, disinfection and sanitization are graphically related to sterilizing processes. Not shown are methods such as filtration processes that may be used to sterilize heat sensitive media. Filtration is discussed in detail in Chapter 12.

pH.   The acidity or alkalinity of a solution, will affect the efficiency of a chemical agent. Bactericides that are acidic (anionic) in character (e.g., organic acids, phenol) are more effective at low pH. Cationic microbicides tend to be inhibited by low pH and by anions. Acid solutions are more likely to be bactericidal if heated since heat tends to increase dissociation of acids.

---

[7]Note caution: DMSO penetrates human tissues very easily and carries within various dissolved, possibly undesirable and toxic chemicals.

Supplementary Reading

(See the list of readings following Chapter 15.)

Sterilization by Heat, Radiation, Chemicals, and Filtration

12

DRY HEAT

INCINERATION. This is an excellent procedure for disposable materials such as soiled dressings, soiled paper mouth wipes, sputum cups, and garbage. One must remember that if such articles are infectious, they should be thoroughly wrapped in newspaper with additional paper or sawdust to absorb the excess moisture. Special, inexpensive, disposable plastic liners for waste-containers are commercially available; these may be easily closed on top and so prevent scattering of refuse. The wrapping protects persons who must empty the trash cans; it also assures that the objects do not escape the fire. But it may also protect the microorganisms if incineration is not complete!

Adequate instructions should be given to workers responsible for burning disposable materials to insure complete burning. For example, a sputum cup containing secretions from a patient who has active tuberculosis is filled with paper or sawdust to absorb excess moisture. The cup is then placed in a plastic bag with shredded absorbent paper to prevent spilling. If it is burned only on the outside, a soggy mass of infective material is left on the inside. This mass of material is certainly dangerous. Other possibilities will occur to the imaginative student.

OVENS. Ovens (Fig. 12–1) are often used for sterilizing dry materials such as glassware, syringes and needles (Fig. 12–2), powders, and gauze dressings. Petrolatum and other oily substances must also be sterilized with dry heat in an oven because moist heat (steam) will not penetrate materials insoluble in water. Figure 12–3 shows the times required to sterilize glassware (syringes) and materials usually not sterilized in an autoclave.

In order to insure sterility the materials in the oven must reach a temperature of 165 to 170 C (329 to 338 F), and this temperature must be maintained for 120 or 90 minutes, respectively. This destroys all microorganisms, including spores; however, the oven must be maintained at

195

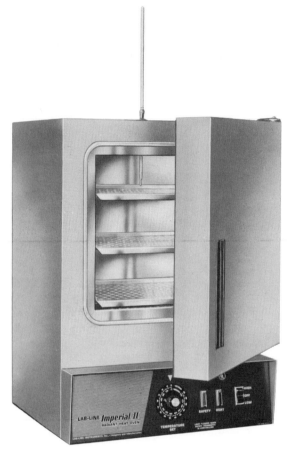

Figure 12–1

A type of sterilizing oven for microbiology. A motor in the bottom of the oven (not visible) forces streams of hot air through the chamber. (Courtesy of Lab-Line Instruments, Inc., Melrose Park, Ill.)

that temperature for the entire time. This means that the oven door must remain closed during the sterilizing time. Opening the door will cool the articles below effective temperatures so that sterilization cannot be assured. Also, *hot* glassware will shatter immediately in contact with cool air. It is usual practice in a microbiology laboratory to let an oven cool completely before it is opened. A home oven, set at 330 F (moderate temperature), can be used as well as an oven built for laboratory or hospital equipment. It is wise to check the temperature in the oven with an oven thermometer. These are available at household supply stores.

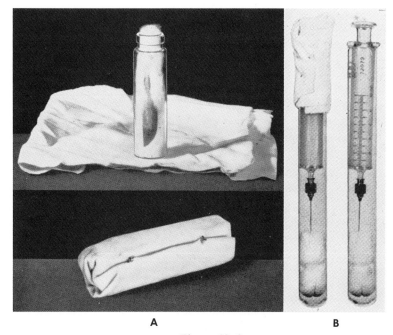

A   **B**

Figure 12–2

A, Method of preparing a scalpel blade for sterilization in the hot air oven or by autoclaving. A small medicine bottle is used containing a wisp of gauze to prevent contact of the blade with the glass. Use a light cotton stopper to close the bottle, and wrap the bottle in muslin as shown.

New blades can be sterilized once only in the hot air oven at 170 C for one hour. Repeated sterilization will destroy the temper.

For autoclaving, the preferable method is to place the bottle on its side to permit air to escape and sterilize 15 minutes at 121 C. (*Surgical Supervisor.* Courtesy of American Sterilizer Co.)
B, This method of preparing syringes for oven sterilization is recommended by Dr. Helen M. Scoville, Pathologist, Pittsfield General Hospital, Pittsfield, Massachusetts. The assembled syringe with needle attached is placed in a Pyrex test tube of such diameter that the barrel of the syringe is a loose fit, with the flange resting on the top or rim of the tube. (*Surgical Supervisor.* Courtesy of American Sterilizer Co.) Many syringes are now made of plastic, sterilized after packaging, with or without a needle attached, and entirely disposable.

MOIST HEAT

BOILING WATER.   Boiling water can never be trusted for absolute sterilization procedures because its maximum temperature is 100 C (at sea level). As indicated previously, spores can resist this temperature. Boiling water can generally be used for contaminated dishes, bedding, and bedpans, however, because for these articles neither sterility nor the destruction of spores is necessary except under very unusual circumstances. All that is desired is disinfection. Exposure to boiling water kills all pathogenic microorganisms in 10 minutes or less, but not bacterial spores or hepatitis viruses. At altitudes over 5000 feet the boiling time should be increased by 50 per cent or more because water there boils at temperatures of only about 95 C or below.

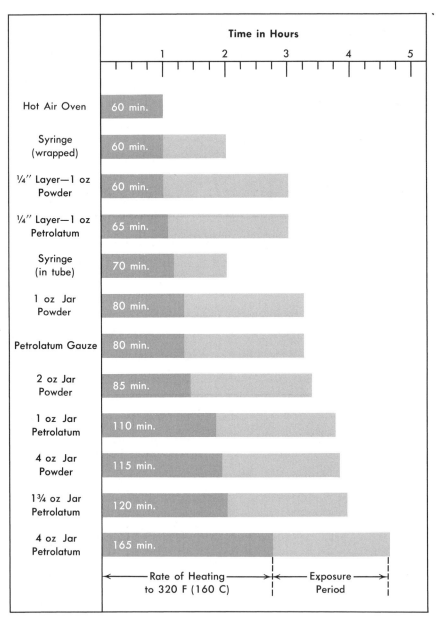

Figure 12–3

Time required to heat specific quantities of materials from room temperature of 75 F to 320 F in a hot air sterilizer. The lightly shaded section of each bar represents the exposure period after the material has reached a temperature of 320 F. The total time consumed in the heating process is equal to the entire length of each bar. (Courtesy of J. J. Perkins: Principles and Methods of Sterilization. Springfield, Illinois, Charles C Thomas, Publisher, 1965.)

LIVE STEAM.   Live steam (free flowing) has been used in the laboratory in the preparation of culture media, or in the home for processing canned foods. It must be remembered that steam does not exceed the temperature of 100 C unless it is under pressure.

To use free flowing steam effectively for sterilization, the fractional method must be used. Fractional sterilization, or tyndallization (mentioned in Chapter 11), is a process of exposure of substances (usually liquids) to live steam for 30 minutes on each of three successive days, with incubation during the intervals. Spores germinate into vulnerable vegetative forms during the incubations and these vulnerable forms are killed during the heating periods. This is a time-consuming process and is rarely used in modern laboratories. The use of membrane (Millipore) filters or similar rapid methods makes the preparation of heat-sensitive sterile solutions much easier.

COMPRESSED STEAM.   In order to sterilize with steam certainly and quickly, steam under pressure in the autoclave is used (Figs. 12–4 to 12–6). An autoclave is essentially a metal chamber with a door that can be closed very tightly. The inner chamber, after allowing all air to be replaced by steam, is filled with steam until the pressure reaches the desired point.

Figure 12–4

Diagrammatic illustration of steam jacketed autoclave. Steam enters the *jacket,* a double-walled shell, at *source of steam* beneath the cylinder. It passes out the top through a pipe to which are attached a wheel valve admitting the steam to the inner *chamber,* a *safety valve,* and a gauge showing *pressure in the jacket.* The steam enters the inner chamber at the right of the diagram, filling the upper portion. Its pressure registers on the *chamber gauge.* It may be allowed to escape rapidly by the *exhaust valve.* If this is closed, steam pushes the cooler air in the lower portion out at the bottom (left), where the *thermometer* registers proper temperature only when the air is gone and is followed by the hot steam. The escaping steam may be allowed to flow out without building up any pressure if the *by-pass valve* is fully opened. If the by-pass valve is closed and the *shut-off valve* is opened, steam passes through the *thermostatic trap,* where the heat shuts off all but a pinhole opening. This causes pressure to build up in the chamber, yet prevents stagnation by permitting a constant minute flow of steam through the apparatus (Courtesy of American Sterilizer Co.)

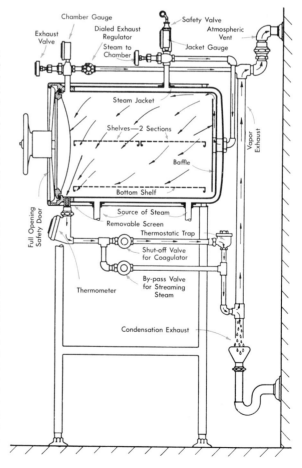

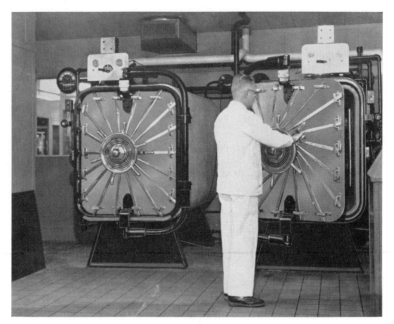

Figure 12–5

Rectangular autoclaves for steam sterilization in a large pharmaceutical manufacturing establishment. Note the heavy steel doors swinging easily on trunions, the steel door-fasteners simultaneously manipulated by the central wheel, and the gauges recording time, temperature, and pressure. Operation is almost wholly automatic and electrically controlled. These enormous autoclaves are no different in principle from the physician's tiny office model seen in Figure 12–6. (Courtesy of Wilmot Castle Co., Rochester, N.Y.)

When steam is compressed its temperature rises far above that of boiling water or of live steam. The temperature depends on the pressure, commonly expressed in pounds to the square inch. Steam under pressure hydrates rapidly and therefore coagulates very efficiently. Also, it brings about chemical changes somewhat like digestion, called *hydrolysis*. These characteristics give it special advantages in sterilization.

Substitution of an autoclave for an oven by admitting steam only to the jacket and keeping the chamber dry is not advisable when sterilization is necessary because the temperature thus achieved (100 C) does not kill spores. The dryness of such an atmosphere may actually preserve some pathogens that would be quickly killed in a moist atmosphere.

Indicators. Many institutions always include some sort of indicator inside bundles being sterilized. These may be: (1) *Dyes* that change color if the necessary temperature has been maintained for the required time. For example, on glassware and bundles, labels are placed that read NOT STERILE before autoclaving or after insufficient autoclaving but read STERILE if sterilization has been fully effective. Another device, similar in principle, is cellulose tape having on it a chemical indicator that changes color when properly heated in the autoclave. (2) *Wax pellets* that melt only at the necessary temperature but that may not indicate lapse of time. (3) Strips of paper containing *bacterial spores*. In method 3, after the sterilizing procedure the strips are dropped into broth in culture tubes. If the sterilizer has been properly operated, these broth cultures should remain

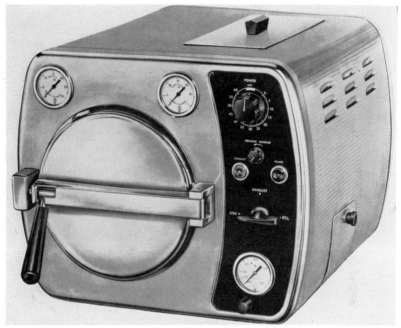

Figure 12–6

A small, rapidly acting autoclave for the physician's or dentist's office. This is controlled by a single knob and has automatic timing. The thermometer is in the waste steam line where the lowest temperatures occur, thus allowing a margin of safety in measuring autoclaving temperature. The door cannot be opened if there is any steam pressure inside. Operation is almost entirely automatic and electrically controlled. (Courtesy of Pelton and Crane Co., Charlotte, N.C.)

sterile, even after seven days of incubation, since all the spores have been killed. This method does not give immediate indication of faulty operation, but it does constitute an absolute and permanent record.

Some modern autoclaves have a self-recording thermometer that plots the temperature the instrument has reached and the time of sterilization required for each "load." A permanent record provided in this way often proves to be very valuable.

By first allowing all the air in the chamber of the autoclave to escape and be replaced by the incoming steam, the spaces in the interior of masses of material may be brought quickly into contact with the steam. The escape of air is more than merely important, it is absolutely essential since sterilization depends on the water vapor. Whenever air is trapped in the autoclave, sterilization is inefficient. One must be sure that:

1. All the air is allowed to escape and is replaced by steam.
2. The pressure of the steam reaches at least 15 pounds to the square inch and remains there. (In most automatic autoclaves it is now 18 pounds, permitting less time of actual sterilization.)
3. The thermometer reads at least 121 C without downward fluctuation for at least 15 minutes. (Less time is required when 18 pounds pressure is used.)

If these conditions are met and if the masses or bundles are well separated and not too large, the autoclaved material will be sterile.

WRONG METHOD

RIGHT METHOD

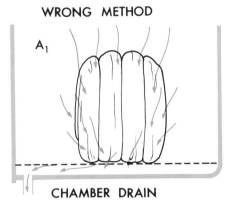

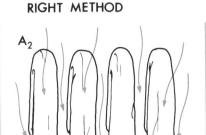

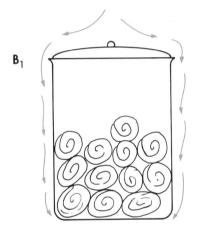

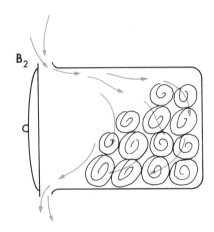

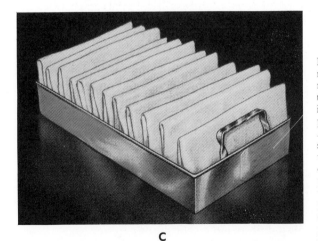

C

Figure 12–7

Figures A_1, A_2 and C show arrangements in the autoclave. B_1 and B_2 may be in the autoclave or another type of packs sterilizer. A_1 shows improper arrangement of four packs, tightly held together, while A_2 shows the same packs slightly separated from each other. Steam will now permeate the entire mass quickly, and in the much shorter period of exposure needed there will be no oversterilized outer portions. B_1 and B_2 indicate the correct and the incorrect ways of placing jars of dressings in the sterilizer. Right side up, even with the cover removed, all air is trapped within the jar. Resting on its side, with the cover held loosely in place, air will drain out and steam will promptly take its place, as indicated by the arrows. (*Surgical Supervisor.* Courtesy of American Sterilizer Co.) C, the instrument sterilizer tray with wire-mesh bottom makes an excellent container for gloves. The glove packs should rest on edge in the sterilizer, stacked loosely, never more than one tier deep. (Underwood: Textbook of Sterilization. American Sterilizer Co.)

The actual amount of water present as steam in the pressure chamber is usually small; consequently, the articles sterilized are not wet with much condensed steam when they are removed from the autoclave. Many autoclaves are arranged so that all the steam may be removed by vacuum after the sterilization period, thus preventing dampening the articles inside.

The modern automatic autoclave, as shown in Figure 12–5, or with a round chamber as used in most smaller laboratories, has the following settings:

1. Manual—used when the electrical power is off. The operator must then set and time all cycles.
2. Slow exhaust—used for a *wet load*, for media.
3. Fast exhaust—used for killing microorganisms quickly on glassware that is to be washed.
4. Fast exhaust and dry—used for pipettes, Petri plates, or dressings, a so-called *dry load*.

After he closes the door tightly, the operator sets this autoclave to the desired setting (e.g., to fast exhaust, to kill organisms, before washing glassware), to the time interval that is desired for the maximum preset temperature and pressure, and to ON. Lights go on as the autoclaving moves from pretimed cycle to cycle. Finally a bell rings and the operator turns the setting to OFF and opens the door carefully.

The exhaust trap inside the autoclave must always be cleaned before starting a load since dirt in the trap may delay the time needed for the various cycles.

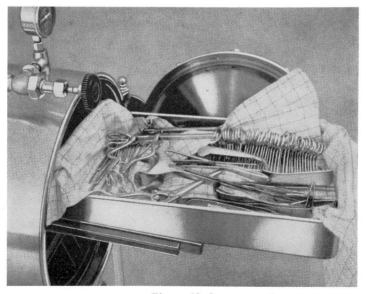

Figure 12–8

One method for preparation of instruments for autoclave sterilization. The muslin sheet or towel in the bottom of the tray provides a soft resting place for delicate scalpel blades and other small instruments. The protection thus afforded justifies the effort. (*Surgical Supervisor*. Couresty of American Sterilizer Co.)

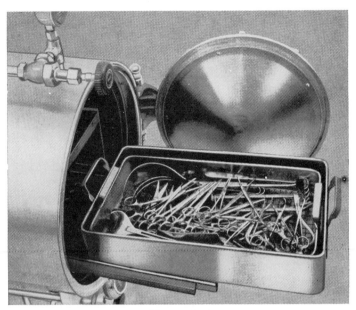

Figure 12–9

Method of sterilizing and washing used instruments. The lower tray is filled with water. The instruments in the perforated tray thus soak in hot water while being autoclaved. At expiration of the autoclaving time the pressure is suddenly released, permitting the water to boil violently, thus subjecting the instruments to a strong flushing action. (*Surgical Supervisor*. Courtesy of American Sterilizer Co.)

Since the effectiveness of an autoclave is dependent upon the penetration of steam into all articles and substances, the preparation of packs of dressings is very important and the correct placement of articles in the autoclave is essential to adequate sterilization (Figs. 12–7 and 12–8).

Cleaning Instruments.   When sterilizing solutions, the pressure must be allowed to fall gradually so that the solutions will not boil. If the pressure falls rapidly, violent boiling occurs. Advantage is taken of this fact in autoclaving used surgical instruments. They are immersed in water in a perforated tray. After autoclaving the pressure is reduced suddenly. The water boils violently and washes the instruments clean (Fig. 12–9).

CLEANING BY ULTRASONIC ENERGY.   Machines are now available for cleaning surgical instruments, syringes, and so on, by extremely rapid (ultrasonic) vibrations. These can clean and dry hundreds of instruments (perfectly) every five to ten minutes. They do not sterilize.

STERILIZATION WITHOUT HEAT

For many years heat was the only dependable and practicable means of destroying bacterial endospores. At least three other means of killing microorganisms and bacterial endospores have been developed to the stage of practical application. These are the gas *ethylene oxide*, the vapors of *beta-propiolactone*, and certain *electromagnetic radiations* (especially electron beams or cathode rays). The method of ultrasonic vibrations, although quite effective in destroying certain microorganisms, is not a practical means for large scale sterilization. Besides, it produces a heating effect. At present, we can only dream of an ultrasonic "dishwasher" that sanitizes dirty dishes, preferably without any water!

Sterilization with Radiations

Some of the electromagnetic radiations mentioned in Chapter 8 are in use or are being developed for general sterilization purposes.

ULTRAVIOLET LIGHT. This is satisfactory for sterilization of air in some operating rooms and on smooth surfaces. It has virtually no power of penetration. Ultraviolet lamps are used to suppress surface-growing molds and other organisms in meat packing houses, bakeries, storage warehouses, and so on. Sunlight is also a good, inexpensive source of ultraviolet rays. It can induce genetic mutations in microorganisms. In excess, it can cause cancer.

X-RAYS. X-rays penetrate well but require very high energy and are relatively costly and inefficient for sterilizing. Their use is therefore mostly for medical and experimental work and the production of microbial mutants.

NEUTRONS. Neutrons are very effective in killing microorganisms but are expensive and hard to control, and they involve dangerous radioactivity.

ALPHA RAYS (PARTICLES). Alpha rays are effective bactericides but have almost no power of penetration.

BETA RAYS (PARTICLES). Beta rays have a slightly greater power of penetration than alpha rays but are still not practical for use in sterilization.

GAMMA RAYS. These rays are high-energy radiations now mostly emitted from radioactive isotopes such as Cobalt[60], which is a readily available by-product of atomic fission. Gamma rays resemble x-rays in many respects. The U.S. Army Quartermaster Corps has used gamma rays and other radiations to sterilize food for military use. X-rays or gamma rays must be applied in 2 mrad* to 4 mrad doses to become a reliable sterilizing treatment of foods. Foods exposed to effective radiation sterilization, however, undergo changes in color, chemical composition, taste, and sometimes even odor. Only slowly are these problems being overcome by temperature control and oxygen removal.

CATHODE RAYS (ELECTRONS). They are used mainly to kill microorganisms on surfaces of foods, fomites and industrial articles. Since electrons have limited powers of penetration, they are at present of only minor usefulness for surgical sterilization. However, as a result of research on proper dosage and packaging, cathode rays are being developed for general purposes such as food processing. This may completely revolutionize the food canning and frozen food industries as well as surgical sterilization techniques.

Pharmaceutical and medical products are adequately sterilized by treatment with a radiation dose of 2.5 mrad. The Association of the British Pharmaceutical Industry has reported that benzylpenicillin, streptomycin sulfate and other antibiotics are satisfactorily sterilized by this method.

---

*One mrad is 1/1000 of a rad. A rad is 100 ergs of absorbed energy per gram of absorbing material (retained by matter).

In addition, package radiation at dose levels of 2.5 mrad has become common procedure for the sterilization of disposable syringes, needles, rubber gloves, tubing, and so on.

Sterilization with Chemicals

ETHYLENE OXIDE.   This is a gas with the formula CH_2CH_2O. The gas is applied in special autoclaves under carefully controlled conditions of temperature and humidity. Since pure ethylene oxide is explosive and irritating in use, it is generally mixed with carbon dioxide or other diluent in various proportions: 10 per cent ethylene oxide to 90 per cent carbon dioxide (sold as Carboxide); 20 per cent ethylene oxide to 80 per cent carbon dioxide (sold as Oxyfume); 11 per cent ethylene oxide to 89 per cent halogenated hydrocarbons (sold as Cryoxcide and Benvicide). Each preparation is effective when properly used. Oxyfume is very rapid in action but is more inflammable and more toxic than Carboxide; however, Carboxide requires high pressure. Cryoxcide is more toxic and more expensive, but it is more convenient and requires less pressure. All cost more and take longer than autoclaving with steam.

Ethylene oxide is generally measured in terms of milligrams of the pure gas per liter of space. For sterilization, concentrations of 450 to 1000 mg of gas/liter are necessary. Concentrations of 500 mg of gas/liter are generally effective in about four hours at approximately 130 F (58 C) and a relative humidity of about 40 per cent. Variations in any one of these factors require adjustments of the others. For example, if the concentration of gas is increased to 1000 mg/liter the time may be reduced to two hours. Increases in temperature, up to a limit, also decrease the time required. At a relative humidity of 30 per cent, the action of ethylene oxide is about ten times as rapid as at 95 per cent. The use of ethylene oxide, although as simple as autoclaving, generally requires special instruction centering around each particular situation. Manufacturers provide specific instructions for the use of their products. At present ethylene oxide is used largely by commercial companies that dispense sterile packages of a variety of products.

In general, seven steps are involved after loading and closing the sterilizing chamber:

1. Draw out nearly all air with a vacuum pump.
2. Admit a measured amount of water vapor.
3. Admit the required amount of ethylene oxide gas mixture.
4. Raise the temperature to the required degree.
5. Hold for required time; turn off heat.
6. Draw out gas with vacuum pump.
7. Admit filtered and sterilized air to the chamber.

A fully automatic ethylene oxide autoclave requiring only proper supervision is available (Fig. 12–10).

BETA-PROPIOLACTONE (BPL).   At about 20 C this substance is a colorless liquid. It has a sweet but very irritating odor. It is unstable at room temperatures but may be stored at 4 C (icebox) for months without deterioration. Aqueous solutions effectively inactivate some viruses, including poliomyelitis and rabies, and also kill bacteria and bacterial spores. The vapors, in a concentration of about 1.5 mg. of the lactone per liter

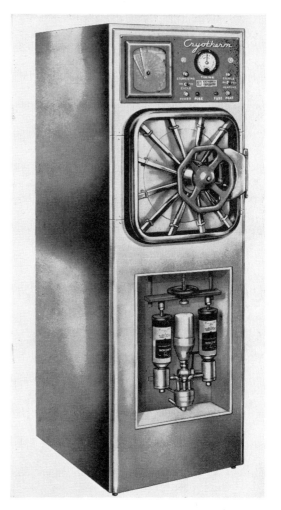

Figure 12–10

Autoclave arranged for sterilization by sporicidal ethylene oxide gas (Cryoxcide). Below the steel door are seen the containers of gas and a water inlet so arranged that the vapors can be mixed and humidified (much as gasoline, air, and water vapor are mixed in a modern automobile carburetor) before admission of the sterilizing vapor mixture to the chamber of the autoclave. Above the door are the dials controlling sterilizing temperature and time, vacuum pump, gas and humidity inlet, and a maximum and minimum recording thermometer. The operation is almost completely automatic. (Courtesy of American Sterilizer Co.)

of air with a high relative humidity (75 to 80 per cent), at about 25 C kill spores in a few minutes. Decrease in temperature, humidity, or concentration of the lactone vapors increases the time required to kill the spores.

Beta-propiolactone is not inflammable under ordinary conditions of use. It is, however, very irritating and may cause blisters if allowed in contact with skin for more than a few minutes. It is not injurious to most materials. It appears to act by forming chemical compounds with cell proteins. The necessity for high humidities during its use and also its cost are disadvantages. Its activity at room temperatures is a distinct advantage. It does not penetrate as well as ethylene oxide and is therefore more suitable for disinfecting surfaces, such as in rooms, buildings, and furniture, by fumigation.

Aqueous solutions of BPL can be used to sterilize biological materials such as virus vaccines, tissues for grafting and plasma.

Sterilization by Filtration

Many fluids may be sterilized without the use of heat, chemicals, or radiations. This is accomplished mechanically by passing the fluids to be

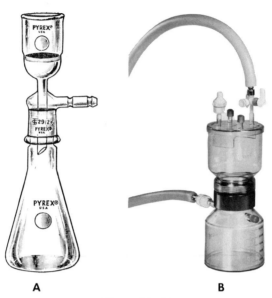

A   B

Figure 12–11

A, Bacteriological filter of the sintered-glass type. (Courtesy of Corning Glass Works.) B, Sterifil aseptic filtration system. C, Sterifil aseptic filtration system disassembled, showing all parts of the unit. D, Solutions may be introduced from a syringe by inserting a needle through a rubber cap covering one of the ports. E, Solutions may be introduced aseptically through a sterilized 2-way valve inserted in a port and connected by an adapter to sterilized ¼ tubing. F, As an alternate to a vacuum pump, a metal syringe may be used to pull solutions through the filter. One Receiver Flask side arm is stuffed with cotton in the conventional manner, the other is capped. (B-F, Courtesy of Millipore Filter Corporation.)

(Figure 12–11C on opposite page; D, E, F, on page 210.)

sterilized through very fine filters. Only fluids of low viscosity that do not contain numerous fine particles in suspension (silt, erythrocytes, and so on), which would clog the filter pores, can be satisfactorily sterilized in this way. The method is applicable to fluids that are destroyed by heat and cannot be sterilized in any other way, such as fluids and medications for hypodermic or intravenous use, culture media, especially tissue culture media and its components such as serum.

Several types of filters are in common use. Of these, the Seitz filter, consisting of a mounted asbestos pad, is perhaps best known. Other filters consist of diatomaceous earth, the Berkefeld filter; porcelain, the Chamberland-Pasteur filters; and sintered glass of several varieties. A widely used sintered glass filter is shown in Figure 12–11. Some sintered-glass-type filters consist of a tubelike arrangement that sucks up fluid around all sides of the tube into a teflon-hose-connected receiving flask. The advantage of this is that the filter is very inexpensive and can be thrown away when it clogs up.

A widely used and practical filter is the membrane, or molecular, or Millipore filter. It is available in a great variety of pore sizes, ranging from 0.45μm for virus studies to 0.01μm. These filters consist of paper-thin, porous membranes of material resembling cellulose acetate (plastic). One common form of these special filters is shown in Figure 9–12. In general, the porcelain, clay, paper, or plastic filtering element is held in some

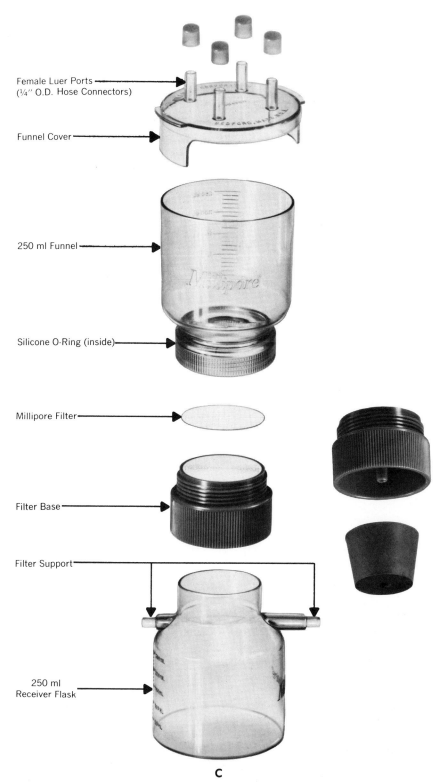

Female Luer Ports
(¼" O.D. Hose Connectors)

Funnel Cover

250 ml Funnel

Silicone O-Ring (inside)

Millipore Filter

Filter Base

Filter Support

250 ml
Receiver Flask

C

Figure 12–11C

D   E

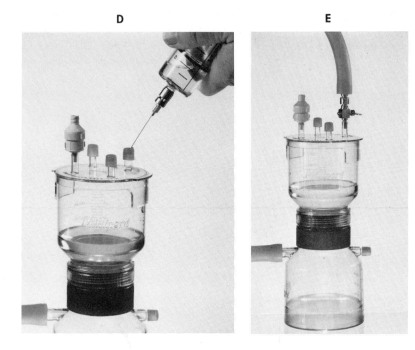

F

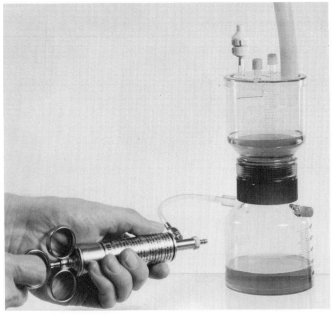

Figure 12–11, D, E, F

supporting structure and the fluid to be filtered is forced through the filter into a receptacle by a vacuum or by pressure. The filter, support, and receptacle are assembled and autoclaved before use. Further details concerning these procedures need not be given here, since sterilization by filtration is rarely used without adequate information pertaining to the specific filtration problem, which in itself would show the advantages of one type of filter over another.

Supplementary Reading

(See the list of readings following Chapter 15.)

Disinfection

13

It would be impossible to include here a discussion of all the chemicals used for disinfection. There are too many, and new ones are brought to the market every day. An attempt will be made to group some of these chemicals and to discuss those most commonly used.

Table 13–1 shows an evaluation of common types of germicides against bacteria. The chart may be useful to the reader, who should remember that, in general, pure compounds have been used in the studies on which Table 13–1 is based, whereas in commercial usage disinfectants are often compounded and mixed for greater effectiveness.

Table 13–1. Partial List of Commonly Used Antiseptics and Disinfectants*

NAMES	REPRESENTATIVE PREPARATIONS	USES
Halogens		
Chlorine	Gaseous element	Disinfection of drinking water.
Chlorinated lime	Bleaching powder	Excreta, etc.
Diluted sodium hypo-chlorite (NaOCl)	Dakin's solution	Wound lavage.
Halazone†	4 to 8 mg/liter	Disinfection of drinking water.
Iodine	2% aqueous solution (with KI)	Topical; abrasions, etc.
	2 to 7% alcoholic solution	Topical; abrasions, etc.
Povidone-iodine (Betadine†)	Surfactant iodophore; 1% aqueous solution	Topical.
Heavy Metals		
Ammoniated mercury	5% ointment	Topical; skin infections.
Merbromin (Mercuro-chrome†)	1 to 2% aqueous solution	Topical; skin and mucous membranes.
Phenylmercuric nitrate	1:1,500 solution or ointment	Topical; skin.

Table 13–1 continued on opposite page.

Table 13–1.   Partial List of Commonly Used Antiseptics and Disinfectants*
(Continued)

Nitromersol (Metaphen†)	1:1,000 aqueous solution	Environmental.
	1:1,500 aqueous solution	Topical; skin and mucous membranes.
	1:2,500 alcoholic solution	As above.
Thimerosal (Merthiolate†)	1:5,000 aqueous solution	Environmental; skin infections.
	1:1,000 alcoholic solution	Mucous membranes.
Fused silver nitrate (AgNO₃)	"Styptic pencil"	Topical; caustic.
Silver nitrate	1% aqueous solution	Topical; prevents ophthalmia neonatorum.
Silver protein conjugate (Argyrol†)	3 to 5% aqueous solution	Topical; skin and mucous membranes.
(Protargol†)	0.05 to 5.0% aqueous solution	As above.
(Neo-Silvol†)	5% aqueous solution	As above.
Oxidizing Agents		
Hydrogen peroxide (H₂O₂)	2 to 4% aqueous solution	Topical: skin and mucous membranes
Potassium permanganate (KMnO₄)	1:5,000 aqueous solution	As above.
Sodium perborate	2% (saturated) solution	Topical; oral antiseptic.
Phenolic Compounds		
Saponated cresol (Creolin†)	2 to 5% aqueous solution	Environmental only.
	0.25 to 0.5% aqueous solution (surfactant)	Skin. Wash with water promptly.
Hexachlorophene (pHisoHex†)	0.5 to 3.0% soaps	Topical; handwash, etc. Wash with water promptly.
Quaternary Ammonium Compounds	(Disinfectant surfactants) 1:1,000 to 1:5,000 aqueous solution; ointments; lotions	Environmental; also skin and mucous membranes; microbistatic; rinse well after use.
Benzalkonium chloride (Zephiran†) Cetylpyridinium Cl (Ceepryn† Cl)		
Alcohols		
Ethanol, Isopropanol	70% aqueous solution	Topical; skin. Utensils injured by H₂O.
Undecylenic Acid		
Copper undecylenate (Decupryl†)	Ointment, topical	For the skin, especially for fungal infection.
Undecylenic acid (Undecap†)	1 to 10% ointment, topical	
Zinc undecylenate (Desenex,† Undesol†)	5% ointment, alcoholic solution, powder, topical	
Various Dyes		
Crystal violet, etc.	0.5 to 1.0 aqueous solution	Topical; skin and mucous membranes

THE HALOGENS

The halogens get their name from a Greek word (*halos*) meaning salt; hence, *halogen* means salt-former. They readily form salts, e.g., sodium chloride. Three of the halogens (chlorine, iodine, and bromine) are among the best bactericidal agents. They act mainly by forming protein-halogen (saltlike) compounds in living cells and they kill quickly. Bromine is rarely used because of its cost and toxicity. In a special category is the most reactive of the halogens, namely, fluorine. As sodium fluoride it is frequently used as an additive in community water supplies to prevent dental caries. It is not commonly used for disinfectant purposes.

Halogens are effective as oxidants. For example,

$$Cl_2 + H_2O \rightleftharpoons HCl + HOCl$$

Hypochlorous acid (HOCl) is a strong oxidizing agent.

Chlorine

CHLORINE GAS.   Although highly effective, Cl_2 is very toxic and requires special equipment for its use. It is widely used to disinfect municipal water supplies and swimming pools.

CHLORIDE OF LIME.   Chloride of lime, or calcium hypochlorite (CaOCl), is used in a 1 to 5 per cent aqueous solution and it is an excellent general disinfectant. It releases chlorine, which when free in appreciable concentrations is toxic for all living things. Although the presence of extraneous organic material somewhat decreases the efficiency of chloride of lime (why?), it is still effective to use on feces from a patient who has an intestinal infection. Usually a 5 per cent solution is used. It is mixed with an estimated equal amount of feces or urine. The mixture is allowed to stand in a covered container (such as a pail) for one hour, before being discarded into the sewer.

Although some local and state health authorities permit the disposal of excreta from patients with enteric infections directly into the sewerage system, it seems a better practice to disinfect the excreta before disposal because of the danger of spattering and of possible leaks or other defects in plumbing systems.

SODIUM HYPOCHLORITE.   Sodium hypochlorite (NaOCl) solution (5.25 per cent) is available in every grocery store as a laundry bleach. (Clorox and Purex, or crystals of Comet are representative products.) This is one of the most generally useful, convenient forms of chlorine, and it is a highly efficient disinfectant and deodorant. Unless diluted, it is irritating to skin and mucous membranes and is used mainly for laundry, floors, and inanimate objects of all sorts. It can be used to disinfect drinking water, to deodorize, and for many other purposes. Manufacturers generally give full details for use on the label. It may leave an odor on the hands.

ORGANIC COMPOUNDS OF CHLORINE.   Azochloramide and chloramine-T, unstable organic compounds of chlorine, and monochloramide (NH₂Cl) are for many purposes more convenient than chloride of lime or sodium hypochlorite. Their action is slower. They and several other similar compounds that give off free chlorine are useful for general

Chloramine-T

sanitization in dairies, restaurants, and similar places. The manufacturers' directions for use are reliable.

Iodine

This is a very useful and effective bactericide. Iodine in the form of an alcoholic solution (tincture) is often used for cuts and abrasions, disinfection of clinical thermometers, and preparation of the skin for surgery. For the latter purpose a strong skin antiseptic with low surface tension is used: 10 g of I_2 with 5 g of KI in 5 ml of H_2O and 90 ml of 95 per cent alcohol. Although aqueous solutions of iodine have a high surface tension, they appear to be very effective for skin abrasions, and the irritating effect of alcohol is avoided. A commonly available preparation for such uses is 2 per cent iodine in 70 per cent alcohol (mild solution of iodine).

Iodine is very poisonous and can cause serious burns of the skin unless used properly. The 2 per cent alcoholic solution should be applied in one coat, allowed to air dry, and then covered with sterile gauze. When used for surgery, iodine solution should not be allowed to run down the sides of the body so that it can concentrate under the patient. If the patient is lying on a rubber mat on an operating room table, this concentration of iodine on the back can cause serious burns.

ORGANIC COMPOUNDS OF IODINE.   Like chlorine, iodine is available in organic combination. This is sold in solutions containing a surface-tension reducer. These may serve for most of the purposes for which solutions of chlorine are used. Being less volatile, the iodine remains longer, and has less odor, and one can tell by the color of the solution approximately how much iodine remains in it. In so-called *iodophors*, organic compounds, iodine is loosely combined with some surface-active agent. *Wescodyne* and *Ioclide*, representative iodophors, are not irritating to the skin (except in cases of iodine hypersensitivity) but may cause a slight, temporary tan discoloration if used in strong solutions. These products are probably sporicidal under certain conditions of use. Other iodophors are *Betadine*, *Hi-Sine*, and *Iosan*.

Fluorine

In the form of sodium fluoride (NaF), fluorine is used in the treatment of dental caries. It is also often added to otherwise deficient water supplies (fluoridation) to reduce tooth decay in children. We find fluorine also in the Freons (as coolants in refrigeration) or in plastics such as Fluon or Teflon. There are many ways by which fluorine reacts with and disintegrates organic compounds and thus destroys microorganisms, especially fungi. Yet, except for the incidental use in water, fluorine is not practical for disinfection purposes. Thus, only two of the halogen elements, chlorine and iodine, are commonly used as antiseptics and disinfectants.

COMPOUNDS OF HEAVY METALS

Heavy metals are commonly used in two forms of compound: inorganic and organic. Examples of each follow.

BICHLORIDE OF MERCURY.   This is a common inorganic form of mercury compound. It was formerly widely employed in dilutions of between 1:1000 and 1:5000, but has been generally replaced by other, more efficient disinfectants.

ORGANIC COMPOUNDS OF MERCURY.   Several organic compounds of mercury are used for disinfection of skin and for superficial applications. Among these are *Mercurochrome, Merthiolate, Metaphen*, and phenyl-mercuric nitrate. These organic forms of mercury are less irritating and less coagulative than bichloride of mercury. They act mainly bacteriostatically, especially when the amount of mercury is small. Their action can be reversed by agents that precipitate mercury, especially sulfur compounds like sodium thioglycollate and hydrogen sulfide:

$$H_2S + Hg = H_2 + HgS$$

No doubt the artificial red color of some organic mercurials makes a child feel proud of his "battle scars," but many bacteriologists question the actual benefit derived from the application of these disinfectants to a wound.

SILVER NITRATE.   Silver nitrate is most frequently used as a 1 per cent aqueous solution in the eyes of newborn babies to prevent gonorrheal (and other) infection (ophthalmia neonatorum). The excess silver nitrate solution must be carefully removed from the eyes by washing with physiologic saline solution after instillation. If the silver nitrate is allowed to remain, it may cause serious irritation to the delicate membranes of the eye. The use of silver nitrate has markedly decreased the number of cases of blindness caused by ophthalmia neonatorum. In some cities the use of penicillin has been substituted for or combined with silver nitrate, with promising results. The use of one or the other is generally required by law for newborn infants.

Fused silver nitrate is also used in the form of a pencil as a styptic, to stop bleeding. This is a fine way to keep your minor cuts aseptic.

ORGANIC COMPOUNDS OF SILVER.   *Argyrol* is an example of an organic (protein) compound of silver. It is used occasionally in 5 to 20 per cent aqueous solutions for the treatment of infections of the mucous membranes of the eye, nose, and urethra. In the concentrations mentioned it is nonirritating on mucous membranes. Other organic silver compounds sometimes used are *Silvol, Neo-Silvol*, and *Protargol*.

DETERGENTS AND QUATERNARY AMMONIUM DISINFECTANTS

Most household detergents are surface-tension reducers. For their activity, these depend on their ability to emulsify lipids (i.e., grease). Exceptions are certain "dry cleaners" that dissolve, adsorb, or decompose lipids. On the basis of their chemical structure the surface-tension reducing (surfactant) detergents are divided into three main groups: anionic, among which are *soaps* and some organic (alkyl) sulfates such as sodium lauryl sulfate, in which the surface-tension reducing property resides in the negatively charged part of the molecule, the anion; nonionic, mainly complex ethers and polyglycerol soaplike compounds represented by Tween 80; cationic, the *quaternary ammonium chloride derivatives*, commonly called "quats," among which are such compounds as Zephiran, Ceepryn, Phemerol Chloride, Diaparene Chloride, C.T.A.B., and Roccal. Some of the anionic detergents have limited disinfectant properties, but the most important detergents, when disinfection is the consideration, are the cationic quats. These combine both disinfectant and surface-tension reducing properties in the cation.

$$\left[\begin{array}{c} R_1 \\ | \\ R-N-R_2 \\ | \\ R_3 \end{array} \right]^+ \cdot Cl^- \qquad \left[\begin{array}{c} O \\ \| \\ H_{25}C_{12}-S-O- \\ \| \\ O \end{array} \right]^- Na^+$$

I   II

I, General formula for cationic ammonium chloride derivatives (quats). In ammonium chloride, the central nitrogen (N) of ammonia has four hydrogen atoms attached, but in the quats these are replaced by various organic radicals (R) such as $-CH_3$, and a chlorine atom is added. II, Formula of an anionic detergent, sodium lauryl sulfate.

The quaternaries are used principally for general external purposes as disinfectants and sanitizing agents. They have many other important properties: they are only slightly injurious to animal tissues, they seem to be effective against many microorganisms in high dilutions, they are stable, they have no odor, they do not stain, they are not corrosive, they dissolve easily in water, and they are inexpensive.

In practice, the cationic quaternaries should never be mixed with anionics such as soaps because of the incompatible charges of the ions. For this reason quats are much less effective in "hard" waters and iron-rich waters; however, they tend to retain their activity in the presence of organic matter like pus, blood, or feces. There is good evidence that alcoholic solutions (tinctures) of quats are very effective against tubercle bacilli. Quats are of little known value against most fungi; some viruses rich in lipids may be susceptible to them.

SOAP

Household soap is a good detergent or cleansing agent, largely because it is a powerful surface-tension reducer. It is a highly effective emulsifier of fats and oils. It thus aids in the mechanical removal of bacteria, especially from oily surfaces like the skin. Many of the currently widely advertised detergents are not soap, but surface-tension reducers. Tide, Cheer, and Electra Sol (used in automatic dishwashers) are representative. They have cleaning and emulsifying properties like those of soap but are not disinfectants. An important ingredient in most of them was the potent surface-tension reducer alkyl benzene sulfonate ("ABS"). This refused to be decomposed by the microorganisms in sewage disposal plants. The result was pollution of rivers and lakes with detergents, as evidenced by excessive foaming, a major problem in sanitary engineering. First in Great Britain and then in the United States, the manufacturers of detergents were quietly urged by their governments to stop using "microorganisms-resistant" chemicals in their products. Today, the "foaming cleanser" actually foams less and is also inferior to the earlier product. It can, however, easily be decomposed by sewage microorganisms (i.e., is "biodegradable"), and can be safely disposed of by running the washing machine water into the sewer—our eventual fresh water supply. Polyphosphates such as sodium tripolyphosphate were subsequently used in many preparations sold on the market. However, phosphates too were found to be undesirable pollutants and are now being replaced.

Soap, in addition to being a surface-active detergent, is bactericidal to some degree. It is especially effective against *Treponema pallidum,* the cause of syphilis. This organism is rich in lipids. The disinfectant value of a soap depends to a great extent on the chemical nature of its fatty acid radical; i.e., what kind of fat it was made from.

PHENOLIC DISINFECTANTS

Phenol ("carbolic acid") is an efficient bactericide in a 1 to 2 per cent solution; however, it is so very corrosive to animal tissue, and, if used in the pure form, is so expensive that it is rarely used as such. Many derivatives of phenol are now available on the market. They are mainly coagulative in action. Pure phenol is used mainly as a standard for testing disinfectants. *"Crude carbolic,"* an impure phenol product, is useful for general purposes. It is apt to cause brown stains.

PHENOL DERIVATIVES. There are scores of these compounds, some of which have wide usefulness as disinfectants; others are too corrosive, too expensive, or otherwise not so useful. Most of these act in somewhat the same manner as phenol, i.e., probably by combined coagulative, toxic, and dissolving action. The exact mechanisms are not clear and differ with different compounds and probably with different species of microorganisms. Many of these compounds are surface-tension reducers and tend to remain adsorbed as thin films on surfaces to which they are applied. Their action is therefore prolonged compared with that of alcohols or halogens, which tend to volatilize quickly. Two general classes of phenol derivative may be noted: the *cresols,* which are like phenol with methyl ($-CH_3$) groups attached, and *bis-phenols,* which are composed of two phenol groups or phenol derivatives joined directly or through some other radical.

Cresols. These are more effective than pure phenol for most general purposes. Saponated solution of cresol (used in a 1 to 5 per cent solution) is a good example of an effective cresol disinfectant. The soapy solution

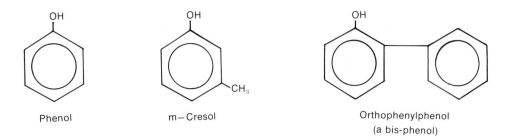

Phenol   m—Cresol   Orthophenylphenol
                                                      (a bis-phenol)

of cresol has a far lower surface tension than does the aqueous solution. This disinfectant is used for feces, soaking contaminated instruments, and general cleaning and disinfecting purposes. Cresols, like phenol, are corrosive to living tissue and are not used in prolonged contact with tissues. Several proprietary preparations similar to saponated cresol (for example, Lysol) are on the market. One great advantage of Lysol over some cresols commonly used is that it does not foam when used in 2 per cent solution for scrubbing and washing surfaces (see formulas above).

Bis-phenols.   Like the cresols, these retain much of their disinfectant action in the presence of soap and other surface-tension reducers and are commonly used in preparations containing surface-active compounds. Prominent among the bis-phenolic disinfectants are several made with hexachlorophene (see formula below). Various proprietary combinations of hexachlorophene with soap and other ingredients are Gamophen, Hex-O-San, pHisoHex, Surgi-Cen, Surofene, and so on. Hexachlorophene has been used in a great number of commercial antiseptics. pHisoHex, Fostex, pHisoderm, Hexagerm, and others are sometimes used as skin washes and shampoos. In some hospitals hexachlorophene took the place of topically used alcohol. For nurses or dentists who must wash their hands many times every day, or for patients' body care, hexachlorophene-containing preparations are less unpleasant to use than many more irritating, but perhaps more effective, antiseptics. Recent investigations concerning the high toxicity of hexachlorophene indicate that it is *absorbed through the intact skin* and may reach a level of 0.38 ppm in blood when used extensively on the body as in bathing babies. It has been shown to cause brain damage in rats. It is not advisable to use hexachlorophene in vaginal deodorants, nor to bathe infants in hexachlorophene washes. At least, it seems now that its use may become as controversial as that of DDT.

HEXACHLOROPHENE

Orthophenylphenol is used in proprietary mixtures such as *O-Syl. Chloro-thymol* is another phenol derivative that has disinfectant properties similar to those just mentioned. These bis-phenol preparations are said to be effective after surgical washup because they tend to sustain the disinfectant action on the skin. Opinions are divided on this. The use of any disinfectant must always be regarded as a supplement to, and not as a substitute for, cleanliness and aseptic technique.

DISINFECTANT SOAPS.   As stated earlier, phenol derivatives, especially cresols and bis-phenols, are often mixed with soaps. Such combinations appear to be fairly effective and there are several on the market. Several contain hexachlorophene; however, since hexachlorophene has relatively little effect on gram-negative bacteria, e.g., those that cause typhoid fever and various forms of infant enteritis, such preparations have limitations, especially in hospital nurseries and similar places. Soap, if present in excess, may coat the bacteria, displacing the disinfectant, and thus protecting the bacteria! Some residual surface action of the phenol derivative is maintained by daily use of the preparation. However, it is quickly removed by ordinary soap and water and alcohol washes. Phenolic compounds must not remain long in contact with the skin or other tissues, especially over large areas.

ALCOHOLS

ETHYL ALCOHOL.   This is used very widely as a skin disinfectant, for "cold sterilization" of instruments, and as a disinfectant for thermometers. It does not sterilize. When used mixed with water for disinfection, the most effective concentration of alcohol is near 70 per cent. The presence of water hydrates and thus aids coagulation by the alcohol, its principal action. It should be noted that near 100 per cent (200 proof), ethyl alcohol is not a good disinfectant, either externally or internally. Like bichloride of mercury, it forms protective coatings of coagulum around microorganisms.

The rapid application of ethyl alcohol to the skin prior to a hypodermic injection probably accomplishes nothing more than cleaning the area and removal of some of the surface bacteria. The time is undoubtedly too short for disinfection. An alcohol rinse or soak, following scrubbing of the hands before surgery, probably reduces the numbers of bacterial inhabitants to some degree. The use of ethyl alcohol as a solution for "cold sterilization" of instruments, syringes, or needles should not be practiced, except for special purposes, because spore-forming organisms or resistant viruses may be present. If thermometers are adequately wiped, or washed with soap and water to remove all organic material, and if these thermometers are then completely immersed for a minimum of ten minutes in 70 per cent ethyl alcohol, they will probably not transmit the bacterial pathogens commonly occurring in the mouth or rectum, especially if the alcohol contains 0.5 to 1.0 per cent iodine or one of the quaternary ammonium compounds. They are not necessarily sterile.

ISOPROPYL ALCOHOL.   Isopropyl alcohol ("rubbing alcohol") is commonly used in a 70 per cent solution and is as effective as ethyl alcohol for ordinary purposes, especially if fortified with iodine or another suitable disinfectant as mentioned. It is cheaper and more easily obtainable than ethyl alcohol.

PINE OIL

Derived by steam distillation from weathered pine boles and roots, this product is emulsified in water with soap or resin. It is effective against many gram-negative bacteria such as *Salmonella typhi* (phenol coefficient of 5), but has very limited bactericidal action against certain gram-positive pathogens. It is sometimes used for janitorial or household purposes on floors, walls, and bathrooms and has a pleasant piny odor. Several proprietary products containing it are available at household supply stores.

DYES

Dyes have been used as antibacterial agents for many years. Their effectiveness depends greatly on the concentration. In general, crystal violet or malachite green inhibits most gram-positive organisms, but not gram-negative bacteria. Crystal violet is also used as an antifungal agent. Acridine dyes (acriflavine) have a wide spectrum of antibacterial action; they are useful against infections caused by gram-positive organisms. Antibacterial dyes are commonly employed in selective culture media for preferential growth of the tubercle bacillus, *Escherichia coli, Brucella* species, and so on.

Dyes as disinfectants are not as practical as was once expected; however, their use led to the formulation of chemotherapy by Ehrlich (pages 223, 224) and the therapeutic applications of the sulfonamides, which originated with the dye Prontosil, employed first by Domagk (1895–1964; Nobel prize winner) in 1935.

FORMALIN

Formaldehyde is marketed in an aqueous solution of 37 to 40 per cent as Formalin. We do not think of Formalin as a disinfectant but rather as a preservative of dead animals in the laboratory. As such it is very effective but at times it is quite corrosive to the skin tissues of the hands of the students.

OXIDIZING AGENTS

Other useful antiseptics are H_2O_2 (hydrogen peroxide), used in 3 per cent solution for a mouthwash or gargle, and another oxidizing agent, potassium permanganate ($KMnO_4$). Since peroxides are strongly mutagenic, their use in the mouth should be discouraged; instead, plain salt water is highly recommended as a gargle. Warm salt water is very effective in oral hygiene. Sodium perborate and zinc peroxide are other oxidizing agents, used as antiseptics in the mouth and on the skin respectively.

AEROSOL SPRAYS

Not to be forgotten are "instant first-aid sprays" like Medi-Quik, UnBurn, Bactine, and others. Read the label of contents of these medications; the chemicals mentioned will be familiar if you have read this chapter.

STRENGTH OF DISINFECTANTS

PHENOL COEFFICIENT. One often hears a disinfectant spoken of as "strong" or "weak" or "mild." What do these terms mean? Do they refer to odor, caustic action, or bactericidal power? Certain kinds of disinfectants, especially aqueous solutions of substances chemically related to phenol, are often rated according to their bactericidal activity as compared with phenol itself. According to this system they are said to have a certain *phenol coefficient.* In the determination of a phenol coefficient the conditions of time, temperature, and concentration during the comparison are very carefully standardized according to specifications of the United States Food and Drug Administration. The standard procedure is based upon the rate at which a certain dilution (1 in 90) of pure phenol (carbolic acid) kills the cells of a certain strain of *Salmonella typhi* at 20 C in 10 minutes. If, under the standard conditions, a given disinfectant kills *S. typhi,* in a dilution of 1 in 180 as compared with phenol dilution of 1 in 90, it is said to have a phenol coefficient of 2 ($180 = 2 \times 90$) or, as a formula:

$$\text{phenol coefficient} = \frac{\text{dilution of disinfectant}}{\text{dilution of phenol}}$$

If a phenol coefficient is greater than 1, the disinfectant tested is better than phenol under the conditions of the test; if it is less than 1, the disinfectant is not as good as phenol.

This procedure is useful but gives a very limited and often inexact idea of the value or activity of a disinfectant. It does not test under "field conditions." For example, a given disinfectant may be 50 times as active as phenol against typhoid bacilli, yet almost worthless against staphylococci. Also, it may be very effective in aqueous solution, yet blood, sputum, or feces may completely inactivate it. Further, if the substance disinfects through corrosive action, is it safe to rely upon its effectiveness as compared with phenol, which acts largely through coagulation? Thus there are many problems connected with the evaluation of disinfectants.

"Practical" tests are more valuable procedures since they simulate practical conditions. For example, the disinfectant may be tested in feces or blood instead of in distilled water; it may be required to act against staphylococci, streptococci, anthrax bacilli, or other organisms instead of *Salmonella typhi.* It may be used at very low temperatures or at body temperatures, instead of at exactly 20 C, and it may be given little time or many hours to act instead of 5, 10, or 15 minutes. What would be its "phenol coefficient," or effectiveness, then?

Supplementary Reading

(See the list of readings following Chapter 15.)

Chemotherapy and Antibiotics

14

INTRODUCTION

One of the most important means of controlling microorganisms is by inhibition or complete suppression of their growth without quickly killing them as is done in sterilization by heat or in vigorous disinfection. When applied to bacteria, prolonged inhibition of growth is called *bacteriostasis;* to fungi, *fungistasis*, and so on. Inhibition of microorganisms is the basis of million-dollar industries and is of much value in clinical medicine. We may consider inhibition of microorganisms in three categories:

1. Inhibition of spoilage microorganisms by nonspecialized but ancient and reliable means such as the drying of foods, making hay, preserving foods in brines and syrups, refrigeration, and addition of acetic acid (vinegar) and other preservatives to certain foods.

2. Inhibition of contaminating microorganisms in culture media so that the organisms causing infections in the patient may be isolated and grown in the diagnostic laboratory. This has previously been discussed as *selective bacteriostasis*. Dyes and certain chemicals are commonly used as microbistatic agents in such situations. In cultivating viruses in cultures of living tissue cells, antibiotics such as penicillin, cycloheximide, and streptomycin are often added to the culture media. These have no effect on viruses but inhibit contaminating bacteria and fungi in the cultures.

3. Inhibition of microorganisms in the body of humans or lower animals (or plants) so that the normal defensive mechanisms, especially phagocytic cells of animals, can more readily clear the body of the invading microorganisms. This process is part of the general field of *chemotherapy* and is used in human and veterinary medicine and in horticulture.

CHEMOTHERAPY

As generally used today, this term means the treatment of infections by means of substances ("chemicals") or drugs that (ideally) in relatively minute concentrations kill or inhibit the growth of the infecting microorganisms but do not adversely affect the host. The term chemotherapy

223

was coined by Paul Ehrlich, the discoverer of the first antibacterial chemotherapeutic agent, active specifically against the spirochete, *Treponema
pallidum*, the cause of syphilis. The drug was an organic arsenic compound,
sold as salvarsan (606, or dioxydiaminoarsenobenzene dihydrochloride).

MECHANISM OF CHEMOTHERAPY.   Whereas older drugs such as
quinine (for malaria) and arsenic (for syphilis) were used on an entirely
empirical basis, most modern chemotherapeutic drugs depend on the fact
that the drug combines specifically with chemicals directly involved in
protein (enzyme) synthesis essential to the pathogen. In many instances
the enzyme, instead of combining with its normal substrate, combines
instead with the drug. The drug, to be effective in this way, must so
closely resemble the molecular form of the normal substrate (or *metabolite*) of the enzyme that the cell is "fooled" into accepting the drug instead
of the normal metabolite. The drug is said to be an *antimetabolite* or an
antagonist of the normal substrate.

As an example of a *metabolite antagonist* consider the chemical structure
of the drug sulfanilamide in comparison with para-aminobenzoic acid,
or PABA (Fig. 14–1). PABA is a normal portion of the molecule known
as the vitamin *folic acid*. Folic acid is in turn a vital part of an important
enzyme in many microbial cells. The structural resemblance between
PABA and sulfanilamide is perfectly clear even to one who is not an organic chemist. When sulfanilamide is given to a patient, the drug antago-
nizes (replaces) PABA in the folic acid in the cells of the infecting microorganism. The enzyme of which folic acid is a part "stops in its tracks"!
This is because the sulfonamide drug is an imposter. It takes the place of
PABA but cannot carry on its functions. The cell stops growing; however,
it remains alive. It is in a state of *microbistasis*. The result of this for the patient is explained later on.

The blocking action of the drug can often be reversed by providing,
for example, a generous dose of PABA, if the reversing agent is not too
long delayed. Clearly the organism is not dead, since it can be reactivated.

Although the action of some chemotherapeutic agents, including antibiotics, is not yet as fully clarified as the action of sulfonamide drugs,
many are known, on experimental bases, to act in a similar manner, i.e.,
through specific molecular combinations that produce microbistatic effects.
Each drug, however, probably acts on a different chemical entity in the
cell, and each drug is highly discriminatory in its action on different species
of cells.

CHEMOTHERAPY AND PHAGOCYTOSIS.   In spite of the fact that many
chemotherapeutic agents do not immediately *kill* the infecting organisms,
they are effective because *inhibition* of the microorganisms permits phagocytes to overpower them. Since the action of phagocytes is greatly facili-
tated and enhanced in the presence of specific antibodies, the value of
chemotherapeutic drugs is said to be heightened if the patient has some
specific antibodies in his blood. He may have them as a result of previous
infection or vaccination or because of the purposeful injection of specific
antiserum along with the chemotherapeutic drug.

This "pinpointed" sort of attack on microorganisms is in contrast to
the indiscriminate, broad combining power of nonspecific, general disinfectants like iodine, chlorine, or the cresols. These tend to form physicochemical combinations with almost anything and everything, from feces
and stable floors to human blood and tissues and will kill the host as readily
as the parasite.

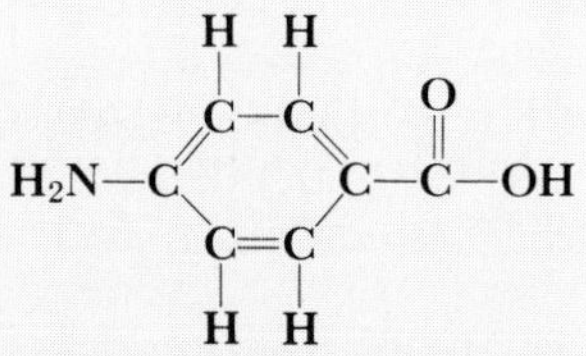

Para-aminobenzoic acid

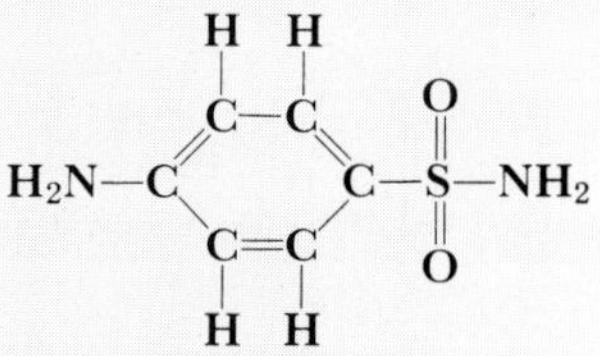

Sulfanilamide

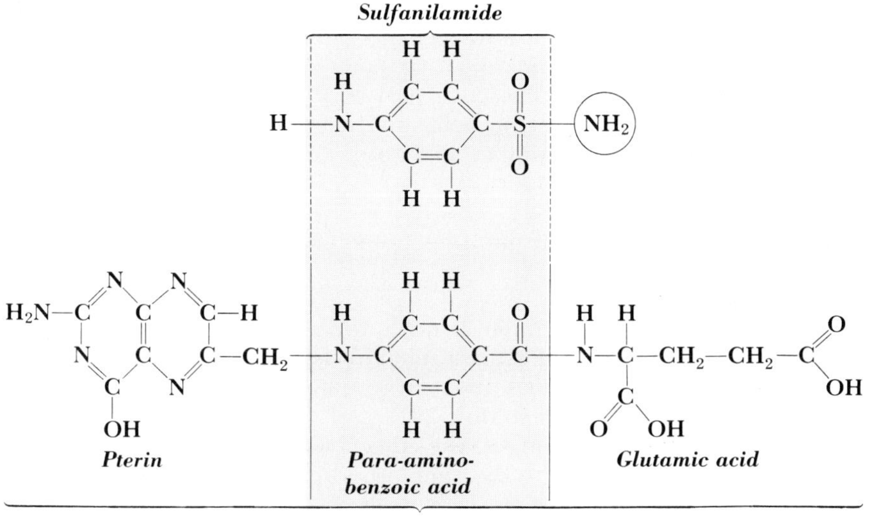

Sulfanilamide

Pterin

*Para-amino-
benzoic acid*

Glutamic acid

Folic (Pteroyl glutamic) acid

Figure 14-1

Structural resemblance between molecules of para-aminobenzoic acid (PABA) and sulfanilamide (above), and the potential antagonism of PABA by sulfanilamide in the folic acid molecule (below).

When sulfonamide replaces PABA in the folic acid molecule (pteroyl glutamic acid), the enzymic functions involving folic acid cease.

TOXIC EFFECTS. It is to be emphasized that chemotherapeutic agents that have been released for general use by the Food and Drug Administration generally are (fortunately!) much more toxic for the parasite than for the host. Thus, in minute doses that have insignificant, or at least not fatal, effects on the host, they help destroy the parasites. It is to be borne in mind, however, that excessive or improperly timed doses of antibiotics or other chemotherapeutic agents (including "miracle drugs") or administration by improper routes or without medical supervision in some instances can produce severe illness or death.

Some antibiotics are allergens (page 310) and patients may have severe allergic responses to them. Penicillin is notable but not by any means unique in this respect. Physicians generally inquire of patients whether they have had any previous bad reactions before giving antibiotics.

CHEMOTHERAPEUTIC AGENTS

There are many antimicrobial chemotherapeutic agents on the market. Today the most widely used are the sulfonamides (synthetic) and the antibiotics (obtained first from living organisms).

Sulfonamides

These were discovered about 1935 by Gerhard Domagk, a German chemist, who investigated the poisonous action of a certain aniline (coal tar) dye, Prontosil. This substance, in staining bacteria, eventually killed them. Sulfanilamide (from which virtually all sulfonamide drugs are derived) was found to be the active part of Prontosil. Although not a dye, sulfanilamide is derived from benzene (from coal tar) like many dyes, and acts in much the same way as Prontosil, i.e., by metabolite antagonism. Fundamentally, sulfonamides are a type of wholly synthetic antibiotic. The antibiotics so-called are, with few exceptions, obtained from bacteria, molds, and other living organisms. Some are artificially modified ("semisynthetic").

The group of "sulfa drugs," as they are often called, includes sulfathiazole, sulfadiazine, sulfamerazine, and many others. One of their chief drawbacks at first was their toxic side effects, but forms are now available that avoid these difficulties to a large extent (sulfisoxazole [Gantrisin], sulfaethylthiadiazole, and so on).

The discoveries leading to the clinical use of sulfonamide drugs gave an entirely new impetus to the chemotherapeutic treatment of infections. Many infections that previously had always been fatal or that always required a prolonged nonspecific treatment followed by a long convalescence could be cured rapidly with these drugs. In general, sulfonamides are more effective against gram-positive than against gram-negative organisms, but there are important exceptions, notably the gram-negative *Neisseria* (gonococcus, meningococcus). Usually sulfonamides are ineffective against viruses, rickettsias, fungi, and protozoa. Since the end of World War II sulfonamide drugs have been superseded by the antibiotics (such as penicillin, to be discussed) in many clinical situations, but they still have important uses, especially in urological infections, e.g., cystitis, and illustrate basic principles of chemotherapy.

DRUG-RESISTANCE OR DRUG-FASTNESS. As previously explained, microorganisms often undergo genetic mutations. These mutations generally result in alterations in enzyme production in the mutant cells. Let us suppose that mutation occurs in a few of the cells of a species of microorganisms (say, *Staphylococcus aureus*) that is multiplying in a patient being treated with penicillin. The mutation may (and, unfortunately, frequently does) so alter a few cells that they are no longer susceptible to the action of the penicillin. They are said to be *antibiotic-resistant* or *drug-fast*. Resistance may similarly develop in many species of microorganisms to any chemotherapeutic drug. The resistant cells proceed to grow, and finally predominate in spite of the drug. This predomination is very dangerous for the patient and for everyone around him who may acquire the organisms. The danger has been dramatically and tragically illustrated by the development of sulfonamide-resistant gonococci, streptomycin-resistant tubercle bacilli, penicillin-resistant staphylococci, and others.

The emergence of such drug-resistant microorganisms can be avoided to some degree by using adequate doses. This keeps a sufficient quantity of the chemotherapeutic drug in the bloodstream to affect even the most resistant members of the infecting organisms before they can start growing. Drug-fastness of infecting bacteria can be detected and measured by laboratory tests as described farther on.

MAINTENANCE OF BLOOD LEVELS. Since many chemotherapeutic drugs tend to be eliminated from the blood and tissues rather rapidly, the amounts in the blood (*blood levels*) tend to fall to levels at which the resistant individuals among the infecting bacteria can grow, unless the dose is repeated at proper intervals. If delayed, the patient soon has to combat a drug-fast infection. He may not survive. It is of the greatest importance, therefore, that any person responsible for giving repeated doses of such drugs sees that the patient receives the drug on time, in order that his blood levels may not fall dangerously low.

Antibiotic Substances[1]

The name antibiotic means "against life." Since antibiotics are most widely used to combat microorganisms, it might be more accurate to call them "anti*micro*biotics." The principal action of some antibiotics (e.g., penicillin) is bactericidal. Others (e.g., chloramphenicol) are bacteriostatic, as are the sulfonamides; they stop the growth of pathogenic microorganisms in infected animals so that phagocytes and other defensive mechanisms, with the help of antibodies, can dispose of the pathogens.

SOURCE OF ANTIBIOTICS. Unlike the artificially synthesized sulfonamide drugs, most antibiotics are produced in culture media during the growth of certain microorganisms, principally species of *Streptomyces* and *Bacillus*, and molds in the genera *Penicillium* and *Aspergillus*. Some well known antibiotics, with the names of the organisms from which they are obtained, are listed in Table 14–1. New antibiotics are constantly being sought and found in many plants and animals, terrestrial and marine (Table 14–2). In the manufacture of antibiotics the desired antibiotic-producing organism is cultivated in large tanks of suitable liquid medium at specified temperature, pH, aeration, etc., for a predetermined length of time. The culture is then centrifuged and filtered to remove the organisms. The filtered fluid, containing the antibiotic, is then subjected to purification and concentration processes. At length, these yield crystals of the pure antibiotic, which is tested for potency and sterility, then packaged and distributed. Later on, the organic chemist learns how to make many of the antibiotics synthetically.

USE OF ANTIBIOTICS. The action of the antibiotics varies greatly. Some may be given by mouth only; some are used in ointments only; others are suitable for intravenous or subcutaneous injection; and some are suitable for any route of administration. Some are effective chiefly against gram-positive organisms, some against gram-negative. Several have a wide range of activity. These last are called *broad-spectrum antibiotics*.

The specific uses, dosage, contraindications, and so on, of antibiotics are given in courses in pharmacology and materia medica, and will not

---

[1] A number of important bacteria are mentioned in this discussion, but it is not necessary that the student become familiar with them at this time. For quick reference look them up in the index.

Table 14–1.   Some Commonly Used Antibiotics*

ANTIBIOTICS†		CHARACTERISTICS‡	SOURCE
Common Name	Trade Name		
Penicillin	Penicillin G	Gram-positive bacteria;	*Penicillium notatum* and
	Oxacillin	*Treponema; Neisseria*	*Penicillium chrysogenum*
	Ampicillin		
	Methicillin		
Fumagillin		*Entamoeba histolytica*	*Aspergillus fumigatus*
Paromomycin	Humatin	*E. histolytica*	*Streptomyces rimosus*
Streptomycin		*Myco. tuberculosis;*	*Streptomyces griseus*
		Gram-negative bacteria	
Dihydrostreptomycin		Like streptomycin	Streptomycin; also some
			species of *Streptomyces*
Tetracycline	Achromycin	Broad-spectrum	Chlortetracycline
Oxytetracycline	Terramycin	Broad-spectrum	*Streptomyces rimosus*
Chlortetracycline	Aureomycin	Broad-spectrum	*Streptomyces aureofaciens*
Chloramphenicol	Chloromycetin	Broad-spectrum	*Streptomyces venezuelae*
Erythromycin	Ilotycin, Erythrocin	Broad-spectrum (not	*Streptomyces erythreus*
		Enterobacteriaceae)	
Carbomycin	Magnamycin	Like erythromycin	*Streptomyces halstedii*
Oleandomycin	Matromycin	Broad-spectrum	*Streptomyces antibioticus*
Neomycin B	Flavomycin	Mycobacteria	*Streptomyces fradiae*
Viomycin	Viocin	Like penicillin	*Str. floridae; Str. funiceus*
Oligomycin		Fungi of plants	*Str. diastatochromogenes*
Amphotericin B	Fungizone	*Candida* sp. &	*Streptomyces nodosus*
		other fungi	
Kanamycin	Kantrex	Broad-spectrum	*Streptomyces kanamyceticus*
Nystatin	Mycostatin	Pathogenic fungi	*Streptomyces noursei*
Cycloheximide	Actidione	Saprophytic fungi	*Streptomyces griseus*
Griseofulvin	Grifulvin	Pathogenic fungi	*Streptomyces griseus*
Bacitracin		Like penicillin	*Bacillus subtilis*
Polymyxin B	Aerosporin	Gram-positive bacteria	*Bacillus polymyxa*
Pyocyanin§		Miscellaneous	*Pseudomonas aeruginosa*
Novobiocin		Staphylococci, *Proteus*	*Streptomyces niveus*
Colistin (Polymyxin E)	Coly-Mycin	Gram-negative bacteria	*Bacillus colistinus*
Ristocetin	Spontin	Resistant staphylococci	*Nocardia lurida*
Vancomycin	Vancocin	Resistant staphylococci	*Streptomyces orientalis*
Demethylchlortetracycline	Declomycin	Broad-spectrum	{ Synthetic; also from { *Streptomyces aureofaciens*
Cephalosporin	Keflin (cephalothin)	Against gram-pos. and	*Cephalosporium*
		gram-neg. bacteria	mold
Isoniazid	Nydrazid	Specific against	Synthetic
		tubercle bacillus	

*Several not listed here are valuable commercially, agriculturally and horticulturally.
†Several of these antibiotics are in reality mixtures consisting of related compounds such as the penicillins, polymyxin A, B, C, D, carbomycin A and B, the rifamycins, cephalosporins, and so on.
‡Not necessarily the only activity.
§Not used medicinally. One of the first known antibiotic substances.

be detailed here. However, the student should be aware of several factors that may cause failure of a particular antibiotic or "antibiotic drug combination" to help the patient to overcome infection. These are: (1) Insufficient or wrong dosage; (2) drug resistance of the microorganism; (3) bacterial "persistence;" (4) poor host defense; (5) drug inactivation by the host's protein or flora; (6) poor penetration of the drug into tissues or cells; (7) toxicity; and (8) allergy to the drug.

Table 14-2 Some Antimicrobial Agents Not Yet in General Use

NAMES	SOURCES AND CHARACTERISTICS
Trimethoprim (Diaminopyrimidine)*	Synthetic from guanidine; inhibits dihydrofolic reductase; effective against gram-positive cocci and *Neisseria.*
4-Homosulfanilamide HCl (Sulfamylon, Mafenide)	Synthetic from sulfanilamide; broad-spectrum; prevents infections in burns and cold injuries.
Carbenicillin (Pyopen)*	Semisynthetic from penicillin; valuable for its effect against *Pseudomonas aeruginosa.*
Epicillin*	Semisynthetic similar to carbenicillin and ampicillin.
Cephalexin (Keforal)	A new cephalosporin; effective against pneumococcus and *Staphylococcus aureus.*
Gentamicin (Garamycin)	From *Micromonospora purpurea*; broad-spectrum, effective against drug-resistant staphylococci but *not* against pneumococci or *Neisseria.*
Rifamycin (Rifampicin, Rifampin)*	From *Streptomyces mediterranei*; inhibits pox viruses and adenoviruses, *Chlamydia* of trachoma; useful against *Pseudomonas* species and in tuberculosis.
5-Fluorocytosine (Ancobon)	Very effective antifungal agent, especially against *Candida albicans, Aspergillus* species, etc.

*Investigational in United States.

CLASSES OF ANTIBIOTICS.   For convenience of discussion, antibiotics may be grouped in various ways. For example, some are more bactericidal than bacteriostatic in the concentrations generally used:

Penicillin
Streptomycin
Bacitracin
Polymyxin B
} When used together, these are often synergistic;[2] never antagonistic. For example, penicillin and streptomycin combined are valuable in bacterial endocarditis.

if both together are less effective than individually, or separate.

Others are more definitely bacteriostatic, especially in the low concentrations generally used in therapy:

tetracyclines
Chloramphenicol
Erythromycin
Carbomycin
Neomycin
Oleandomycin
Novobiocin
} These are neither antagonistic nor synergistic. They sometimes work well in combination with antibiotics of the first group.

Antibiotics of the second group are generally of the broad-spectrum type. There are many other broad-spectrum antibiotics, and new ones appear on the market frequently.

[2]The combination is more effective than the sum of both.

Table 14–3. Response of Some Microorganisms to Antibiotics

MICROORGANISM	USUAL RESPONSE TO PROPER ANTIBIOTIC TREATMENT	FREQUENCY OF APPEARANCE OF RESISTANCE IN STRAINS IN PATIENTS
Pneumococcus Meningococcus Gonococcus Beta streptococci *Shigella Haemophilus Treponema*	Rapid	Rare
Staphylococcus	Rapid	Frequent
Alpha and gamma streptococci Coliforms *Proteus Pseudomonas* Tubercle bacilli	Slow or incomplete	Frequent
Brucella Salmonella typhi Rickettsias	Rapid. Frequent relapses require repeat treatments.	Rare

Two important properties of microorganisms in relation to antibiotics are their usual response to antibiotic therapy, and the probability that they will become drug-fast or antibiotic-resistant. Some of these properties are shown in Table 14–3.

Some Representative Antibiotics

Nystatin or *fungicidin* (Mycostatin) is of particular interest because it is one of the very few therapeutically useful antibiotics that are effective against pathogenic fungi. It is often combined with broad-spectrum antibiotics.

Cycloheximide (Actidione), another antifungal antibiotic, is effective against *Cryptococcus neoformans*, a pathogenic yeast, and many destructive fungi of plants. Cycloheximide is also used in the laboratory to suppress saprophytic fungi that contaminate cultures of bacteria and viruses.

Griseofulvin is a fungistatic agent that has proved to be quite effective against superficial mycoses (diseases of the hair, the skin, and the nails caused by molds). Its action is due to nucleic acid interference by the drug.

Penicillin, the first clinically effective antibiotic, was discovered by Sir Alexander Fleming in 1929 (Nobel Prize winner, 1945, with Florey and Chain) (Fig. 14–2). As produced in cultures of *Penicillium notatum* or *Penicillin chrysogenum*, it is generally a mixture of related substances called penicillins X, G, F, dihydro F, and K. Penicillin G, or a derivative, is mostly used. In addition to the five natural penicillins just mentioned, a number of valuable derivatives have been produced by chemical and biosynthetic processes. Among these are benzathine penicillin G, benzathine penicillin V, and penicillin G procaine. Unlike natural penicillin G, these forms are not so readily excreted from the body and are not destroyed by the acidity of gastric juice. They therefore maintain high blood levels and are suitable

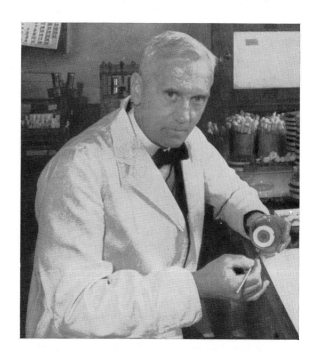

Figure 14–2

Sir Alexander Fleming, penicillin discoverer and Nobel Prize winner, points with his inoculating needle to a giant colony of *Penicillium notatum*, the organism that produces penicillin, on agar in a Petri dish. (Courtesy of Pfizer *Spectrum*.)

for oral administration. In addition there is benzylpenicillin sodium, suitable especially for injection. Several semisynthetic penicillins (e.g., methicillin and cloxacillin, also called oxacillin) have also been developed which are effective against certain strains of *Staphylococcus* resistant to ordinary penicillin. Ampicillin is used orally in bacterial meningitis, salmonellosis, and enterococcal infections.

Penicillin is very effective against infections with most gram-positive organisms. It is also very effective against the gram-negative gonococcus and certain spirochetes, especially those causing syphilis and the related tropical diseases called yaws and bejel.

It is important to know that some penicillin solutions, as well as the dry powder, are relatively unstable and rapidly deteriorate on exposure to air, sunlight, and warmth. Such penicillin preparations should not be dissolved or opened until needed and should be kept in the refrigerator in the dark.

Some forms of penicillin are excreted rapidly from the body in the urine so that repeated large doses are necessary. In order to prolong the effect of a dose and prevent its prompt excretion, it may be combined in peanut oil or other preparations designed to delay absorption by the tissues.

Streptomycin, discovered by Selman A. Waksman (Nobel Prize winner), and *dihydrostreptomycin*, a derivative, are among the most valuable antibiotics, since they are effective against human strains of tubercle bacilli. The drugs are used as an adjunct to bed rest and other medical and surgical therapy in the treatment of tuberculosis. Streptomycin is also effective against several species of gram-negative bacteria that are unaffected by penicillin: *Brucella* (cause of undulant fever), *Shigella* (dysentery bacilli), and others. It also controls some gram-positive species.

Chloramphenicol (Chloromycetin), discovered by Paul R. Burkholder,

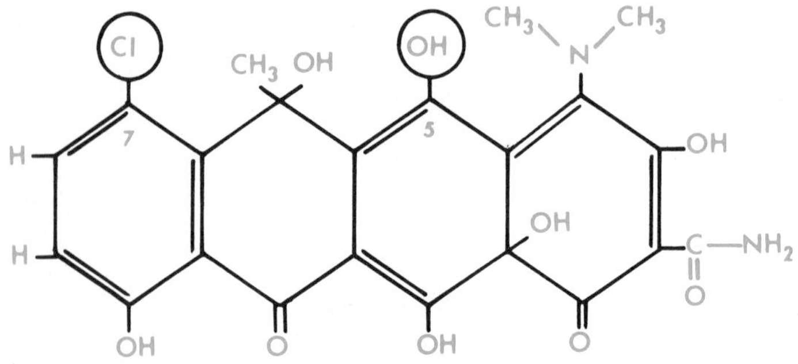

Figure 14–3

Composite formula of the tetracycline group of antibiotics. In tetracycline each of the numbered carbon atoms (5 and 7) has an attached hydrogen atom. In chlortetracycline, chlorine (circled) replaces the hydrogen of the number 7 carbon atom; in oxytetracycline an OH group (circled) replaces the hydrogen of the number 5 carbon atom.

is effective against a large number of bacterial infections, both gram-positive and gram-negative. It has been found of particular value in typhoid and paratyphoid infection, as well as in the treatment of some rickettsial and a few chlamydial diseases. There is evidence that it adversely affects the blood-forming organs. Its use should therefore be carefully followed by appropriate daily examinations of the blood.

Tetracycline Group. The antibiotics called *Achromycin, Terramycin,* and *Aureomycin* are chemically related. All belong to the tetracycline group of compounds. Their chemical relationship and structures are explained in Figure 14–3.

Although each is derived from a different species of *Streptomyces,*[3] they all have similar, but not identical, antibiotic properties. They are effective against many gram-negative and gram-positive species of bacteria, some chlamydias and some rickettsias. They are typical of the broad-spectrum antibiotics and have similar ranges of therapeutic activity. In spite of their similarities, however, in any given patient, any one of these drugs may at times show surprising irregularities, giving unexpectedly brilliant results or failing. This is a very important fact to remember about all antibiotics.

EFFECTS OF EXCESSIVE OR IMPROPER USE. These antimicrobial substances, although often referred to as "miracle drugs," are not without their disadvantages. The danger of antibiotic-resistance has already been discussed. Sensitivities or allergies that cause serious reactions to the drugs may develop in human beings. This is especially true of penicillins. Several produce serious toxic side effects if their administration is not carefully controlled.

One unfortunate side effect of the administration of antibiotics in large, prolonged dosages is seen in a disturbance of the normal host-parasite relationships. Microorganisms that ordinarily remain restricted harmlessly to the skin or mucous membranes find an opportunity to set up an infection, possibly because competing microorganisms that ordinarily hold them in check are suppressed by the antibiotic, or for other

---

[3]Tetracycline is now derived commercially mainly by artificial alteration of the chlortetracycline molecule.

reasons that are entirely obscure. Fungi, especially *Candida albicans*, often harmlessly present in the normal intestine or vagina, sometimes cause distressing gastrointestinal or vaginal *superinfections* in such circumstances. For this reason drugs like amphotericin B and 5-fluorocytosine are of great importance. Staphylococci, ordinarily not important in the intestine, sometimes grow there excessively, producing severe and even fatal enteritis when competing microorganisms of the gut are suppressed by antibiotics in preparation for surgery of the gastrointestinal tract. Antibiotics are not harmless and should not be used without medical supervision.

Antibiotics should be used only when definitely indicated and not for any and every infection. In some critical cases, the doctor may have to make a diagnosis on the basis of the clinical picture before laboratory reports are available. In these cases, the doctor may have to choose the antimicrobial agent most likely to be effective before the causative agent is known. Even in these cases, however, it is advisable to attempt to find the causative organism rather than to continue to treat blindly. It is also essential to know whether the particular strain of organism causing the infection is or is not wholly resistant to the drug chosen for use. This can be determined in the bacteriology laboratory by procedures called "sensitivity testing."

Sensitivity Testing

TUBE DILUTION METHOD.   In this method the drug to be tested against an infectious organism is added, in a series of dilutions (1:5, 1:10, 1:20, and so on), to test tubes containing an appropriate culture medium for the bacterium under examination. Each tube is then inoculated with the organism whose resistance to the drug is being tested. After incubation of all the tubes, a comparison of the growths is made and the resistance of the organism under investigation to each drug is evaluated (Fig. 14–4).

DISK PLATE METHOD.   In this procedure, an agar plate of suitable medium is heavily inoculated with the infecting microorganism whose sensitivity is in question. Previously prepared disks, saturated with various concentrations of several antibiotics, and available commercially, are released from an automatic disc dispensor onto the agar surface. The plate is then incubated. The drugs diffuse from the paper disks into the agar. If the organism is not resistant to the drugs, zones of complete inhibition of the growing organism are found around the disks containing the effective drugs (Fig. 14–5).

AGAR DILUTION METHOD.   This is similar to the tube dilution method in principle. The antibiotics are diluted, not in tubes of broth, but in tubes of melted, cooled (45 C) agar. The agar dilutions are poured into plates. When the agar is solid, the organisms to be tested, perhaps several on a single plate, are streaked on segments of the agar surfaces and the plates are incubated. Effectiveness of an antibiotic is indicated by failure of a bacterial culture to grow (Fig. 14–6).

SIMPLIFIED DISK PROCEDURE.   Sterile filter paper disks are saturated with a suspension of live bacterial spores and a harmless dye, like methylene blue, which is decolorized when reduced by bacterial growth in a closed chamber. The disks are dried. For use, one or more disks are laid on a glass or plastic strip and wetted with a few drops of sterile water (Fig. 14–7). Air is excluded by enclosing the disks in a small, tight glass chamber or covering with transparent plastic tape. When incubated, the spores germinate in one to three hours and their growth reduces the methylene blue, which becomes colorless. If the disk is wetted with some test fluid that contains enough of an antibiotic to which the organism is sensitive, then no growth occurs and the disks remain bright blue. By various experimental adjustments the method may be made roughly quantitative.

BLOOD-AGAR PLATE METHOD.   This rapid and effective procedure is representative of several basically similar methods that use sensitive indicators of bacterial growth. In this example, blood is used as the indicator. These procedures depend on the drug's suppressing the discoloring effect of growing bacteria on fresh blood, or on whatever alternative indicator is used. If blood is the indicator, sterile blood is mixed with melted agar of suitable nutrient composition, at 45 C.

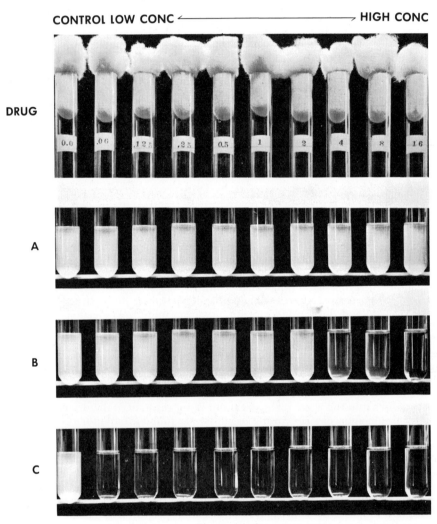

CONTROL LOW CONC ◄—————————————————► **HIGH CONC**

DRUG

A

B

C

Figure 14–4

Testing sensitivity of a bacterium to antibiotics or other chemotherapeutic agents by the "tube dilution" method. In the top row, tubes of broth culture contain an antimicrobial "Drug" in increasing amounts, as shown by the figures on the tubes. The second row contains "Agent A" in the same amounts, while the third row contains "Agent B" in the same quantities. The bottom row contains graded amounts of "Agent C". All tubes were inoculated with "Organism X" from the same patient and the same culture at the same time, and incubated together. Growth, as shown by white turbidity, has occurred even in the highest concentration of Agent A, showing that Organism X (perhaps from a patient very ill with this infection) is not in the least affected by this drug. The drug of choice will be Agent C, which prevents growth of Organism X even in the lowest concentration. Agent B is slightly effective. The left-hand tube in each row is a "control," containing medium but no antibiotic. (Courtesy of Abbott Laboratories, North Chicago, Ill.)

CL — Coly-Mycin
AM — Ampicillin
TE — Terramycin
P — Penicillin
C — Chloramphenicol
PB — Polymyxin B
N — Neomycin
Fd — Nitrofurantoin
T — Tetracycline
K — Kanamycin
LR — Cephaloridine
GM — Garamycin
SSS — Triple Sulfa
CB — Carbenicillin
NA — Nalidixic Acid

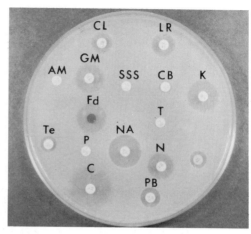

Figure 14–5

Testing sensitivity of a bacterium to antibiotics or other chemotherapeutic agents by the "disk method." The entire surface of agar medium in a Petri plate is inoculated with the organism to be tested. Paper disks of uniform thickness containing graded amounts of the agent to be tested (or the same amount of different agents if a comparison is desired) are then placed on the surface of the agar. The agent diffuses into the agar and prevents growth of the bacterium in a zone around the disk. The width of the zone indicates, roughly, the sensitivity of the organism to the agent or agents being tested, though the *presence* or *absence* of a zone is of greater significance. (About one-half actual size.) (Courtesy of Linda Kaye Hickey).

This mixture is poured into a Petri dish to a depth of about 2 mm and allowed to solidify. This is the blood or *base layer*. A thick suspension of the bacteria to be tested is mixed in a separate tube with similar fluid agar but without blood. This mixture is poured on the base layer. When solidified it forms the *seed layer*. Sterile disks of paper saturated with desired antibiotics are spaced at suitable intervals on the surface of the seed layer, as in the disk plate method. The plate is then incubated.

Examined after two to six hours, the action of an effective antibiotic is seen in zones of bright red, unchanged blood under and around the disk containing the effective antibiotic. Elsewhere the blood is discolored and may be hemolyzed (erythrocytes destroyed) because of uninhibited growth of bacteria. This is a very rapid test because the effect of the bacterial cells on the blood color is readily visible many hours before the growth itself is visible.

In a simplified adaptation of this principle filter paper pads containing dried medium, antimicrobial, and an indicator dye are inoculated with about 0.5 ml of aqueous suspension of the microorganisms under investigation. Growth (or inhibition of growth) is indicated after a few hours of incubation, by change (or no change) in the color of the indicator dye.

Bacteriocins

Bacteriocins are bactericidal proteins, or polypeptides, produced by certain species of bacteria. They exert their lethal action against other bacteria of the same family. *Colicins* produced by *Escherichia coli* are one type of bacteriocin. Many other organisms produce these apparently specific antibiotic substances, for example, *megacins* from *Bacillus megaterium* and *pyocins* from *Pseudomonas aeruginosa* (formerly called P. pyocyanea). Bacteriocins resemble bacteriophages in many respects. They

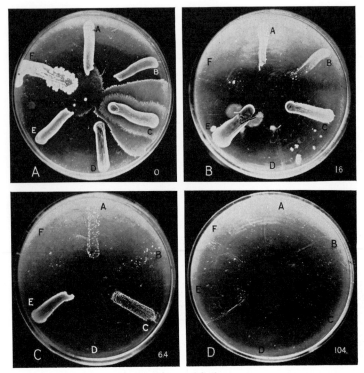

Figure 14–6

Testing sensitivity of several species of bacteria to three different concentrations of streptomycin by the agar-dilution method. Plate A contains no antibiotic and is inoculated with (*A*) *Escherichia coli*, (*B*) *Salmonella typhi*, (*C*) *Proteus* sp., (*D*) *Klebsiella pneumoniae*, (*E*) *Pseudomonas aëruginosa*, (*F*) *Mycobacterium tuberculosis*. In Plate B, containing 1.6 mg of streptomycin per ml of agar, organisms *D* and *F* have been virtually eliminated. Larger amounts of the antibiotic, as shown in Plates C and D, successively eliminate all but a few resistant colonies of the other organisms. (What is the significance of these resistant colonies?) Note the great sensitivity of this strain of *M. tuberculosis* to streptomycin. (Courtesy of Merck & Co., Inc.)

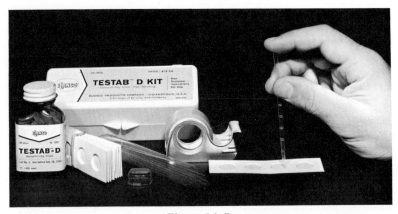

Figure 14–7

Simplified procedure for antibiotic detection or assay. For explanation see page 233. (Courtesy of Elanco Products Co., Indianapolis, Ind.)

may be incomplete bacteriophages. They constitute a type of antibiotic agent that may become important in the treatment of certain diseases when we understand more about their structure as opposed to the genetic code of the pathogen and host cells. Bacteriocin production is controlled by an episome, a Cf or Col factor, analogous to the F or fertility factor.

Supplementary Reading

Anderson, E. S.: The ecology of transferable drug resistance in the enterobacteria. *Ann. Rev. Microbiol.*, 1968, *22*:131.

Basch, H., Erickson, R., and Gadebusch, H.: Epicillin: In vitro laboratory studies. *Inf. Immun.*, 1971, *4*:44.

Becker, Y., and Zakay-Rones, Z: Rifampicin—a new antitrachoma drug. *Nature*, 1969, *222*:851.

Bodey, G. P., and Stewart, D.: In vitro studies of semisynthetic α-(substituted-ureido) penicillins. *Appl. Microbiol.*, 1971, *21*:710.

Bodzansky, M., and Perlman, D.: Peptide antibiotics. *Science*, 1969, *163*:352.

Clark, H., and Turck, M.: In vitro and in vivo evaluation of cephalexin. Antimicrobial Agents and Chemotherapy. Proceedings of the Eighth Interscience Conference on Antimicrobial Agents and Chemotherapy. 1968, Baltimore, The Williams & Wilkins Co., for the American Society for Microbiology, p. 296.

Crofton, J.: Some principles in the chemotherapy of bacterial infections. *Brit. Med. J.*, 1969, *1*:137.

Dulaney, E. L., and Laskin, A. I. (Editors): The problems of drug-resistant pathogenic bacteria. *Ann. N.T. Acad. Sci.*, 1971, Vol. 182.

Editorial: Rifampin—a major new chemotherapeutic agent for the treatment of tuberculosis. *New Eng. J. Med.*, 1969, *280*:615.

Falconer, M. W., Norman, M. R., Patterson, H. R., and Gustafson, E.: The Drug, the Nurse, the Patient. 4th Ed. 1970, Philadelphia, W. B. Saunders Co.

Falconer, M. W., Patterson, H. R., and Gustafson, E.: Current Drug Handbook 1972–1974. Philadelphia, W. B. Saunders Co.

Garrod, L. P., and O'Grady, F. (Editors): Antibiotic and Chemotherapy. 2nd Ed. 1968, Baltimore, The Williams & Wilkins Co.

Hobby, G. L. (Editor): Antimicrobial Agents and Chemotherapy. 1972, 11th Proceedings, Interscience Conference on Antimicrobial Agents and Chemotherapy. Baltimore, The Williams & Wilkins Co., for the American Society for Microbiology.

Hurwitz, N.: Predisposing factors in adverse reactions to drugs. *Brit. Med. J.*, 1969, *1*:536.

Krupp, M. A., Sweet, W. J., Jawetz, E., and Biglieri, E. G.: Physician's Handbook. 15th Ed. 1968, Los Altos, California, Lange Medical Publications.

McCabe, W. R.: Septicemia. *In* Conn, H. F. (Editor): Current Therapy 1969. Philadelphia, W. B. Saunders Co.

Mitsuhashi, S. (Editor): Drug Action and Drug Resistance in Bacteria. 2 Vols. 1972, Baltimore, University Park Press.

Morgan, C., Rosenkranz, H. S., Carr, H. S., and Rose, H. M.: Electron microscopy of chloramphenicol-treated *Escherichia coli. J. Bact.*, 1967, *93*:1987.

Newton, B. A.: Mechanisms of antibiotic action. *Ann Rev. Microbiol.*, 1965, *19*:205.

Newton, B. A., and Reynolds, P. E. (Editors): Biochemical studies of antimicrobial drugs. 16th Symposium. *Soc. Gen. Microbiol. (London)*, 1966.

Riva, S., and Silvestri, L. G.: Rifamycins: a general review. *Ann. Rev. Microbiol.*, 1972, *26*:199.

Sherris, J. C.: IX. Antibiotic susceptibility testing. *In*: Clinical Microbiology Laboratories Manual, Bacteriology. University of Washington Hospital, July, 1969.

Simon, H. J., and Yin, E. J.: Microbioassay of antimicrobial agents. *Appl. Microbiol.*, 1970, *19*:573.

Snell, J. F. (Editor): Biosynthesis of Antibiotics. Vol. 1. 1967, New York, Academic Press.

Stratford, B. C.: Treatment of infections due to *Pseudomonas aeruginosa* with carbenicillin (Pyopen). *Med. J. Aust.*, 1968, *2*:890.

Tassel, D., and Madoff, M. A.: Treatment of *Candida* sepsis and *Cryptococcus* meningitis with 5-fluorocytosine. *J.A.M.A.*, 1968, *206*:830.

Umezawa, H. (Editor): Index of Antibiotics From Actinomycetes. 1967, Baltimore, University Park Press.

Weisblum, B., and Davies, J.: Antibiotic inhibitors of the bacterial ribosome. *Bact. Rev.*, 1968, *32*:493.

Zähner, H., and Mass, W. K.: Biology of Antibiotics. 1972, Springer Verlag, New York.

Sterilization and Disinfection in Health Care

15

In this chapter we shall describe some procedures that illustrate the application of principles underlying disinfection and sterilization in the practice of nursing and related activities of health personnel.

IN THE MEDICAL AND SURGICAL WARDS OF A GENERAL HOSPITAL

HANDWASHING. All health personnel should wash their hands carefully: after the care of each patient, before serving food, before preparing and pouring medicines, before doing each surgical dressing, after dressing an infected wound, after handling bedpans and urinals, and before going to the dining room for their meals.

The manner in which handwashing is done is far more important than the time taken for the procedure. Adequate soaping, care in washing all areas of hands, mechanical friction, and frequent rinsing and resoaping are all-important factors in good handwashing to prevent transfer of microorganisms by means of hands. Nurses sometimes say that they "do not have time to wash their hands." These same nurses would not say that they did not have time to scrub their hands before assisting with a surgical operation.

THERMOMETER TECHNIQUE. There seems to be little justification for attempting to take temperatures on a 30 bed ward with fewer thermometers than there are patients. Yet unfortunately this is sometimes necessary. Whether thermometers are left at the bedside or kept in a central location on each ward depends on availability and individual organization of nursing care. Let us not forget that what may seem simple and common at one place may not really be so at other locations. Would you put two patients into one bed? A former nursing student wrote back to us that this is exactly what she encountered when she returned to her own country.

Oral Thermometers. A recommended procedure for disinfecting oral thermometers is: wipe the thermometer clean with gauze or cotton saturated with a mixture of equal parts of tincture of green soap and 95 per cent ethyl alcohol, rinse well with clear water, and immerse the entire thermometer in a solution of 0.5 to 1 per cent iodine in 70 per cent ethyl or isopropyl ("rubbing") alcohol for ten minutes. Plain 70 per cent alcohol may be used with good results, but it is not as effective without the iodine. Possibly the organic iodine disinfectants referred to previously would be as effective, though further experience with them is needed. Formaldehyde, bichloride, and phenolic disinfectants should not be used because they have been shown to be less effective against tubercle bacilli. Tinctures of quaternaries appear to be as good as the alcoholic iodine solutions. They are effective against tubercle bacilli. After disinfection, the thermometers should be thoroughly rinsed. They may then be kept in a clean, dry container until used again. They are not infectious but are not necessarily sterile (why?). Improved, electronically registering thermometers have disposable plastic covers over the bulb.

Rectal Thermometers. These should be lubricated before use with a water-soluble lubricant. Petrolatum or other oily lubricants are difficult or impossible to remove with soap and cool water. After use, rectal thermometers can be cleaned and disinfected in the same way that oral thermometers are treated. Petrolatum and oils entirely prevent proper cleaning and disinfection. Where facilities are available, well wiped thermometers may be sterilized with germicidal vapors.

SYRINGES AND NEEDLES. These articles are used for intramuscular or intravenous injection or for withdrawal of venous blood or at times even for arterial blood. Most of the syringes now in use are presterilized, nontoxic, nonpyrogenic, *disposable plastic syringes* (Fig. 15–1). They are quite inexpensive, come in all sizes that are in common use, and are supplied either with attached needles or with separate needles

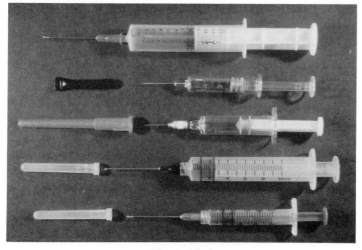

Figure 15–1

Photograph of several different disposable syringes and needles.

individually packaged for easy connecting to needle-less syringes. At all times these presterilized syringes and needles are safe to use, since they are never used more than once. This also assures that the needles are sharp, quite a relief to anyone who ever was injected with a needle having a hook at the tip resulting from "resharpening" a needle poorly. The older type glass syringes are frequently boiled rather than autoclaved, or sterilized in the hot air oven. Boiling is not the method of choice, since spores and some viruses, especially those of epidemic hepatitis and of homologous serum jaundice, may resist boiling for indefinite periods.

All syringes should be handled carefully so that the plunger and inside of the barrel remain sterile. In mounting a separately sterilized needle on a syringe, the sterile needle is carefully held by the shank, or better placed mechanically on the syringe without handling. The shaft and point of the needle are preferably in a sterile tube. It is not good technique to moisten sterile gauze with disinfectant, handle it with fingers (depositing numerous organisms from the hand), and then place this moist gauze over the sterile needle.

A small bottle of skin disinfectant (such as 1 per cent iodine in 70 per cent alcohol) should be carried, with the loaded syringe and the properly mounted and protected needle, to the patient. The sterile syringe and needle need no contact with a disinfectant if properly protected with a sterile glass tube or gauze (Fig. 12–2).

An excellent method of handling sharp instruments that cannot be sterilized by heat is to mount them on convenient racks in jars (Fig. 15–2) containing a disinfecting solution such as the Bard-Parker germicide (Parker, White and Heyl, Inc., Danbury, Conn.): isopropyl alcohol, 65.26 per cent; methyl alcohol, 2.75 per cent; formaldehyde, 8 per cent; hexa-

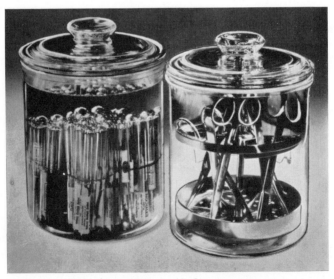

Figure 15–2

Method of maintaining sterility of instruments and of disinfecting suture capsules by mounting in convenient racks and soaking in disinfectant in covered jars. (Courtesy of Bard-Parker Co., Inc., Danbury, Conn.)

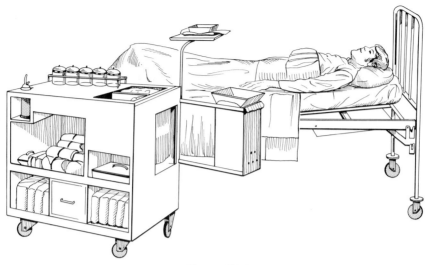

Figure 15–3

A surgical dressing cart for use at patient's bedside. Note wide-mouthed opener fitted over paper bag to receive soiled dressings. (Why?) Note tray that can be held above patient to provide a sterile field for instruments and dressings. Soiled instruments are discarded into the instrument pan. They are later decontaminated, cleaned, and resterilized. There should be no confusion between sterile and unsterile equipment. (Redrawn from: Walter, Carl W.: The Aseptic Treatment of Wounds. The Macmillan Co.)

chlorophene, 0.5 per cent; water, and so on, 23.49 per cent (patented). This solution is said to kill spores in about three to five hours.

SURGICAL DRESSINGS.   Dressings from all wounds, whether aseptic or infected, should never be removed by hand because organisms may easily have penetrated the outer layer of the gauze. These dressings should be removed with sterile gloves to a plastic or paper bag or newspaper, carefully wrapped, and either placed directly in the incinerator or put in a covered trash can for incineration later. Before sterile and disposable gloves were generally available, sterile forceps were used for the changing of dressings. These forceps were discarded into a covered container until they could be boiled, cleaned, and resterilized in the autoclave or hot air oven. A new sterile dressing is applied over the infected wound, preferably with sterile gloves, sterile forceps or by hand, in either case carefully touching only the outer layer of the dressing (keeping the layer that touches the wound uncontaminated until the moment of contact).

Dressings removed from clean (noninfected) wounds may be removed by touching only the outer layers of the gauze. The health worker's hands should never touch any cut, incision, or wound without sterile gloves because of the possibility of infecting the wound with potential pathogens nearly always present on the hands and, conversely, of infecting the health worker's hands.

THE DRESSING CART.   An instrument that was used extensively, before the general use of sterile gloves, present on a surgical dressing cart (Fig. 15–3) or tray was the transfer forceps (Fig. 15–4). Used correctly, this instrument greatly increased the efficiency of the surgical dressing procedure. If used incorrectly, it became a source of gross contamination. The

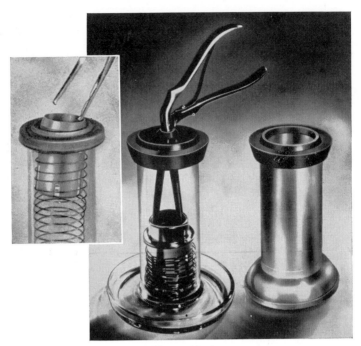

Figure 15–4

An excellent type of transfer forceps. As the instrument is withdrawn from the holder the submerged collar rises on a spring, above the top of the jar, to surround and protect the forceps from contamination by the lip of the jar (see insert). (Courtesy of Bard-Parker Co., Inc., Danbury, Conn.)

transfer forceps is a sterile instrument and was used only to transfer sterile instruments or dressings from one sterile field to another. If at any time this instrument touched unsterile surfaces or objects, it had to be discarded until resterilized. The transfer forceps was kept in a tall jar with enough chemical disinfectant present in the jar to cover adequately any part of the instrument that came in contact with sterile instruments or dressings (Fig. 15–4). Not only have sterile gloves replaced transfer forceps, but even more widespread is the use of individually (or in packages of 2 or 4) wrapped sterile instruments, which greatly facilitate the work of the health worker. Disposable materials have simplified many procedures and certainly are safer to use.

CATHETERIZATION.   The equipment for catheterization (removal of urine from the urinary bladder) is sterilized in the autoclave. The hands are washed thoroughly immediately before carrying out the procedure of catheterization, and sterile gloves are always worn. The external meatus is washed gently with a mild disinfectant solution. This mechanically removes a large percentage of the organisms that may be present; it does not sterilize. The rubber or plastic (glass and metal are no longer used) catheter is adequately lubricated with sterile, water-soluble lubricant and then gently inserted into the urethra. Anything that may traumatize these delicate tissues will increase the possibility of infection.

REVERSE PRECAUTIONS.   In certain medical conditions the doctor will request to have his patient put on "reverse precautions." This order indicates that the doctor wants special precautions taken to protect the *patient* from any kind of infection. He will order reverse precautions for a premature baby, a patient with anuria who has a transplanted kidney, a patient with severe and extensive burns, or a debilitated patient. Patients on steroids (i.e., patients who are receiving tissue or organ transplants) are more susceptible to infections. In brief, reverse precautions will be ordered for any patient whose resistance is low and who is very susceptible to infection. To someone who understands what needs to be accomplished, the procedures for establishing this routine become obvious. All personnel wash their hands thoroughly before entering the room; gowns, masks, and caps are worn by everyone who comes in contact with the patient. Visitors are restricted; no one who has the slightest infection is permitted to be in contact with the patient. Everything that enters the room is either sterile or scrupulously clean. Cleaning and dusting are done with a vacuum cleaner or with moist, disinfectant-soaked mops and cloths, to avoid stirring up and disseminating the dust.

Modern techniques sometimes enclose the patient and his bed and equipment entirely within a plastic cubicle or "bubble." Access to the patient is via built-in plastic arm covers, air tubes, telephone, and so on. Such procedures have been used in heart transplant work and so on.

TERMINAL DISINFECTION

After any patient is discharged from the hospital, especially a patient with a communicable disease, the room or ward unit should be cleaned, the bed washed with soap and water or disinfectant solution, bedside equipment sanitized by boiling and cleaning, the linen autoclaved, washed with hot water and detergent, or both, and then ironed with steam ironers, the mattress and pillow autoclaved, the blankets washed, autoclaved, or both, and the unit re-equipped with clean linens and utensils. Insofar as possible, each private room and each ward unit should have individualized equipment. In hospitals that do not have facilities for autoclaving mattresses and pillows, these articles should be protected with special covers that can be removed and laundered (or cleaned) after the discharge of each patient. There is no excuse for the exchange of undisinfected blankets between patients. Much of the transfer of antibiotic-resistant staphylococci in hospitals, now recognized as a constant serious danger, has been attributed to carelessness in regard to these several precautions.

IN THE OPERATING ROOM

All objects or substances that are to come in contact with a surgical wound must be sterile. Instruments, linens used for drapes, gowns, and gloves should all be sterilized by autoclaving or in the hot air oven. A few instruments used in surgery would be ruined by heat sterilization. Chemical disinfection must therefore be used. (See sections on ethylene oxide and beta-propiolactone.) Notable in this group are delicate instruments for surgery of the eye. Some sutures in nonboilable packages may not be subjected to heat. These are disinfected with gas, radiation, or a chemical solution (phenol, 2 per cent; ethyl alcohol, 70 to 75 per cent, and so on). The package is opened in a sterile towel and the sutures are transferred to the sterile field with sterile forceps.

In preparing for a surgical operation or for a delivery, the nurse must thoroughly clean all instruments, open instruments that are hinged so that all surfaces will have contact with the gas, steam, or dry heat, and sterilize by gas, autoclaving, or in the hot air oven. The nurse is responsible for the sterilization of linens and dressings and for her own technique. She carefully covers her hair with a cap so that no hair or dandruff escapes; she covers her nose and mouth with a gauze mask to prevent infecting the patient and she scrubs her hands and forearms with soap for 10 minutes, being sure to wash each area thoroughly. Soap containing hexachlorophene, 3 per cent, may still be used routinely in many hospitals. Its use is now restricted to special situations (see warning on page 219).

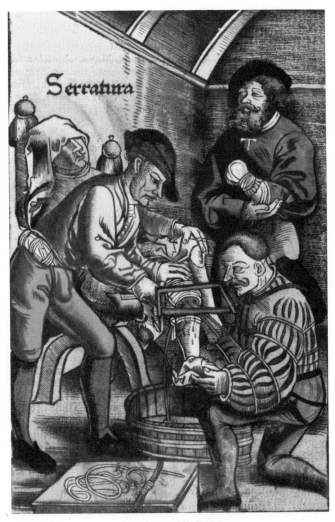

Figure 15–5

First illustration of amputation, from Von Gersdorf. Bandages constrict, at most, superficial veins. Two arteries are spurting uncontrolled. Man in background is wearing Gersdorf's pig's bladder dressing over his forearm stump. Bacteria had a field day under such conditions! (From Hans von Gersdorf's Feldtbuch der Wundt Artzney, Frankfort, 1551. Trent Collection, Duke University Medical Center Library.)

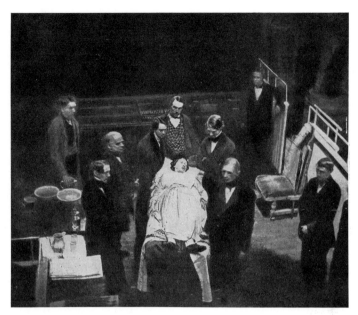

Figure 15–6

How an operation was performed in preantiseptic days. The frock coats were often hung on pegs in the operating room and used by successive visitors and surgeons at different (often infectious) operations! This patient had a tumor of the jaw. The picture is of historical interest. It shows one of the first public demonstrations of ether anesthesia in the Massachusetts General Hospital, October 16, 1846. (From J. Collins Warren: The Influence of Anesthesia on the Surgery of the Nineteenth Century.)

Some hospitals have omitted the use of the scrub brush because of excessive irritation and depend entirely on friction produced by gauze or by the hands. Following the soap and water scrub, all soap should be thoroughly rinsed from the hands and forearms with clear running water. If hexachlorophene was not used, the hands and arms may be immersed in a mild disinfectant solution (70 per cent ethyl alcohol, aqueous Zephiran, 1:1000, or others). The nurse puts on a sterile gown and sterile rubber gloves and is ready to assist in setting everything up (instruments, linens, etc.), and she dresses the surgeons and helps with the operation as needed. She must be alert at all times to maintain sterility on the sterile field; she must guard against contamination and report to the surgeon any breaks in technique that have been unobserved by other members of the operating team (Figs. 15–5 to 15–8).

From the viewpoint of microbiology, the patient is prepared by thoroughly washing the skin of the operative area with soap and water, shaving this area to remove all hairs, and applying ether or acetone to remove fatty skin secretions. In the operating room, the area is again washed well with a detergent solution for 10 minutes, or with soap and water. Then an antiseptic agent is applied (1.5 to 3 per cent alcoholic iodine solution, organic mercurial, organic iodine disinfectant, or other suitable substance). It is important to remember that the cleaning of an operative area of the skin is probably more effective in the removal of microorganisms than the chemical disinfectant is in killing them. The actual cleaning process not only removes microorganisms but removes superficial organic material so that the penetration of the disinfectant is improved. As early as 1882

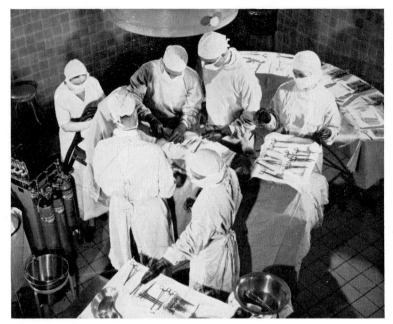

Figure 15-7

Modern surgery. Note the sterile masks, caps, gowns, rubber gloves, and sheets. The instruments have all been sterilized. (St. John's Hospital, Brooklyn. Courtesy of Ewing Galloway.)

Lister disinfected the field of surgical operations by maintaining a fine spray of dilute phenol (carbolic acid) over the area (Fig. 1–8).

As is evident, no attempt has been made to cover in detail the field of operating room and delivery room technique. The health team worker who has an understanding of the principles of microbiology as related to transfer and control of microorganisms will quickly see numerous other examples of the relation of this science to his or her role in the operating room.

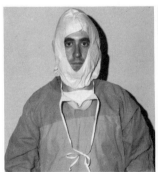
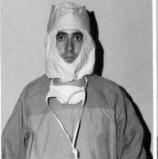
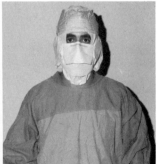

Figure 15-8

Modern surgical face masks. These masks are designed to accommodate present-day hair styles and beards. (Courtesy of Jan F. Fuerst, M.D., Harbor General Hospital, Torrance, California).

IN THE COMMUNICABLE
DISEASE UNIT OR HOSPITAL

When a patient has a communicable disease, the microbiologic problems are mainly those of keeping the infecting organisms confined to one patient and to his unit or cubicle, and of preventing transfer of pathogenic organisms from patient to patient, patient to health personnel, and patient to visitors or the outside world.

BEDSIDE EQUIPMENT. It is essential that the same bedside equipment (such as bedpans and thermometers) be used for the entire infectious phase of the disease. Equipment used only occasionally must be adequately disinfected or sterilized between patients. There is rarely excuse for using stethoscopes, otoscopes, and other instruments for examining successive patients without disinfecting these objects after use. Adequate immersion in a disinfectant, or boiling, is far more effective than merely wiping with 70 per cent isopropyl or ethyl alcohol; however, not all instruments can be boiled or immersed. Thorough wiping with saponated cresol solution (0.5 to 1 per cent) followed by a wipe with clean water and drying is a useful method for handling such instruments, though the cresol may impart an odor to hands and instruments and leave an irritating residue. Gas sterilization is recommended when applicable.

DISHES. The dishes of *all* patients, and certainly those of any patient who has a communicable disease, should at least be scraped to remove uneaten food, boiled 5 to 15 minutes to destroy pathogenic organisms, and washed for the next use. This is of course best done with the electric dishwasher. The food may be contaminated and should also be burned or disinfected before disposal as garbage. Other waste from patients' trays should also be burned. Some communicable disease units and hospitals have adopted attractive paper plates, cups, and other dishes to eliminate the time-consuming problem of disinfecting dishes. The paper dishes are burned and only the silverware, if not also disposable, needs disinfection and washing. Patients with diseases caused by spore-forming bacteria or hepatitis viruses require special care.

SECRETIONS AND EXCRETIONS. If a disease-causing microorganism is known to be transferred by respiratory secretions, paper tissue is used by the patient to receive the secretions (Fig. 15–9) and then the wipes are burned. If the respiratory secretions are copious, as in tuberculosis, they are received into a covered watertight container and the entire container is carefully wrapped and burned. In some instances, sawdust, fine newspaper strips, or another absorbent material, may be used in the container to absorb the excess moisture. If a container other than a plastic liner is used (glass or metal), the container and contents are immersed in saponated solution of cresol, 5 per cent, or strong chlorine bleaching solution for at least one hour. The containers may then be washed and reused. Containers to receive specimens for microscopic examinations should be *new* (Why?).

Many hospitals now use disposable plastic bags inside bedside trash cans and also for large garbage cans.

Urinary or intestinal excretions from a patient with a communicable disease may be disinfected in a tightly covered pail (so that insects cannot touch the infectious matter) by contact with chlorinated lime 5 per cent, strong chlorine bleaching solution, or 5 per cent saponated solution of cresol, for at least one hour. The contents should be disposed of in a

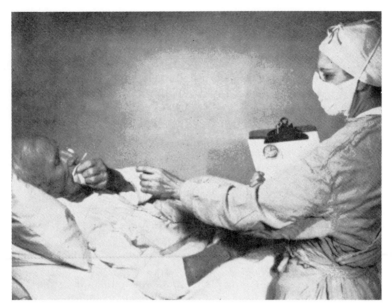

Figure 15-9

Nurse receiving a thermometer from a patient who has a transmissible respiratory infection (e.g., tuberculosis). Note the nurse's cap, gown, and mask. Patient has wiped saliva and sputum from the thermometer with paper wipe so that thermometer can be easily read and nurse does not need to touch contaminated end of thermometer. The patient is ready to protect the nurse from possible cough by covering his mouth and nose with a paper wipe. (Courtesy of Esta H. McNett: *Am. J. Nursing*, Vol. 49, No. 1.)

sewerage system if available. The bedpan or urinal should then be autoclaved or at least boiled for 5 to 15 minutes so that the pathogenic organisms will be destroyed. A very convenient device, available in many hospitals, is the bedpan flusher. This washes the pan and then throws jets of steam upon it, which disinfect if allowed sufficient time for action, but do not sterilize!

Dressings from infectious skin lesions should be burned. Bed and body linens used by patients who have communicable diseases are probably adequately disinfected by processing through routine laundry procedures if the water is hot enough and sufficient contact is allowed. If there is any question about the adequacy of linen disinfection, it should be soaked in saponated cresol 2 per cent or laundry bleach solution overnight, autoclaved or boiled.

Other applications of the principles of disinfection and sterilization will be apparent as the health worker becomes more familiar with methods of transfer of organisms, portals of entry and exit, and other factors involved in transmission of communicable disease. These are discussed farther on.

Details of sterilization of instruments and other hospital supplies are tabulated in Appendix C.

NOTE ON BOILING

Boiling (at 100 C) for ten minutes kills the vegetative or actively multiplying cells of all pathogenic bacteria, chlamydias, PPLO, and rickettsias and appears to inactivate virtually all viruses[1] if they are fully exposed and not protected by clots of blood, masses of food, feces, mucus, and so on. This period of boiling also appears to kill or severely injure cysts of protozoa, ova of helminths, spores of pathogenic yeasts, and conidia of molds.

Boiling for 10 minutes, or even 100 minutes, however, does not guarantee safety when bacterial spores (especially of tetanus, gas gangrene, and anthrax bacilli) and the highly thermoduric hepatitis viruses are concerned. Spores of tetanus and gas gangrene organisms can be assumed to be present in all soil, feces, and dust and on instruments or bandages contaminated with dust, blood, exudates, or exposed materials of any kind. Anthrax spores are rare except in areas where animals infected with these organisms live. The virus of epidemic (so-called "infectious") hepatitis can be assumed to be present in feces and sewage and anything (including hands!) contaminated therewith; the virus of serum hepatitis can be assumed to be present in any undisinfected blood, exudates, serum, or plasma or on instruments and the like contaminated therewith.

Where these spores and these viruses are *known* not to be present, boiling for ten minutes at 100 C is a reasonably safe means of disinfection (not sterilization) of glassware and instruments if they are not grossly soiled with blood, feces, food, and the like. Boiling for 30 minutes greatly increases the margin of safety. These facts may be summarized as follows:

Boiling at 100 C for 10 minutes inactivates or kills:

1. Vegetative forms of all bacteria and fungi pathogenic for man
2. Rickettsias and chlamydias pathogenic for man
3. Helminths and their ova
4. Many viruses (except hepatitis viruses)
5. Bacterial toxins (except staphylococcal enterotoxin)

Boiling at 100 C for 10 minutes does not inactivate or kill:

1. Bacterial spores
2. Hepatitis viruses (possibly some others)
3. Ascospores and conidia of some fungi pathogenic for man[2]
4. Staphylococcal enterotoxin

Care and well informed judgment must be exercised in deciding when boiling may be used with safety and how long it should be continued. Factors such as the source, amount and nature of soiling or contamination, uses to which the boiled articles are to be put, altitude above sea level, and pH of suspending fluid, if any, must influence the decision.

When in doubt, autoclave! (Or use sporicidal gases or chemicals if necessary and feasible.)

---

[1]It does not destroy the viruses of epidemic hepatitis or serum hepatitis.

[2]Accurate data not available for all species. Many fungal spores and conidia may be killed by less than 100 C.

DISINFECTION IN COMMUNITY HEALTH PRACTICE

The principles of microbiology that have been discussed relative to practice in the hospital apply equally to the care of the patient in the home. The community health worker is usually more aware of the importance of hand-washing after visiting each patient than is the worker in the hospital, because the former must go from home to home between patients. The community health worker, however, as well as the hospital worker must be sure to wash all areas of his or her hands thoroughly so as not to be a carrier of infection from one patient to another.

For the visiting worker starting from headquarters, syringes and needles, unless in preassembled, packaged, and presterilized units (plastic units available commercially), should be sterilized by autoclaving or in a hot air oven and carried in sterile containers in the worker's bag. In an emergency, away from hospital or headquarters facilities, syringes and needles may be disinfected for ordinary purposes by boiling in a covered saucepan for 30 minutes. A home oven sterilizes as well as a hospital oven, and a pressure cooker holding as little as one or two quarts of water can serve perfectly in lieu of an autoclave. There is no justification for simply rinsing syringes and needles with a disinfectant solution before their use for injection. Presterilized, packaged, disposable needles and plastic syringes are now in general use.

Obviously the community health worker cannot carry a thermometer for each patient visited. A satisfactory procedure is to carry a screw cap tube of glass or metal cushioned with cotton at the bottom and around the inside. This tube is then filled with 70 per cent alcohol (or other suitable disinfectant) into which the thoroughly washed and wiped thermometer may be placed until used again. The worker may carry two such outfits in order to provide longer disinfection for each thermometer.

Pasteurization may be carried on at home or in camp very easily. A double boiler or similar arrangement of buckets is adapted so that water in the outer container is heated to about 70 C and the temperature of the milk in the inner container held at between 63 and 65 C for 30 minutes. The milk is then cooled rapidly and refrigerated. Babies' bottles may be heated in an inexpensive apparatus purchasable in most department stores.

Isolation technique can be set up admirably in the home if the principles of microbiology and disease transmission are understood by the health worker. The patient with a communicable disease is isolated in a unit (preferably in one room) and equipment is kept inside that room for that person only. Any objects, such as dishes, are removed from the unit in a covered container and are disinfected by boiling for 30 minutes, by soaking in 5 per cent saponated solution of cresol for one hour, or by other effective methods. Linens and bedding are rolled tightly, with soiled surface inward, and placed in plastic or tightly closable bags. Members of the family can usually be taught the principles of isolation technique, and if the principles are clearly understood by them, they can safely care for patients.

IMPROVISATION TECHNIQUES. An ingenious public health worker can use the simple domestic equipment at hand to accomplish the desired results. (One must have a clear idea of what the desired results are!) We have already mentioned substituting a pressure cooker for an autoclave, the oven of a cooking stove for a laboratory oven, a covered pan of boiling water for disinfection of dishes, and laundry bleach for disinfectant. One may also adapt a wash boiler containing disinfectant or boiling water for disinfection of linen, use a covered pail for disinfection of body secretions or excretions, and make numerous other adaptations limited only by the resourcefulness and knowledge of the worker, and without sacrificing safety.

Supplementary Reading

Bartlett, P. G., and Schmidt, W.: Surfactant-iodine complexes as germicides. *Appl. Microbiol.,* 1957, *5:*355.

Benenson, A. S. (Editor): Control of Communicable Diseases in Man. 11th Ed. 1970, New York, American Public Health Association.

Falconer, M. W., Norman, M. C. R., Patterson, H. R., and Gustafson, E. A.: The Drug, the Nurse, the Patient. 4th Ed. 1970, Philadelphia, W. B. Saunders Co.

Falconer, M. W., Patterson, H. R., and Gustafson, E. A.: Current Drug Handbook 1970–1972. Philadelphia, W. B. Saunders Co.

Finland, M., Jones, W. F., Jr., and Barnes, M. W.: Occurrence of serious bacterial infections since introduction of antibacterial agents. *J.A.M.A.,* 1959, *170:*2188.

Harding, W. le R., Balcom, C. E., and Van Belle, G.: Control of Infections in Hospitals. 1968, Toronto, University of Toronto Press.

Lawrence, C. A., and Block, S. S.: Disinfection, Sterilization and Preservation. 1967, Philadelphia, Lea & Febiger.

Perkins, J. J.: *Principles and Methods of Sterilization.* 2nd Ed. 1966, Springfield, Ill., Charles C Thomas, Publisher.

Rockwell, V. T.: Surgical hand scrubbing. *Amer. J. Nurs.,* 1963, *63:*75.

Sommermeyer, L., and Frobisher, M.: Laboratory studies on disinfection of oral thermometers. *Nurs. Res.,* 1952, *1:*32.

Sommermeyer, L., and Frobisher, M.: Laboratory studies on disinfection of rectal thermometers. *Nurs. Res.,* 1953, *2:*85.

Sykes, G.: Disinfection and Sterilization. 2nd Rev. Ed. 1965, Philadelphia, J. B. Lippincott Co.

Top, F. H. (Editor): Control of Infectious Diseases in General Hospitals. 1969, New York, American Public Health Association.

U.S. Department of Health, Education, and Welfare (Center for Disease Control): Investigation of hospital use of hexachlorophene and nursery staphylococcal infections. *Morbidity & Mortality,* Vol. 21, Nos. 5 and 30, 1972.

Wade, N.: Hexachlorophene: FDA temporizes on brain-damaging chemical. *Science, 174:* 805–807, 1971.

Brochures

Beta-propiolactone (BPL). 1959, Wilmot Castle Co., Rochester, N.Y. 14618.

Data on membrane filters. The Millipore Filter Corporation, Bedford, Mass.; also, Karl Schleicher, and Schull, Keene, N. H.: AG Chemical Co., P.O. Box 65C, Pasadena, Calif. (Bibliography included.); Arthur H. Thomas Co., P.O. Box 779, Philadelphia, Pa., 19105

Wade, N.: Hexachlorophene: FDA temporizes or brain-damaging chemical. *Science* 1971, *174:*805–807.

Stierling, H., Reed, L. L., and Billick, I. H.: Evaluation of Sterilization by Gaseous Ethylene Oxide. 1962, Washington, D.C., U.S. Dept. of Health, Education, and Welfare, Public Health Monograph No. 68.

Infection, Immunity and Allergy

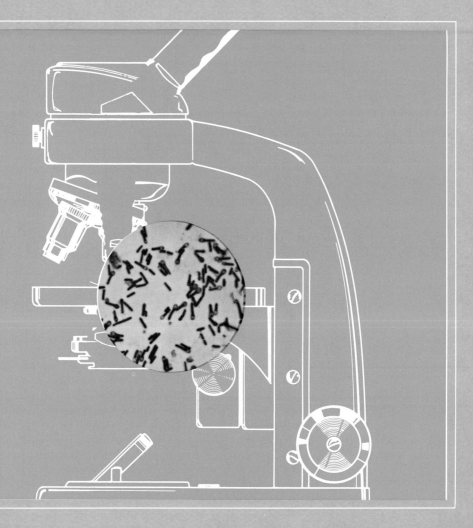

Section Four

Components of Normal Blood and Their Role in Microbiology

16

The blood is of fundamental importance in the production, transmission, diagnosis, prevention, and cure of conditions and diseases caused by microorganisms. Therefore, in order to have an adequate understanding of these processes, it is necessary that we review the composition of, and some other details concerning, blood. The blood, either directly or indirectly, serves as a means of intercommunication among the various cells and tissues in the body, transporting food, hormones, oxygen, carbon dioxide, and other important substances to and from cells, and removing waste products. It may even indirectly carry destruction to tissues if bacteria or their poisons invade the body. Blood also contains substances and living cells that help the body combat disease caused by bacteria and other microorganisms.

THE COMPOSITION OF BLOOD

The body of an average adult male, weighing about 160 pounds, contains about 5.8 liters of blood; the body of a female contains about one liter less. Of this, the blood cells constitute about 2.7 liters, and the liquid (plasma) about 3.1 liters. The cells and plasma may be measured and separated by adding an anticoagulant (e.g., sodium oxalate) and centrifuging in a calibrated, flat-bottomed, tubular vessel called a *hematocrit*. The cells are heavier and settle to the bottom; their volume may be read on the calibrations on the tube. The clear, oxalated or citrated, supernatant plasma may be drawn off into a separate vessel.

PLASMA. The fluid portion of blood (the plasma) is a yellowish, transparent fluid, and is a complex mixture of proteins and other substances: food for the body tissues, and waste products excreted from the tissues. It consists of about 91 per cent water, 1 per cent minerals (CO_2, salts of Na, K, Ca, Mg, P, and minute amounts of several others), 7 per cent proteins, and about 1 per cent of various organic substances, such as uric acid, urea, amino acids, glucose, lipids (fats and fatlike substances), and hormones.

254

Table 16–1.   Major Protein Fractions of Human Blood as Determined by Electrophoresis. (See accompanying diagram.)

PLASMA PROTEIN FRACTION	PERCENTAGE OF TOTAL PROTEIN
Albumin	52.0–68.0
α_1 globulin	2.4– 4.4
α_2 globulin	6.1–10.1
β globulin	8.5–14.5
γ globulin*	18.7–21.0

*Contains the antibodies.

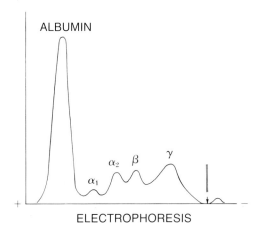

Important among the proteins are albumin and various globulins, which, together with electrolytes and other components, help maintain the water balance of the body (Table 16–1). Of the protein components, *gamma globulins* are exceedingly important since all specific antibodies (Chapter 19) are gamma globulins. *Fibrinogen*, another plasma protein, plays an important role in the blood-clotting mechanism, being converted from its normally soluble state to insoluble *fibrin*, which will be discussed later in this chapter. Plasma, which makes up approximately 55 per cent of whole blood, serves as the fluid medium for the transportation of the formed elements: red cells, white cells, and platelets, which together make up the remaining 45 per cent. The normal pH of plasma is 7.4, and of whole blood between 7.35 and 7.45.

Figure 16–1

Drawing of a smear of blood stained with Jenner's stain, showing common forms of blood cells. *A, B,* and *C,* Polymorphonuclear leucocytes with two-, three- and four-lobed nuclei, respectively. *D,* Eosinophil showing lobular nucleus and prominent, eosinophilic (red-staining) granules. *E,* Lymphocyte. *F, G,* and *H,* Various forms of monocytes ("large lymphocytes"), *I,* Lymphocyte with horseshoe-shaped nucleus ("transitional cell"). *J,* Erythrocytes (red blood cells); note biconcave disk shape, thin at center. *K,* Platelets. (Magnification about ×1000.)

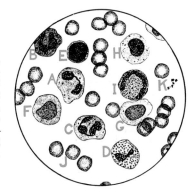

Table 16–2. Blood Cells*

HEMATOPOIETIC TISSUES					
				CIRCULATING BLOOD	
Rubriblast———	Prorubricyte———	Rubricyte———	Metarubricyte———	Diffusely——— Basophilic Erythrocyte	Erythrocyte
Megakaryoblast———	Promegakaryocyte———	Megakaryocyte———	Metamegakaryocyte———		Thrombocyte
		E. Myelocyte———			Eosinophil
Myeloblast———	Promyelocyte<	N. Myelocyte———	N. Metamyelocyte———	Neutrophil——— Band	Neutrophil Segmented
		B. Myelocyte———			Basophil
Monoblast———	Promonocyte———				Monocyte
Lymphoblast———	Prolymphocyte———				Lymphocyte
Plasmoblast———	Proplasmocyte———			Plasmocyte	

(Undifferentiated Stem Cell)

*From Diggs, Sturm, and Bell: The Morphology of Human Blood Cells. 1970, Chicago, Abbott Laboratories.

THE RED BLOOD CELLS (RBC'S).   These are also called erythrocytes (from Greek, *erythros*, red, and *kytos*, cell). They are formed mainly in the bone marrow and float in the plasma (Fig. 16–1). The red color of the blood comes from hemoglobin, which the erythrocytes contain. Hemoglobin is an iron-containing pigment of the class known as *respiratory pigments*. These have the property of forming a loose chemical combination with oxygen when exposed to air (as in the lungs) and of releasing the oxygen to body tissues that need it. Hemoglobin acts, therefore, as an oxygen carrier. Bacteria do not contain hemoglobin, but many species have a yellowish, iron-containing respiratory pigment of similar function called *cytochrome* (Greek, *kytos*, cell, and *chroma*, color).

All blood cells originate from undifferentiated mesenchymal cells. From these "stem cells," clones of cells differentiate and ultimately appear in the circulating blood as red cells, platelets and various types of white cells. The earliest cells of each cell line have similar morphologic characteristics and cannot be differentiated one from the other by appearance alone. They are given specific names such as "myeloblast," "lymphoblast," or "rubriblast," depending on the tissue in which they are found, the cells with which they are associated and the definitive cell that they are destined to produce (Table 16–2).

The red cells of mammals are formed mainly in bone marrow. They are initially nucleated cells called *proerythroblasts*. These develop into *normoblasts* and finally into erythrocytes.

Human erythrocytes, circulating in the blood, are non-nucleated, biconcave disks about 7.5 microns in diameter with a limited life span (approximately 130 days). They are constantly being replaced from hemopoietic tissues in bone marrow. In the normal adult male, erythrocytes number approximately 5.3 million per cubic millimeter of blood, and in women, about 4.3 million per cubic millimeter.

When red cells break up, the hemoglobin escapes into the surrounding fluid. This process is called *hemolysis* (Greek, *haima*, blood; *lysis*, to disrupt or dissolve). Certain bacterial toxins (poisons) have the power of hemo-lyzing red corpuscles both in the body (producing an anemia) and in the test tube. As we shall see later, this capacity to produce hemolysis is used in the laboratory as one method of identifying certain organisms, espe-cially those (*Streptococcus pyogenes*) that cause scarlet fever and "strep throat" (tonsillitis).

THE WHITE BLOOD CELLS (WBC'S).   These cells, of which there are several types, contain no hemoglobin and are collectively called leucocytes (Greek *leukos*, white). They are larger and less numerous than RBC's (Fig. 16–1). There are between 5000 and 9000 per cubic millimeter of normal blood. Some types (the *granulocytes:* polymorphonuclear neutro-philic, eosinophilic and basophilic) are derived from bone marrow cells (*myelocytes*). Other leucocytes originate in the thymus (*thymocytes*), and still others (*lymphocytes*) from lymphoid tissues such as spleen, adenoid tissues, and lymph nodes ("lymph glands").

GRANULOCYTES.   The granulocytic myelocytes, especially polymor-phonuclear neutrophils ("polys" for short), have an important function as scavengers and "policemen" in the blood. The first part of the name, "poly-morphonuclear," means "with a many-lobed nucleus." The nucleus, when stained, is seen to consist of two to four large, connected lobes and is very distinctive. The cell designation "neutrophil" indicates that certain stain-able granules in the cell do not exhibit special affinity for either acidic or basic stains. Other granulocytes have large, round nuclei and contain granules that are either strongly basophilic (basophilic leucocytes) or acido-philic (eosinophilic[1] leucocytes). These *basophils* and *eosinophils* are rela-

---

[1]Eosin is one of the acidic dyes, i.e., it tends to dye the more basic (generally, the cyto-plasmic) parts of the cell.

Figure 16–2

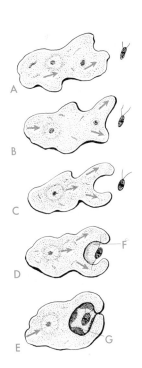

Diagrammatic representation of an ameba ingesting a flagellate (unicellular animal). In *A*, the ameba is moving toward the flagellate by means of a pseudopod (indicated by arrow). In *B* the pseudopod has divided into two smaller pseudopodia preparatory to sur-rounding the flagellate. The process is completed in *C, D,* and *E. F* and *G* show the formation of a vacuole around the flagellate. Any other portion of the ameba could have extruded itself around the flagellate as well as that indicated in the picture. Leucocytes behave in the same manner. (From Schaeffer: Ameboid Movement. Princeton University Press.)

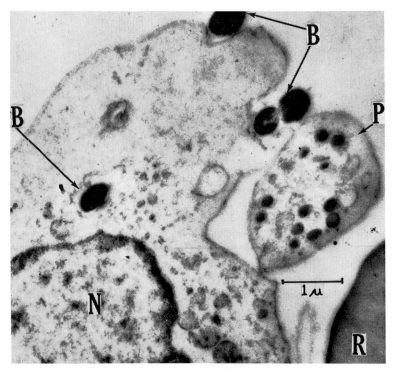

Figure 16–3

Electron micrograph of an ultra-thin (around 350Å) section of a part of a human polymorpho-nuclear leucocyte, showing phagocytosis of virulent *Staphylococcus aureus*. *N* is part of one lobe of the nucleus of the leucocyte; note the well-defined nuclear membrane. *B* are cells of *S. aureus*; note that one bacterium is undergoing fission. The bacteria at the upper right are just being sur-rounded or grasped by the finger-like pseudopodia of the leucocyte. The bacteria will be "ingested" or drawn completely inside the leucocyte. They will be surrounded by a vacuole wall such as is seen to be forming around the bacterium at the left of center. Note the granular structure of the cytoplasm of the leucocyte and its differentiation from the nucleoplasm. *P* is a platelet; *R* is part of a red cell. Note the line (*μ*) indicating 1 micrometer. (×27,500.) (Courtesy of Drs. J. R. Goodman and R. E. Moore, V. A. Hospital, Long Beach, Calif.)

tively rare in the blood, except in certain diseases. Any foreign particles, such as bacteria or dead tissue cells that enter the blood or tissues, are promptly engulfed by the "polys" and certain other cells of the vessel linings that also have the power of ingesting solid particles directly (Figs. 16–2, 16–3).

The polymorphonuclear leucocytes are remarkably like the class of protozoa called amebas, which can be found in soils, sewage, stagnant waters, and the like. They have no constant shape and can move about by sending out temporary swellings or thin, finger-like cytoplasmic ex-tensions called pseudopodia ("false feet") and then flowing into them (ameboid movement; Chapter 3). They can thus intrude themselves into minute crevices (such as exist between tissue cells of the body). They are often called *wandering cells*. Most importantly, from the standpoint of natu-ral defense against disease, they can extend pseudopodia around minute particles, draw them in, and engulf them. The particle passes through the cell membrane to the leucocyte's interior. If the particle is a bacterium, it may be killed there and liquefied by digestive enzymes inside the white cell. However, leucocytes are often destroyed by bacteria. The whole process of ingestion by these leucocytes and also by certain *reticuloendothelial cells* that line the blood vessels (*fixed phagocytes*) is called *phagocytosis*.[2]

By means of ameboid movements, leucocytes are able to move out of the blood vessels, passing between the cells lining the vessels. They can thus travel about through the tissues. When some undesirable particles (as bacteria in a boil or a splinter of wood) set up inflammation, the leucocytes are attracted to the spot by certain substances in the affected tissue. They congregate there, sometimes in enormous numbers. The white, creamy material in a boil or other infected spot consists largely of dead leucocytes ("pus cells"), dead bacteria, some of the tissue cells, and lymph and serum from blood and tissues, all mixed up together. This material is called pus (Fig. 16–4).

Monocytes and *lymphocytes* (large and small) are white blood cells with round nuclei, commonly seen in inflammatory exudates. The former are active in phagocytosis; the small lymphocytes and certain monocytes (plasma cells) are important in the production of specific antibodies (gamma globulins) (Fig. 16–1).

In normal adult blood the proportions of the different types of WBC's are as follows:

	Normal Values (%)
Polymorphonuclear leucocytes (also called granulocytes)	
1. Eosinophils	1–4
2. Basophils	0–1
3. Neutrophils	60–70
Agranular leucocytes	
1. Large lymphocytes	0–3
2. Small lymphocytes	25–30
3. Monocytes	4–8

[2]*Phago* is from the Greek *phagein*, to eat. Phagocytosis, therefore, is the process of being eaten by a cell. A *phagocyte* is a cell that eats cells and other particulate matter.

Figure 16–4

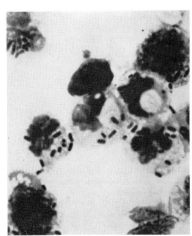

Stained smear of pus from lung of mouse inoculated with a species of pathogenic bacilli. The bacilli are seen to have been engulfed by the leucocytes (phagocytized) in large numbers. This is an excellent illustration of one of the most important defensive measures. (×1000.) (Courtesy of M. R. Smith and W. B. Wood, Jr., Washington University School of Medicine, St. Louis, Mo. In *J. Exp. Med.*, Vol. 86.)

LEUCOCYTE COUNTS.   Leucocytes may vary in kind and numbers. An increase in the percentage of polymorphonuclear leucocytes indicates infection or inflammation or toxin absorption. Noninfectious conditions, some of a normal nature, such as labor or exercise, and some not so normal, such as convulsions or vomiting, also tend to increase the neutrophil percentage.

The percentage of lymphocytes increases in mumps, brucellosis, whooping cough, influenza, tuberculosis, goiter, certain mycoses, and often after exposure to excess sunlight.

A relative increase in monocytes is most distinctive of typhoid fever, but also arises in certain parasitic infestations, or in Rocky Mountain spotted fever, Hodgkin's disease, and some types of microbial intoxication.

Eosinophil percentages increase in many helminthic and protozoal infections, allergic conditions such as bronchial asthma, myelogenous leukemia, scarlet fever, and others.

Not much is known about basophils, but their percentage may increase with myelogenous leukemia. They play a role in allergy.

In some infectious processes, acute appendicitis, for example, the number of white blood cells increases from the normal 5,000–9,000 per cubic millimeter to 15,000 or even 20,000 per cubic millimeter. An increased number of leucocytes in the blood is called a *leucocytosis.*

The *differential count* (percentages of the various types of WBC's) also changes during infectious processes. The proportion of polymorphonuclear leucocytes especially increases, sometimes to 80 or 90 per cent, and others diminish in proportion.

Certain infections always cause a leucocytosis. The organisms causing such infection are said to be pyogenic (Greek, *pyon*, pus; *gennan*, to produce). Others do not increase the leucocyte counts. Among the pyogenic group are the infections caused by staphylococci, gonococci, streptococci, and pneumococci; in the nonpyogenic group, there are typhoid fever, measles, influenza, tuberculosis, and syphilis. In some diseases in the second group, typhoid fever and influenza, for example, there is a diminution of leucocytes below normal numbers. Such a condition is not uncommon in disease and it is called *leucopenia* (Greek, *leukos*, white [white cell]; *penia*, scarcity of).

BLOOD PLATELETS.   These are non-nuclear, irregularly shaped bodies (Fig. 16–1), varying in size, but being much smaller than erythrocytes, and occurring in low numbers, about 300,000 per cubic millimeter of blood. They are derived by fragmentation from the largest cells of the bone marrow, which are called megakaryocytes. They play a role in the process of coagulation of blood by producing thromboplastin, one of the components of fibrin. They are sometimes called *thrombocytes.* Because platelets easily stick together (agglutinate), they may plug up small breaks in the circulatory system, and thus prevent seepage of blood.

BLOOD CLOTTING.   Blood plasma contains several substances, among them fibrinogen, which causes blood to *clot* when it leaves the body. Inside the body, certain substances in the plasma normally keep the blood in a fluid condition. Once the blood escapes, however, the coagulation mechanism is initiated and the clot forms. The clot is composed of *fibrin*, an elastic, spongy, interlacing network of protein fibers in which the red and white blood cells become enmeshed (Fig. 16–5). As it shrinks (clot retraction), it pulls the red and white cells with it, exuding a clear, straw-

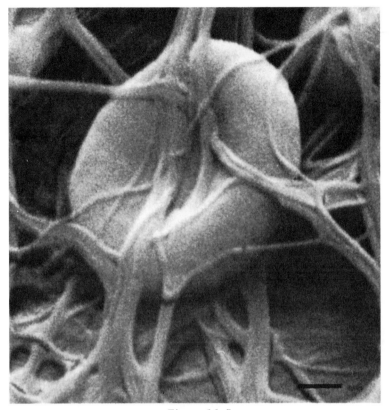

Figure 16–5

Scanning electron micrograph of an erythrocyte enmeshed in fibrin. Part of a thrombus (blood clot) found on the inner surface of an intravenous catheter implanted proximal to the heart (about ×20,500.) (Emil Bernstein and Eila Kairinen, Gillette Company Research Institute, Rockville, Maryland.)

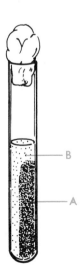

Figure 16–6

Tube with clot *(A)*, which has shrunk, enmeshing virtually all the blood cells, leaving the pale yellow serum *(B)* quite clear.

colored fluid, which is plasma minus the components of the clot, and which is called *serum* (Fig. 16–6).

Substances important in blood clotting are:

1. Prothrombin—found in blood plasma
2. Antiprothrombin—found in blood plasma
3. Calcium—found in blood plasma
4. Fibrinogen—found in blood plasma
5. Thromboplastin—from tissue fluid and platelet disintegration

Prothrombin, antiprothrombin, fibrinogen and thromboplastin, together with albumins globulins, etc., are among the "blood proteins" (Table 16–1).

Normally antiprothrombin combines with prothrombin and forms *bound prothrombin* in the blood, but when tissues are injured and platelets are disintegrated in a wound, the following processes occur:

Wound or cut

Vitamin
K $\longrightarrow$ releases

Thromboplastin + antiprothrombin $\longrightarrow$ bound antiprothrombin formed

Now free prothrombin is available:

Free prothrombin + calcium $\longrightarrow$ thrombin
thrombin + fibrinogen (soluble protein) $\longrightarrow$ fibrin (insoluble protein)
fibrin + blood cells $\longrightarrow$ blood clot (normally in 2–6 min.)

If, however, heparin or sodium oxalate or citrate is used (in the syringe or test tube), the calcium of the blood reacts with these chemicals and is not available to react with the free prothrombin; no thrombin is formed. In this case, the fibrinogen does not become fibrin and, consequently, the blood does not clot.

FUNCTIONS OF THE BLOOD

The blood and its arterial and venous networks constitute the great transportation system and supply lines of the body. Blood is pushed continuously through the arterial system by the left ventricle of the heart under normal arterial blood pressure (about 130 to 150 mm of Hg). In the smallest, most remote branches of the system, the microscopic *arterioles* and *venules*, or *capillary vessels*, the walls of the blood vessels are only one cell in thickness. Through these thin, membrane-like walls, nutrients, hormones, and other substances pass by diffusion and filtration with, and to, the fluid (*lymph*)[3] that surrounds the capillaries and the tissue cells. The lymph (or interstitial or tissue fluid) constitutes a sort of culture

---

[3] Latin *lympha*, water.

medium for the tissue cells. Lymph is actually blood plasma minus most blood proteins; thus it consists of the fluid from about 2.8 l of liquid plasma. The nutrients are brought from the gastrointestinal tract and liver by the arterial blood and passed into the lymph.

Waste metabolic products (acids, carbon dioxide, and other substances) from the tissue cells diffuse into the lymph and from the lymph into the bloodstream and are carried back to the right auricle of the heart via the capillary venules and venous system, which are a direct continuation of the arterioles—a "return route."

The blood is then forced through the lungs by the right ventricle. Oxygen from the air is taken up by the red cells, carbon dioxide is given off by both red cells and plasma, and other important exchanges occur. The blood is then returned to the left ventricle and circulated to the tissues again. As previously noted, lymph seeps into a sort of drainage system— the lymphatic channels—passes through a system of filters (*lymph nodes*) where particles such as cell detritus, bacteria and the like are phagocytized by lymphocytes and similar cells, and is returned to the venous blood via a large lymph channel, the thoracic duct.

The physiology of the blood is very complex and need not be further detailed here. The relation of the capillary blood vessels to tissue cells and to the tissue fluids surrounding them is shown diagrammatically in Figure 16–7. One leucocyte is shown passing between the cells of the capillary wall by *diapedesis* (Greek, *dia*, through; and *pedis*, a foot; hence, "to walk through").

Figure 16–7

Relationships between intercellular lymph or tissue fluid *(F)*, the tissue cells *(T)*, and the blood plasma *(P)*. At *A*, soluble food passes from the plasma, through the microscopically thin wall *(W)* of the capillary blood vessel or arteriole into the tissue fluid and thence into the tissue cells. (Blood flow in this drawing is from left to right.) At *C*, wastes from the tissue cells are leaving in the reverse manner. At *B*, oxygen brought by the erythrocytes *(E)* is diffusing through the arteriole wall and lymph to the tissue cells and, at *D*, carbon dioxide from the tissue cells is leaving in the same manner via a venule. Leucocytes are seen at *L*. One of these is moving out of the capillary into the tissue space by passing between two cells that compose the capillary wall, illustrating the phenomenon of diapedesis. (Modified from Hegner and Stiles: College Zoology, The Macmillan Co.)

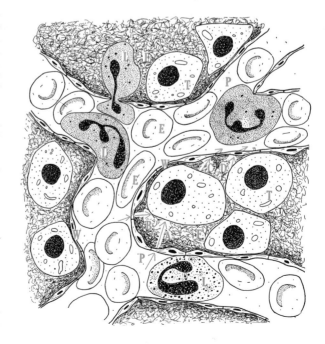

THE HUMAN BLOOD GROUPS

Every human individual is born with a blood type of the A, B, AB, or O blood group series that is inherited from his parents. There are numerous other blood group factors or substances: Le^a, Le^b, MN, P, S, Rh, and so on. Since 23 chromosomes of each set of 46 are transmitted normally from the mother and one set of 23 from the father, the genes on two homologous chromosomes determine the genotype of an individual for any trait. This trait, or phenotype, also applies to blood groups. For simplicity purposes, in the A, B, and O groups three alleles (different expressions of a gene) have been postulated to explain this inheritance; they are I^A, I^B, and I^O. In reality, subtypes of these alleles are known and play an important role in genetics. Some cause difficulties to the offspring somewhat like those resulting from the Rh factor, which will be discussed later in this chapter. Table 16–3 shows a simple diagram explaining the inheritance of these blood types. We may assume that a person's own *serum* does not contain agglutinins against his own erythrocytes, but only against the absent agglutinogen(s). Isohemagglutinins do not agglutinate (clump) one's own RBC's. As can be seen from Table 16–4, serum from a person with blood type A produces isohemagglutinins[4] (antibodies) against type B erythrocytes (anti-B); O serum contains anti-A and anti-B antibodies; however, AB serum contains no antibodies against any RBC's at all. The term *iso* implies that these hemagglutinins (antibodies) are inherited, i.e., are from the same species, and not formed as the result of previous exposure, immunization, and so on.

Table 16–3. Inheritance of Human Blood Types

BLOOD GROUP OF INDIVIDUAL AS DETERMINED BY BLOOD TYPING	PRESENCE IN ERYTHROCYTE OF AGGLUTINOGENS (ANTIGENS)
PHENOTYPE	GENOTYPES *
A	$I^A I^A$ or $I^A I^O$
B	$I^B I^B$ or $I^B I^O$
O	$I^O I^O$
AB	$I^A I^B$

*It should be noted that one I gene comes from the mother and one I gene from the father. It is impossible to transmit a gene to one's natural offspring if one does not have that gene.

A person's blood group is a physiologic constant determined by the basic Mendelian laws of inheritance. By properly selecting donors and recipients of compatible groups, it is possible to avoid hemagglutination following transfusions. Most hospitals have blood or a list of donors of various groups available. Blood banks consist of citrated blood donations already grouped and held in the refrigerator until needed. A cross match between the patient's RBC's, serum or plasma, and the donor's RBC's and serum is always advisable.

---

[4]These agglutinate erythrocytes of another individual of the *same species*.

Table 16–4. Isohemagglutination. International System of Blood Groups*

SERA FROM PERSONS OF BLOOD GROUP: (CONTAIN ANTIBODIES AGAINST RBC's)	AGGLUTINATE THE ERYTHROCYTES OF PERSONS OF BLOOD GROUP:**			
	AB	B	A	O
AB (contains no antibodies)	−	−	−	−
B (anti-A)	+	−	+	−
A (anti-B)	+	+	−	−
O (anti-A and anti-B)	+	+	+	−

*This table is an oversimplification, since blood subtypes exist in this system like A_1 or A_2, in A_1B, A_2B, and the "Bombay type." For example, A_2B may occasionally form anti-A_1 antibodies.

**+ means agglutination occurs; − means agglutination does not occur.

BLOOD GROUPING. *Cells* of the recipient, usually prepared by adding a drop of the patient's blood to a small amount of physiologic salt solution (0.9 per cent NaCl), are mixed on a microscope slide (or white porcelain plate) with specially prepared rabbit sera containing pure anti-A or anti-B antibodies. Agglutination, if any, is usually prompt and readily visible (Fig. 16–8).

If the cells of the recipient are agglutinated by both anti-A and anti-B rabbit sera, the cells are of group AB; if the cells are agglutinated by neither serum, they are of group O. If anti-A serum agglutinates them and anti-B serum does not, the cells are of group A; if anti-B serum agglutinates them and anti-A does not, the cells are of group B.

The *serum* of the recipient is then tested against the red cells of the donor blood to be sure that no mistake has been made and to eliminate certain irregularities in reaction that sometimes occur.

The microscopic reactions are shown schematically in Figure 16–8.

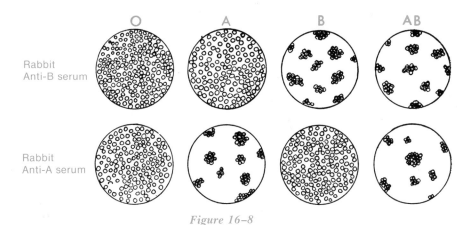

Figure 16–8

Diagram of hemagglutination in blood grouping (blood typing in the laboratory). Anti-B serum and anti-A serum have been mixed on glass slides with erythrocytes of groups O, A, B, and AB. Anti-B serum agglutinates erythrocytes of persons of groups B and AB: anti-A serum agglutinates erythrocytes of persons of groups A and AB.

Note that in this diagram agglutination is by specially prepared rabbit sera, containing antibodies against group A or group B antigens in the cells of persons of group A or group B, respectively.

"Universal (?)" Donors. A person of group O is sometimes inaccurately (and unfortunately) called a "universal" donor because his cells are not usually agglutinated by serum of recipients of any other group, but he must receive only O blood because his serum agglutinates cells of all other groups in the A-B-O system.

Actually, there is no such thing as a safe "universal" donor (without direct cross matching between recipient and donor), because although the erythrocytes of a person of group O do not contain A or B antigens (i.e., are not agglutinated by A or B group sera), there are several other antigen-antibody systems in human bloods such as the Rh factor, M-N-S types, P types, and so on, which may cause serious transfusion reactions regardless of the A, B, O, or AB group (See Table 16–4).

H Antigen. While typical O cells have neither A nor B isoagglutinogens, the serum of O type persons contains both A and B antibodies. The I^A gene determines the A antigen, the I^B gene the B antigen. While the I^O gene determines neither A nor B, O cells nevertheless have a specific heterogenetic or *H* agglutinogen that reacts (like the heterogenetic Forssman or heterophil antigen) with sera from several species of lower animals as well as with sera from man. When the H antigen (also A and B antigens) are absent from certain unusual O type persons first observed in Bombay ("Bombay types"), the serum contains not only A and B antibodies but also H antibodies that agglutinate O cells.

Rh Factor. In 1940 it was discovered that if erythrocytes of *Rh*esus (Rh) monkeys were injected into rabbits, the serum of the rabbits soon contained anti-Rh agglutinins. These antibodies could also agglutinate the erythrocytes of 85 per cent or more of human beings. The antigen in the red cells of humans with which the anti-Rh rabbit serum reacted was designated as the Rh agglutinogen, and individuals containing it as Rh positive (+). The remaining 15 per cent, i.e., persons with red cells that do not react with the anti-Rh rabbit serum, because of the absence of the Rh agglutinogen, are designated as Rh negative (−). Later studies showed that the Rh agglutinogen is a complex one, corresponding to several antibodies or *blood factors*, the most important of which is called the **Rh₀** (**Rh**) factor. (Some of the other, related factors are: **Hr₀, hr′, rh′, hr″, rh″**, and so on.) Here we need consider only the **Rh** factor as being representative.

Nomenclature. Some confusion in names has arisen because of the use of various symbols and ideas to express these antigen-antibody relationships. A widely used system of symbols is that of Fisher, the C-D-E system. The Wiener Rh-Hr system and the C-D-E system, although based on different theories, and not properly interchangeable, are nevertheless sometimes used as approximate equivalents:

	WIENER (*Blood Factors*)	FISHER (*Agglutinogens*)	FREQUENCY IN CAUCASIAN POPULATION
Rh Factors	**Rh₀**	D	85%
	rh′	C	70%
	rh″	E	32%
Hr Factors	**hr′**	c	80%
	Hr₀		63%
	hr″	e	97%

In the Fisher system a person with one gene D (not d) is Rh positive, while dd would be Rh negative. Thus, an individual could be genotype CcDDee or ccDdEe, or any other possible combination, as long as he (or she) has six determining genes for the Rh factor.

Rh FACTOR AND TRANSFUSION. If an Rh negative person receives a blood transfusion from a person who is Rh positive, the recipient develops antibodies (in about two weeks) that agglutinate the red cells of all Rh positive persons. Now, if a subsequent transfusion is given from an Rh positive donor and the Rh antibody concentration (titer) of the recipient is sufficiently high, all the red cells of the donor are agglutinated and later hemolyzed, and a severe transfusion reaction occurs, often with a fatal outcome. Thus, it is of vital importance to determine the Rh status as well as the blood group (A, B, etc.) of donors and recipients before each transfusion.

Erythroblastosis Fetalis. If an Rh negative woman becomes pregnant by an Rh positive man, the chances are good that the child will inherit Rh antigen in its blood cells. During pregnancy, if the child is Rh positive, fetal red cells often cross the placental barrier and pass into the blood of the mother. Acting as an antigen, the Rh+ cells from the fetus may then stimulate the maternal tissues to produce Rh antibodies. These antibodies, as soluble components of blood plasma, freely diffuse back into the fetal circulation. In an *initial* pregnancy, the mother's Rh antibody titer may be too low to produce any harmful effects in the fetus. With subsequent pregnancies, however, the increase in concentration of Rh antibodies may be sufficient to destroy the red cells of the fetus. Thus the child, possessing both the Rh antigen (i.e., Rh+) and Rh antibodies may be born dead (uncommon) or with hemolytic disease of the newborn (erythroblastosis fetalis), which is not uncommon. A similar situation may occur if the mother, being Rh negative herself, has previously received a transfusion from an Rh positive donor.

If the Rh agglutinogen should represent a complicating factor in pregnancy, a precautionary measure frequently employed is the periodic examination of the maternal blood for a *rising titer* of Rh agglutinins. A newborn child with erythroblastosis fetalis receives what is called a "blood exchange." Actually this process is a slow dilution procedure in which a small amount of blood is withdrawn from the baby to be replaced by the same type of blood as the child's, but without the Rh antibodies in it. This process may be repeated for hours, as long as is necessary. Some uninformed students visualize blood exchange as draining the baby of all blood and replacing it with new blood. If this were done, the baby would be dead.

Rh immune globulin (RhIG), now available, is derived from human donors whose blood is rich in Rh antibodies. Injected intramuscularly into Rh negative women whose blood is devoid of Rh antibodies, within 72 hours after delivery of an Rh positive infant or an abortion, the antibodies suppress the formation of Rh antibodies during a *subsequent* Rh positive pregnancy or abortion. The protection may be needed for each subsequent pregnancy or abortion.

Supplementary Reading

Biology Data Book. 1964, Washington, D.C., Federation of American Societies for Experimental Biology.

Blood Group Antigens and Antibodies as Applied to Compatibility Testing. 1967, Ortho Diagnostics, Raritan, N.J.

Blood Group Antigens and Antibodies as Applied to the Hemolytic Disease of the Newborn. 1968, Ortho Diagnostics, Raritan, N.J.

Blood Group Antigens and Antibodies as Applied to the ABO and Rh Systems. 1969, Ortho Diagnostics, Raritan, N.J.

Carpenter, P. L.: Immunology and Serology. 3rd Ed. 1972, Philadelphia, W. B. Saunders Co.

Clarke, C. A.: The prevention of "Rhesus" babies. *Sci. Amer.*, 1968, *219*(Nov.):46.

Faulkner, W. R., King, J. W. and Damm, H. C. (Editors): CRC Handbook of Clinical Laboratory Data. 2nd Ed. 1968, Cleveland, The Chemical Rubber Co.

Gilmore, C. P.: The Scanning Electron Microscope: World of the Infinitely Small. 1972, New York, New York Graphic Society.

Gershowitz, H., and Neel, J. V.: The blood group polymorphism: Why are they there? Blood and Tissue Antigens. 1970, New York, Academic Press.

Kieth, L., Cuva, A., Houser, K., et al.: Suppression of primary Rh-immunization by anti-Rh. *Transfusion*, 1970, *10*:142.

Levine, P.: Prevention and treatment of erythroblastosis fetalis. *Ann. N.Y. Acad. Sci.*, 1970, *169* (Art. 1):234.

Morgan, W. T. J.: Molecular aspects of human blood-group specificity. *Ann. N.Y. Acad. Sci.*, 1970, *169* (Art. 1.):118.

Oatley, C. W.: The Scanning Electron Microscope: Part I, The Instrument. 1972, Cambridge, Cambridge University Press.

Queenan, J. T. (Ed.): The Rh problem. *Clin. Obstet. Gynecol.*, 1971, *14*:491.

Race, R. R., and Sanger, R.: Blood Groups in Man. 4th Ed. 1962, Springfield, Ill., Charles C Thomas, Publisher.

Wiener, A. S.: Elements of blood group nomenclature with special reference to the Rh-Hr blood types. *J.A.M.A.*, 1967, *199*:985.

Wiener, A. S.: Modern blood group nomenclature. *J. Amer. Med. Technol.*, 1968, *30*:174.

Blood In Relation to Infections

BLOOD AND DISEASE. Many species of pathogenic microorganisms can enter the tissues, the blood, or both, and grow,[1] often with fatal effects to the victim. Sometimes microorganisms present in infected tissue may enter leucocytes and "hitchhike" to other tissues, carried by the blood. If blood circulates through tissues in which pathogenic microorganisms are producing poisonous substances (toxins), as in diphtheria and tetanus, or some diseases caused by streptococci, the toxins enter the blood and are distributed, with detrimental effects, to all the tissues in the body.

In diseases in which the microorganism causing the condition are transported by blood or cells, the pathogen may establish itself in other organs as well, causing various complications, such as brain abscesses, osteomyelitis, and middle-ear infections (otitis media). We shall point out later how numerous blood-borne diseases (malaria, yellow fever, plague, and others) are regularly transmitted by various extraneous means, especially mosquitoes, from person to person over large geographic areas.

BLOOD AND DEFENSES. Certain cells, especially *plasma cells* derived from *small lymphocytes* that originated in the thymus early in life, respond to infection by producing *antibodies*. Antibodies are soluble protein molecules of the type called *gamma globulins*. There are several forms of gamma globulins. These have been designated alphabetically as γG, γA, γM, γD. In most normal and hyperimmune individuals over 85 per cent of the immunoglobulins are γG type proteins. These have been further subdivided into heavy chain (H) and light chain (L) subunits. The chemistry and physical properties of these proteins have been extensively investigated, but they are too complex to discuss here.

That differences in molecular structure of the various antibodies (immunoglobulins or Ig's) are of great practical as well as simple theoretical interest is illustrated, for example, by the fact that a perfectly healthy, newborn baby of a syphilitic mother may have syphilitic IgG in its serum, the IgG having been derived transplacentally from its mother.

---

[1]This condition is called *septicemia* (Greek, *septikos*, microbial destruction, and *haima*, blood; hence "blood poisoning").

269

In contrast, if the baby's serum contains syphilitic IgM, it shows that the neonate has active spirochaetal infection (congenital syphilis). IgM of the baby is not derived from the mother because IgM cannot pass the placental membrane. The two forms of Ig may be differentiated by a special technique of the FTA-ABS fluorescent antibody test for syphilis.

The gamma globulins act as a defensive barrier against microorganisms and their toxins. This action will be explained in Chapter 19. The blood transports antibodies and defensive phagocytic blood cells throughout the tissues, like a supply train that distributes soldiers and ammunition to an embattled army. Other, stationary phagocytic cells called *histiocytes* line the inside of the blood vessels and, like snipers in war, destroy invaders (microorganisms) or other foreign substances that pass by. These cells constitute the *reticuloendothelial system*. Tests made with antibodies and with blood cells are of immense importance in the diagnosis—and consequently the treatment—of disease. An important role in the activities of both antibodies and phagocytes is played by a group of blood proteins that together constitute the substance (or *activity*) called *complement*. Complement and various other blood components will be discussed later.

The blood also obligingly carries antibodies and drugs injected or swallowed to combat infection.

INFECTION

Host-Parasite Relationships

In the course of evolution many species of living organisms, forced to coexist, have established a variety of interrelationships. Like many other environmental factors, these relationships are also investigated in studies in *ecology*. In some environments living organisms are mutually helpful (*symbiosis* or *mutualism*); some are mutually antagonistic (*antibiosis*). Others involve various degrees of mutual tolerance or intolerance. Some organisms thrive at the expense of others (*predation* and *parasitism*). Most of the infectious diseases represent the latter type of ecologic relationship.

When one creature (e.g., a *parasite*) attempts to thrive at another's (e.g., a *host's*) expense, the host nearly always reacts in some manner to evade, remove, or kill the parasite. If evasion, removal, or killing fails, host and parasite often become mutually adapted (sometimes only after generations of contact and dwindling antagonism) and establish a sort of armed truce in which they live, more or less peaceably, side by side (*commensalism*). Many curious host-parasite relationships and adaptations are exhibited in the processes we call *infection, the carrier state, immunity,* and *allergy*.

There is nothing vindictive or purposeful in microorganisms, any more than the growth of weeds or poison ivy in a flower garden is vindictive or purposeful. For convenience in discussion, however, an infectious disease may be regarded as a struggle between an attacking force (the parasite) and a defending body (the host). Both combatants have their means of "offense" and "defense." We shall first consider the struggle from the side of the parasitic microorganisms.

Microorganisms may gain entrance to the tissues of the body and grow in or on them, injuring them and producing a reaction in the host. This is an *infection*.[2] The sensed or demonstrable (clinical) aspects of this reaction to infection are commonly fever, chills, nausea, and headache. Some infections are so mild that they cause hardly any discomfort; others are fatal. A pimple, for example, is a trivial reaction to an infection of the skin; typhoid fever is a serious and — without antibiotic treatment — often fatal infection of the blood, intestine, and other organs.

Factors in Infection

DOSE OF INFECTING ORGANISMS. An important factor in determining whether infection shall or shall not occur is the number of infecting organisms. A single coccus or a single bacillus, even though highly virulent, alone might not be sufficient to establish a foothold in the healthy body. If a hundred or a million such organisms were to be implanted, they might well overcome even a strong resistance. Mildly virulent or even supposedly harmless organisms may set up an infection if their number is sufficiently large, especially if tissue resistance is lowered by other factors, such as disease, fatigue, drugs or alcoholism.

VIRULENCE OF ORGANISMS. Virulence is the ability of a microorganism to establish, maintain, and extend an infection and to damage the body (thereby producing a disease). Virulence depends upon at least two other properties: *aggressiveness* and *toxigenicity*. Each of these is a resultant of a number of other properties. Actually, exact knowledge of all the factors, and their interrelationships, that comprise the property of virulence is still incomplete.

Aggressiveness. An aggressive organism is one that is not unfavorably affected by the normal resistance of the body or too rapidly ingested by wandering cells or histiocytes and can enter the blood or tissues and grow there vigorously at the expense of the victim. Degrees of aggressiveness vary greatly. For example, the mucous membranes of the upper respiratory tract are inhabited by large numbers of bacteria that are not equipped to penetrate the normal, unbroken membrane or overcome normal resistance. Many are potentially dangerous pathogens. They remain on the surface without causing an infection because they are readily held in check by the normal protective mechanisms of the body. Once these organisms gain entrance to the deeper tissues, because of injury or weakening of the defensive mechanisms by age, disease, and so on, they may exhibit great "aggressiveness" simply because they find conditions favorable to good growth, like weeds in a fertile field, and because there is nothing to oppose them. Other, more aggressive bacteria require only a very slight opportunity in order to gain a foothold even in normal and healthy tissues, and can invade the tissues in spite of the protective agencies opposing them.

---

[2]Some authors distinguish between *infection* and *disease*, the former term being used to describe the mere presence of organisms, the latter term designating the detrimental effect upon the host. The need for such a distinction in terminology is based upon the more or less widespread use of the phrases "inapparent (or *subclinical*) infection" or "latent infection," in which no detrimental effect is detectable.

Organisms initially of relatively low aggressiveness may rapidly become highly aggressive by means of their own reaction to the defensive mechanisms of the host. They appear to undergo various physiological and biochemical changes, some known (such as genetic mutations and enzyme induction), others unknown, that enable them to evade the host's defensive mechanisms. One of the most readily demonstrable of these changes is the formation of a sort of protective armor in the form of a thick, usually viscous, polysaccharide capsule, often referred to as SSS (soluble specific substance). Thus, microorganisms in the blood or body fluids of patients are particularly likely to be highly dangerous. This is of vital importance to visitors in hospitals and to nurses, laboratory technologists, bacteriologists, physicians, and other health personnel.

Toxigenicity. This is the capacity to produce a toxin or poison. For example, if a bacterium is poisonous, or if it secretes a poisonous substance, then it need not be very aggressive (i.e., invasive) in order to be virulent. It can damage the body by means of its toxin and can paralyze or destroy the powers of resistance of the body cells in which it localizes. It may lack aggressiveness almost entirely and not be able to invade beyond very superficial tissues. Yet, if only a few very toxigenic organisms lodge in the throat on the tonsils or in small foci, such as abscesses at the roots of the teeth, or in the wound made by the puncture of a nail, they may, by producing their poison—which is absorbed and carried all through the host's system—kill their victim.

This is exactly what happens in diphtheria and in tetanus ("lockjaw"). The bacteria that cause these diseases lack aggressiveness almost entirely. Yet by maintaining a slight foothold, as in the crushed, dead tissues of a mangled limb (tetanus), or on the surfaces of the tonsils (diphtheria), they can fatally poison the patient. They are extremely virulent because of their toxigencity, not because of their aggressiveness. Highly invasive or aggressive organisms, such as the streptococci that cause septicemia ("blood poisoning"), and the staphylococci that cause such diseases as meningitis and osteomyelitis, are particularly virulent because they produce several kinds of toxins, some of which destroy leucocytes. Some produce an enzyme that destroys penicillin (*penicillinase*). Many other such pathogenic agents, e.g., lipid-digesting enzymes (*lecithinases*), and enzymes that digest intercellular "cement" substance (*hyaluronidases*) are produced by a variety of virulent microorganisms.

Toxins

Toxigenic microorganisms produce their toxic effect in one or both of two ways.

ENDOTOXINS. Some microorganisms synthesize components of the cell structure that are extremely poisonous. Such toxins, being inside the cell (i.e., part of the cell structure itself), are called *endotoxins* (Greek, *endon*, inside). For example, in the group of bacteria (Enterobacteriaceae) represented by typhoid bacilli (*Salmonella typhi*) and gram-negative bacteria generally, the endotoxins are the lipopolysaccharides of the cell walls. Other examples of endotoxin-producing bacteria are gonococci (*Neisseria gonorrhoeae*) and tubercle bacilli (*Mycobacterium tuberculosis*).

EXOTOXINS. Toxigenic bacteria may also form toxic proteins that diffuse out from the cell. They pass out as waste substances through the cell membrane and wall. Such toxins are called *exotoxins* (Greek, *exo*, outside). Examples of bacteria that produce exotoxins are *Corynebacterium diphtheriae* and *Staphylococcus aureus.* Some bacteria form both exotoxins and endotoxins.

Most exotoxins are proteins or substances much like proteins. Just how they injure the tissues of the body is not yet fully understood. Some evidently combine with certain vital tissues: nerves, heart muscle, liver, and so on, in some noxious manner. Others injure the phagocytes. Some are types of digestive enzymes and digest living cells or parts of cells. Some of these cause destruction of erythrocytes (*hemolysis*). It should be noted that the production of toxic substances is not limited to microorganisms, but is frequently observed in representatives of both the plant kingdom (such as some "toadstools," e.g. *Amanita phalloides*) and the animal kingdom (e.g., poisonous fish, and spider and snake venoms).

SPECIFICITY OF TOXINS. The toxin of each microorganism differs chemically from all others. Thus, diphtheria toxin, an exotoxin, injures the kidneys, nervous tissues, and heart particularly. Tetanus toxin (also an exotoxin) injures certain nerves and thus produces the spasms of lockjaw. As noted previously, staphylococci produce several toxins. One of these, called enterotoxin, which happens to be an exotoxin, produces violent vomiting and diarrhea when swallowed (staphylococcal food poisoning). The term *enterotoxin* implies that the poison acts in the intestine.

staph. is killed very easily by heat, but not its toxin, since it is heat resistance.

Variations in Virulence

Virulence may vary. A highly pathogenic organism may become attenuated or lessened in virulence (or pathogenicity) by growing in certain unfavorable situations, by contact with certain substances, or because of genetic mutations. Bacteria maintained in laboratory culture media may lose some or all of their virulence for animals or human beings. Like hothouse plants, they lose their native power to fend for themselves because of a protected and pampered existence in an artificially suitable environment. As has been stated earlier, bacteria generally lose their capsular material on cultivation on media in the laboratory; they also are less smooth and eventually become rough in their colony-type formation capacity. There is so much irregularity in this, however, that one can never safely say that an organism has entirely lost its virulence unless very careful and extensive tests have been made to establish this fact. Also, by passing organisms of relatively low virulence from one animal or person to another, their virulence may be enormously increased. These apparent changes in microbial virulence probably result from faster growth of, and eventual predominance by, certain individual mutants among the millions of bacterial cells, such mutants being the most capable of multiplying under the condition of cultivation (or infection or chemotherapy) to which the entire microbial population is subjected.

In the next two chapters two types of resistance to infection will be discussed: *nonspecific* resistance (Chapter 18), and *specific* resistance or "immunity," (Chapter 19).

Supplementary Reading

Ajl, S. J., Montie, T. C., et al.: Microbial Toxins, Vol. 2A: Bacterial Protein Toxins. 1971, New York, Academic Press.

Bernheimer, A. W.: Cytolytic toxins of bacteria. *Science*, 1968, *159*:847.

Burrows, W.: Textbook of Microbiology. 19th Ed. 1968, Philadelphia, W. B. Saunders Co.

Caldwell, J. G.: Congenital syphilis: a non-venereal disease. *Am. J. Nursing*, 1971, *71*:1768.

Davis, B. D., Dulbecco, R., Eisen, H. N., Ginsberg, H. S., and Wood, W. B.: Microbiology. 1968, New York, Hoeber Medical Division, Harper & Row.

Joklik, W. K., and Smith, D. T. (Editors): Zinsser Microbiology. 15th Ed. 1972, New York, Appleton-Century-Crofts.

Schwartzman, S., and Boring, J. R., III: Antiphagocytic effect of slime from a mucoid strain of *Pseudomonas aeruginosa. Inf. Immun.*, 1971, *3*:766.

Smith, H.: Biochemical challenge of microbial pathogenicity. *Bact. Rev.*, 1968, *32*:164.

Smith, I. M.: Death from staphylococci. *Sci. Amer.*, 1968, *218*:84.

Villee, C. A.: Biology. 6th Ed. 1972, Philadelphia, W. B. Saunders Co.

Nonspecific Resistance to Infection

18

GENERAL DEFENSIVE MECHANISMS

Although *immunology* is an all-inclusive term, *immunity* is commonly used to imply action of *specific* antibodies. Resistance, like immunology, is a more general term, and includes mechanical barriers, interferons, and so-called "natural" and nonspecific, antibody-like substances, such as various lysins and possibly properdin.

The human race and other species of animals have survived these many centuries because they are equipped with various defensive physiologic mechanisms. These tend to prevent damage by biologic agents such as microorganisms or their toxins that gain entrance to the spaces or tissues of the body. Some of these defensive mechanisms are of a general nature and serve to protect against many types of harmful agents. They are the basis of *nonspecific resistance* and are discussed in this chapter. Other defensive mechanisms are specific in that each is effective against a certain noxious agent and no other. The latter mechanisms are spoken of as *specific resistance*, or *specific immunity*. These will be discussed in the next chapter.

The various kinds of defensive mechanism of the mammalian body (especially the human body) are outlined in Figure 18–1. Unless we are born with immunity (nonspecific, congenital) to a certain disease, we may *acquire* resistance to it either by being infected or receiving maternal antibodies *in utero* or, artificially, from being vaccinated against it, or injected with antitoxin. Acquired resistance may be *active* artificial (resulting from vaccination), when the individual produces his or her own immune response, or *passive* artificial (on injection of antitoxin), when another individual or another species (horse, etc.) has produced the antitoxin.

Species or Racial Resistance

Some species of animals have certain diseases that are peculiar to them, and are resistant to infective conditions that affect only animals of

275

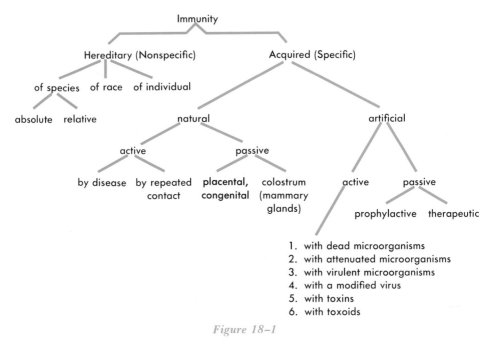

Immunity
Hereditary (Nonspecific)
of species   of race   of individual
absolute   relative
absolute   relative
natural
active   passive
by disease by repeated   placental,   colostrum
            contact   congenital   (mammary
                                        glands)

Acquired (Specific)
artificial
active   passive
            prophylactive   therapeutic

1. with dead microorganisms
2. with attenuated microorganisms
3. with virulent microorganisms
4. with a modified virus
5. with toxins
6. with toxoids

Figure 18–1

Classification of Immunity. (After Professor Andrés Soriano. Adapted from Smith, D. T., Conant, N. F., and Overman, J. R.: Zinsser Microbiology, 13th Ed. New York, Appleton-Century-Crofts.)

some other species. For example, the lower animals never have measles or typhoid fever under natural conditions. Birds are resistant to the kind of tubercle bacilli that infect cattle or human beings. Again, human beings rarely or never become infected with the bird (avian) type of tubercle bacilli or with fowlpox. Under natural conditions none of the lower animals contracts either syphilis or gonorrhea. This blessing is reserved for man.

Species resistance against many mammalian diseases, especially in birds and fish, is probably due largely to differences in body temperature, although chemical and physiologic variations in diverse animals undoubtedly also play a part. A microorganism adapted to living and multiplying in one species often finds it difficult or impossible to adapt itself to life in another, finding there an unfavorable environment. It is virulent with respect to the one, and harmless with respect to the other.

An individual of any race or species, plant or animal, because of general health and robust condition, may be resistant to certain diseases to which members of that race or species are usually susceptible. This is largely a relative resistance, entirely nonspecific; it may vary from day to day and constitutes a resistance not to any specific disease but to disease in general. For example, a man in robust health may resist infection by pneumococci or influenza viruses discharged onto his face by a coughing patient. If, however, he becomes exhausted and weakened by starvation, cold, overwork, or some chronic disease, he may readily succumb to these and a variety of other infections that he could easily resist if he were healthy. Tuberculosis is an excellent example of this type of infection. Because of the interplay of so many factors that determine resistance and immunity, it is almost impossible to resolve what determines an infective dose of a specific microorganism.

The First Line of Defense

The first line of defense against infective microorganisms is the mechanical barriers of the body. The *unbroken skin*, for example, is a good mechanical protection against most microorganisms; with few exceptions, they cannot get through it. Not only is the skin a thick, scaly covering, but in addition the secretions of the skin are bactericidal. If, however, the skin is injured or torn, even microscopically, microorganisms may enter the underlying tissues. Here they may find favorable conditions for growth and then multiply, causing an inflammation, usually with the formation of pus. The danger of neglected accidental wounds and cuts is that they may be the starting point of a serious infection, especially in personnel in the health fields who come into contact with infectious material from patients.

THERAPY FOR BURNS OF THE SKIN.   Damage caused by fire to an extensive area of the body impairs the skin's ability to function effectively in two critical roles for the following reasons: water rapidly escapes from the body, and bacteria, finding warm, moist, and nutritious conditions, maintain an alarmingly high rate of proliferation. As little as 16 hours after a severe burn, dense colonization by *Staphylococcus aureus* and pathogenic gram-negative bacteria has begun. By 24 hours after injury, the bacterial count per gram of eschar (scab, crust) may be as high as 100 million. At the New York Academy of Sciences Conference on Early Treatment of Severe Burns (1967), methods of treatment incorporating both water retention and bacteriostasis were the subjects of many of the papers presented.

Silver nitrate, in a concentration of 0.5 per cent, has been used in the past on wounds infected with *S. aureus* and *Pseudomonas aeruginosa*, two pathogens frequently associated with severe burns. Penicillin and oxacillin are administered to all patients as a precaution against lymphangitis from *Streptococcus pyogenes* and *S. aureus*—both being organisms that multiply in the lymphatic vessels.

In another method of treating burns, Sulfamylon,[1] a drug effective against most of the bacteria commonly found in burn wounds, is utilized as a 10 per cent emulsion in a cream base. Initially, patients are covered twice daily with the cream; no other dressing is used. Daily the wound is cleansed and loosened eschar is removed. Deep dermal wounds, which previously would have been converted to full-thickness injury by infection, can now be kept relatively free of infection without having to resort to skin grafting. Burn wound sepsis has been relegated to a minor role in burn mortality by the use of topical Sulfamylon therapy.

A logical way to provide a substitute for the two important functions of skin destroyed by burns is to give the victim a temporary synthetic skin. The best skin substitute is a double layer of Velour. The double-layer graft is flexible and easily applied. Prosthetic skin has remained in place as long as eight months without evidence of sepsis or rejection.

---

[1] 4-Homosulfanalamide.

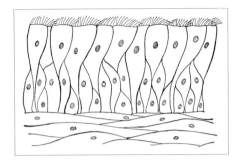

Figure 18–2

Section through the wall of a bronchus, showing the ciliated epithelial cells. These cilia are in constant waving motion, carrying dirt and bacteria upward toward the mouth. The walls of the trachea and nasal sinuses are similarly lined with ciliated epithelium. (About ×1000.)

The *conjunctivae* are protected by the motion of the eyelids and the constant washing of the tears, which carry microorganisms down into the nose. Tears contain a bactericidal substance or enzyme, lysozyme, which presumably helps protect the eyes. Certain bacteria, however, may find the conjunctivae a portal of entry. Gonococci sometimes infect the eye, as do certain organisms of the so-called influenza or hemophilic group that cause "pink-eye." Influenza bacilli and occasionally pneumococci and chlamydias infect the conjunctivae.

The *lungs* are safeguarded by the complicated arrangement of the nasal passages, with their moist mucous membrane. The mucous membranes are covered with a slimy secretion in which dust, bacteria, and other foreign particles are caught like flies on flypaper. The secretion is then removed by sneezing or other means. Leucocytes that have engulfed bacteria may usually be found in the normal nasal secretion. The bacteria that get by and pass into the lungs are generally carried out again by mucus and coughing and by the action of the cilia of the cells lining the trachea and bronchi (Fig. 18–2). If the bacteria are virulent respiratory pathogens, they may evade these defensive mechanisms.

The *gastrointestinal tract* is protected to some extent by the acidity of gastric juice and by other secretions, such as mucus and bile. The acidity of the stomach, however, is often much diminished temporarily by foods such as milk and eggs, so that its protective action may be circumvented. In the intestine, phagocytosis and mucus are important defensive mechanisms. Bile is lethal to many bacteria.

The *mucous membranes of the genitalia* are protected from most bacteria by a rather thick layer of epithelium (skinlike cells) and by acid and mucous secretions. Several organisms can, however, invade the body by means of the genital surfaces. Among these are, of course, the organisms of gonorrhea (*Neisseria gonorrhoeae*) and syphilis (*Treponema pallidum*), as well as *Streptococcus pyogenes, Diplococcus pneumoniae,* and even *Corynebacterium diphtheriae.*

Phagocytosis and Enzymes

One of the most important defensive mechanisms comprises leucocytes (wandering cells) and certain phagocytic tissue cells. The leucocytes and the process of phagocytosis have already been described.

As previously stated, the phagocytic tissue cells are often called *histiocytes* (Greek, *histio,* tissue). They differ from leucocytes in being relatively fixed in the tissues; they do not travel about freely. Histiocytes belong to a large group of cells lining the blood vessels and are present in the spleen, the liver, and the bone marrow. These fixed phagocytes are called the *reticuloendothelial system.* All phagocytic cells ingest many things besides bacteria—bits of harmful or of useless material of various kinds, such as inhaled coal dust or the remains of red blood cells.

Leucocytes may dispose of a comparatively large mass by removing it piecemeal. The "core" of a boil is gradually carried off by the leucocytes, as are also silk and catgut ligatures and, in part, the exudate in various inflammatory conditions. The leucocytes are attracted by anything abnormal or unusual in a tissue or in the blood, such as bacteria, a slight injury, a hemorrhage, the presence of a poison, any dead or useless tissue, or a foreign body. This attraction is probably of a chemical nature and is sometimes called *chemotaxis.* Some phagocytes secrete enzymes that enable them to reduce digestible foreign matter to harmless liquids or in other ways dispose of it. It is probable that phagocytes of all kinds constitute a second line of defensive mechanisms of the body, after the mechanical barriers.

The Properdin System

This is a group of serum components that together apparently play an important role in primary, nonspecific resistance to infection. There are three components in the system: (1) *properdin,* a serum protein, (2) *magnesium* ions, and (3) *complement,* a complex of about 11 interrelated and interacting serum proteins (designated as $C'1$, $C'2$, $C'3$, $C'4$, and so on) that are very important in complementing the action of specific antibodies. Complement is discussed more fully in Chapter 19.

Properdin itself is an enzyme-like agent. It appears to be closely related to, if not an actual part of, the complement complex. The amount of properdin in the blood seems to be directly related to the degree of nonspecific resistance to numerous agents. It is thought to participate in the destruction of certain bacteria, the lysis of certain red cells, and the inactivation of viruses. Injection of properdin-rich serum from animals having naturally high levels of properdin in their serum increases resistance to infection. Injection of certain carbohydrate complexes (*zymosan*) found in the cell walls of certain bacteria and yeasts greatly reduces properdin levels, and with them resistance to infection. Electromagnetic irradiations (this includes visible light, infrared, ultraviolet, X-ray and gamma-ray radiations and also radio frequencies) and infection with certain bacteria also lower properdin levels.

For properdin to affect microorganisms, it is necessary that magnesium ions and complement be present. The exact nature and mechanism of the action of properdin are not yet fully understood. The present evidence indicates that properdin may be a sensitizing agent or one of several nonspecific factors present in serum: immunoglobulin-like substances, enzymes (e.g., lysozyme) or poorly defined bacteriostatic or lytic substances (e.g., beta lysins; basic polypeptides), phagocytin, and the like. These substances are not specific in their action and are generally present at birth in the absence of any known antigenic stimulus.

This type of nonspecific resistance is sometimes called "natural immunity." The term "natural antibody" is sometimes used for the more or-less specific immunoglobulin-like substances mentioned above. These may or may not result from unknown infection or antigenic stimulus. Their exact status seems unclear.

INTERFERON

Interferon is the name given to any or all of a group of closely related proteins (first described in 1957 by Isaacs and Liebermann) of relatively low molecular weight (20,000 to 100,000) that are produced by animal cells in response to the entrance of *double*-stranded viral DNA or RNA (or certain other agents; see below) into the cell either by infection or artificial introduction. Viral infection appears to stimulate new synthesis of interferon; nonviral agents may release preformed interferon of a slightly different nature.

Neither the mode of induction nor the mode of action of interferon is fully understood. Interferon was at first thought to interfere (hence its name) with replication of the virus in the cell, probably by blocking an early eclipse activity of the viral mRNA synthetase system. It is now also thought that interferon evokes synthesis of a second protein that may or may not be antiviral per se. Interferon has no effect whatever on extracellular virus or on intracellular replication of the virion once it has developed beyond the early eclipse phase.

Interferon is neither an enzyme nor a coenzyme. Unlike specific antibodies, it is not an immune globulin (Ig) and is not specific in its action against any particular virus but acts against viruses in general. It has no immunologic relationship to the inducing virion or other inducing agent. The only specific aspect of any interferon is the apparent limitation of its protective activity to animals of the same species as the animal whose cells produced it, although interferons from evolutionarily closely related species (e.g., some primates and man) will cross protect to some extent. Interferon released by an infected cell is taken in by other cells of the same species and thus tends to limit spread of the infection: in the body, in a tissue culture or in a passive recipient of the interferon-containing fluid.

Interferon can be induced by a number of nonviral agents, some microbial (e.g., bacterial lipopolysaccharide endotoxins and certain intracellular parasites), and some synthetic. Important synthetic inducers are double-stranded synthetic homologues of viral nucleic acids such as certain polynucleotide complexes; e.g., polyribocytidylic-polyriboinositic acid (poly C:poly I) and polyriboadenylic-polyuridylic acid (poly A:poly U).

Interferon removed from animals or from tissue cultures (exogenous interferon) has been used both prophylactically and therapeutically in

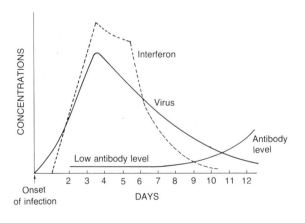

Figure 18–3

Note that appearance of interferon in the blood is almost immediate and its increase rapid. It quickly prevents further virus concentration. Antibodies form much later and more slowly.

animals, with encouraging results. The injection of inducers into animals at the time of, or just prior to, infection with a virus, with a view to stimulating the cells to produce their own protective or curative interferon (endogenous interferon), has also given very promising results. Problems arise from technical difficulties in obtaining large amounts of interferon exogenously; from the necessity of using the greatest caution in dealing with materials derived from human cells that may be infected with oncogenic or other agents; and from the extreme toxicity of some of the inducers, especially the synthetic inducers, endotoxins, and viral nucleic acids. With respect to clinical usefulness of interferons, data from animal studies are abundant and in general are encouraging; however, much human research needs to be done, since the present knowledge is still inconclusive.

INFLAMMATION

Inflammation is a defensive response of living body tissues to any irritating or injurious agent. The inflammatory reaction is a complex process involving several physiologic processes that tend to remove the cause of the irritation, and to repair the damage done, i.e., to heal the wound or lesion. Injury or irritation resulting in inflammation may be due to mechanical factors (such as blows, cuts, breaks), to chemical agents (acids, excessive applications of mustard, bee stings, pepper, certain war gases and the like), to physical agents (such as excessive heat or cold, ultraviolet light), or to living agents (pathogenic microorganisms, worms, and so forth).

The four obvious features of any acute inflammation, frequently referred to as its "cardinal signs," are *redness* or hyperemia (rubor), *swelling* (tumor), *heat* (calor), and *pain* (dolor). These may be observed readily in a boil or in an inflamed joint. The redness results from the increased amount of blood in the dilated local blood vessels; the pain is caused by compression and injury of the sensory nerve branches in the tissue. The swelling (often called *edema*) is caused by the dilatation and increased permeability of the local blood vessels, resulting in the collection of fluid under some slight pressure in the spaces between the tissue cells (inflammatory exudation of fluid).

HYPEREMIA.   Because of the increased blood, an inflamed area is said to be *hyperemic*. The dilatation of the vessels locally causes the blood flow to slow down in that particular area, and in severe injury blood flow may actually be stopped. Then it forms clots, or *thrombi,* in the tiny vessels all around the point of injury. These often act to prevent the entrance of microorganisms and their poisons from the inflamed site into the general blood circulation.

PUS FORMATION.   As the blood slows or stops, the leucocytes, constantly arriving, leave the vessels and begin to make their way into the area of damage, passing between the cells of the vessel walls by the process of ameboid motion called diapedesis. As previously pointed out, these leucocytes become *pus cells*. Inflammation, especially if acute and intense, is therefore usually accompanied by the formation of pus. A mild inflammation may heal without the production of visible pus. In an intense inflammation, such as the venereal disease gonorrhea, very large amounts of pus appear.

TEMPERATURE CHANGES.   The increased heat of inflammation is more apparent than real, being essentially the warmth of the deep body blood brought rapidly to the surface by local dilatation of the capillary blood vessels. Thus, the inflamed area actually feels hot as compared with the usual cool temperature of the body surface. Complicated chemical changes go on in the infected sites, and these may also contribute to the warmth of the inflamed area.

DEFENSIVE FIBRIN. The inflammatory exudate referred to previously is an important defensive factor. Like plasma, which it closely resembles, it contains fibrinogen and other important elements needed in the formation of the blood clot. The inflammatory area is thus soon filled and surrounded by a continuous network of fibrin fibers. At the periphery of the infected area, connective tissue cells (*fibroblasts*) begin to grow among these fibers. The entire inflammatory area is therefore soon surrounded by a wall or sac of fibrin and fibrous connective tissue that tends to confine the inflammatory process and prevent its spread. The area is said to be "walled off." A closed sac of this type, filled with pus and microorganisms, is called an *abscess*, pimple, boil, or furuncle. Several coalesced or inter-communicating abscesses are called a *carbuncle*.

ENZYMES. Various microorganisms produce or activate enzymes that tend to digest the fibrin obstruction. The fluid portion of the exudate in the inflammatory area or sac also contains enzymes and antibodies from the blood that help combat the microorganisms. These enzymes may eventually digest the wall of the abscess nearest the exterior, finally making an opening through which the abscess drains. A boil "coming to a head" is a good example of this process.

Types of Inflammatory Process

An acute inflammation is of short duration, lasting perhaps for a number of days. It is usually, but not always, fairly intense.

A chronic inflammation is usually thought of as lasting for weeks, months, or years. It may be either mild or severe, extensive or restricted. *Catarrhal inflammation*, which may be either acute or chronic, is a form that affects principally a mucous surface. It is marked by discharge of mucopus and epithelial debris as in colds or influenza.

Fibrinous inflammation is that in which the inflammatory exudate contains fibrin in large amounts. It is seen often in very intense and acute inflammations and is characteristically found on certain inner surfaces, such as the lining of the abdominal cavity (peritoneum), the covering of the heart (pericardium), or the coverings of the lungs and lining of the thoracic or chest wall (pleurae). The fibrin strands may cause roughness of the surfaces with resultant pain on motion, as in pleurisy. Fibrin may also cause adherence (fibrous *adhesions*) between structural surfaces or following surgery, with resulting disturbances of function.

In *serous inflammation* there is more of the serum-like fluid and less of the fibrin. Sanguino- (bloody) serous and other combined types of exudate may occur. The blood seen in such exudates may have escaped from local capillary vessels injured by the pathogenic agent.

If much pus is formed, we may describe the process as *purulent* or *suppurative*. A fluid may be *sanguinopurulent* or *fibrinopurulent*, and so on.

Healing and Scar Formation

As soon as fibrin forms and other defensive mechanisms begin to bring the infection or injury under control, tissue cells (fibroblasts) and other tissue elements (blood vessels, and so on) begin to grow into the area of healing from the periphery, and to form new, healthy tissue. This early healing process is called *organization*, and the tissue it forms is solid, tough, connective tissue when mature. This tissue, in repair situations, constitutes *scar tissue*. The process of scar formation is called *cicatrization*.

Supplementary Reading

Berry, L. J., Smythe, D. S., Colwell, L. S., Schoengold, R. J., and Actor, P.: Comparison of the effects of a synthetic polyribonucleotide with the effects of endotoxin on selected host responses. *Inf. and Immun.*, 1971, *3*:444.

Carpenter, P. L.: Immunology and Serology. 3rd Ed. 1972, Philadelphia, W. B. Saunders Co.

Colby, C., and Morgan, M. J.: Interferon induction and action. *Ann. Rev. Microbiol.*, 1971, *25*:333.

De Clercq, E., and De Somer, P.: Antiviral activity of polyribocytidylic acid in cells primed with polyriboinosinic acid. *Science*, 1971, *173*:260.

Fitzpatrick, F. W., and Di Carlo, F. J.: Zymosan (reproperdin). *Ann. N.Y. Acad. Sci.*, 1964, *118*(Art. 4):233.

Hanna, M. G., (Editor): Contemporary Topics in Immunobiology. Volume 1. 1972, New York, Plenum Press.

Herrmann, E. C. Jr., and Stinebring, W. R. (Editors): Second Conference on Antiviral Substances. *Ann. N.Y. Acad. Sci.*, 1970, *173*(Art. 1):1–844.

Hirsch, J. G.: Phagocytosis. *Ann. Rev. Microbiol.*, 1965, *19*:339.

Kabat, E. A.: Structural Concepts in Immunology and Immunochemistry. 1968, New York, Holt, Rinehart & Winston, Inc.

Kazar, J., Gillmore, J. D., and Gordon, F. B.: Effect of interferon and interferon inducers on infections with a nonviral intracellular microorganism, *Chlamydia trachomatis. Inf. and Immun.*, 1972, *3*:825.

Spector, W. G. (Editor): The acute inflammatory response. *Ann. N.Y. Acad. Sci.*, 1964, *116* (Art. 3):747.

Specific Resistance to Infection

ACTIVE IMMUNITY

An individual may become immune to certain infectious diseases by actually contracting them and recovering. The resulting immunity is entirely *specific;* that is, a person who recovers from diphtheria is usually immune to subsequent attacks of diphtheria, but this does not prevent him from contracting typhoid or smallpox.

The following question concerning resistance to infection is frequently asked by students. "What diseases induce permanent immunity in the patient who recovers from them?" A complete reply would include a considerable list of diseases. Among the well known diseases of man, lasting immunity usually results from measles, chickenpox, whooping cough, bubonic plague, poliomyelitis, smallpox, Rocky Mountain spotted fever, diphtheria, scarlet fever, tularemia, typhus fever, typhoid fever, and yellow fever, among others. Second (confirmed) cases of yellow fever, smallpox, and measles have rarely been reported, though some second cases have been reported to occur following diphtheria, scarlet fever, cholera, typhoid fever, mumps, and several other diseases. In some of these the diagnosis of either the first or the second case has been questioned; in other cases, there is no doubt of the repetition. The implication is that immunity can vary and is not necessarily either absolute or unchanging. Little if any lasting immunity results from the group of infections called "common colds" or from influenza, erysipelas, furunculosis, gonorrhea, septic sore throat, herpes simplex, or pneumococcal pneumonia (if caused by a strain of *Diplococcus pneumoniae* other than that which induced the initial infection). The immunity is, in large part, a result of the production by plasma cells and probably others of soluble protein molecules called *antibodies* or *immunoglobulins* (see page 255).

In some diseases, the stimulus by the infecting organism is long-lasting (see page 270), so that the antibody-producing cells continue to produce the antibodies long after the infection has disappeared, sometimes during the entire life of the patient. In some instances this may be due to continuous subclinical infection. The antibodies can often be found in the blood many years after recovery from clinical disease by appropriate test methods, some of which will be described later. In other infections (for example, typhoid fever) detectable antibody production subsides completely and the plasma cells that produced the specific antibodies revert to a sort of "dormant" state as small lymphocytes, though they remain "alert" or conditioned to react with the specific antigen that engendered them. On renewed contact with the specific antigen, they quickly become reactivated and multiply rapidly as plasma cells. Within a few hours they produce large amounts of the required specific antibody (in this case, antityphoid antibodies). Because they appear to "remember" the typhoid bacilli (or any other specific antigen), the small lymphocytes that become specifically reactivated to antibody-producing plasma cells are sometimes called "memory cells."

SUBCLINICAL OR INAPPARENT INFECTIONS.   In order to acquire specific active immunity against a disease one need not contract that disease in a severe (or *clinical*) form. On the contrary, many persons develop immunity to such diseases as diphtheria and scarlet fever and, in the tropics, to yellow fever, without ever being aware of any definite attack of illness. Their youth, health, or racial stock may have enabled them successfully to withstand the invaders to the extent that no severe illness occurred, yet the body cells were sufficiently stimulated to produce antibodies. Possibly the organisms may have been somewhat less virulent than usual. Either way, this antibody response in the absence of recognizable clinical symptoms is usually ascribed to a *subclinical, latent,* or *inapparent* infection.

Specific Antibody Formation

The formation of specific antibodies is a response of lymphocytes and probably other cells of the body to certain substances that are of particular chemical composition and that, except for certain rare cases, come from sources outside the body proper. The foreign substances that stimulate antibody formation are given the general name of *antigens*. These must be discussed before we can understand antibodies and antibody formation.

ANTIGENS.   Any substance that, when it gains entrance to the blood or tissues of the body, stimulates the production of *antibodies* with which it will react is called an antigen (or *immunogen*). As already noted, the body responds to antigens with the production of antibodies, which act as specific "antidotes" to the antigens and react with them to destroy or remove them. It should be explained that, unless otherwise noted, the discussions of antigens, the reaction of body cells to antigens, and the formation and role of antibodies in Chapters 18 through 20 refer to *initial contact* of the body cells with antigen. This contact, in addition to inducing specific immunity or tolerance, may also induce a state of *hypersensitivity* or *allergy* on later contact with the same antigen (see Chapter 21).

Until recently it was thought that, with a few important exceptions, the only substances that could act as antigens were water-soluble *proteins* or nonprotein substances combined (conjugated) with proteins, and that if a substance was a protein or a protein conjugate, it could probably act as an antigen. Indeed, proteins and protein conjugates are the most active of all antigens. It is now recognized, however, that *carbohydrates*, such as pneumococcal polysaccharides, carbohydrate-amino acid compounds, the yeast polysaccharide zymosan, synthetic *polypeptides*, or even *lipoidal* substances (e.g., sterols or lecithin), may be antigenic in certain animals or man. Even *nucleic acids* such as DNA and RNA have been shown to be antigenic in rabbits, most likely because of specific functions of the purine and pyrimidine bases.

Antigens need not be poisonous or of microbial origin. Such substances as egg white, serum, milk, snake venom, dead or living bacteria, bacterial exo- and endotoxins, plant or animal tissues or their derivatives, chiefly proteins or protein conjugates, may act as antigens when introduced into the deeper body tissues, or subcutaneously. Most substances taken into the normal gastrointestinal tract as food do not act as antigens because their molecular structure is quickly destroyed by the digestive juices. To act antigenically the substance must gain entrance to the blood and other tissues in a chemically unaltered state. Entrance is commonly by infection, injection, or parenterally (Greek, *para*, beyond or outside of; *enteron*, intestine), i.e., by routes other than by the gastrointestinal tract. There are certain exceptions such as food allergies (Chapter 21).

ANTIBODIES.   Antibodies are globulins released by certain cells of the blood and tissues into the blood in response to antigenic stimulation. They have been discussed in Chapter 16. Antibodies may act in one or more of several different ways as described below.

Opsonic Action.   Some antibodies appear to have no directly injurious effect on microorganisms, yet seem to render the microorganisms more susceptible to phagocytosis. They appear to alter the surfaces of the organisms so that the phagocytes more readily engulf them. It was once thought that special antibodies called *opsonins*[1] were involved. It now appears that several of the antibodies to be discussed perform this function. It is perhaps more correct, therefore, to speak of the *opsonizing effect* (or *opsonic action*) of antibodies. As previously stated, phagocytosis is one of the most (if not the most) important defensive mechanisms. Since opsonic action greatly enhances phagocytosis, it, also, is seen to be of major importance.

Haptens.   As shown by Landsteiner, Pauling, Boyd and others, numerous substances not ordinarily thought of as antigens (i.e., not immunogenic), including various drugs such as aspirin and penicillin, synthetics such as perfumes, and rubber, that lack the chemical structure and molecular weight to make them antigenic per se, can, nevertheless, become conjugated with proteins and thus become fully and specifically antigenic. As a class, such substances are called *haptens* or *partial antigens* or, if derived from larger molecules, *residue antigens*. Many of them, even if entirely separated from the protein that made them antigenic, can combine with the specific antibodies. In such combinations they do not typically cause a precipitin or other demonstrable antigen-antibody reaction; however, their combination with antibody inhibits combination of the antibody with the true, complete, specific antigen. This is called *hapten inhibition*. As will be discussed in Chapter 21, many haptenic substances can be of great importance as inducers of the *allergic state*, i.e., as *allergens*.

Antitoxins.   Plant, animal, or bacterial *exotoxins* that are *proteins* and *soluble in water* stimulate the formation of antibodies called *antitoxins*. These, by means of a physicochemical interaction, inactivate or neutralize

---

[1] The name is based on the Greek word *opsonein*, meaning a cook, or one who prepares food.

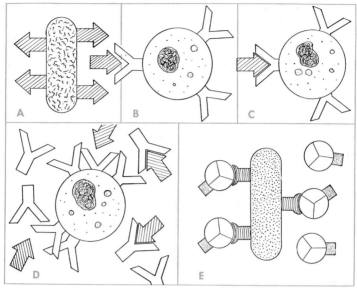

Figure 19–1

Type of diagram used to illustrate part of Ehrlich's side chain theory. *A* represents a bacterium secreting molecules of exotoxin, which are represented as dart-shaped bodies. *B* is a body cell with chemical affinities represented by Y-shaped portions ("side chains"), *antibodies* or *receptors*. *C* represents the combination of the exotoxin molecules with the cell antibodies or receptors due to the correspondence of shape (chemical structure) of the points of the darts and the indentation of the side chains. This cell is poisoned. *D* represents a cell, stimulated by toxin, giving off Y-shaped side chains that represent molecules of specific *antitoxin*. These combine with the toxin molecules (darts) before they reach this or other cells. *E* represents a bacterium with fixed side chains representing endotoxin. These have been completely neutralized by antibodies from tissue cells. Specificity is represented by the fact that antigens (in this case exo- and endotoxins) and antibodies fit together. If the endotoxin molecules in *E*, for example, were convex instead of concave, the disk-shaped antitoxin bodies could not fit onto (combine specifically with) them and the bacterium would remain poisonous.

It is now known that antibodies are produced principally by lymphocytes and plasma cells. It is thought that each antigen promotes growth of plasma cell variants especially adapted to that specific antigen (clonal selection hypothesis).

the exotoxins that stimulated their formation. For example, when diphtheria organisms establish themselves in the throat and grow there, they excrete a powerful exotoxin into the blood. The antibody-producing cells of the body respond by producing *diphtheria antitoxin*. An analogous reaction occurs with all other soluble protein toxins, no matter how they gain entrance (undigested) to the blood—by infection, by hypodermic injection, or by absorption. Each toxin, however, stimulates the production of antibodies only against itself and not against some other toxin. For example, the poison of the cobra will engender antitoxin (antivenin) only against the cobra venom and not against diphtheria toxin or tetanus toxin. Each antibody is strictly specific against its own antigen.

IMMUNOLOGICAL SPECIFICITY. In an attempt to explain this specificity, Paul Ehrlich, the famous German physician and medical immunologist, tried to express the specific relations of antigens and antibodies graphically. He thought of these substances as particles or complex protein molecules having chemical groups called side arms or "side chains," which could mutually fit together only by complex chemical interactions. An example of the type of Ehrlich's diagrams of his side chain theory is given in Figure 19–1. Today Ehrlich's basic idea is still applicable, but we now know that the chemical side chains as conceived by Ehrlich include in addition all chemical, physical, atomic, and electrical configurations of the molecular surfaces and structures. Some of these chemicophysical relationships between antigen and antibody are very complex—much like a complicated Yale lock and the elaborately shaped and highly specific key needed to unlock it. Specificity is characteristic of all immunologic reactions and enzyme functions. The molecular basis of antigen-antibody specificity is beyond the scope of the present discussion. The subject is fascinating, however, and interested readers will find guides in the list of Supplementary Reading following Chapter 20.

Sensitizers and Complement

There are thousands of different antibodies. Not all, however, are antitoxins. The antigen-antibody combinations of some of them become manifest in a variety of other ways. One of the best known of these is due to the type of specific antibodies called *sensitizers*. The manifestation of their reaction with antigen is a little more complicated than that of the antitoxins since, instead of reacting with soluble molecules of protein (exotoxins), sensitizers react with antigens that are parts of whole cells.

CYTOLYSINS. A good illustration of sensitizers is the type of antibody called cytolysin (Greek *cyto*, cell; *lysin*, dissolves). The production of sensitizing antibodies is stimulated by organized structures such as living bacterial cells (as contrasted with unorganized matter such as soluble toxins, cobra venom, egg white, and serum). The cytolysins, as their name indicates, help dissolve the cells that stimulated their production.

In causing the destruction of cells such as red blood cells of another species, the cytolysin must first combine with the specific "side chain" portion (or *antigenic determinant*) of the cell. The antibody is said to be *adsorbed* by the cells; this is a specific physicochemical surface combination. This combination is not by itself sufficient to dissolve or lyse the cells. It sensitizes them, however, to the action of substances called the *complement* complex previously referred to on page 279.

COMPLEMENT. This thermolabile serum fraction has also been called alexin and (originally) cytase. It is enzyme-like in activity and is always present in fresh, normal blood. Complement is not produced as a result of the introduction of an antigen. It complements the work of lysis, hence its name. It is nonspecific because it assists any and all cytolysins, and some other antibodies (e.g., opsonins), to complete their work.

Complement cannot produce cytolysis alone, but must act through the intermediation of the specific sensitizer. No matter how many different specific sensitizers are produced, the same nonspecific complement functions with all. Complement consists of several substances that are generally recognized as factors $C'1$, $C'2$, $C'3$ (which is now subdivided into six proteins: $C'3$, $C'5$, $C'6$, $C'7$, $C'8$, and $C'9$), and the heat stable $C'4$ component. Other components are known, but are still being studied.

HEMOLYSINS. If an animal is injected several times with the erythrocytes of another species of animal, the serum of the recipient animal acquires the power of destroying the RBC's of the donor species. This is due to the formation of cytolysins that combine with the donor red cells and sensitize them to complement in the blood of the recipient. Further reactions are very complex. They involve stepwise incorporations of complement fractions (proteins) and enzyme-like cofactors. The red blood cell, or bacterial cell, develops small holes, each 100 Å in diameter, through which the hemoglobin (or bacterial cell contents) escapes into the surrounding fluid. Lysis then occurs. This process is called *cytolysis* or, in the case of RBC's, *hemolysis*. The hemolytic cytolysins are called *hemolysins*. Similarly, the specific sensitizing antibodies that mediate the dissolution of bacterial cells are designated *bacteriolysins*. Gram-positive bacteria, including mycobacteria, are not susceptible to the action of complement.

FIXATION OF COMPLEMENT. When complement is involved in a reaction between antigen and antibody, it combines with them, presumably by adsorption on the surface of the combined antigen and antibody molecules. It is apparently used up or "fixed." *Complement fixation* (CF) is said to have occurred.

The *Wassermann test* (or Kolmer-Wassermann test) is an outstanding application of CF for diagnostic purposes. The German bacteriologist and physician August von Wassermann (1866–1925) showed that the organisms of syphilis, like other bacteria, engender specific sensitizers. These sensitizers, like others, "fix" complement when combined with their antigens, the syphilis organisms, or, as we shall see later, a nonspecific cardiolipin antigen. The fixation of complement can then easily be demonstrated by a simple test (hemolysis) for free (unfixed) complement. The CF technique has many other diagnostic and research applications. For example, it may be used to diagnose infections with the TRIC agents, the *Chlamydia* of trachoma inclusion conjunctivitis, or to determine antibodies present in individuals infected with adenoviruses, arboviruses, influenza or rickettsial diseases, and so forth.

IMMOBILIZING ANTIBODIES. Once infection with the spirochete *Treponema pallidum* occurs, syphilis develops. In the absence of drug therapy, as the disease progresses specific antibodies appear in the blood. These can be demonstrated by CF tests, as just mentioned. They can also be demonstrated by mixing a little serum from the patient with a suspension of living *T. pallidum*. The spirochetes, ordinarily characterized by an active twisting, undulating, corkscrew-like motion, are seen to lose this mobility within a short time in the presence of syphilitic serum. They die soon afterward. The test is entirely specific and is highly reliable when properly performed. Similar specific immobilizing antibodies can be shown to occur in numerous other infections.

It is of particular interest to note here that: the *Treponema pallidum* immobilization (TPI) test was the first practical and specific blood test for syphilis; complement is a necessary component of the immobilization test. This suggests that the immobilization antibody is of the nature of a sensitizer, but the true nature of the antibody is not yet clear.

THE IMMUNE-ADHERENCE PHENOMENON. Bacteria of several widely different species, in the presence of specific, sensitizer-like antibody and complement, adhere to the erythrocytes of the host as though the microorganisms had become sticky. This immune-adherence phenomenon is of importance because when the sticky bacteria are thus held by the erythrocytes, they fall an easy prey to the leucocytes. The immune-adherence phenomenon is thus seen as a specific opsonic function, aiding an important defensive mechanism as well as offering a good diagnostic test.

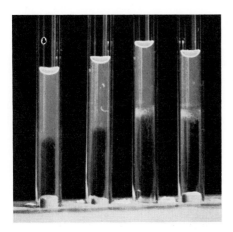

Figure 19–2

Precipitin test in narrow-bore glass tubes. The antigen solution is the cloudy zone above; the antiserum is the clear zone below. At the interface between them, in the two right-hand tubes, a definite white floc or precipitate has formed, representing a reaction between specifically related antigen and antibody. The same antigen fails to react with a different (nonspecific) serum in the two left-hand tubes. (×5.) (Preparation by Dr. Elaine L. Updyke. Photo courtesy of the Communicable Disease Center, U.S. Public Health Service, Atlanta, Ga.)

PRECIPITINS. In addition to the antibody reactions already described, there are antitoxins and antitoxin-like antibodies that combine with molecules of soluble proteins and cause the protein molecules to gather in minute but visible flakes or granules, bringing about a cloudiness in the fluid in which they are suspended. This flocculent turbidity is called a precipitate (Fig. 19–2). Antibodies that act in this way against protein molecules are called *precipitins*, and the antigen-antibody reaction itself is termed *precipitation*. These reactions, like all antigen-antibody reactions, are specific. Although not essential to precipitate formation, complement is fixed if it is present. This is because complement is readily adsorbed by any minutely particulate matter, such as soot and clay.

The Unitarian Hypothesis of Antibodies. It is important to note that precipitins are engendered by the sorts of antigens that also engender antitoxins, i.e., soluble (noncellular) proteins or protein complexes, such as toxins, serum, and egg white. Antitoxins and precipitins are very much alike in many ways. They may be identical.

Chemically pure antigens are uncommon in nature. Any living or active antigen (e.g., a virus or bacterial cell, or even serum) is really a mixture of antigens. On injection of, or infection by, any such antigen, several types of antibodies are generally formed. Of these, some may react in only one kind of milieu to cause only one manifestation of antigen-antibody reaction (e.g., precipitation); the same, or others, may cause a different manifestation, depending on the antigens, the types of antibodies engendered and the physicochemical conditions of the milieu. The apparent diversity of antibodies may actually represent milieu-determined reactions of only a few types.

Precipitin Reactions. These are used for many purposes when the identity of a protein antigen or antibody is in question. For example, if we have on hand a group of known antigens, we may use them to detect unknown antibodies in a patient's serum and, thus, diagnose his disease. We may also have available a collection of sera, each containing a known type of precipitin for a different protein, and use these antibodies to identify organisms and also various protein substances. For example, in legal medicine, it is possible to determine whether a blood stain is of human or animal origin. If it is human blood, an extract made from it gives a precipitate when the serum of an animal immunized by repeated injections

Table 19–1.   Scheme for a Complete Precipitin Test*

	TUBE NUMBER									
	TESTS					CONTROLS				
	1	2	3	4	5	6	7	8	9	10
UPPER LAYER (ANTIGEN)	Extract 1:HT	Extract 1:10T	Extract 1:T	Extract 1:H	Extract 1:10	Extract 1:H	0.9% NaCl	Substrate extract	Heterologous blood 1:T	Known human blood 1:T
LOWER LAYER (ANTIBODY)	Antiserum	Antiserum	Antiserum	Antiserum	Antiserum	Normal rabbit serum	Antiserum	Antiserum	Antiserum	Antiserum
EXPECTED RESULTS						−	−	−	−	+

*H standing for hundred and T for thousand are common abbreviations used in bacteriology for designating certain dilutions. Thus, 1:HT represents a 1:100,000 dilution, 1:T stands for 1:1,000, and so on. The controls as shown must give the expected results or the tests will not constitute valid data. For example, if the antigen is human blood on a man's shirt in medicolegal testing, tubes 6 and 7 would test for the antibody specificity, tube 8 for the possibility that a piece of the man's shirt could be responsible for a false-positive test (this has to be ruled out), tube 9 would be blood from other than human sources, and known human blood would be the positive control in tube 10.

of human blood is added to the solution of the stain. The test is very delicate and may be done even many years after the stain has dried. If the blood spot has come from other than human sources, it will not give a precipitate with the serum of an animal immunized against human protein. Table 19–1 shows a typical scheme for a complete precipitin test with controls.

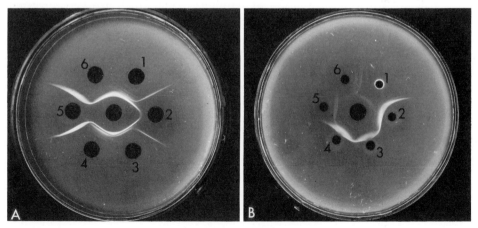

Figure 19–3

A, Immunodiffusion pattern using Auto-Gel 7 mm size cutters. Goat anti-human serum in the central cup; (1) and (4) normal human serum, (2) goat anti-human gamma G, (3) and (6) human urine, (5) goat anti-human albumin. B, Immunodiffusion pattern using Auto-Gel 4 mm size cutters. Normal human serum in the central cup; (1) goat anti-human alpha^2 macroglobulin, (2) and (4) goat anti-human serum, (3) goat anti-human albumin, (5) goat anti-human gamma globulin, (6) goat anti-human glycoprotein. (Courtesy of Grafar Corp., Michigan.)

The Precipitin Test in Agar.   The test is often done in a Petri dish by placing serum that contains precipitins in a depression in the surface of a layer of agar, near a depression containing fluid antigen. The antigen and antibodies diffuse outward, in the agar, from their respective depressions. Along the line where they come into contact a white precipitate appears in the agar if antigens and antibodies are mutually specific (Fig. 19–3). This is the basis of the "Ouchterlony" method. There are various modifications of this procedure, using gels in test tubes: single diffusion, double diffusion, and so on. Widely used are the Oudin procedure, the Preer method and the Oakley-Fulthorpe diffusion in one dimension. Often the precipitin reaction in agar is combined with mobility studies of the proteins (antibody, antigen) in one electric field. This technique is called "immunoelectrophoresis" (Fig. 19–4). It permits the identification of each constituent with great resolving power and has unlimited applications in immunochemistry research.

AGGLUTININS.   Agglutinins are similar to precipitins in their action, but they bring about the clumping of entire organized cells rather than molecules of protein. Under the influence of agglutinins the bacterial or other cells act as though their surfaces had become sticky so that they are glued together in clumps—hence *agglutination.* This reaction, due to the much larger antibody-antigen complex, is macroscopic, whereas the precipitin reaction particles are almost at the microscopic level of visibility. The connecting of cells by "bridges" of coupling antibody molecules has an opsonic effect, since aggluntinated cells are more rapidly and readily engulfed by phagocytes than single cells. The production of agglutinins can be stimulated by injections of various kinds of cells; among those that have the greatest practical importance to the diagnostician are bacteria and erythrocytes.

A number of useful diagnostic tests are based on bacterial agglutinins. For example, if a person has typhoid fever, his blood will be found to contain agglutinins against typhoid bacilli. By mixing a little of his serum with a culture or suspension of typhoid bacilli, which are kept growing in the laboratory for such tests, the action of the agglutinins can be observed. After a short interval all the bacilli, evenly distributed throughout the culture at first, become gathered together into fairly large clumps and flocs and settle to the bottom of the test tube, leaving the suspending fluid clear (Figs. 9–15, 9–16).

Diagnosis of various undetermined infections can be made in this way. If a patient's serum agglutinates a certain kind of organism, then

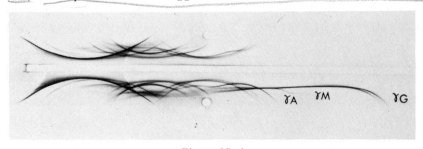

Figure 19–4

Immunoelectrophoresis of serum (*A*). *Top,* Congenital agammaglobulinemia. Note complete absence of γM, γA and γG bands. *Bottom,* Normal serum showing normal amounts of γM, γA and γG. (Bellanti: Immunology. W. B. Saunders Co., Philadelphia, 1971).

he probably has, or has had, an infection with that organism. Sometimes a person's serum gives an agglutination reaction, not because he has an infection at present, but because he has previously received injections (vaccine) of the organism that his serum agglutinates.

Diagnostic Importance of Rising Titers. In order to distinguish between antibodies of any kind due to present infection and those due to past infection or to vaccines given long since, it is necessary to take two specimens of the patient's serum, one near the onset of the infection and one 10 to 12 days later. If the patient's cells are producing antibodies in response to the present infection, the *titer* (concentration of antibodies in the serum) will be low in the first specimen and definitely higher in the second. If few or no antibodies are present in either specimen, the patient is failing to produce any, because of a congenital defect (agammaglobulinemia), excessive radiation, or other immunosuppressive measures or because his infection is due to some organism other than that being used as antigen. If antibodies are present but fail to show any change in titer between first and second specimens, then they were probably present before the infection began and are unrelated to it.

Hemagglutination. In addition to the specific agglutination of bacteria described in the preceding pages, there are some curious and important agglutination phenomena called *hemagglutination* because they are related to red blood cells. These may be considered under four headings: *cold hemagglutinins, passive or indirect hemagglutination, viral hemagglutination,* and *isohemagglutinins.*

COLD HEMAGGLUTININS. These are substances that appear in the blood of persons with certain respiratory diseases, such as certain "atypical" pneumonias of mycoplasma (*M. pneumoniae*) origin, and also in the blood of those infected by certain protozoan parasites (trypanosomiasis). These hemagglutinins are of unknown significance beyond the fact that, since they rarely appear in association with other diseases, they are of value in aiding diagnosis. The sera of the patients, in dilutions as high as 1 : 10,000, agglutinate their own erythrocytes (autohemagglutinins) when cooled to 2 C but do not do so at 37 C. This agglutination at low temperature gives rise to the name *cold hemagglutination.*

INDIRECT (PASSIVE) HEMAGGLUTINATION REACTION. This very useful procedure illustrates the fact that antigens at the surface of a cell determine its immunological specificity. Erythrocytes (sheep, in this example) are washed free from their serum. The cells are treated with tannic acid or formaldehyde to solidify them and toughen the surfaces. The erythrocytes are again washed and then suspended in a saline solution containing any desired *soluble* antigen—for example, an antigen extracted from tuberculosis bacilli. This antigen is adsorbed by the surfaces of the erythrocytes and covers them as a coating. The cells are again washed to remove excess antigen and suspended in saline solution.

A series of dilutions is now made with serum containing antibodies specific for the antigens with which the erythrocytes are coated (in this example tuberculosis antigen). Into each serum dilution is introduced a drop of the saline suspension of antigen-coated erythrocytes. In this example they behave as though they were tubercle bacilli. Within a short time the coated sheep erythrocytes are specifically agglutinated. Tuberculosis antibodies have no visible effect whatever on the uncoated, tannic-acid-treated erythrocytes of a sheep. It is interesting that totally inert particles of plastic, gum arabic, latex, and so on can be similarly coated with antigen and agglutinated by specific antibodies. The method is very accurate and is being widely adapted for diagnostic purposes, e.g., in syphilis.

VIRAL HEMAGGLUTINATION.   Agglutination of red cells of chickens is brought about by several respiratory viruses, such as the influenza virus. Note that this is not antibody agglutination. The virus itself appears to adhere to the red cells of the chick at about 5 C and agglutinate them. It can be separated (eluted) from them by mixing them with saline solution followed by incubation for two hours at 37 C. Still other viruses, such as those of yellow fever and encephalitis (mosquito-borne viruses), cause agglutination of avian erythrocytes at temperatures around 30 C. These hemagglutination tests, which may involve the use of red cells derived from many different species, are important in the study of viruses and in the diagnosis of viral diseases.

In some infections antibodies may occur that prevent viral agglutination of erythrocytes. They are called hemagglutination-inhibition (HI) antibodies. They are of great practical importance in diagnostic virology, being one of the principal means of identifying infecting viruses (Fig. 19–5).

ISOHEMAGGLUTININS.   These remarkable and important antibodies occur genetically in the serum of most normal persons. Isohemagglutinins are responsible for the A, B, AB and other blood groupings discussed in Chapter 16.

FLUORESCENT[2] ANTIBODY STAINING.   This method, sometimes

---

[2]By fluorescence is meant the property of reflecting light rays having a color (wavelength) differing from that of the incident rays. Fluorescent objects are particularly brilliant in ultraviolet light.

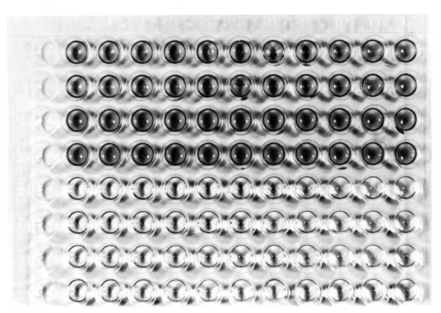

Figure 19–5

Tests for hemagglutination-inhibiting (HI) antibodies against influenza virus. HI antibodies were present in the sera tested in the four lower rows of tubes (viral hemagglutination completely inhibited); viral hemagglutination occurred in all other tubes (no influenza HI antibodies present). The bottoms of the tubes are viewed from directly above.

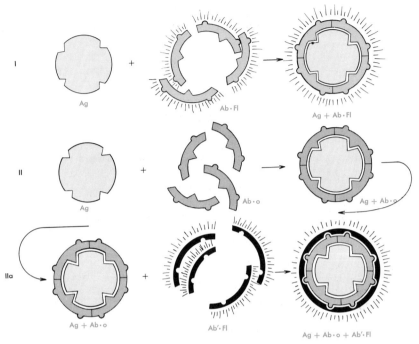

Figure 19–6

Direct and indirect fluorescent-antibody staining. In the direct method (I) antigen (Ag) is allowed to react with its specific antibody which has previously been conjugated with a fluorescent dye (Ab·Fl.) When viewed in the microscope with ultraviolet illumination the antigen-antibody combination (probably on the surface of bacteria or virus particles) glows brilliantly.

In the indirect method (II) the antigen is combined with ordinary (nonfluorescent) specific antibody (Ab·o). Viewed with ultraviolet light no fluorescence is seen. It is impossible to say whether specific combination of Ag and Ab has occurred. The invisible Ag + Ab·o combination is now treated (IIa) with fluorescent antibody specific for *any* gamma globulin (from a different species of animal) (Ab'·Fl). All antibodies including Ab·o, are gamma globulins. Ab'·Fl therefore combines with Ab·o on the surface of Ag, causing the particles of Ag + Ab·o + Ab'·Fl to glow in ultraviolet light.

called FA staining, is one of the most interesting and valuable advances in the field of microbiology. It involves the fluorescent labeling of antibodies so that their combination with specific antigens may be detected visually and immediately. This is in contrast to the time-consuming antigen-antibody tests previously described.

Although the FA staining procedure is technically complex, the principle involved is relatively simple. The first step is the separation and concentration of specific antibody globulins from the serum in which they occur. These globulins are then combined with a fluorescent dye, commonly fluorescein isothiocyanate or rhodamine B. The antibodies are then said to be *labeled* or *conjugated*. When illuminated with ultraviolet light they emit a brilliant glow (Fig. 19–6). Various labeled antibody preparations may be obtained commercially.

Let us suppose that a bacterial smear, section of tissue, or tissue culture containing a particular antigen (such as virus, rickettsia, bacterium) is flooded with a solution of fluorescent-labeled antibody specific for the antigen. The antibody combines as usual with the corresponding antigen.

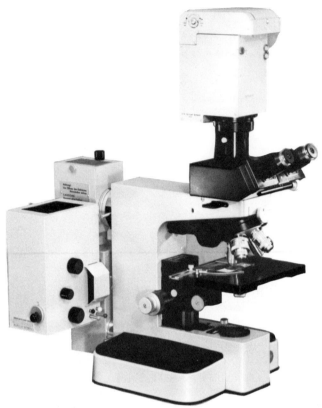

Figure 19–7

Leitz ORTHOPLAN microscope set up for transmitted and reflected fluorescence microscopy, as well as bright field observations. Attached to the back of the microscope are two lamp housings. The larger one contains a mercury burner HBO 200 (for transmitted light) and the smaller one the HBO 100 (for reflected light). On top of the fluorescence microscope is the automatic 35 mm ORTHOMAT W camera. (This illustration was provided through the courtesy of Mr. Albert Heydemann and the E. Leitz Co., Rockleigh, N.J.)

The preparation is then washed to remove excess (unattached) antibody. When the smear or section is viewed with a microscope using ultraviolet light as a source of illumination, the presence of the antigen, with the fluorescent antibody combined with it, is revealed as a brilliantly fluorescent particle glowing on a relatively dim or dark background (Fig. 19–7).

This staining procedure has many variations, including the direct method, an indirect method (Fig. 19–6), and the detection of complement fixed in situ, where the antigen-antibody reaction has taken place. It has greatly simplified problems of medical diagnosis and research by making it possible to detect, and localize quickly, extremely minute amounts of antigen, even virus particles inside of infected cells.

Supplementary Reading

(See the list of readings following Chapter 20.)

Active and Passive Immunity

20

ACTIVE ARTIFICIAL IMMUNITY

As described in the preceding chapter, immunity that is actively acquired in the ordinary course of life (i.e., as a result of clinical or subclinical infectious disease) is generally very effective and often durable. However, if one wishes to acquire a certain kind of immunity at a particular time, one can never be sure whether such natural processes will occur, when they will occur, or whether the infection necessarily involved will cause severe or fatal disease. It is often desirable to develop immunity safely, with certainty, at certain times, in certain people. For this purpose man has developed *artificial* processes such as vaccination, which simulate nature but which are adapted to meet practical requirements and are under human control. Several types of such processes are used, as follows.

Injection of Living, Attenuated or Harmless Organisms

Active specific immunity may be acquired "artificially" by imitating nature's method of mild, or subclinical, infection. Living organisms are actually injected, or otherwise put into the body, but they are either previously weakened (*attenuated*) by various processes so that they cannot cause a severe infection or, alternatively, a less virulent species, so closely related to the actual disease agent that both share the immunogenic properties, may be used. Either method induces only a very mild disease but one that produces the desired immunity. A good illustration of these types of immunization is the use of attenuated rabies (hydrophobia) virus for immunization of domestic animals against this disease. In the modern, effective immunizing treatment for prevention of rabies in dogs, active, attenuated rabies virus is commonly used (see page 301). Active but attenuated viruses are also used in vaccination against smallpox, the Sabin oral vaccine against poliomyelitis, the more recently developed measles vaccine of Dr. J. F. Enders and other workers, and the mumps and rubella vaccines

297

that came into wide use early in 1968. Other active virus vaccines are applied in veterinary medicine.

VACCINATION AGAINST SMALLPOX.   The virus that causes smallpox in human beings appears also to produce in cows a mild disease called cowpox, or *vaccinia,* which causes a pustular eruption on the udder. Although the virus of cowpox (called vaccinia virus) is distinct from that of smallpox, nevertheless the two are immunologically very closely related. It is thought by many investigators that smallpox virus, when inoculated into cows, changes its character and produces the mild disease cowpox. Be this as it may, when vaccinia virus (whether modified cowpox virus or modified smallpox virus is not certain) is transmitted to man, as is done in vaccination, it causes, not smallpox, but the mild condition seen in vaccination and called *vaccinia.* This is sufficient to give protection from smallpox for one to 10 years or longer, depending on the individual and his environment.

The relationship between cowpox and smallpox, and the fact that inoculation with material from the eruption of cowpox would protect against a later inoculation with the virus of smallpox, were demonstrated by *Edward Jenner,* an English country doctor. Jenner noted that persons working around cows that had cowpox developed sores on their fingers like those on the cow's udders, and that these persons never caught smallpox during an epidemic. He published his observations in 1798, after he had been studying and experimenting on the subject for 20 years. He introduced on a large scale the practice of inoculating people with the material from the eruption of cowpox. This, in an improved form, is what we now call vaccination (from the Latin, *vacca,* cow). To Jenner, therefore, belongs the credit of giving vaccination to the world. Smallpox, which in Jenner's time was widely prevalent, has been a scourge of humanity since antiquity. In older times, and even recently in some areas, it has killed hundreds and thousands — even millions — in vast epidemics. Vaccination is taken so much for granted now that we are in danger of forgetting how valuable the protection is. Nevertheless, the United States Public Health Service no longer advocates routine vaccination of American youngsters as formerly.

Vaccination is now recommended only for persons proceeding to or returning from endemic or epidemic areas or persons at special risk (e.g., certain health personnel). The decision is based on the greatly reduced probability of importation of cases (only one in, and since, 1949) from foreign countries, the effectiveness of measures to detect and prevent spread of imported cases, and complications and risk of vaccination. In 1968 there were, in the United States, 16 cases of postvaccinal encephalitis, 11 of vaccinia necrosum, 126 cases of eczema vaccinatum and numerous less serious complications, some requiring hospitalization. There were nine deaths among 14.2 millions of persons vaccinated. Most of the cases resulted from careless or improper technique.

By surveillance and control measures, with vaccination only in special areas, the World Health Organization (WHO) expects to eradicate smallpox from its last strongholds in the world in Ethiopia, Sudan, India, Nepal, Pakistan, Afghanistan, and Indonesia by 1976.

Constant surveillance will now be necessary. An enormous nonimmune population will soon develop and may demand a crash defensive program if even one case of smallpox should enter the country unrecognized.

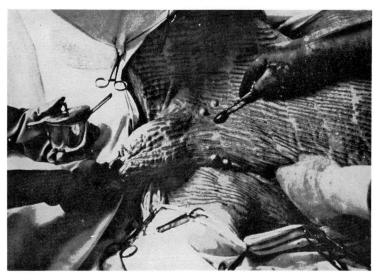

Figure 20–1

The collection of cowpox lymph from the skin of a calf. The skin has been shaved, cleaned, disinfected, and inoculated in long parallel scratches (clearly seen in the picture) with cowpox lymph. Typical pustules have developed along the scratches and the lymph from these is being collected with surgical cleanliness. (From Monteiro and Godinho.)

Vaccine virus is commonly prepared by inoculating perfectly healthy calves with living cowpox organisms either from an animal previously inoculated with vaccine virus or from a human vaccination sore. In a few days the calf develops vesicles or sores similar to those following vaccination in human beings. The material from these is scraped out and mixed with glycerin (see Fig. 20–1). Freshly prepared vaccine of this sort always contains bacteria. It is therefore disinfected with phenol which, curiously, does not inactivate this particular virus. The virus is tested for bacterial contamination and for its immunizing power (*antigenicity*) by animal experimentation. These safety controls are maintained by the National Institutes of Health in Bethesda, Maryland. In England, a similarly prepared glycerinated lymph vaccine, obtained from sheep, is used for immunization.

A single dose of virus is put up in a small, hermetically sealed tube. This is cleaned with alcohol gauze before use, broken while being grasped with sterile gauze, and emptied by means of a small rubber bulb. To prevent rapid deterioration, it is advisable to store the virus at temperatures of about 1 C until it is used. Any alcohol or disinfectant gaining entrance to the tube from gauze or from the patient's skin will inactivate the virus. For some purposes frozen and dried (*lyophilized*) vaccine (reconstituted with fluid for use) is very useful.

One major disadvantage in the use of these vaccines prepared from animals is the presence of bacterial contaminants. This has been overcome by the use of preparations in which the virus has been propagated on the chorioallantoic membrane of the developing chick embryo or in tissue culture. These preparations are currently undergoing field tests, pending wider use.

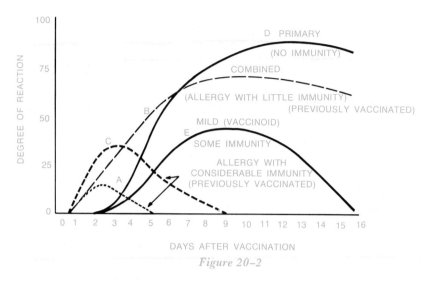

DAYS AFTER VACCINATION

Figure 20–2

Types of reaction to smallpox vaccination. Curves A and C represent rapid, superficial reactions beginning during the first 24 hours, sometimes showing small vesicle formation, but terminating rather quickly after a mild course, without scar formation. These occur only in previously vaccinated persons (or in those convalescent from smallpox), and the quick reaction of short duration and mild degree is characteristic of immunity with allergy to the smallpox virus, active or inert. Allergy may exist when immunity has all but lapsed, as shown in curve B. This begins as an allergic reaction but goes on to a real "take" with papule, vesicle, pustule and eventual scar formation, much like the primary "take" in a wholly susceptible person without allergy, shown in curve D. Curve E is a milder reaction in a person without allergy but with a considerable degree of immunity. This is a "vaccinoid" reaction, usually without scar formation. Note that the reactions in the absence of allergy (curves D and E) do not begin until the second or third day. It is occasionally difficult to differentiate the types of reaction. (Adapted from M. Mitman, River Hospitals, Joyce Green, Dartford, Kent, England. In *Monthly Bull. Minist. Health*, 2:100.)

In using smallpox vaccine it is essential that fresh, properly stored material be used; otherwise, no "take" will be obtained. Sometimes this failure to take is erroneously thought to represent immunity in a previously vaccinated person.

Immune Reaction in Vaccination.   In an immune person there is usually a more or less mild, rapidly developing and transitory (about 24 to 96 hours) reaction recognized as probably allergic in nature (Fig. 20–2).

Pasteur's Preventive Immunization Against Rabies.   As developed by Pasteur about 1885, immunization against rabies consisted of a series of 7 to 14 daily antigenic injections of live, *attenuated* rabies virus in the form of dried spinal cord of rabies-infected rabbits, the virus being attenuated by propagation in rabbits and by the drying process. Later, the Pasteur method of immunization for human beings (now less often used) consisted of injections of rabbit cord containing phenol-inactivated virus (Semple vaccine). These rabbit tissue vaccines sometimes cause the development of an allergic response to the rabbit tissues carrying the virus, with distressing, sometimes fatal, demyelinating encephalomyelitis. Also, there is little viral antigen in them in relation to the bulk of rabbit tissues.

Avianized Rabies Vaccines.   To avoid the allergic response just described, an attenuated virus (the Flury strain) is cultivated repeatedly in successive, live, embryonated[1] avian eggs, now more often of ducks than of chickens. After the contents of the eggs (containing large amounts of virus) have been collected, the virus is inactivated (for human use) by various means (formalin, ultraviolet irradiation, phenol) and finally is dehydrated. This material, reconstituted with fluid, is used as vaccine more safely and effectively than rabbit-tissue vaccine. For persons frequently exposed to rabies (veterinarians, dog handlers, and so on), an initial series of several immunizing doses of vaccine, followed by booster doses[2] repeated at intervals and immediately after any known exposure, is recommended. For dogs and other animals, active virus attenuated by long propagation in live avian embryos is widely used to protect against rabies. It is highly effective. For cats, a high-egg-passage or HEP (many egg passages) of active Flury virus is used. Tests of such active vaccines in humans have given results that indicate their possible use for humans as well as for lower animals.

The techniques and principles discovered by Pasteur do not constitute a therapeutic procedure but an immunizing measure, used after bites by suspect animals, to develop immunity before rabies has time to develop.

Antirabies Serum. In cases of severe bites by known rabid animals, especially bites near the head, face, and hands, the use of serum (hyperimmune) containing ready-formed antirabies antibodies is of great value and can prevent the horrible death from rabies when the action of vaccines would be far too slow. Such serum is available commercially. When the injection of serum is followed, after an interval of some days, by a course of vaccine treatment, the protection obtained is excellent. Note that hyperimmune antirabies sera must be given immediately if possible; at latest within 72 hours of the bite. Part of the dose should be injected below and around the bite(s).

The use of immunologic preparations however, does not preclude the necessity for local treatment of the bites. Such treatment as prompt, thorough, washing with soap or detergent and the cauterizing of puncture wounds are frequently the most important steps in preventing the development of the disease.

Control of Rabies. After symptoms of rabies have developed, death was considered inevitable until 1971, when a boy, bitten by a bat and *believed to be* infected with rabies, was treated with many specific drugs to prevent each symptom before it occurred. This careful attention to all disease details saved his life. Still the best way to control rabies is to vaccinate and control all pet dogs and cats, destroy all stray dogs and cats, and require that others be kept from wandering at large. This sounds like a simple program, but it is at present impossible in the United States. In Great Britain it is an accomplished fact. Wild mammals of most species, including several species of bats, can also contract and spread rabies and should be controlled.

BCG VACCINATION. The effectiveness, safety, and value of vaccine consisting of live tubercle bacilli which have low virulence for human beings, as an immunizing agent against tuberculosis, were first demonstrated by Calmette and Guérin, two French scientists, who introduced this method in 1925 in France. The material injected consists of cultures

---

[1]Incubated long enough (eight to 14 days) to contain a partly developed chick or duckling.

[2]"Booster" doses restimulate antibody production and reinforce immunity that has waned with passage of time. Booster doses will be explained more fully later in this chapter. They are widely used in artificial immunization, such as vaccination against polio.

of tubercle bacilli grown in a special medium containing bile, which lowers the virulence of the bacilli. It is called BCG (Bacille Calmette Guérin) vaccine. It should be noted here that the use of BCG is still controversial. Its use is definitely not indicated in tuberculin-positive individuals (see Chapter 31). Large scale studies conducted in England, Puerto Rico, among the North American Indians, and in other places proved the BCG vaccine to be between 13.4 and 83.0 per cent effective as an immunizing agent. It is used especially for groups frequently exposed to the disease i.e., nurses, doctors, and inhabitants of areas where tuberculosis is highly prevalent. Its use will be discussed further under tuberculosis. BCG is one of the few examples of living bacterial vaccines used for human beings. Veterinary use of attenuated bacterial vaccine includes *Brucella abortus* to prevent contagious abortion or Bang's disease in cattle, and cultures of attenuated *Bacillus anthracis*, the efficacy of which was first demonstrated by Pasteur in 1881.

BCG is available as fluid or dehydrated (lyophilized) cultures. The latter are reconstituted with appropriate sterile fluid. Either type of culture is usually injected very superficially into the skin of the deltoid region by a multipointed needle (*multiple puncture method*). The WHO statement on tuberculosis indicated that only the intradermal route assures that an effective dose of vaccine is given. In addition, in hot climates freeze-dried BCG heat-stable vaccine must be used.

Injections of Dead Organisms

In a second method of producing active artificial immunity, the actual organisms that cause the disease are injected into the person needing the protection, whose defensive mechanisms react as usual by producing antibodies. In the particular procedure under discussion, however, the microorganisms, instead of being attenuated, weakened, or of low virulence, as just discussed, have been killed or inactivated by heat or some chemical disinfectant.

BACTERINS. Immunizing preparations consisting of suspensions of killed bacteria are properly spoken of as *bacterins*, but are more frequently called *bacterial vaccines* or simply vaccines.[3]

Many types of bacterial vaccine are used. The commonest are typhoid vaccine and whooping cough (pertussis) vaccine. Typhoid vaccine is prepared by cultivating fully virulent typhoid bacilli on broad agar surfaces. The fresh young growth is washed from the agar with physiologic salt solution, and the suspension of bacilli thus obtained is heated at a temperature of approximately 60 C for about one hour. In some laboratories, the bacilli are killed with formaldehyde instead of heat. The suspension is then diluted to a suitable concentration (to contain about one billion organisms per milliliter); a small amount of disinfectant (tricresol or phenol, 0.25 per cent) is sometimes added as an additional precaution, and the bacterin is put up in ampules. It is ready for injection after suitable tests to prove that the bacteria are dead, that no extraneous bacteria are present, and that the vaccine produces immunity in animals. It is customary to

---

[3]The term "vaccine" can, from its Latin derivation, be properly applied only to the cowpox material used for immunization against smallpox. However, it is widely used for any artificial immunizing procedure.

give three successive injections of this vaccine at intervals of about a week and an annual "booster dose" (see page 304).

Mixed Vaccines. Sometimes several kinds of bacteria are mixed together in a single suspension. This is usually done with typhoid vaccines; preparations are available containing also dead paratyphoid bacilli of two types. In some countries dysentery bacilli and the vibrios of cholera are included. Vaccines containing more than one kind of organism are spoken of as *mixed vaccines*. In preparing whooping cough vaccines, it is common practice to mix antigens for diphtheria and for tetanus, and sometimes other antigens, e.g., inactivated (Salk) polio virus, with the pertussis bacilli. There exists at least one effective vaccine with these four components. It is called the "quad" vaccine of the WHO of the United Nations. It is prophylactic against whooping cough, diphtheria, polio and tetanus. This is not only effective but also saves many extra "shots," or injections. Also, each antigen in the mixture helps the others to be more effective. The exact reason for this is not clear. It should also be noted that vaccines consisting of active viruses, e.g., Sabin polio, measles (rubella and rubeola), mumps, yellow fever, and smallpox vaccines, require different time sequences of immunization and cannot be given mixed with other vaccines.

Sensitized Vaccines. Sometimes organisms intended for use in a vaccine are treated before injection with the serum of a person or animal who is immune to those bacteria. The bacteria combine with the antibodies in the serum so that they are acted upon quickly by the blood, tissues or phagocytes of the person into whom they are injected and presumably immunize more rapidly and advantageously. Such a vaccine is called a *sensitized vaccine*.

Autogenous[4] Vaccines. It sometimes seems advisable to prepare a vaccine from organisms isolated from the patient himself. This is often done with staphylococci isolated from boils. Such a vaccine is called an *autogenous vaccine*. In staphylococcal infections that are resistant to all available antibiotics, this is the only really effective way to clear up the condition, which may have spread all over the body.

VIRAL VACCINES. Three of the best known immunizing agents made with inactivated viruses (instead of with live, attenuated viruses as in rabies, smallpox, and Sabin's poliomyelitis oral vaccine) are the vaccine against influenza (especially the so-called "Asiatic flu"), inactivated measles vaccine, and the Salk vaccine against poliomyelitis. Many persons who have visited areas in which yellow fever occurs have received active, attenuated (17D) yellow fever vaccine, one of the most effective. All these vaccines are good illustrations of the principles just outlined.

One of the newest and best active-virus vaccines is that against rubella (German measles) which, when it occurs in women during the first three or four months of pregnancy, causes death or defects in the fetus. The United States Public Health Service Advisory Committee on Immunization Practices (1972) recommends the active vaccine for all children between the ages of one year and puberty, and for all older females of child-bearing age who are susceptible by serological (agglutination-inhibition) test and who are cautioned not to become pregnant during the two months following vaccination. Males of any age over one year may be vaccinated to pre-

---

[4] *Auto* is from a Latin word meaning self. For example, an automobile is a self-moving vehicle.

vent spread of the virus to nonimmune pregnant women during epidemic periods. Vaccination of *pregnant* women is absolutely contraindicated because the virus can infect and damage the fetus.

Injection of Bacterial Exotoxins

A third method of producing active immunity artificially differs from the two preceding methods in that no organisms, living or dead, come into contact with the body. In certain diseases, for example diphtheria and tetanus, the principal damage is done by the exotoxins that the bacteria give off into the blood. These toxins engender antibodies (antitoxins) very readily. Therefore, if a person receives carefully controlled injections of small amounts of toxin, he will soon be able to withstand large doses of the same toxin. His body develops antitoxin just as though he had had the disease naturally. There is danger from the toxin, however, even when mixed with antitoxin (T.A.T.), as was the practice at the turn of the century.

TOXOIDS. Rather than inject these potent and dangerous toxins, it is now the custom to inject substances derived from toxins by heating and by combining the toxins with formaldehyde. These modified toxins are called *toxoids*. They are not poisonous, but act as specific antigens. They are among the most widely used immunizing agents.

Primary and Secondary Antigenic Stimuli

In most of the processes of active artificial immunization described, several injections of the immunizing agents are used. These immunizing agents, whether living organisms, dead organisms, or exotoxins, are collectively spoken of as *antigens* or *immunogens,* since they stimulate antibody production. The response of the body to initial contact with most antigens (a so-called *primary stimulus*) is relatively slow, requiring two to ten weeks to reach fully effective antibody titers. The antibodies and the immunity of a person who has been immunized may decline to a very low level with the passage of several years. It is then desirable to reimmunize. This reimmunization is called a *secondary stimulus*. It has been found that the body cells, on reimmunization, respond very much more rapidly than at first, often within a few hours (Fig. 20–3). For this reason only a small, single dose of the antigen (a so-called "booster dose") is needed to reestablish high-grade immunity.

BOOSTER DOSES. Examples of the practical use of this rapid reaction to secondary stimuli are seen in the methods of preventing polio, tetanus, diphtheria, and salmonellosis. Persons having once received an initial course of three 0.5 ml subcutaneous injections of typhoid (*Salmonella*) vaccine need only take an annual booster dose of about 0.1 ml *intracutaneously*. This tiny intracutaneous dose very rarely produces sore arms or severe general reactions. The fourth and later injections of Salk vaccine are based on the same principal. Similarly, personnel on induction into military service, and others, including children, receive an initial immunization against tetanus consisting of injections of tetanus toxoid. If these persons are later wounded, they immediately receive a small booster dose of tetanus toxoid, which helps prevent tetanus. Together with prompt surgical treatment of wounds, the use of antibiotics, and other treatment,

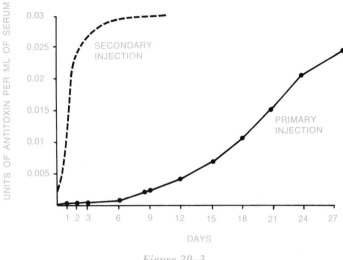

Figure 20–3

Curves showing rate of antitoxin production following a primary injection and following a secondary injection. Note that after the secondary injection antibody production is much more rapid and extensive than after the first or primary stimulus. The rate and extent of the secondary reaction vary with different individuals, antigens, and species.

the booster dose procedure has reduced the incidence of tetanus among our population to a very low level.

SLOW RESPONSE TO PRIMARY STIMULUS.   Because the production of antibodies after primary antigenic stimuli is relatively slow, the primary injections must be commenced weeks or months before a person is likely to be exposed to disease, e.g., on starting school. Active immunization is therefore too slow to be of value as a *therapeutic* measure once disease is established, or as a preventive measure in the face of *immediate* exposure. There are, however, methods of developing immediate immunity to some diseases. They are called *passive immunization* and will be discussed next.

PASSIVE IMMUNITY

Artificial Passive Immunity

NEED FOR PASSIVE IMMUNITY.   In cases of exposure to such diseases as diphtheria and tetanus, it is necessary that a large supply of antibodies appear in the blood immediately. The chief damage in these diseases is caused by the bacterial exotoxins in the body of the patient. The poisonous action is very rapid. When the patient is already ill, there is no time to lose in waiting for him to develop an active immunity, natural or artificial. The patient must immediately receive an ample supply of ready-made antibodies. Immunity resulting from injections of these ready-made antibodies is called *passive immunity* because the patient passively receives them and his tissues have no part in actively producing them.

It is now possible to purchase, at all well stocked pharmacies and health departments, syringes or ampules already filled with antitoxic serum, prepared for just such emergencies. Such antibody-containing serum is obtained from animals, usually horses, that weeks or months previously had received repeated injections of the special antigen against which antibodies are desired.

PREPARATION OF THERAPEUTIC SERA.   Among the most important therapeutic sera are those against the diphtheria and tetanus bacilli. Innumerable lives have been saved by their use. The use of immune, antiviral serum to help combat rabies has already been mentioned. Passive immunity is also used in dealing with measles, viral hepatitis, and several other diseases.

A common method of making therapeutic antitoxic sera is as follows: A horse (or rabbit) is injected subcutaneously or intravenously, at intervals of five to seven days, with gradually increasing amounts of broth in which the desired organisms have grown, and which contains either their dead cells, their toxins, or both. The horse is the animal usually chosen for antitoxins since, because of its size, it yields a large amount of desired serum. The first injected dose of toxin is very small, not enough to make the animal sick. By the end of the treatment the animal may take, without symptoms, many times what would have been a fatal dose at the beginning. At the end of three or four months, when the horse has developed a large amount of antibody in its blood, it is bled with aseptic precautions from the jugular vein; six to eight quarts of blood are removed at one time. The blood serum separates from the clot on standing and contains the antitioxic gamma globulins used in medical practice. The horses used for the production of curative sera are kept under the best hygienic conditions and remain well and comfortable throughout the treatment, which is not painful. Toxoids are now often used as antigen instead of the dangerous toxin.

Sera must be kept in a dark, cool place, as they gradually lose their strength when exposed to light and warmth. Under suitable conditions their potency is retained for a year or more. A difficulty with the use of such sera is that the equine proteins act as antigens and induce a marked allergic state toward any proteins from horses.

In order to reduce the number and severity of *allergic protein reactions*, processes have been devised to remove as much of the nonspecific and unneeded proteins—i.e., *horse* (equine) proteins as contrasted with *antitoxin* (gamma globulins)—from therapeutic sera and leave as much of the antitoxin as possible. Such purified material is called *concentrated* or *purified antitoxin* or *immune serum globulin(s)* (ISG). It is much superior to the unconcentrated serum and is the preparation generally sold as antitoxin.

Injections of antibody-containing sera into an infected patient, before the toxin or virus or other microorganisms in the patient have done too much damage, practically always result in an improvement of condition and usually a cure. It is extremely important to remember that therapeutic sera will stop the damaging process but will not repair damage already done. Sera given very late in any disease are practically without effect and may then do harm.

In the United States the production and sale of therapeutic sera, bacterins, smallpox vaccine, and other immunizing agents for human use (also for use in animals) are regulated by law. The establishments which manufacture these agents are licensed, and samples of the products for human use are tested at the National Institutes of Health at Bethesda, Maryland. Products that do not come up to the standards set for them are not allowed to be sold. The U.S. Food and Drug Administration, in laboratories located in many states, also checks these types of medications upon requests of consumers. Also, the State Departments of Health may assure that the laws of the state are not being violated. All of these laboratories will collaborate if necessary. Veterinary products are similarly controlled.

PASSIVE IMMUNITY IN THE PREVENTION OF DISEASE.   Passive immunity is used in the prevention, as well as in the cure, of disease. For example, if it is known or suspected that a person is soon likely to become exposed or has very recently been exposed to certain diseases, it is under some circumstances (to be determined by the physician) an excellent plan to inject a small quantity of serum, or some derivative of serum containing the appropriate antibodies, as a preventive or prophylactic[5] measure. Diseases against which this form of prophylaxis is commonly used are measles, diphtheria, and tetanus. Effective sera are also available for some other infections (e.g., rabies and viral hepatitis). Still others are yet under investigation.

Before the immunizing value of tetanus toxoid had been widely demonstrated, it was a routine measure in most hospital accident wards to inject tetanus antitoxin in order to prevent the development of this disease in persons injured in street and farm accidents. This was because in these accidents, dirt containing spores of tetanus bacilli get into the wound where the tetanus bacilli can grow and produce their toxin. Today toxoid immunization and booster doses are used more than antitoxin in preventing tetanus.

The use of immune serum in the prevention of hydrophobia in human beings, along with the Pasteur prophylactic series of injections, is now recognized as essential in serious bites by dogs suspected of having rabies, and so forth.

If a child who is susceptible to diphtheria has to live in the same house with another member of the family who has the disease, it is sometimes advisable to give the well but susceptible child about 2000 units of antitoxin, unless an allergic sensitivity to horse serum exists. The slower but more enduring active immunization with toxoid can come later or be started at the same time.

ALLERGY IN PASSIVE IMMUNITY.   If a susceptible individual is not allergic to horse serum, the injection of antitoxin will produce such allergy. This is a serious deterrent to the indiscriminate use of horse serum, either therapeutically or prophylactically. The next chapter will deal with this type of response and similar induced allergic conditions.

HUMAN GAMMA GLOBULINS.   To avoid the use of serum from lower animals, with resulting allergic complications, and also because certain antibodies are more readily available from human sources, human blood is often used to provide therapeutic and prophylactic antibodies. The immune globulins are separated from the blood of adult (or immune) humans and, as we have indicated, are often injected into other persons to provide *passive immunity* against several diseases: especially measles and infectious hepatitis, and less often, herpes zoster, pertussis, and others.

---

[5]Greek *pro,* before; *phylassein,* to guard or protect. Prophylaxis is generally thought of as being used in advance, to prevent disease or infection.

For example, very young or "delicate" children and pregnant women, in whom measles is a dangerous disease, often receive gamma globulin of some child or adult who is convalescing or who has recently recovered from measles. This prevents or modifies the disease in the expectant mother, and in the young or fragile child until he is older and can better withstand the infection. Usually this sort of passive protection is used during epidemics, times of special danger, or just before long journeys. Artificial active immunization is certainly preferable if time permits.

Human ISG is of special value for patients whose immune response is being suppressed, as in heart and other organ transplantation.

AGAMMAGLOBULINEMIA.[6] Some persons suffer from a genetic difficulty (or total inability) to form gamma globulins. They therefore have the condition called *agammaglobulinemia*. As a result, they lack antibodies and are often extremely susceptible to infectious disease and may not respond well, or at all, to vaccinations. A similar condition results from *hypoglobulinemia*, or reduced amount of globulin in the blood.

Natural Passive Immunity

An expectant mother who has antibodies against infectious diseases confers a share of these antibodies on her unborn child through the placenta. This is *natural passive immunity*. Of the various types of gamma globulins, the γG molecules, being the smallest (lowest molecular weight, 150,000), can pass the placenta, and consequently they are found in the blood of the infant at birth. They have two important advantages over commercial antibodies such as diphtheria or tetanus antitoxins prepared from the serum of immunized horses. First, as already noted, antibodies from animal sources make the recipient allergic to the proteins of the animal. Second, such antibodies are completely rejected and destroyed in the body within two to four weeks. Human maternal antibodies do not cause allergy and remain in the body of the recipient for many months. Thus, they serve to protect the child long after birth (six months to one year). After that, the child becomes susceptible to many infectious diseases. It is therefore advisable to begin active immunization of the child early (second month to sixth month) against pertussis and diphtheria. Tetanus toxoid may be given either simultaneously or later; and still later (or simultaneously) immunization may be begun against other diseases, including poliomyelitis. The use of combinations of several antigens (but not active viruses) in one or two "shots" is now common and effective.

It is important to note that immune gamma globulins (IgG) in the young infant imply immunity in the mother. The woman who anticipates becoming pregnant but who does not have good antibody titers to diphtheria, tetanus, pertussis, poliomyelitis, rubella, and possibly salmonellosis, would do well to become actively immunized before pregnancy in order to confer passive immunity on her child.

---

[6]This formidable word is really a graceful Latin phrase: *a*, without, or lacking; *gamma globulin* has already been explained; *emia*, in the blood. Pronunciation is just as the word is divided here, and spoken thus comes trippingly from the tongue!

In hypoglobulinemia, the prefix *hypo*, meaning little or "below par," is obviously substituted for *a* in the preceding word, and *gamma* is left out.

Supplementary Reading

Beutner, E. H. (Ed.): Defined Immunofluorescent Staining. *Ann. N.Y. Acad. Sci.,* 1971, *177.*

Boyd, W. C.: Fundamentals of Immunology. 4th Ed. 1967, New York, Interscience Publishers, Inc.

Carpenter, P. L.: Immunology and Serology. 3rd Ed. 1972, Philadelphia, W. B. Saunders Co.

Current Topics in Microbiology and Immunology, Vol. 40. 1967, New York, Springer-Verlag.

Eichhorn, M. M.: Rubella: Will vaccination prevent birth defects? *Science,* 1971, *173:*710.

Friedman, H. (Ed.): Immunological Tolerance to Microbial Antigens. *Ann. N.Y. Acad. Sci.,* 1971, Vol. 181.

Frobisher, M.: Fundamentals of Microbiology. 8th Ed. 1968, Philadelphia, W. B. Saunders Co.

Grubb, R.: The Genetic Markers of Human Immunoglobulins. *Mol. Biol. Biochem. Biophys.,* 1970, Vol. 9. New York, Springer-Verlag.

Holborrow, E. J. (Ed.): Standardization in Immunofluorescence. 1970, Philadelphia, F. A. Davis Co.

Humphrey, J. H., and White, R. G.: Immunology for Students of Medicine. 2nd Ed. 1964, Philadelphia, F. A. Davis Co.

Kawamura, A., Jr., (Ed.): Fluorescent Antibody Techniques and Their Applications. 1969, Baltimore, University Park Press.

Kochwa, S., and Kunkel, H. G., (Eds.): Immunoglobulins, *Ann. N.Y. Acad. Sci.,* 1971, *190.*

Public Health Service Advisory Committee on Immunization Practices. *Morbidity and Mortality,* 1972, *21:*25.

Tunevall, G.: Periodicals Relevant to Microbiology and Immunology: A World List 1968, 1971–1972, New York, John Wiley & Sons.

Weir, D. M.: Handbook of Experimental Immunology. 1967, Philadelphia, F. A. Davis Co.

WHO Expert Committee on Rabies. 5th Report. 1966, Geneva, World Health Organization, Technical Report Series, No. 321.

WHO Expert Committee on Tuberculosis. 8th Report. 1964, Geneva World Health Organization, Technical Report Series, No. 290

Wiener, A. S.: Elements of blood group nomenclature with special reference to the Rh-Hr blood types. *J.A.M.A.,* 1967, *199:*985.

Allergy

21

INTRODUCTION

Before the many aspects of allergy are discussed, it should be emphasized that allergy is one of the most important defensive mechanisms of the body against infectious disease.

The word allergy is derived from two Greek words: *allos*, altered or changed, and *ergon*, action. It refers to an increase in reactivity or sensitivity that develops in certain tissue cells toward an antigen 10 to 15 days after the first contact with (or injection, or dose of) that same antigen. This dose of antigen is commonly called a *sensitizing dose*. There is no *perceptible* change or reaction following the sensitizing dose. A second dose, given intravenously 10 to 15 days later, if large enough, typically precipitates a violent allergic reaction and is accordingly called a *toxic* or *shocking dose*.

The increased reactivity induced in tissue cells by a sensitizing dose[1] of antigens, such as toxoids, vaccines, and also actual infections such as smallpox and active-virus polio vaccines, though differing in mechanism, as discussed farther on, is a very beneficial aspect of the allergic response, because it is the basis of booster doses, previously referred to. Unfortunately, in some instances the increase in sensitivity and reactivity is excessive. Allergy is, accordingly, often referred to as *hypersensitivity*. Substances inducing allergy are often called *allergens*.

The phenomenon of allergy brings to the mind of the average individual nothing but distressing thoughts of hay fever, hives, gastroenteritis, asthma, and other unpleasant, disagreeable, and sometimes fatal reactions. As noted previously, however, allergy is one of the most valuable of the defensive mechanisms against infectious disease. It must be admitted that,

---

[1] Included in this term are the usual two to four small subcutaneous doses of various vaccines given one to six weeks apart.

in some instances and in some individuals, it appears to do more harm than good. This is when it is inadequate, overactive, or misplaced, like an overzealous servant who, attempting to warm the living room with a good fire, burns the house down. Further, as is true of drug idiosyncrasies, certain individuals, said to be *atopic*, are congenitally more prone to undesirable allergic reactions than others.

It should be remembered that allergy does not constitute a disease condition; rather the individual who suffers from hypersensitivity is more than normal in his response to foreign substances or organisms that invade his body. Usually these people do not become ill from infections as often as other individuals.

TYPES OF ALLERGY

Allergic reactions may be classified under two general headings, *immediate* and *delayed*. Although the underlying mechanisms are different, both are related to immunity and to the response of certain tissue cells to antigens or haptens. Because the "immediate" reactions are sometimes deceptively slow, and the "delayed" reactions are sometimes not delayed very much, it is customary to speak of the delayed-*type* or the immediate-*type* reaction rather than to the rates at which they occur.

All allergic reactions exhibit a high degree of specificity. In the immediate-type reaction, the presence of *precipitins*, or of antibodies like precipitins circulating in the blood, is essential. In the delayed type, circulating antibodies have not been demonstrated. The *antigens*, or *inducers*, of the delayed-type reaction appear to combine directly with specific, antibody-like molecules (sometimes spoken of as *reagins*) or groups (receptor sites) that remain firmly attached to certain specifically sensitized lymphocytes. That macrophages (wandering cells) are especially involved in delayed-type hypersensitivity is shown by the fact that on contact of sensitized lymphocytes with the specific antigen in vitro, the macrophages (normally actively motile) cease their migrations. The inhibition of motility results from a cytotoxic substance released by the sensitized lymphocytes.

PASSIVE ALLERGY.   One of the striking differences between the delayed-type and immediate-type allergy is that immediate-type allergy is caused by antibodies that can circulate in the blood and, therefore, can be transferred, like passive immunity, in serum from a sensitized animal to a normal animal. In an hour or so the antibodies in the serum from the donor animal will have attached themselves to reactive cells in the recipient, making him also hypersensitive to whatever specific antigen is involved. In marked contrast, serum of an animal having delayed-type hypersensitivity will not transmit delayed-type hypersensitivity at all. Delayed-type allergy is transferable from the sensitized animal to a normal one only by means of lymphocytic cells (or parts of them), which have the necessary, specific, combining sites for the antigen or allergen.

Whether immediate or delayed, the basic explanation of virtually any allergic manifestation is that a reaction has occurred in the body between an antigen—or, in delayed-type hypersensitivity, an inducer—and its specific antibody or receptor site. Occurring *only in the blood*, this reaction would cause no allergic response and is the normal defensive process. The antigen-antibody complexes circulating in the blood stream are quickly engulfed by phagocytic cells or otherwise removed from the blood. The situation that results in allergy is that the antigen-antibody combination occurs in or *on certain tissue cells*. The type of allergic reaction which then results is determined by several factors, important among which are: kind of antigen or inducer, kind of antibody (precipitin or reagin), concentrations of antigen and of antibody, location and kind of tissue cells involved, and type of animal involved.

Immediate-Type Allergy

Immediate-type allergy results from a *precipitin* reaction occurring in or on certain tissue cells, mainly mast cells (basophil-like granulocytes), platelets, and possibly some other cells. The immediate-type reaction is well exemplified by the painful itching bumps or wheals known as "hives" such as those that may appear after eating certain foods or that may be seen in patients after they received injections of therapeutic serum. Intense gastroenteritis, coming on within a few minutes after eating certain foods to which the victim is allergic, and asthma (constriction in the chest and difficulty in breathing), resulting almost immediately after contact with certain animals or pollens, are other manifestations.

Since immediate-type allergic reactions are due to specific antigen-antibody (precipitin) reactions in or on tissue cells, it is evident that (with some exceptions, which need not be considered at this point) the person having the allergic reaction must have had previous immunizing or sensitizing contact with the antigen causing the allergic response. This contact must have occurred long enough previously (about ten days at least) for precipitins to have formed. As previously noted, antigens responsible for precipitin formation are, in general, water-soluble proteins: serum, egg white, proteins from various fish, meats, crustacea, vegetables, and so on. However, allergens in certain pollens, animal hairs or feathers, and plant fibers or derivatives such as poison ivy toxin can also give rise to antibodies and to immediate allergic responses, hives, hay fever, gastroenteritis, and the like.

SHOCK TISSUES. The signs, symptoms, and appearance of any immediate-type allergic reaction depend upon which tissue cells are affected. Tissues that suffer are known as "shock tissues." The most important effects of an immediate-type allergic reaction result from several physiologically active substances: *histamine, heparin, serotonin*, certain enzyme-activating agents (still under investigation) called *kinins*, and a *slowly reactive substance* designated as SRS-A (Table 21–1). These various substances, produced by mast cells and similar basophilic leucocytes, and by platelets, cause strong contractions of smooth muscles (abundant in blood vessels, gastrointestinal tract, uterus, bronchioles, and so on), exudation of fluid from local vessels with edema and swelling, various effects secondary to contractions of smooth muscles, dilatation of some capillary blood vessels, edema, and lowered coagulability of blood due to release of heparin (an anticoagulant).

If the shock tissues affected, consisting of smooth muscle fibers and capillary vessels, are in the gastrointestinal tract, diarrhea and cramps result; if in the gravid uterus, abortion results; if in the bronchioles, asthma results; if in the walls of cutaneous blood vessels, hives result, and so on.

Table 21–1. Substances that Produce Anaphylactic Reactions in "Shock Tissues"

PHARMACOLOGICALLY ACTIVE AGENT		SOURCE	CHEMICAL PRECURSOR	IN SPECIES
Name	*Structure*			
Histamine*†	$N—CH$ $\parallel$ HC $N—C—CH_2—CH_2—NH_2$	Mast cells, platelets, basophilic leucocytes, etc.	L-histidine	Guinea pig Rabbit Dog Man
Serotonin (5-hydroxytryptamine)	HO $CH_2—CH_2—NH_2$ (indole ring) N H	Mast cells, platelets, enterochromaffin cells	L-tryptophane	Rabbit Rat Mouse Dog?
Heparin	A polysaccharide polymer consisting of hexosamine, hexuronic acid, and sulfuric acid ester groups	Mast cells	Heparin	Dogs Other species?
Bradykinin*† Lysyl-bradykinin*†	Arg-pro-pro-gly-phe-ser-phe-arg Lys-arg-pro-pro-gly-phe-ser-pro-phe-arg	Plasma salivary glands, some tumors	α-Globulin in plasma	Guinea pigs Rabbit Rat Mouse Dog Man?
SRS-A* (slowly reactive substance-anaphylaxis)	Possibly a lipoprotein	May come from mast cells?	Unknown	Guinea pig Rabbit Man

*Found in man in shock (the kinins?).
†Action blocked by antihistamines.

It takes only a knowledge of the distribution of the shock tissues and their location in the body to suggest other possibilities.

Smooth muscle contraction is not the only manifestation of immediate-type allergy. Edema and inflammation are characteristically present in both immediate- and delayed-type allergy, though in different degrees of intensity. Edema and inflammation may occur on any of the mucosal surfaces. When the edema, as sometimes happens in immediate-type reactions, occurs in tissues around vital passages, such as the larynx and glottis, rapid death from asphyxiation can ensue. Stings of bees and hornets are notorious in this respect. Injections of 0.5 to 1 ml of 1 : 1000 epinephrine (Adrenalin), a potent *antihistamine* (inhibitor of histamine) and a vasoconstrictor and decongestant, quickly reduce these swellings. The drug should always be immediately available when administering biologicals hypodermically, especially serum and vaccines, some antibiotics, and similar preparations containing proteins and certain haptenic substances (e.g., some drugs). Numerous antihistamines are being sold in tablet form, some even without a physician's prescription. Since they give only symptomatic relief, it is best to follow the advice of your physician if you suffer from allergy.

ANAPHYLAXIS.   This term was devised by Richet, about 1902, to describe what was then viewed as a sort of immunologic betrayal, i.e., increased susceptibility as the result of immunizing injections instead of increased resistance (Greek, *ana*, against; *phylaxis*, protection; opposite of prophylaxis). The anaphylactic reaction is the most dramatic of the several manifestations of the immediate-type allergic reaction.[2] Fortunately, it is not common in man, but is well illustrated by the guinea pig. A protein, for example, egg white, is usually entirely harmless when injected the first time (except that it produces a state of allergy or hypersensitivity; i.e., it is a *sensitizing dose*). It may produce severe and sometimes fatal reactions called *anaphylactic shock* in guinea pigs or rabbits if injected a second time, that is, as a *toxic* or *shocking dose,* about two weeks later. Anaphylactic shock in the guinea pig is characterized by a lowered body temperature, difficult breathing, weakness, and finally convulsions and death. Guinea pigs show this phenomenon with particular violence. Other animals may present a very different picture, depending on numerous anatomic and physiologic differences. If the second (shocking) dose of the protein is given before the end of the two week period—during the so-called *"refractory period"*—no anaphylactic reaction is produced. This is the period during which precipitins are being formed.

DESENSITIZATION.   In immediate-type allergy, including anaphylaxis, if the hypersensitive animal (or person) survives the second injection (the toxic dose) he is temporarily insensitive because the precipitins available for an immediate reaction have been used up in the anaphylactic response. More precipitins may or may not be produced. The animal or person is said to have been *desensitized* by the second inoculation and can then safely receive large injections of the protein for the time being. The allergic state often reappears if more precipitins are produced. Desensitization is often accomplished easily and safely by the physician by giving a series of very small cutaneous doses of the antigen several hours apart. These combine with the precipitins in several small steps, and "let the pa-

---

[2]Others are Arthus's phenomenon and serum sickness.

tient down" gradually. In delayed-type allergy, desensitization is difficult and often impossible.

SERUM REACTIONS. These occur in two forms: One is the *acute* and serious form, resembling anaphylaxis, accompanied by collapse and dyspnea, and coming on a few minutes after the injection of therapeutic serum (such as diphtheria antitoxin) into a hypersensitive person. The other is a milder, delayed form, known as *serum sickness*. Both are dependent on precipitins in the patient; i.e., both are immediate-type allergic reactions.

Either type of serum reaction is due to the animal proteins in therapeutic serum, not to the specific antitoxin. The patient may have a chill, nausea, and sometimes extensive, painfully itching hives or serum rash. These reactions can end in fatal anaphylactic shock. This is preventable with epinephrine. However, although they are undesirable, the reactions seldom end fatally unless the patient is in a serious stage of his disease and in a weakened condition. As these reactions are most likely to occur in patients who have, or have had, asthma or pulmonary inflammation, or previous injections of serum, investigation is made on these points before injecting serum.

Delayed Serum Reactions. Serum sickness may not appear for ten days to two weeks after a therapeutic dose of serum. This is not a delayed-type reaction. Precipitins have been accumulating in the tissues during this period. When they reach a certain concentration, they react with the proteins of whatever residual portion of the therapeutic serum may still remain in the body. The result is an immediate, precipitin-mediated, allergic reaction, though modified in severity. It is characterized by itching hives (urticaria), fever, joint pains (arthralgia), and some lesser discomforts. If serum is to be given parenterally, a preliminary skin test for hypersensitiveness to horse serum may be made. If the test is positive, the patient should be *desensitized* by giving him a number of tiny (0.1 to 1 ml) doses of the serum at intervals of an hour or so before the main injection. The possible shock to the patient is materially lessened. Persons who have had previous injections of serum usually require desensitization. Serum reactions may occur also in persons not known to have had previous injections of serum.

Delayed-Type Allergy

In delayed-type allergy there is no shock and the tissue response appears many hours or even days after contact between the allergen and the sensitized tissue cells. There is local inflammation, sometimes a febrile reaction, with general malaise (ill feeling), and sometimes local necrosis. The anaphylactic type of response does not ordinarily appear. No precipitins can be demonstrated. The reaction subsides slowly.

THE TUBERCULIN REACTION. Delayed-type allergy is best illustrated by the tuberculin reaction and is often called the tuberculin type of allergy. Persons infected by tubercle bacilli, whether perceptibly ill or not, become allergic to proteins in tubercle bacilli. Their hypersensitive state can be demonstrated by injecting a minute amount of sterile protein (tuberculin) derived from tubercle bacilli, intracutaneously into the forearm. This constitutes the *tuberculin test* and is widely used in the study of tuberculosis. Tuberculin preparations are of two main types: "O.T." (old tuberculin) and "P.P.D." (purified protein derivative). The local swelling, inflammation, and, rarely, necrosis, resulting from the intradermal test for allergy to tuberculin, appear only after a delay of 36 to 48 hours; the area is characterized by being firmly indurated, in great part due to large numbers of lymphocytes. These do not appear in immediate-type reactions. Several other cytologic details of the delayed-type reaction are very different from the hive-like reaction seen in immediate-type allergy. Further, the dermal swelling of the tuberculin-type reaction persists for five to ten days, while the hive-like swelling of the immediate-type reaction disappears in an hour or so, especially with the aid of antihistamines, which do not affect delayed-type reactions.

Many other slowly progressive bacterial infections besides tuberculosis (notably syphilis, yaws, leprosy, brucellosis, tularemia) induce the same sort of delayed allergy. For this reason delayed-type allergy is often called infection-type allergy. Pollens (e.g., ragweed), poison ivy, and other nonbacterial antigens may also act as delayed-type allergens. Some may cause either delayed-, immediate-, or combined-type reactions, depending on individuals, antigens, and other little understood factors.

CORTISONE AND ACTH. Because histamine and related substances are largely responsible for the signs and symptoms of immediate-type allergy, antihistamines are of great benefit in controlling reactions, including some conditions such as hay fever, that are in part due to immediate-type allergy. In delayed-type allergy the signs and symptoms are unrelated to histamine or similar substances, and principally comprise inflammation, cellular infiltration, and vasodilation with edema. Drugs commonly used with marked effectiveness in delayed-type allergy, and some combined conditions, are cortisone or the pituitary adrenocorticotrophic hormone (ACTH), which stimulates production of cortisone by the adrenal cortex. Cortisone suppresses inflammation and edema. It is useful in rheumatic fever, which presumably is an infection-type allergy, especially of heart muscle, due to unknown antigens of beta-type hemolytic, group A streptococci (*S. pyogenes*, see Chapter 28). Similarly, cortisone gives relief (but does not cure) in certain conditions thought by some to be delayed-type allergy to one's own tissues, the so-called *auto-* (self) *immune diseases:* rheumatoid arthritis, multiple sclerosis, lupus erythematosus, and so on. The inciting tissues in such conditions are called *autoantigens.* Caution against excessive use of cortisone is urged since, among other undesirable side effects, cortisone can entirely suppress antibody production.

ISOANTIGENS. Another manifestation of allergic response is the tissue-rejection or *homograft reaction.* Unless tissues for transplantation (skin grafts, hearts, kidneys) are "self," i.e., derived from one's own body (difficult in the case of heart transfer!) or from an identical (monozygotic) twin, the immune mechanisms of the body tend to reject them sooner or later. In general, tissues (or any antigens) from any source other than one's own body are immunologically "resented" by the body as "not self."

Any immune response may be delayed by various immunosuppressive measures that prevent antibody and lymphocyte production: x-radiation, treatment with cobalt–60, DNA base analogues, cortisone, and so forth. Organ or tissue transfer patients so treated may retain the transplant for some time but are constantly prone to infection and must be constantly guarded against it. "Not-self" antigens from a donor animal of the same species as the recipient animal are called *isoantigens* (see also blood groups). "Transplanted" hearts have not lasted as long as five years. At this state of "the art" the immunosuppressive treatment permits infections to become too dangerous to the patient with the "big new heart." Yet for some reason, not quite clear, kidney transplants have been proved much more lasting and practical.

IMMUNE TOLERANCE. Animals may be made tolerant, thus unresponsive to, various antigens by injecting the antigen into newborn animals or into the fetus in utero. The "immature and naive" tissues of animals so treated seem to accept such antigens as "self." Immunologic unresponsiveness of this type is called *induced tolerance.*

ATOPY. Some individuals inherit, not allergy itself, but a certain increased tendency to form reagins and thereby to develop allergic reactions, such as asthma and hay fever, and perhaps liability to certain forms of arthritis and rheumatic heart disease. These persons are of a group sometimes called *atopic* (and *always* called unfortunate!).

DRUG IDIOSYNCRASIES. Certain plant perfumes, cosmetics, drugs, rubber goods, dyes, and so forth, may also cause immediate allergy-like responses such as hives, dermatitis, and asthma. These immediate reactions, although closely simulating allergy and sometimes actually due to allergic mechanisms, may often be basically different from true allergy and not primarily dependent on specific antibodies at all. Such reactions are usually limited to certain individuals. These allergy-like reactions are often referred to as *drug idiosyncrasies.* The exact mechanism underlying such reactions is not fully understood. One should always differentiate between *drug hypersensitivity* and *drug intolerance.* Drug hypersensitivity is true allergy and is often induced by antibiotics such as penicillin, the sulfonamides, aspirin, and barbiturates and reactions are the result of previous sensitization to the drug. Sensitivity to penicillin increases at a steady rate in our population; however, the drug is still given too freely, too often when the patient could do without it. Drug intolerance is a physiologic, metabolic response of the body, and is of greater intensity than normal, but within the expected pharmacologic activity of the drug. This is not an allergy.

SKIN TESTS FOR HYPERSENSITIVITY

When a small quantity of the sensitizing antigen is scratched or injected into the skin of a person or an animal hypersensitive to that protein, a large, red, swollen area will develop after an interval; the time, type of reaction, and duration depend on whether one is dealing with delayed (slow reaction) or immediate (rapid reaction) type allergy. These reactions persist for an hour or two in immediate-type allergy, and for several days in delayed-type allergy. Such local allergic reactions are extremely useful in determining what antigen is causing a patient's trouble. Tests for hypersensitivity to horse serum and many other antigens are made in this way.

The most widely used test for bacterial allergy is the tuberculin test already discussed (see also Chapter 31). Analogous tests for allergy to certain fungi (*Histoplasma, Coccidioides*) are also widely used (see also Chapter 37).

APPLICATION TO HEALTH

Knowledge about allergy helps to understand untoward reactions when certain individuals come into contact with antigenic (allergenic) substances, such as serums, antibiotics, some drugs, vaccines and some foods. With this knowledge a person can sometimes be successful in preventing a severe allergic reaction following injection of an antigenic substance, and may save a life. For example, if a patient is allergic to eggs, and the physician, not knowing this, has ordered a viral vaccine that has been prepared in chick embryos, e.g., yellow fever vaccine, the person giving the injection should immediately inform the doctor about the allergy to avoid a severe, possibly fatal, allergic reaction. Also, if a patient receives a dose of antitoxic serum that has been prepared in horses, and especially if the patient has had previous injections of horse serum, he may have a severe and even fatal reaction to the serum, which, although given to provide him with immediate protection against a specific disease, is really for him a potentially deadly dose since he is allergic to horses. It is important to note that the patient's reaction to the antitoxic serum is not due to the antibodies in it *per se* but to the equine proteins in the serum. He would react to any horse serum, whether antibodies were present in it or not.

The person who is knowledgeable about such potentialities of allergic response will always have a supply of epinephrine or other antihistamines readily available whenever antigens or antibodies are being given by injection (*parenterally*), since such drugs control immediate allergic reactions. Patients must be observed constantly for immediate- and delayed-reactions to antigenic or allergenic substances. If a patient reacts allergically to any substance, he should be informed so that he may avoid future injections of this particular substance.

Supplementary Reading

Allergy Foundation of America: Allergy: Its Mysterious Causes and Modern Treatment. 1967, New York, Grosset & Dunlap, Inc.

Becker, E. L., and Austen, K. F.: Anaphylaxis. In: Mueller-Eberhard, H., and Mischer, P.: Immunopathology. 1967, Boston, Little, Brown & Co.

Chase, M. W.: The allergic state. In: Dubos, R. J., and Hirsch, J. G.: Bacterial and Mycotic Infections of Man. 4th Ed. 1965, Philadelphia, J. B. Lippincott Co.

Craven, R. F.: Anaphylactic shock. *Amer. Jour. Nurs.* 1972, *72*:718.

Epstein, W. L.: To prevent poison ivy and oak dermatitis. *Amer. J. Nurs.,* 1963, *63*:113.

Hellström, K. E., and Hellström, I.: Immunological enhancement as studied by cell culture techniques. *Ann. Rev. Microbiol.,* 1970, *24*:373.

Krahlenbuhl,, J. L., Blaykovec, A. A., and Lysenko, M. G.: In vivo and in vitro studies of delayed-type hypersensitivity to *Toxoplasma gondii* in guinea pigs. *Inf. and Immun.,* 1971, *3*:260.

Levine, B. B.: Immunochemical mechanisms of drug allergy. *Ann. Rev. Med.,* 1966, *17*:23.

Leskowitz, S.: Immunologic tolerance. *Bioscience,* 1968, *18*:1030.

Milgrom, F., Centeno, E., Shulman, S., and Witebsky, E.: Autoantibodies resulting from immunization with kidney. *Proc. Soc. Exp. Biol. Med.,* 1964, *116:*1009.

Milstein, C., and Munro, A. J.: The genetic basis of antibody specificity. *Ann. Rev. Microbiol.,* 1970, *24:*335.

Nakahara, W.: Recent Advances in Human Tumor Virology and Immunology. 1972, Baltimore, University Park Press.

Notkins, A. L., Mergenhagen, S. E., and Howard, R. J.: Effect of virus infections on the function of the immune system. *Ann. Rev. Microbiol.,* 1970, *24:*525.

Ruddle, N., and Waksman, B. H.: Cytotoxic effect of lymphocyte-antigen interaction in delayed hypersensitivity. *Science,* 1967, *157:*1060.

Shaffer, J. H., and Sweet, L. C.: Allergic reactions to drugs. *Amer. J. Nurs.,* 1965, *65:*100.

Uhr, J. W.: Delayed hypersensitivity. *Physiol. Rev.,* 1966, *46:*359.

Pathogenic Microorganisms

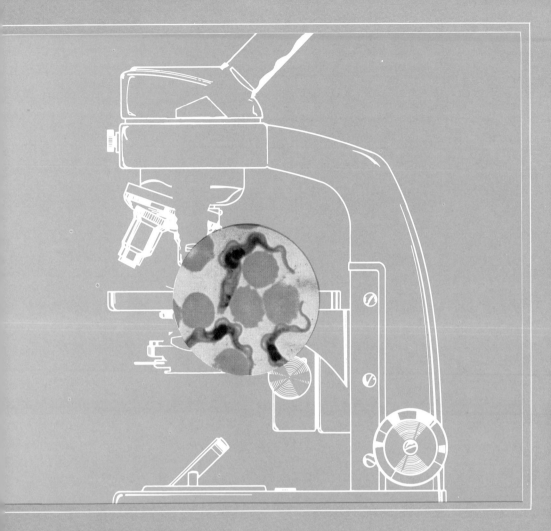

Section Five

Factors in Transmission of Communicable Diseases

22

The occurrence of communicable disease implies: (1) a source of infection, i.e., the presence of active pathogenic agents in or on some sort of transmissible matter, animate or inanimate; (2) a vector, animate or inanimate, capable of transmitting those agents to a host capable of harboring them; (3) some means of egress or *portal of exit* of the pathogenic agent from the infected body; (4) the arrival of the pathogenic agent at a place where it can gain a foothold in a new host. The last statement implies a *portal of entry*.

PORTALS OF ENTRY

These are certain routes or pathways by which some microorganisms normally enter the body and cause infections. There are other portals through which they cannot, or do not ordinarily, enter (see next paragraph). The particular route in a given instance depends on the kinds of microorganism and, to some extent, the kind of vector involved. The most important portals of entry are through cuts or abrasions in the skin, including those due to bites of arthropods and other animals, and through mucous membranes of the respiratory tract (nose, throat, tonsils, and lungs), the eyes, the mouth and gastrointestinal tract, and the genitourinary tract.

ABNORMAL PORTALS OF ENTRY. In presenting the evidence here, it is stipulated (or mutually understood and agreed) that in this discussion only normal and natural portals of entry are considered. Many microorganisms, even so-called harmless saprophytes, may cause a rapidly fatal infection if injected with a hypodermic needle into the brain, for example, or the peritoneal cavity, or if sprayed into the nose and lungs. Such treacherous doings, while valuable experimentally, are like admitting a hostile army through a secret postern gate into a walled city, bypassing the normal portal of entry.

Many disease organisms have their *obligate* portals of entry and can cause an infection only if they enter via such a portal. Thus dysentery ba-

323

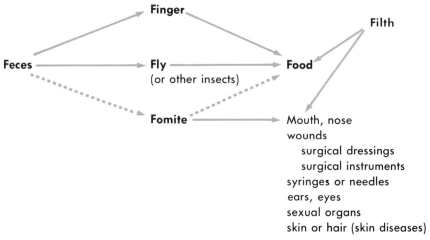

Figure 22–1

Transmission of disease-causing microorganisms from feces to food with fomites as vectors in our daily life. Fomites are nonliving objects — inanimate vectors that transmit pathogens. Examples of fomites are: money (coins or paper money), pencils, pens, ballpoints, eating utensils, plates, forks, glasses or bottles (soft drink), toys (especially dolls), postage stamps, stationery, door handles, bed linens, pillows, towels, thermometers, books, magazines, newspapers, dentists' and physicians' instruments, toilet items, men's, women's and children's clothing, and many other objects used in daily life. Filth has been added because in our present society pollution of the environment is not our only problem. We are also "stuck" in our own *filth* — dirt in food establishments, in the kitchens, below counters, behind refrigerators; dirt from animal droppings and dead insects; dust. In general, filth carries microorganisms but is neither a true fomite nor an insect.

cilli rubbed into a wound of the skin would probably not be responsible for any infection, whereas the same organisms, if swallowed, might produce fatal dysentery. Conversely, cocci that cause boils do not produce infections when swallowed, whereas if rubbed into the skin or a wound, they can produce a severe, even fatal, infection. Some microorganisms can enter the body tissues through almost any portal.

PATH OF ORGANISMS IN THE BODY. From the various portals of entry or sites of initial infections, organisms may pass into the circulating blood and start a secondary or *metastatic* infection in some of the internal organs or in the membranes of the brain and spinal cord (spinal meningitis). Organisms entering through the nose or mouth may take one of several paths. They may be swallowed and thus reach the stomach and intestines. In most instances they will be killed by bile and other digestive juices. If they are pathogens of the intestinal tract (*enteric pathogens*), such as those which cause typhoid fever, dysentery, cholera, or poliomyelitis, they will survive contact with the gastrointestinal juices and gain entrance to the tissues via the gastrointestinal tract, especially in the presence of foods that temporarily reduce acidity of the gastric juice.

If they are respiratory pathogens, such as pneumococci, diphtheria bacilli, tubercle bacilli, scarlet fever and septic sore throat streptococci or the bacilli of whooping cough, they may locate in and on the tonsils, as in the case of diphtheria and "strep throat" or scarlet fever; or they may pass on to the lungs, as they do in pneumonia and tuberculosis (Fig. 22–2).

The organisms of syphilis and gonorrhea find their principal portal

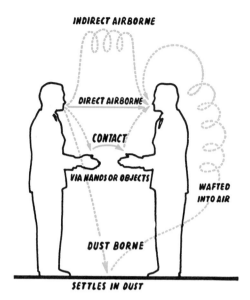

INDIRECT AIRBORNE

DIRECT AIRBORNE

CONTACT

VIA HANDS OR OBJECTS

WAFTED
INTO AIR

DUST BORNE

SETTLES IN DUST

Figure 22–2

Transmission of infectious agents from the respiratory and oral tract of one person to another by direct contact or indirectly via airborne particles. Among the agents of disease thus transmitted are viruses of influenza, colds, measles, and mumps; streptococci; pneumococci; meningococci; tubercle and diphtheria bacilli; some fungi; and occasionally other pathogens such as plague and anthrax bacilli. Every educated person should visualize these pathways of transmission and create obstructions (such as effective gown and mask technique, correct hand washing, correct food handling procedures, correct sputum disposal, and proper sweeping methods) to protect himself and others against diseases transmitted via these and other routes. (After F. Schwentker. Courtesy of American Sterilizer Co.)

of entry in the mucosal surfaces and glands of the genitourinary tract, though they not infrequently infect the eyes (gonorrheal ophthalmia), lips and oral cavity (syphilis) and are transmitted via these portals.

It is tragic when several young people use a single nonsterile hypodermic needle to inject drugs into each other via a blood vessel, after the same needle has been used by a person with hepatitis or malaria. This "drug scene" is truly bad medicine!

PORTALS OF EXIT

Equally important is the portal by which microorganisms leave the body on their journey from one host or patient to another. How can any person attending a patient with infectious disease protect himself and his environment if he does not know when and where the microorganisms of the disease are leaving the patient and how to deal with them? In the course of an infectious disease, microorganisms often follow a devious and complicated path through the host and may leave from a portal different from that by which they entered. Indeed, infectious organisms may be conveniently grouped on the basis of their usual portals of entry and exit. These are more fully discussed later in this unit.

VECTORS

Vectors of infectious organisms may be animate or inanimate.

INANIMATE VECTORS. These may be food, the discharges (feces, saliva, pus, and the like), to be described, and also water, bandages, dressings, instruments, hypodermic needles, bedding, eating utensils, and other inanimate objects (fomites) contaminated with infectious discharges. When one knows the portal of exit of any pathogen, the possible vectors are almost self-evident.

ANIMATE VECTORS. These vectors are generally arthropods or mammals. Thus anopheline mosquitoes are notorious vectors of malaria; dogs and other mammals are vectors of rabies. The *hands* of patients, doctors, nurses, and other persons in contact with an infectious patient or his fomites may also be classed as animate vectors. Other animate vectors will be described farther on. The control of each type is a specialized study in itself. Of course, man himself may be regarded as one of the most dangerous vectors of disease because he cannot be eliminated with DDT or muzzled and put on a leash. For example, he is the only significant living vector of such diseases as poliomyelitis, infectious mononucleosis, measles, and syphilis, and he is the most frequent live vector of tuberculosis of man.

The whole philosophy of communicable disease management, and indeed of the entire profession of preventive medicine as it relates to communicable disease, is based largely on knowledge of these three factors (portals of entry, portals of exit, and vectors) and their ramifications. The nurse or other health worker who grasps these simple basic principles will be well prepared in the field of communicable disease control.

PREVENTION OF DISEASE TRANSMISSION

It is evident that the transfer of microorganisms from one person to another may be blocked at one or more of three points just mentioned:

PORTAL OF ENTRY. The entrance of pathogens into the body is (theoretically) always preventable if their portal of entry is known. For example, the respiratory portals may be covered by masks; cuts and scratches on the hand may be covered by bandages or surgical gloves. The alimentary tract is best protected by appropriate selection and disinfection (as by pasteurization of milk, chlorination of water, and cooking) and sanitary preparation of foods. The skin may be protected from biting arthropods by clothing, repellents, and screens. The tissues and blood may be made resistant by vaccination and by the prophylactic use of antibodies and of chemotherapeutic drugs.

PORTAL OF EXIT. Unless the vector is a blood-sucking arthropod, the transmission of most infectious agents may be stopped at the portal of exit by immediate collection and proper disposal of whatever bodily excretions, secretions, discharges, tissues, and so forth, may contain the pathogens: feces, urine, saliva, mucus, pus, tissue drainages, bandages, and the like. Details concerning each are given farther on.

All of these matters will be discussed more in detail in following chapters. In Appendix D various pathogens are listed according to their portal of exit, which is the point at which one can most effectively block routes of disease transmission.

VECTOR. Transmission of infection may theoretically be entirely blocked by effective vector control. In some cases this has been dramatically effective, as when yellow fever and malaria were abolished from certain areas such as Cuba and the Panama Canal Zone by elimination of the vector mosquitoes. The transmission of such enteric diseases as cholera and typhoid fever by municipal water supplies has been completely blocked in the Western Hemisphere and Europe by expert sanitation of water supplies and sewage disposal. Cholera, once a world-wide scourge, no longer exists in endemic form in these areas. Water-borne typhoid fever is virtually extinct in the United States. Other examples of large scale prevention of disease transmission will occur to the thoughtful student.

Supplementary Reading

(See list of references at end of each of the other chapters in Section V.)

Pathogens Transmitted
from the Intestinal
and/or Urinary Tracts

Salmonellosis, Shigellosis
and Cholera

23

THE FAMILY
ENTEROBACTERIACEAE

GENERAL DESCRIPTION.   The name of this family of bacteria is derived
from the fact that nearly all species in it more or less constantly inhabit
the intestine of man or animals or both. Important pathogenic members
of the family include the bacilli of typhoid and paratyphoid fevers (salmonellosis), of bacillary dysentery (shigellosis) and some related bacilli,
notably *Escherichia coli*. The Enterobacteriaceae are gram-negative, nonspore-forming straight rods, facultative aerobes, ranging in dimensions
from 1 to 2 μm in diameter by about 3 to 10 μm in length. All species
ferment glucose. Microscopically, the various species in the family are
indistinguishable. Most species are motile with peritrichous (not polar)
flagella; however, the dysentery bacilli (*Shigella*) are characteristically nonmotile. Several strains of *Salmonella, Shigella, Escherichia, Klebsiella, Entero-
bacter*, and *Proteus* possess fimbriae or pili.[1] All these bacilli grow readily
on simple, blood-free culture media, including many common foods,
such as milk, salad dressings, and sandwich fillings, over a range of temperatures from 15 to 40 C. Most of them can resist cold well and survive
in soil, sewage, ice, water, milk, and foods for periods varying from hours
to weeks, depending on species and environment. Since they do not form
spores, however, they are readily killed by five minutes of boiling, by the
commercial processes of pasteurization and by standard disinfectants.
Drying and direct sunlight destroy them fairly quickly.

    SUBDIVISIONS.   These gram-negative enteric bacilli are classified
here by a system based on, and almost identical to, one proposed by
Edwards and Ewing, differing from the classification given in the seventh
edition of *Bergey's Manual*. Many laboratories now use the system of
Edwards and Ewing. The classification given here agrees in part with the
Edwards and Ewing system and in part with the newer system of the
International Subcommittee on Enterobacteriaceae. The nomenclature
covers both systems.

---

    [1] Pili, as readily seen under the electron microscope, are smaller than flagella. Pili are not
antigenically related to flagella. See page 57.

Table 23–1.   Pathogenic and Potentially Pathogenic Species
in the Family Enterobacteriaceae

Family	IV Enterobacteriaceae	
Tribe	I Escherichieae	
	I *Escherichia*	
	Species 1. *E. coli*	Important as indicators of fecal pollution of water and foods. Certain types of *E. coli* cause enteritis, urinary tract infections, and secondary infections.
Genus	II *Shigella*	
	Species 1. *S. dysenteriae* 2. *S. flexneri* 3. *S. boydii* 4. *S. sonnei*	Cause of bacillary dysentery or shigellosis.
Tribe	II Edwardsielleae	
Genus	I *Edwardsiella*	Generic term used since 1965. May cause diarrhea.
	1. *E. tarda*	
Tribe	III Salmonelleae	
Genus	I *Salmonella*[1]	
	Species 1. *S. typhi*	Cause of typhoid fever (a form of salmonellosis).
	2. *S. paratyphi A* 3. *S. paratyphi B* (or *S. schottmuelleri*) 4. *S. paratyphi C* or (*S. hirschfeldii*) 5. *S. typhimurium* 6. *S. cholerae-suis* 7. *S. enteritidis*	Cause of various forms of salmonellosis other than typhoid fever, especially food infection.
Genus	II *Arizona*[2]	Cause salmonellosis-like conditions.
	1. *A. hinshawi*	
Genus	III *Citrobacter*	
	Species 1. *C. freundii*	Confused with *Salmonella* and *Arizona;* may not be truly pathogenic.
	Species 2. *C. intermedius*	
Tribe	IV Klebsielleae	
Genus	I *Klebsiella*	
	Species 1. *K. pneumoniae*	Pneumonia, enteritis, septicemia, peritonitis, urinary infections etc.
Genus	II *Enterobacter*	
	Species 1. *E. cloacae* 2. *E. aerogenes*	Urinary tract infections. septicemias.
Genus	III *Hafnia*	
	Species 1. *H. alvei*[3]	
Genus	IV *Pectobacterium*	May have become opportunist pathogens.
Genus	V *Serratia*	
	Species 1. *S. marcescens*	
Tribe	V Proteeae	
Genus	I *Proteus*	
	Species 1. *P. vulgaris* 2. *P. mirabilis* 3. *P. morganii* 4. *P. rettlgeri*	*P. vulgaris* and *P. mirabilis* may cause infections of urinary tract. *P. mirabilis* and *P. morganii* cause diarrhea, especially in infants.
Genus	II *Providencia*	Diarrhea, urinary tract infections.

[1]Some authors recognize only *S. typhi, S. cholerae-suis* and *S. enteritidis* as distinct species.
[2]Genus *Arizona* is considered a species of *Salmonella* in a newer classification.
[3]Also called *Enterobacter hafniae.*

The family is here divided into five tribes[2] and ten genera, as shown in Table 23–1. Special emphasis is given to the pathogenic species named in each genus. Most important among these groups are the tribe Escherichieae (named for a German scientist, Escherich) containing some harmless saprophytes, but also some troublesome pathogens: the genus *Shigella*

[2]Bergey's eighth edition will probably also have five tribes in the family Enterobacteriaceae. Part of this classification is shown in Appendix A.

named after the Japanese microbiologist Shiga; the tribe Salmonelleae, (after the American bacteriologist, Salmon) containing the typhoid, paratyphoid, and dysentery bacilli; and the tribe Proteeae (named for the pleomorphic Greek god Proteus) containing some troublesome pathogens and also some species that are occasionally confused with *Salmonella*.

Because of the importance of the Enterobacteriaceae in sanitation and

Table 23–2. Differential Characters of some Enterobacteriaceae*

GROUPS	GENERA	SPECIES	Glucose	H₂S[a]	Indole	Phenylalanine deaminase	Urease	Dulcitol[b]	Lactose[c]	Lysine[d,e] decarboxylase	Simmons Citrate[f]	Ornithine decarboxylase	Motility
Escherichia-	*Escherichia*	coli	⊕	−	+	−	−	v	⊕	−	−	v	±
Shigella	*Shigella*		+	−	∓	−	−	v	−	−	−	∓	−
	Edwardsiella	tarda	⊕	+	+	−	−	−	−	+	−	+	+
Salmonella-			⊕	+	−	−	−	+	−	+	+	+	+
Arizona-			⊕	+	−	−	−	−	v	v	+	+	+
Citrobacter			⊕	+	−	−	v	v	v	−	+	∓v	+
Klebsiella-	*Klebsiella*	pneumoniae	⊕	−	∓	−	+	∓	⊕	+	+	−	−
Enterobacter-	*Enterobacter*	cloacae	⊕	−	−	−	±	∓	⊕	−	+	+	+
Serratia		aerogenes	⊕	−	−	−	−	−	⊕	−	+	+	+
		hafniae	⊕	−	−	−	−	−	∓	+	v	+	+
		liquefaciens	⊕	−	−	−	v	−	v	v	+	+	+
	Serratia	marcescens	⊕	−	−	−	v	−	−	+	+	+	+
Proteus-	*Proteus*	vulgaris	⊕	+	+	+			−	−	−	−	+
Providencia		mirabilis	⊕	+	−	+			−	−	−	+	+
		morgani	±	−	+	+			−	−	−	+	±
		rettgeri	∓	−	+	+			−	−	−	−	+
	Providencia		±	−	+	+			−	−	−	−	+

*+ Positive
− Negative
± Most are positive
∓ Most are negative
v Various biochemical types
⊕ Acid and gas produced

a. *S. enteritidis* (bioserotype *paratyphi A*) and some others may be H₂S negative.

b. Most salmonellae ferment dulcitol in 24 hours; *S. typhi*, *S. enteritidis* (bioserotypes *paratyphi A* and *pullorum*) and *S. cholerae-suis* often ferment slowly or not at all.

c. *Shigella sonnei* ferments lactose only after 24 hours.

d. After 24 hours reactions may become positive.

e. *S. enteritidis* (bioserotype *paratyphi A*) does not decarboxylate lysine.

f. *S. cholerae-suis* utilizes citrate slowly; *S. typhi* and *S. enteritidis* (bioserotype *paratyphi A*) not at all.

†Modified from *Enterotube*®, Roche Diagnostics, Nutley, N.J.

Table 23–3. A Comparison of Four Different Systems of Biochemical
Tests for the Enterobacteriaceae and Closely Related Species

FERMENTATION IN DURHAM TUBES AND OTHER COMMON TESTS*	API-20** TESTS	ENTEROTUBE TESTS***	R/B ENTERIC**** DIFFERENTIAL SYSTEM
1. Lactose	1. Lactose	1. Lactose	1. Lactose
2. Arginine*	2. Arginine		
3. Lysine*	3. Lysine	3. Lysine	3. Lysine
4. Ornithine*	4. Ornithine		4. Ornithine
5. Phenylalanine*	5. Phenylalanine	5. Phenylalanine	5. Phenylalanine
6. Citrate*	6. Citrate	6. Citrate	
7. H₂S formation*	7. H₂S formation	7. H₂S formation	7. H₂S formation
8. Urease*	8. Urease	8. Urease	8. (Urease-additional)
9. Methyl Red*			
10. Indole*	10. Indole	10. Indole	10. Indole
11. V.P.*****	11. V.P.		
12. Gelatin*	12. Gelatin		
13. Glucose	13. Glucose	13. Glucose	13. Glucose
14. Mannitol	14. Mannitol		14. (Mannitol-additional)
15. Inositol	15. Inositol		
16. Sorbitol	16. Sorbitol		16. (Sorbitol-additional)
17. Rhamnose	17. Rhamnose		17. (Rhamnose-additional)
18. Sucrose	18. Sucrose		
19. Melibiose	19. Melibiose		
20. Arabinose	20. Arabinose		
21. Dulcitol		21. Dulcitol	21. (Dulcitol-additional)
	22. Amygdaline		
23. Motility*			23. Motility
24. Raffinose			24. (Raffinose-additional)
25. Maltose			
			26. (Acetate-additional)
			27. (DNase-additional)

*Tests other than fermentation tests.
 **API-20 is a system of 20 test capsules on one card. The test medium is dehydrated in these capsules. Distilled water is used to rehydrate. API-20 was supplied by Analytab Products, Inc., New York, N.Y.
 ***Enterotube is a set of eight media contained in one tube. It was supplied by Roche Diagnostics, Nutley, N.J.
 ****Diagnostic Research, Inc.
 *****V.P. is the abbreviation for the Voges-Proskauer test.

disease, the identification of genera and species is essential. Table 23–2 shows a scheme to differentiate these organisms. Many suppliers of microbiologic media have recently manufactured their own systems for performing the necessary biochemical tests. Three of these commercially available test systems (API-20, the Enterotube, and the r/b system) are listed for comparison with the standard common tests in Table 23–3.

We may simplify our thinking about these organisms by relating them to three general types of clinical conditions as follows:

Salmonella and *Arizona* enteritis infections (salmonelloses):
   Typhoid fever and similar generalized infections by *Salmonella* species
   Gastroenteritis, with infection confined to the bowel (food infections)
Shigella infections (shigelloses):
   Bacillary dysentery
Escherichia and *Proteus* infections:
   Gastroenteritis and infant diarrhea
   Urinary tract infections

LOCATION OF REACTIONS

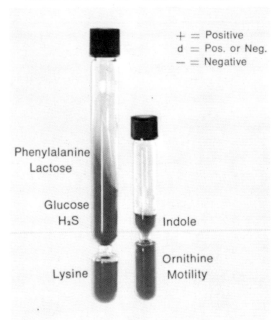

+ = Positive
d = Pos. or Neg.
— = Negative

Phenylalanine
Lactose

Glucose
H₂S   Indole

                       Ornithine
Lysine   Motility

Figure 23–1

Types of tubes used in the r/b system and some of the reactions they can demonstrate. Courtesy Diagnostic Research, Inc., Roslyn, N.Y.

Although the classification of the Enterobacteriaceae in Table 23–1 presents the organisms in different sequence, it is more convenient here to discuss the salmonelloses first, then the shigelloses, and other infections due to Enterobacteriaceae subsequently.

The Salmonelloses

Salmonellosis is the medical term for infection with any species of *Salmonella*. Certain species of *Salmonella* are more likely to invade the blood than others, and to cause the more severe salmonelloses. *Salmonella typhi*, causing typhoid fever, is one of these. Others are *S. paratyphi* and numerous related species. The name *S. paratyphi* A indicates "typhoid-like" and was given to certain salmonellas causing typhoid-like conditions. The term "paratyphoid bacillus" is still often used for nearly all salmonellas except *S. typhi*. Today, except for gradations in clinical severity, the same basic pathogenesis is recognized in all *Salmonella* infections.

The term salmonellosis, therefore, includes typhoid fever and paratyphoid fever, and infection by any of over 1000 very similar species or serotypes of *Salmonella*.

TYPHOID FEVER.   Typhoid fever is a good representative of enteric infections in general: bacterial, viral, and others. It is the type of infection transmitted by feces or urine. With regard to *means of transmission*, what is true of typhoid is, with a few minor modifications, also true of *Salmonella* food-borne infections (often incorrectly called "food poisoning"), bacterial dysentery, epidemic viral hepatitis, and amebic dysentery. Details of the differences as they affect practices of health workers will be given in their proper places. Although typhoid fever is not any longer a common disease in the United States, it was one of the major causes of death five or six decades ago and still is, in some lands. There are good reasons for discussing it. The fact that a disease is now rare is no indication that it cannot again become the scourge that it once was. We are too apt to forget that if the sanitary precautions (sanitary sewerage systems, water purification plants, pasteurization of milk, food and restaurant sanitary regulations), arduously built up over the years because thousands of victims died, are even temporarily neglected (even for an hour!), the pestilence of enteric infections of many sorts is waiting there to strike. With them come dysentery, cholera, amebiasis, hemorrhagic jaundice, epidemic hepatitis, and other formerly terrifying specters of disease or death. It is well, therefore, to know something not only of the causative organisms but also of the structure of environmental sanitation and of the nature of the menace which it holds at bay.

Salmonella typhi has also been called Salmonella typhosa, Eberthella typhosa, or the typhoid fever bacillus. It was discovered by a German physician (Eberth) in 1880, in the spleens of typhoid victims at autopsy. It appears to be a peculiarly human parasite and is rarely or never found in lower animals, unlike many other species of Salmonella. Although the bacillus develops chiefly in the human body, it can survive in the outside world in water, foods, and so on, which are polluted by the excreta of typhoid patients or carriers. It is quite hardy outside the body. Experiments have shown that it may survive for several weeks in river water, 12 days in sewage, four months in butter, and 39 days in ice cream. It is not killed immediately by freezing, and if polluted water is used for making ice, or if these organisms are present in milk used for other dairy products, some of the typhoid bacilli may survive in the food for days. Impure ice or ice cream are therefore real sources of danger. Fresh cheese made of contaminated milk can transmit typhoid bacilli. The typhoid (and other Salmonella) bacilli appear to pass through the stomach uninjured and may multiply in the intestine, shortly afterward infecting patches of lymphatic tissue (Peyer's patches) in the intestinal wall.

Usually S. typhi (and occasionally other Salmonella species) appears in the circulating blood in the first week of the disease. Salmonellosis, especially that form of it caused by S. typhi (typhoid fever), therefore soon becomes a septicemia. In typhoid fever, ulcers of the small intestine are practically always present. The bacilli, especially S. typhi but also other salmonellas if they invade the blood, may localize in the periosteum (membranes covering bones), liver, gallbladder, bone marrow, spleen, or kidney, and may even cause meningitis or pneumonia. These complications are usually the cause of death, rather than the original intestinal involvement of the disease.

Salmonella typhi begins to appear in the stools from the broken-down intestinal ulcers after the first week of the disease. By the second week it is present in stools in enormous numbers. Other Salmonella organisms are usually present in the stools from the first signs of enteritis; much less frequently, and later, in the blood. Billions may be passed in a single bowel movement. The bacilli usually decrease during convalescence and finally die out. In about 10 per cent of patients they continue for eight to ten weeks, and in a small percentage, perhaps 2 to 4 per cent, they persist indefinitely. The first group of persons are temporary convalescent carriers, and the second group, permanent convalescent carriers. The carrier state may also occur temporarily, and possibly permanently, in persons who have no knowledge of having had an attack of salmonellosis, including both typhoid and paratyphoid fevers, since many infections are so mild that they pass without notice. Typhoid Mary is a classic case of a permanent carrier. She was a cook whose trail of employment across the United States was followed by outbreaks of the typhoid fever that she left behind. She was finally forbidden by court order to obtain any employment in which she could transmit her infection to others.

Because of lesions in the urinary tract, *S. typhi* may appear in the urine about the fifteenth day of the disease, often in great numbers. It may continue for weeks, months, and, in rare cases, for years. There are thus urinary as well as fecal typhoid carriers. Species of *Salmonella* other than *S. typhi* rarely appear in the urine.

Transmission of Enteric Infection

All of the Enterobacteriaceae referred to in this chapter are discharged from the body in the feces; *S. typhi* also occurs in the urine. They gain entrance to the body through the mouth by anything (food, water, milk, hands, and so on) polluted with sewage, fecal material, or urine. It is distressing to think how readily and frequently careless, unsanitary people ingest food contaminated by feces and urine and pollute the environment of other people every day in their lives. Each case of enteric infection, including those due to enteric viruses, enteric protozoa, and some helminths, comes from a previous case or from a carrier; that is, the excretions of a diseased person or a carrier are in some way, often hard to trace, taken into the mouth of someone else who in turn becomes infected.

Enteric infection of any kind (viral, bacterial, and others) is frequently spread by close association with the patient. Individuals who care for these patients may soil their hands with contaminated feces and neglect to wash them properly before going to meals or preparing food. Thus, these individuals may infect themselves or transfer enteric disease to others.

Carriers are extremely important in the spread of all enteric (and many other) diseases. They seem to be perfectly healthy. Typhoid carriers have been reported who had recovered from the disease as long as 64 years before they were found to have *S. typhi* in their stools. In typhoid carriers the source of the bacilli in the feces is probably the gallbladder, in which the organisms may sometimes continue to live and multiply for years as comfortably as in a culture tube in the incubator. From the gallbladder they are carried to the intestine with the bile. There is no certain way known at present to prevent a patient from developing into a carrier. There is also no certain successful method of curing carriers, although various kinds of treatment have been tried. Removal of the gallbladder often removes the infection.

Carriers of any intestinal infection are a continual source of danger if they have anything to do with caring for patients (especially infants) or with the preparation of food or milk. Many epidemics of salmonellosis, food infection (incorrectly, food poisoning), have been traced to them. The history of such an epidemic, which occurred in a California town some years ago, illustrates what may happen. Within a few days of one another a large number of typhoid cases broke out in a certain town. It was found that all the patients had attended the same supper about three weeks previously, and the one dish they had all eaten was creamed spaghetti. The woman who had contributed this to the supper had had typhoid many years before, and examination of her feces by the State Board of Health proved that she was still a carrier. In this particular case she had contaminated the spaghetti with typhoid bacilli from her fingers, while preparing it. There were 93 cases of typhoid altogether, including the persons infected from the carrier and those which developed from contact with the first cases. About ten persons died.

A less severe outbreak of *Salmonella* gastroenteritis was traced to a New Year's Eve party at which a buffet dinner was served. Among approximately 540 guests, 116 persons were interviewed for clinical and food histories. Of these, 51 (44 per cent) were ill with watery diarrhea, cramps, vomiting, headache, and fever; three persons were hospitalized. The mean incubation period was 22½ hours and the illness lasted from two to four days. *Salmonella st. paul* was recovered from stool specimens from five of the patients. Food histories clearly incriminated a turkey salad made from commercially prepared, precooked frozen turkey, rolls and salad ingredients, but unfortunately none of the served food was available for culture. The kitchen employees denied symptoms of gastroenteritis, but six of 14 stool cultures obtained from them yielded *Salmonella st. paul*. All six employees with positive cultures had helped prepare the turkey salad and admitted that they had eaten a portion during preparation.

The vast majority of carriers of *Salmonella* and other enteric pathogens are never discovered. As a rule, unless a special search is made by laboratory methods, only those are known who have been proved to be the cause of other cases of the disease.

Flies can act as distributors of salmonellas and other enteric pathogens. In areas without a sewerage system, flies contaminate their feet with infected feces in unscreened privies or other places of convenience to which they have access, then crawl over food, depositing the bacilli on it, or drop into milk and inoculate it with *Salmonella* or *Shigella* (dysentery bacilli), which can readily multiply there. Rats, mice, and many other vertebrates, domestic and wild, frequently harbor and distribute various species of *Salmonella* (except *S. typhi*). Poultry are often vectors.

Milk and other foods contaminated by flies or by actual cases or carriers of enteric bacterial pathogens, or by feces or urine of rats, and so on, account for scattered cases and occasionally for epidemics. *Salmonella* and *Shigella* grow rapidly in milk without changing its appearance or taste. Under improper conditions of milk production (which is the usual state of affairs in many parts of the world), the organisms may get into the milk from the hands of the dairyman or milkman, in case he or any of his family are infected (knowingly or not) or are carriers; the bacilli may also be introduced by washing the cans or bottles in polluted water. All these seem remote dangers, yet the most extensive North American epidemic of typhoid fever of this century occurred in a large Northern city and was believed to be caused by its milk supply. In this epidemic there were 4755 cases of typhoid fever and 453 deaths. It seems that for some reason certain sanitary precautions surrounding the production of the milk failed to function properly for a few hours and the result was this appalling loss of life. Too much stress cannot be laid upon the proper (constantly maintained!) control of public milk supplies and other aspects of environmental sanitation.

Numerous epidemics have also been traced to ice cream, cheese, and butter made from milk containing *Salmonella* bacilli. An outbreak of ty-

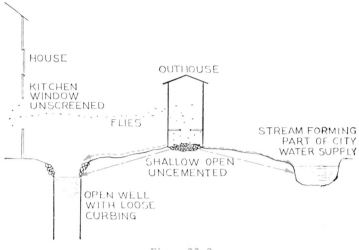

Figure 23–2

How an unsanitary outhouse may be a source of pollution of a city water supply (over-the-surface washings and underground seepage), a household well (surface washings and underground seepage), and a kitchen (flies).

phoid fever among tourists in a fashionable European resort received newspaper publicity in 1963.

Water polluted with sewage was formerly the most frequent source of typhoid fever. Other enteric infections (viral, bacterial, protozoal, and helminthic) may also be transmitted by water. In the United States waterborne epidemics due to *S. typhi* are now virtually nonexistent. Most large North and South American cities have provided themselves with good water supplies. In the United States, typhoid fever or any other enteric infection which may occur in a city is usually due to a carrier, or sources other than water. In country districts and in villages, on the other hand, polluted water still accounts for some cases of this disease as well as other enteric infections. In such places wells and privies are often situated near each other and feces may be washed by rains or carried by animals over the ground and into an open well (Fig. 23–2). Enteric pathogens of various sorts may occasionally be carried into the well through the soil by underground seepage, especially through crevices in rocks. In the United States, streams, lakes, and springs are nearly always polluted.

Diagnosis

In most cases of salmonellosis (also of shigellosis) with early diarrhea, the organisms can be found by the bacteriologist in the feces during the first days of the infection.

In typhoid fever, early enteritis is not as prominent, and the bacilli usually do not appear in the stools first, but rather in the blood. The nurse or health worker may be asked to assist in obtaining specimens for diagnosis and should have some knowledge of what is involved.

Blood Culture. The diagnosis of typhoid fever is made in the first week of the disease by means of a *blood culture*. As already mentioned, in typhoid fever a blood culture may be positive before stool cultures become positive. Blood taken with a 5 ml syringe is transferred to 100 ml of bile broth or other favorable medium. After incubation, plates of nutrient or selective agar are streaked and incubated. Appropriate types of plating media used for blood cultures are bismuth sulfite, Salmonella-Shigella (SS), eosin-methylene blue (EMB) or MacConkey agar. Blood agar may be included. Characteristic colonies are sought and transferred in pure culture for further study. Usually the diagnosis may be made in this way only during the first week, since after seven or eight days the bacilli usually disappear from the blood. The typhoid bacilli may then be cultivated from the stools. In other forms of salmonellosis blood cultures are positive less commonly, and then usually only in later stages.

STOOL CULTURE.   In diagnosing enteric bacterial infections in general, a drop of fresh feces is spread over the surface of plates of agar such as those mentioned in the preceding paragraph. Except blood agar, these contain certain substances, e.g., sodium desoxycholate and citrate, or dyes such as eosin and methylene blue, and other chemicals that inhibit nearly all organisms except Enterobacteriaceae. These media also contain lactose. The inhibitory substances serve two purposes: inhibition of bacteria other than Enterobacteriaceae, and indication of which colonies have fermented the lactose and produced acid. When acid is formed from the lactose, the dyes in the medium change color. The acid-forming (lactose-fermenting) colonies can thus easily be recognized. Reference to Table 23–2 will show that none of the species of Salmonella or Shigella forms acid promptly from lactose. It is therefore easy to differentiate their colorless colonies at a glance from those of Escherichia coli and related nonpathogens, which ferment the lactose promptly and therefore have deeply colored (red or violet) colonies.

The desired colonies (easily recognized) are subcultured on triple-sugar-iron (TSI) agar slants (Fig. 23–3) for more study in pure culture (Table 23–2). As seen in Figure 23–3. TSI agar and other media and tests described there are used for further identification of genus and species of infective organisms.

URINE CULTURE ISOLATION.   About 25 per cent of typhoid fever cases yield Salmonella typhi from urine culture. Other species of the Enterobacteriaceae may also be isolated from this source, such as Escherichia, Proteus, Klebsiella and other Salmonella species. It is recommended to centrifuge urine suspected of containing Salmonella, then to transfer the sediment to enrichment media. Selective and inhibitory plating media are also employed with success.

Carriers are similarly detected by finding the bacilli in cultures from their feces, their urine, or both.

AGGLUTINATION REACTIONS.   In salmonellosis and especially in typhoid fever, antibodies begin to appear in the blood about five days after onset. The antibodies most easily demonstrated are agglutinins. In most cases of salmonellosis an attempt is made to demonstrate the presence of these specific agglutinins in order to confirm the diagnosis. The test is often called the Widal test after the French physician Widal (1862–1929), who first published information on the subject. Diagnostic agglutination reactions have already been described.

The Widal reaction may cause erroneous diagnosis unless the history of the patient is known, because the reaction is often positive in carriers, in persons who have had typhoid fever and also in persons who have been

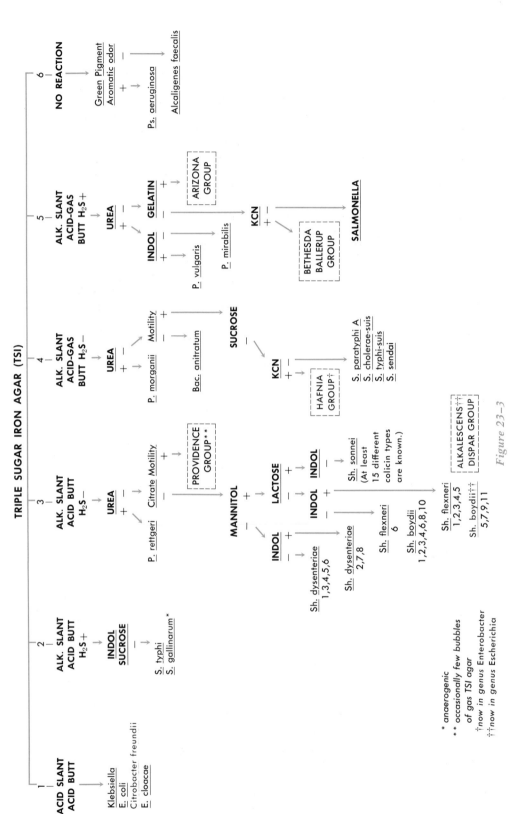

TRIPLE SUGAR IRON AGAR (TSI)

Figure 23-3

Key to partial differentiation of enteric bacilli. TSI agar contains three sugars—glucose, lactose and sucrose—and phenyl red indicator to demonstrate hydrogen sulfide production. (After Smith, D. T., Conant, N. F., and Overman, J. R. (Eds.): Zinsser

* anaerogenic
** occasionally few bubbles
   of gas TSI agar
† now in genus Enterobacter
†† now in genus Escherichia

injected with dead typhoid bacilli (typhoid vaccine) for the prevention of the disease. In those who have had typhoid fever, or who have been immunized against it, a positive Widal reaction may sometimes be obtained during any febrile disease, such as malaria or influenza. Such a nonspecific Widal reaction is said to be an *anamnestic*[3] *reaction.* Similar nonspecific increases in specific antibody titers may also occur in other infectious diseases. Supplementary tests, using separately the antigens of the flagella (H antigens) and of the cell body (O or somatic antigens), are often used to eliminate such errors. The tests are often called "H and O agglutination tests." Increase in O agglutinins is more suggestive of a current *Salmonella* infection; H agglutinins often appear anamnestically.

Agglutinins against the Vi antigens also occur in the blood of typhoid patients, especially during the presence of the bacilli in the body. Vi antigens are somatic antigens of a special type. They are often, but not invariably, associated with *Vi*rulence. The Vi agglutinins which they evoke in the serum of the patient or carrier tend to disappear after the bacilli disappear from the carrier. The detection of Vi agglutinins is therefore of value in detecting carriers. Unfortunately, although generally furnishing good supporting or indicatory information, none of these tests is infallible. Associated with the Vi antigen is the V to W variation. W cells have lost the Vi antigen. The V type of organism is virulent and does not agglutinate with O antiserum. The W form agglutinates in O anti-

---

[3]From the Greek word *anamnesis:* to remember or recall; thus, any antigenic stimulus may reactivate or *recall* a previous antigenic stimulus.

Table 23–4. Some Serotypes of the Kauffmann-White Antigenic Schema

TYPE	O ANTIGENS	H ANTIGENS* Phase 1	Phase 2
S. *paratyphi A*	Group A 1, 2, 12	a	—
S. *tinda*	Group B 1, 4, 12, 27	a	e, n, z_{15}
S. *paratyphi B*	1, 4, 5, 12	b	1, 2
S. *typhi-murium*	1, 4, 5, 12	i	1, 2
S. *heidelberg*	4, 5, 12	r	1, 2
S. *paratyphi C*	Group C_1 6, 7, Vi	c	1, 5
S. *thompson*	6, 7	k	1, 5
S. *newport*	Group C_2 6, 8	e, h	1, 2
S. *typhi*	Group D 9, 12, Vi	d	—
S. *enteritidis*	1, 9, 12	g, m	—
S. *sendai*	1, 9, 12	a	1, 5
S. *oxford*	Group E_1 3, 10	a	1, 7
S. *london*	3, 10	l, v	1, 6

*From Bailey, W. R., and Scott, E. G.: Diagnostic Microbiology. 3rd Ed. 1970, The C. V. Mosby Co., St. Louis.

serum and it is avirulent; it can not be typed with Vi phages. Pigmentations of solid media are also different for V and W colonies.

The Kauffmann-White Schema.   It is interesting to note that there are over 1200 kinds of *Salmonella*, each differing in its content of various antigens. One aspect that may be confusing is that each type of *Salmonella* has a species name, usually representing the place where it was first isolated (Table 23–4). New types are often discovered. They bear such names as *S. manhattan*, *S. california*, *S. heidelberg*, *S. mikawashimia*, and *S. homosassa*. Many are grouped and classified according to a numbered and lettered antigen system, called the *Kauffman-White schema*. They are of great interest to epidemiologists and other professional experts, but all *Salmonella* (and *Shigella*) are transmitted in the same general ways, and diseases caused by them are prevented by the same general precautions and require the same general type of treatment.

Food Infection: Paratyphoid Fever

Important in this country as causes of food-borne enteric *infection* (not food *poisoning*) are *Salmonella paratyphi B*, *S. paratyphi C*, *S. oranienburg*, *S. cholerae-suis*, *S. newport*, *S. enteritidis*, and *S. typhimurium*. Less common in the United States, but often found in Europe and elsewhere, is *Salmonella paratyphi A*.

The usual history of a food infection outbreak due to *Salmonella* parallels the experience with spaghetti previously recounted. A group of people are all infected at the same meal by a certain dish of food prepared by an unsuspected *Salmonella* carrier and left in a warm room for some hours, thus incubating the bacilli. Twelve to 24 hours after the food has been eaten, there develop cases of gastroenteritis of various degrees of severity, ranging from mild diarrhea (common) to severe (uncommon) or fatal (rare) attacks.

As previously noted, hogs, cattle, poultry, and eggs are sometimes infected with *Salmonella* bacilli, and if the improperly cooked flesh or eggs are eaten, infection is apt to occur. Dealers and cooks may be infected by handling the raw meats. Animals such as dogs, rats, and mice are often carriers of paratyphoid bacilli, especially *Salmonella typhimurium*, and thus can be vectors of food infections. *Salmonella* infections, understandably, are frequent.

Immunization Against Salmonellosis

It is possible to produce a certain degree of *artificial active* immunity to salmonellosis by giving injections of dead typhoid or paratyphoid bacilli (bacterin or vaccine). A common procedure consists in giving three doses of such vaccine one week apart, the first of one billion, the second and third of two billion bacilli. The vaccine usually contains a mixture of typhoid and paratyphoid bacilli. It is often called "T-A-B vaccine," in reference to *Salmonella typhi*, *S. paratyphi A*, and *S. paratyphi B*. The injections are often followed within 24 hours by considerable swelling and soreness of the arm. There are sometimes general symptoms, headache, nausea, and a rise in temperature, but these are not serious and they pass off in a day or so. The most suitable time for giving the inoculations is late Friday or Saturday afternoon; the person should remain quiet for the rest of the day and should not undertake hard work on the following day.

The immunity is only relative and is probably transitory. For this reason a booster dose of 0.1 ml given intradermally every two or three years, or oftener if indicated by special conditions of exposure, is recommended by many to bolster waning immunity.

Vaccination is not at any time an absolute protection against salmonellosis, since a recently vaccinated person may develop the disease if he receives a large dose of virulent bacilli. The treatment will, however, give some protection against the moderate doses that one is likely to get in ordinary chance infection. A vaccinated person must not relax any precautions against polluted water, food, milk, patients, and so on, that he would otherwise take. An immunized person should be as scrupulously careful about washing his hands and taking all other measures to protect himself as if he were not inoculated.

Much of the reduction in salmonellosis must be ascribed to sanitation of foods, water and milk supplies, clean sewage disposal, control of carriers, and the like (*environmental sanitation*).

Shigellosis

Dysentery is a pathologic term for any form of diarrhea due to intestinal irritation. It may have several causes, from eating unripe apples to Asiatic cholera.

BACILLARY DYSENTERY. This is an infectious enteric disease caused by dysentery bacilli (*Shigella*). The term *bacillary* is used to distinguish dysentery due to these bacteria from dysentery due to protozoa, commonly called *amebic* dysentery or *amebiasis*, and from viral and other forms of dysentery. A shorter and more specific term for bacillary dysentery is *shigellosis*.

Shigellosis may vary greatly in severity, ranging from a very mild and transitory intestinal disturbance to severe and fatal dysentery. In severe cases, the dysentery bacilli cause ulcers of the large intestine, the appearance of blood, mucus, and pus in the stool, and the most intense and painful diarrhea, nausea, fever, dehydration, and toxic symptoms. *Shigella* organisms do not, as a rule, invade the blood, like some salmonellas, but are usually limited to the large intestine. Shigellas form a potent endotoxin that causes the diarrhea and the consequent prostration and loss of weight associated with the disease. *Shigella* organisms are cast off in large numbers in the stools and may persist for months in convalescents.

Most cases of shigellosis in adults in the United States are relatively mild. Many originate from persons with a transitory diarrhea so mild that they do not suspect the nature of their disease, take no special sanitary precautions, and ascribe their trouble to "something they ate." The same infection may prove fatal to young children. Adults with diarrhea should, therefore, avoid contact with children.

DYSENTERY BACILLI. There are several groups or types of dysentery bacilli. The first species to be described, now called *Shigella dysenteriae*, was discovered by a Japanese physician, Shiga, during an epidemic in Japan in 1898. A similar type, discovered in Europe, is sometimes called *Shigella ambigua* or Schmitz bacillus. Another type was discovered by an American physician, Flexner, in 1906, in the Philippine Islands and is often called the "Flexner dysentery bacillus" or *Shigella flexneri*. A number of similar varieties have since been discovered that are sometimes collectively called *Shigella paradysenteriae*. Still another type, common in the United States, first discovered by Duval and described by Sonne, is now called the Sonne dysentery bacillus (*S. sonnei*). A large group, headed by *S. boydii*, comprises species like that first discovered by a British worker, Boyd.

To simplify matters, four main groups are now recognized: *dysenteriae, flexneri, sonnei*, and *boydii*. They may be differentiated by cultural (Table 23–5) and immunologic tests. For purposes of treating the patient, the differentiation of the organisms is generally not necessary and they may be considered as a single species.

Like other members of the Enterobacteriaceae, *Shigella* species grow well in simple culture media and are easily killed by heat, drying, and disinfectants. They remain alive outside the body on food, cloth, or in the soil or water for only a short time, as compared with *Salmonella*; however, they can grow in milk and other foods without changing appearance or taste.

TRANSMISSION.   The disease is spread in much the same manner as salmonellosis, that is, by feces, fingers, flies, milk, foods, and by any articles that have been in contact with the feces of a patient or carrier. *Shigella* does not survive for long periods in feces or sewage. Thus, although waterborne epidemics of dysentery occur, they are less common than waterborne epidemics of typhoid fever. *Shigella* species are not commonly found in animals as are many species of *Salmonella*.

DIAGNOSIS.   Diagnosis of dysentery in the laboratory is made in much the same manner as the diagnosis of salmonellosis except that blood

Table 23–5.   Biochemical Differentiation of Genus *Shigella**

Acid only in glucose**				
Mannitol negative		Mannitol positive†		
Indole negative	Indole positive	Lactose negative		Lactose positive‡
		Indole negative	Indole positive	Indole negative
Sh. dysenteriae 1	*Sh. dysenteriae* 2			
3	7			
4	8	*Sh. flexneri* 6	*Sh. flexneri* 1	*Sh. sonnei*
5		*Sh. boydii* 1	2	
6		2	3	
9		3	4	
10		4	5	
		6	*Sh. boydii* 5	
		8	7	
		10	9	
		12	11	
		14	13	
			15	

*From Bailey, W. R., and Scott, E. G.: Diagnostic Microbiology. 3rd Ed. 1970, The C. V. Mosby Co., St. Louis; adapted from Edwards, P. R., and Ewing, W. H.: Manual for enteric bacteriology. 1951, Atlanta, National Communicable Disease Center.

***Sh. flexneri* 6 varieties may be aerogenic (Newcastle and Manchester).

†Certain cultures of *Sh. flexneri* 4, *Sh. flexneri* 6, and *Sh. boydii* 6 may not produce acid from mannitol.

‡Lactose fermentation is delayed with *Sh. sonnei* (usually 4 to 7 days). Closure of the fermentation tube with a tightly fitting stopper will hasten the reaction.

cultures are of little value because dysentery bacilli rarely invade the blood. Repeated stool specimens are often necessary. They must be fresh. (Why?) Agglutination tests with patient's serum are not very satisfactory in shigellosis.

Dysentery has not disappeared from modern communities as has typhoid fever, but like other forms of salmonellosis is constantly with us. Both are spread about in great part by the feces-soiled hands of unknowing and unsuspected ambulatory cases and carriers or contaminated wells.

PREVENTION OF SHIGELLOSIS. The methods of preventing the spread of bacillary dysentery in adults are in general the same as for salmonellosis, except that dysentery vaccines are of little value. Certain sulfonamides to eliminate the bacilli have been employed in many cases.

Prevention of Shigellosis in Infants. This depends on encouraging breast feeding, on teaching mothers and hospital personnel correct methods of caring for babies and of preparing their food, and on the general improvement of milk and water supplies and pasteurization of all milk. The breast-fed baby not only gets milk that is especially suited to its needs, but also it gets it in a sterile condition as long as the breasts are kept clean and the mother does not contaminate them with her hands.

For artificial feedings, there are at least four forms of commercial products (such as Similac, Enflo, or other milk preparations called formulas) available besides homogenized milk; two of these have to be mixed with sterilized or disinfected water (boiled for 25 minutes). These preparations are (1) powder, (2) liquid concentrate in a can, (3) canned formula, up to 32 ounces, which requires no additional water, (4) ready-to-use 6- or 8-ounce disposable bottles, to which only a sterilized nipple needs to be attached. For the first three preparations, bottles and nipples still have to be presterilized. In most hospitals, a formula is used from prepackaged bottles fitted with nipples; all one has to do is break the seal and give the bottle to the baby. Warming the milk or formula before giving it to the baby is not considered necessary and has been almost entirely discontinued, but the milk must be brought to room temperature. Such unheated formula may be kept at room temperature for four hours safely. It is peculiar that disposable nipples are not universally used; perhaps the perfect nipple of this type has not yet been invented? The feedings should be prepared by a person with clean hands, and the bottle, after it is prepared, should be kept away from flies and dirt and refrigerated until used. Hospital nurseries generally have very strict procedures for preparing and handling baby formulas. Aseptic technique during the preparation of food for babies in hospitals is essential.

Babies should be kept away from anyone having an intestinal disturbance. A person who is caring for a child with summer diarrhea or "summer complaint" should not prepare food for other children or for adults. The baby's crib and carriage should be screened during the fly season. The diapers of infants suffering from diarrhea should be disinfected at once by placing them in a bucket with a 2 per cent saponated cresol solution or other good disinfectant. Disposable, absorbing diapers with plastic liners are now available in many different sizes, designs and makes, and are purchasable in most drug and department stores.

The children's clinics have been a strong factor in diminishing dysentery in infants. Community health nurses and other health workers connected with these clinics visit the homes and teach the mothers correct methods of preparing the baby's food and the general care of the child.

One practice should be discontinued. It is the use of the unsanitary pacifier. If this need is not established in the baby, it is not necessary later on to break a bad habit. Maybe fewer people would smoke, if oral gratification had not been overly encouraged in early childhood?

The Escherichiae

The organisms of this tribe have the general properties of the Enterobacteriaceae. *Escherichia* may be differentiated from *Salmonella* and *Shigella* by various biochemical tests, especially by rapid (24 to 48 hours) fermentation of lactose, as shown in Table 23–2, and by typical IMViC reactions (++–– for *E. coli*). This means that typical *E. coli* gives a positive *Indol* and *Methyl-red* test, and a negative reaction in *Voges-Proskauer*[4] and *Citrate* tests.[5]

Various species of *Escherichia* are of special importance to medical and sanitation personnel because certain serotypes cause enteric and urinary tract infections and because of their relation to the sanitary bacteriology of water and milk. The genus *Escherichia* contains over 150 O antigenic groups and many of these organisms possess K antigens, which may be of the L, A, or B type. H antigens may also be present. Now included within the genus *Escherichia* is also the former *Alkalescens-Dispar* group. *Escherichia coli* occurs in enormous numbers in normal feces and is widely distributed in the intestinal canal of animals and of man. Ordinarily it does no harm.

Pathogenic Escherichia.   Extensive studies of bacteria in the feces of infants with diarrhea indicate that many cases of infant diarrhea are due to certain particular kinds of *Escherichia coli*. These pathogenic *E. coli* can be distinguished from less harmful varieties by immunologic studies (similar to studies used in establishing the Kauffmann-White schema) of their antigenic structure. Some of these strains of *E. coli* are designated as 026:B, 0111:B4, 055:B5, 0119:B14, 0127:B8, 086:B7, and so on. The numbers and letters refer to antigens in them. Ewing reported 13 such strains in 1963. Now 11 enteropathogenic *E. coli* serotypes are generally recognized. In a study by Rantz it is pointed out that in patients with urinary infections, about 45 per cent of these infections were acquired in the hospital as the result of catheterization. Other studies give even higher percentages.

These organisms are particularly troublesome in children's institutions and nurseries. They are spread about by hands and fomites, as are other enteric pathogens, and at times are very difficult to eradicate. Only the most scrupulous attention to clean technique keeps them under control.

One of the difficulties is the handling of diapers in such situations. In one useful study it was found that for the small hospital or the home a three-step process using home laundry equipment yields an adequate supply of clean, dry, noninfectious diapers, as follows:

1. On removing diaper, drop it carefully into a covered can containing enough Watkin's solution[6] (4 oz to 1 gal of water) to cover it

---

[4]Production of red color with NaOH in peptone-glucose broth, due to acetylmethylcarbinol formation.

[5]Utilization of citrate as a sole source of carbon in a mineral medium.

[6]A mixture of cresols with isopropyl alcohol and soap.

and soak at least two hours. (Probably 2 per cent saponated cresol would serve as well.)
2. Wash in an automatic machine that rinses, washes with detergent and rinses three times.
3. Dry immediately in an automatic dryer.

To overcome the problems associated with diaper handling almost all cities in the United States now have diaper services for mothers and institutions. These commercial services pick up the soiled diapers in plastic bags and return sterile, fresh diapers, at quite reasonable fees. However, the previously mentioned disposable diapers may in time eliminate all reusable diaper services.

SANITARY SIGNIFICANCE OF ESCHERICHIEAE. Since *Escherichia coli* is always present in feces, and since other species of the Escherichieae tribe frequently accompany it and closely resemble it, this tribe is frequently referred to as "the coliform (i.e., *E. coli*-like) group." The presence of any of them in water, milk or food in considerable numbers strongly suggests pollution with feces. They are easily cultivated and recognized and usually remain alive in foods and water for considerable periods of time. The coliform group is therefore commonly sought after in bacteriologic examinations of water, milk, and food as evidence of fecal pollution (and potential infection), rather than *Salmonella* or *Shigella*. These latter may be present only in small numbers, intermittently, and therefore may be difficult or impossible to find. Further, sewage pollution can introduce enteric viruses, protozoa and other intestinal pathogens besides *Salmonella* and *Shigella*.

EXAMINATION OF WATER. Since the coliforms rapidly ferment lactose with the production of acid and gas, measured portions of the suspected water (or other material to be examined) are put into broth containing lactose. Gas is looked for after incubation. If gas is present, however, it is not necessarily due to coliform species. Several other organisms also produce gas from lactose. Plates or tubes of *selective* medium are therefore inoculated from the lactose-broth tubes showing gas. After incubation, colonies resembling those of the coliform group are selected for pure-culture study and are subjected to simple biochemical tests that easily identify them (Table 23–2). This work is carried on in every public health laboratory. For official purposes methods are prescribed by the American Public Health Association and affiliated groups. These tests usually constitute a substantial part of the laboratory work in a course for which this textbook is written; thus, the student will receive proper instructions in older and newer methods in which *E. coli* is used as an indicator of fecal pollution in laboratory methods.

Besides the coliform group, enteric streptococci (*S. faecalis* and so on) are also often used as test organisms in detecting fecal pollution.

Infections of the Genitourinary Tract

In addition to its sanitary and pathologic relationships just mentioned, *E. coli* and several related species of bacteria found in feces are of great importance as the cause of serious infections of the genitourinary tract (Table 23–6).

Proteus species (Tribe Proteeae) are a genus of Enterobacteriaceae occasionally found in the normal intestine but more commonly found in sewage and also decomposing organic matter of nonfecal origin. *Proteus*

Table 23–6. Bacteria Common in Infections of the Genitourinary Tract

BACTERIUM	MORPH-OLOGY	GRAM STAIN	MOTIL-ITY	SPORES	COMMON HABITAT	LAC-TOSE	GLU-COSE	URE-ASE	GELA-TIN	PIGMENT	OTHER DISTINCTIVE CHARACTERISTICS
Escherichia coli	rod	neg.	+	−	intestine	$\oplus$[1]	$\oplus$	−	−	none	
Enterobacter aerogenes	rod	neg.	−	−	intestine	$\oplus$	$\oplus$	±	−	none	encapsulated
Proteus sp.	rod	neg.	+	−	intestine	−	$\oplus$	+	+	none	spreading growth on agar plates
Pseudomonas aeruginosa	rod	neg.	+	−	intestine	−	−	−	+	blue & yellow	
Enterococci (*Streptococcus zymogenes*)	coccus	pos.	−	−	intestine	+[2]	+	−	+	none	beta hemolysis (group D)
Streptococcus faecalis	coccus	pos.	−	−	intestine	+	+	−	−	none	alpha hemolysis ("viridans")
Staphylococcus aureus	coccus	pos.	−	−	skin, nares	+	+	−	+	yellow	

[1]Produces acid and gas
[2]Produces acid or some other distinctive reaction indicated by column heading.

is sometimes found in cases of infant diarrhea. It is distinguished from all other Enterobacteriaceae by rapid (two to four hours) decomposition of urea (production of the enzyme urease) and other characteristics shown in Table 23–2 and Figure 23–3.

Pseudomonas aeruginosa in many respects resembles *Proteus*, as just described, but differs in having polar flagella and in some other details. It is not one of the Enterobacteriaceae, but is classed in the order Pseudomonadales. It is characterized especially by producing two pigments: a water-soluble, yellow, fluorescent pigment, and a chloroform-soluble, sky-blue pigment called pyocyanin (*cyan* is from a Greek word meaning blue; compare with *cyan*otic). The mixed blue and yellow pigments of *Ps. aeruginosa* give cultures of the organism or the pus in which it is growing a blue-green color, hence the older name *Bacillus pyocyaneus* (blue-green pus). Like *Proteus*, it is a frequent invader of any tissue already injured. In fact *Pseudomonas* infections are becoming more and more major problems in hospitals, responding to none of the older antibiotics. Some newer antibiotics give promise of controlling *Ps. aeruginosa*, e.g., tobramycin, gentamycin, butirosin.

Proteus species and *Ps. aeruginosa* are often found on the skin in the perianal regions and around the genitourinary openings. As a result, they are frequently introduced into the urethra and bladder and adjoining organs by instruments such as cystoscopes and catheters and during surgical operations in these regions, in spite of the most careful technique. They may also infect in the absence of instrumentation, especially in patients with strictures or other structural abnormalities of the genitourinary tract.

Many strains of these bacteria have, through long contact with most antibiotics during treatment of patients, become highly resistant to these drugs. Consequently, they cause very stubborn and troublesome infections (such as cystitis, pyelitis, urethritis, and bacteriemia), with a fairly high fatality rate. Other antibacterial chemicals such as the nitrofurans, methanamine, and mandelic acid are sometimes effective in such conditions.

ASIATIC CHOLERA

VIBRIO CHOLERAE. *Vibrio cholerae* (also called *Vibrio comma*) is not one of the Enterobacteriaceae, but is a strongly aerobic, facultatively anaerobic, short, comma-shaped rod with polar flagella (Fig. 23–4). Although classed with the Pseudomonadales, *V. cholerae* resembles *Salmonella* in several respects (Table 23–2) and is included here as an important and dangerous enteric pathogen. *Vibrio cholerae* reduces nitrates to nitrites. Grown in nitrate-peptone broth, it gives a *cholera-red-color* when sulfuric acid is added. The reaction is due to production of nitroso-indol, which gives a red color in the presence of H_2SO_4. Once thought to be distinctive of *V. cholerae*, and therefore called the "cholera-red test," the color reaction is now not considered to be of diagnostic significance.

V. cholerae causes Asiatic cholera, the chief symptoms of which are intense diarrhea, prostration, and emaciation. Death often occurs within two or three days of onset, but may result within hours unless treatment is started in time. It is not unusual for a severe cholera patient to lose 20 liters of water per day. The treatment, consisting of infusion of water and

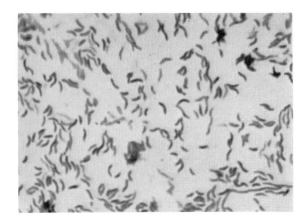

Figure 23–4

A typical *Vibrio*, morphologically like *V. cholerae*, cause of Asiatic cholera. Note the short, comma-shaped rods and the long, wavy forms. The particular species shown here is *V. fetus*, cause of infectious abortion in farm animals. It is closely related to *V. cholerae* (×1500). (Courtesy of Dr. Wayne Binns, Department of Veterinary Science, Utah State Agricultural College, Logan, Utah.)

electrolytes into the veins, results in a quick and remarkable relief of symptoms of the disease.

The vibrio may be cultivated on the same sort of nonselective media (i.e., without dyes, etc.) as are used for Enterobacteriaceae, but special media of alkaline pH (9.0), containing egg and peptone, are preferable. An excellent medium containing thiosulfate, sodium citrate, bile salts and sucrose (TCBS) agar is available commercially. The pH should be near 8.6. The colony morphology of the vibrio is distinctive. On meat extract agar, the organism forms translucent, gray colonies. It is nonspore-forming and, like Enterobacteriaceae, easily killed by boiling, pasteurization, and standard disinfectants. Recent reports by Finkelstein and his colleagues indicate that the cholera vibrios produce an "exo-enterotoxin." This toxin is an antigenic protein, which appears to be a very potent permeability factor. It has been shown to produce clinical manifestations of cholera in laboratory animals as well as in human subjects in the absence of living vibrios. A toxoid has been prepared from the toxin and is presently under trials in southeast Asia and Pakistan. Older vaccines, using killed cholera vibrios, have not been very effective.

CHOLERA AND ITS TRANSMISSION. Asiatic cholera is transmitted from person to person in the same manner as *Salmonella typhi*, and its spread is prevented by the same measures. Like *S. typhi*, it is a distinctively human pathogen. Large outbreaks of cholera are usually water-borne. Like the dysentery bacilli, cholera vibrios do not ordinarily invade the blood, but generally remain within the intestine. The vomitus of cholera patients is infectious, and soiled clothing and bedding remain infectious while damp. This is important in concurrent disinfection. In endemic[7] and epidemic[8] areas food-borne infection is common, and healthy carriers are said to be frequent sources of infection, though there is disagreement on this point. Very mild cases occur which are unrecognized sources of infection, much as are carriers.

Cholera has long been present in India and other Eastern countries. In the past it has many times started from the East along caravan and

---

[7]Always present in a population at a relatively constant rate of prevalence.

[8]An epidemic is a sudden marked increase in prevalence of a disease, which later declines to the usual rate of prevalence.

shipping routes and been carried over almost the entire earth. During the nineteenth century there were five such great epidemics, some of which reached the United States. Millions died. Epidemics of cholera occurred in the Philippines in 1961, and in Taiwan in 1962. The widespread El Tor type cholera began in Southeast Asia during 1961. Clinically, it seemed to be no different from the classic cholera type. The causative El Tor *Vibrio*[9] can be differentiated from the classic *V. cholerae* only by laboratory methods. It is commonly referred to as the El Tor variant. Other types of *Vibrio* less virulent than *V. cholerae* or the El Tor *Vibrio* are known, e.g., the Ubon El Tor type from Thailand and some enteritis-causing, antigenically different groups. Numerous saprophytic species have been described; some species are pathogenic for sheep and other animals. There is no known endemic cholera at present in Europe or the Western Hemisphere. This is true only because of constant watchfulness by the public health agencies in this and other countries. Still, in the first eight months of 1970 the number of registered deaths due to cholera listed in the World Health Statistics Report were: 3577 in Ghana, 19,280 in India, 8066 in Pakistan, but also 293 in Brazil and 5 in the United States—the last being cases imported from Vietnam.

Prophylactic vaccination with killed cultures of the cholera vibrio may be of some value. The immunity lasts for six months or less and is not very potent. The newer cholera toxoid may prove more effective. Antibiotics help but are not curative.

VIBRO PARAHEMOLYTICUS. This organism, closely related to *Vibrio cholerae*, has come into prominence since it was first suspected, by the Japanese microbiologists Fujino, Okuno, and associates, as a cause of *shirasu*, a severe form of gastroenteritis found in Japan, the United States and elsewhere. The disease is associated especially with the eating of marine and estuarine seafoods. It differs from *V. cholerae* in these respects: failure to grow in 1 per cent tryptone broth without about 8 per cent NaCl; production of soluble hemolysin for goat erythrocytes; growth at 42 C. In many ways *V. cholerae* and *V. parahemolyticus* resemble Enterobacteriaceae but do not produce indophenol oxidase. *V. parahemolyticus* is found in the stools of patients and in crabs, shrimp, and so forth.

PREVENTION OF ENTERIC INFECTIONS

It is clear, from what has been said, that infectious organisms from the intestinal tract, such as cholera vibrios, *Salmonella*, *Shigella*, bacilli that cause undulant fever and intestinal tuberculosis, the viruses of poliomyelitis and viral hepatitis, pathogenic protozoa and some worms (helminths), can be controlled most effectively at the bedside as they come from the patient (or healthy carrier), and before they are scattered.

The feces and urine must be disinfected (or otherwise disposed of in an approved manner), as well as everything that could possibly be contaminated with them, such as bed linen, clothing and wash water. Bedpans must be given special attention immediately after use by the patient. If a mechanical disinfecting flusher or other approved means of disposal is not available, the feces or urine should be transferred to a covered vessel,

---

[9]El Tor is the name of a town on the west side of the Sinai peninsula.

then thoroughly disinfected with saponated cresol or chloride of lime, or strong chlorine laundry bleach. The bedpan is flushed and boiled if possible, or soaked in disinfectant solution, after which it is thoroughly washed and returned to the patient. Disposable paper (papier-mâché) bedpans are now available. Special apparatus is required for their disposal. The patient's dishes should be boiled or disinfected in an electric dishwasher. Attractive disposable paper dishes are readily available and currently used in many hospitals that have patients with infectious diseases.

The patient must be isolated as any case of infectious disease; no visitors should be allowed in the sickroom. If the patient is at home and if milk is taken from a dairy using bottles, the milk man is notified not to collect empty milk bottles, as they may carry the infectious organism back to the dairy. The person who cares for the patient should not prepare food for anyone else, even for himself. Cholera, salmonellosis, and shigellosis patients should, if possible, be treated in hospitals in isolation quarters designed to exclude flies. The presence of flies in or around a hospital is evidence of carelessness.

The greatest danger of infection is not, however, from the known *Salmonella* or *Shigella* or cholera patient, but from a person in an infectious stage before a diagnosis has been made and from persons with such mild symptoms that diagnosis is never made. Every patient having any intestinal disturbance associated with fever should be put on enteric precautions until a diagnosis can be made. This measure would help prevent the spread of cholera, shigellosis, and salmonellosis. It is better to isolate unnecessarily than too late.

No convalescent from salmonellosis or shigellosis should be taken out of isolation until consecutive specimens of feces and urine, taken at intervals of six days, and not earlier than one month after onset, have been found to be negative for the causative organisms. This is often difficult, however, because convalescents sometimes continue to harbor enteric bacilli for long periods. These persons may be released with suitable injunctions for protection of others, and under health department supervision. Even with repeated examinations under the most favorable conditions some carriers will be missed.

CONTROL OF CARRIERS. The control of carriers is difficult but very important. The most important point is their occupation. It is imperative that the carrier shall not engage in any occupation requiring the handling of food and milk, that the feces shall be disinfected (or otherwise disposed of in such a manner as to avoid infecting others with them), and that the carrier shall conscientiously and thoroughly wash and, if possible, disinfect the hands after using the toilet. The health authorities keep in touch with known carriers by means of visits and reports.

INDIVIDUAL PRECAUTIONS. For one's individual protection certain precautions should be taken. If one suspects that the water supply is polluted, drinking water should be boiled. Campers, picnickers, and vacationists should be careful about their drinking water.

A good precaution when boiling the water is not feasible is to provide oneself with commercially available tablets of chloramine (e.g., Halozone, Globaline) for disinfecting water. These are available in drug stores or sporting goods stores and are very effective when used as directed. A good emergency substitute is to add 20 to 30 drops of one of the numerous household laundry bleaches that contain about 5 per cent NaOCl, such as Clorox, to a quart of water at least 30 minutes before use. Laundry bleaching fluids or strong solutions of hypochlorite are also excellent general disinfectants for feces, floors, and bedpans. The labels on the bottles give detailed directions for various uses, including infectious disease applications.

Pasteurized milk in one form or another is the only kind available for sale in most states and communities in the United States. In many public eating places, it is approved practice to offer customers milk in the original container (unopened cartons or bottles). These practices and laws have been designed to prevent transmission of infection by milk.

Supplementary Reading

Bailey, W. R., and Scott, E. G.: Diagnostic Microbiology. 3rd Ed. 1970, St. Louis, Mo., C. V. Mosby Company.

Balows, A., Herman, G. J., and De Witt, W. E.: The isolation and identification of *Vibrio cholerae*—a review. *Health Lab. Sci.*, 1971, *8*:167.

Benenson, A. S. (Editor): Control of Communicable Diseases of Man. 11th Ed. 1970, New York, American Public Health Association.

Chambers, J. S.: The Conquest of Cholera. 1938, New York, The Macmillan Co.

Drinking water disinfection. Washington, D. C., Superintendant of Documents, Government Printing Office, Public Health Service Publication No. 387

Edsall, G.: Typhoid fever. *Amer. J. Nurs.*, 1959, *59*:989.

Edwards, W. M., et. al.: Outbreak of typhoid fever in previously immunized persons traced to a common carrier. *New Eng. J. Med.*, 1962, *267*, 15:742.

Eichner, E. R., Gangarosa, E. J., and Goldsby, J. B.: The current status of shigellosis in the United States. *Amer. J. Public Health*, 1968, *58*:753.

Ewing, W. H.: Enterobacteriaceae infections. In: Diagnostic Procedures for Bacterial, Mycotic and Parasitic Infections. 5th Ed. 1970, New York, American Public Health Association.

Ewing, W. H.: *Vibrio cholerae*. In: Diagnostic Procedures for Bacterial, Mycotic and Parasitic Infections. 5th Ed. 1970, New York, American Public Health Association.

Felsenfeld, O.: The Cholera Problem. 1970, St. Louis, Mo., Warren H. Green, Inc.

Finkelstein, R. A., and Peterson, J. W.: In vitro detection of antibody to cholera enterotoxin in cholera patients and laboratory animals. *Inf. and Imm.*, 1970, *1*:21.

Goldschmidt, M. G., Lockhart, B. M., and Perry, K.: Rapid methods for determining decarboxylase activity: ornithine and lysine decarboxylases. *Appl. Microbiol.*, 1971, *22*:344.

Hirschhorn, N., and Greenough, W. B., III: Cholera. *Sci. Amer.*, 1971, *225*:15.

Kauffman, A. F., Hayman, C. R., Heath, F. C., and Grant, M.: Salmonellosis epidemic related to a caterer-delicatessen restaurant. *Amer. J. Public Health*, 1968, *58*:764.

Keusch, G. T., Atthasampunna, P., and Finkelstein, R. A.: A vascular permeability defect in experimental cholera. *Proc. Soc. Exp. Biol. Med.*, 1967, *124*:822.

Smith, P. B., Rhoden, D. L., Tomfohrde, K. M., Dunn, C. R., Balows, A., and Hermann, G. J.: R/b enteric differential system for identification of Enterobacteriaceae. *Appl. Microbiol.*, 1971, *21*:1036.

Vibrio parahemolyticus—Louisiana. Morbidity and Mortality, 1972, *21*(No. 40):341.

Washington, J. A., II, Yu, P. K. W., and Martin, W. J.: Evaluation of accuracy of multitest micromethod system for identification of Enterobacteriaceae. *Appl. Microbiol.*, 1971, *22*:267.

Wasilauskas, B. L.: Preliminary observations on the rapid differentiation of the Klebsiella-Enterobacter-Serratia group on bile-esculin-agar. *Appl. Microbiol.*, 1971, *21*:162.

WHO Expert Committee: Water Pollution Control. 1966, Geneva, World Health Organization Technical Report Series No. 318.

Brucellosis and Leptospirosis

24

The two groups of bacteria discussed in this chapter are not such distinctively "enteric" organisms as *Salmonella* and *Shigella*, and, as will appear, have more than one means of transmission. *Brucella* (cause of brucellosis or undulant fever) is sometimes present in the feces of patients, and *Leptospira*, cause of leptospirosis (hemorrhagic jaundice, canicola fever, Weil's disease, and so on) occurs in the urine of patients. These facts necessitate the same general precautions for control of infections by *Brucella* and *Leptospira* as are used in all feces-borne and urine-borne diseases. Certain species of *Clostridium* are constantly present in feces, but are also common in the soil and are more fully described in connection with the soil-borne diseases, tetanus and gas gangrene (Chapter 36).

GENUS BRUCELLA

Brucella is among the smallest of bacteria. It is a short, often coccoid, nonmotile bacillus, gram-negative, nonspore-forming, microaerophilic, and rather fastidious in its growth requirements. In these respects it resembles the genus *Haemophilus*, described in Chapter 30. It belongs to the same family, Brucellaceae.

Brucella differs from *Haemophilus* in not requiring blood derivatives for growth and in several other biochemical properties. It is much more invasive than the hemophilic group, and generally penetrates to all of the tissues of the infected body and circulates in the blood. In man it causes the disease undulant fever or brucellosis. In cattle, swine, and goats it causes infectious abortion and tends to localize, especially in the udders of lactating animals.

These bacteria were first discovered in 1887 by Bruce, a British scientist, hence the name of the genus. Bruce discovered the bacilli originally in goats and in British soldiers in Malta who had drunk goat's milk. Since then, several varieties of the organism have been found in other parts of the world, causing slightly different diseases, according to whether

352

the organism is of the variety that primarily infects cattle, hogs, or goats. Since it is commonly found in the milk of infected animals, unpasteurized (or *un-Certified*) milk is an important means of transmission. Infected animals often secrete the organisms in milk only intermittently.

SPECIES OF BRUCELLA.   The variety infecting cows characteristically causes abortions in these animals when they are pregnant for the first time and is called *Brucella abortus*. The variety infecting hogs is called *Brucella suis*, and that infecting goats, *Brucella melitensis*.[1] The infectivity is not highly specific. Any of the types may infect other animals, including horses, sheep, and dogs, as well as man. A fourth species, *Brucella neatomae*, was isolated in 1957 from the desert rat. It does not seem to affect man. However, *Brucella canis*, a dog pathogen, has been known to infect laboratory workers. It is sometimes a problem in kennels and similar places.

Characteristics of Brucellas.   When first isolated, the various species of *Brucella* often grow very slowly. Cultures of infectious milk, blood, cerebrospinal fluid, at times even urine or tissues used for diagnosis should therefore be incubated for at least four weeks and subcultured and examined every day or every two days to see if growth has started. *Brucella abortus* will grow at first only in a special atmosphere containing about 5 per cent carbon dioxide. The other varieties of *Brucella* can use carbon dioxide, but can also grow well aerobically. Blood cultures are of special value in diagnosing human cases. The three varieties of *Brucella* pathogenic to man can be differentiated only by very careful laboratory tests. Some of these differentiations are shown in Table 24–1. The best growth may be obtained on tryptose, trypticase, liver infusion or brucella agar at pH 7.0 to 7.2, or slightly more acid, in 5 per cent carbon dioxide.

In the infected body the organisms tend to be removed from the blood by phagocytic cells lining the blood vessels (reticuloendothelial system). Cultures are therefore often made from bone marrow (taken usually from the sternum, or "breast bone") or with material drawn with a trochar from a lymph node. The nurse or health worker should be prepared to assist in obtaining such material for diagnostic culture. It requires local anesthetization.

Brucellosis (Undulant Fever)

The disease in man, most commonly called undulant fever (Malta fever, Mediterranean fever, or Bang's disease), is frequently characterized by a long preliminary stage, lasting days or weeks, during which there is an increasing weakness and later backache, stiffness of the joints, progressive loss of weight, and a long list of other, less definite, and highly variable symptoms. The incubation period may be as long as a month or as short as four or five days. There are usually severe night sweats and remittent daily fever or repeated undulatory attacks of fever, each lasting several days, with remissions between the waves. In its milder forms, which are frequent, the malady may be regarded by the victim as "grippe" or "intestinal flu." About 2 per cent of the cases are acute and fatal, but the great majority of persons afflicted, after being ill for days, weeks, or months, eventually recover.

The bovine type of infection (*Br. abortus*) in man is likely to be mild,

---

[1]Malta was known to the ancient Romans as *Melita* because of the fine *mel* (honey) to be had there; hence *melitensis*, meaning "of Melita."

Table 24-1. Physiological Characteristics of Typical Strains of *Brucella**

SPECIES	PREFERRED HOST**	5% CO_2 REQUIREMENT	H_2S PRODUCTION	HYDROLYSIS OF UREA	SENSITIVITY TO DYES IN AGAR MEDIUM		AGGLUTINATION TESTS
					With Thionine	*Basic Fuchsin*	
*Brucella melitensis*①	Goats	−	− or ± for 4 days	Slow or negative	+	+	Has specific antigens
*Brucella abortus*②	Cows	+	+ for 2 days only	Slow or negative	−	+	Share antigens, but different from
*Brucella suis*③	Hogs	−	+ for 4 days	Rapid	+	−	*B. melitensis*

*Strain variations exist.
**Actually any type may infect other animals or man.
①Biotypes I-III are known.
②Biotypes I-IX are known.
③Biotypes I-IV.

and many cases pass unnoticed and undiagnosed. The porcine and caprine varieties (*Br. suis* and *Br. melitensis*) cause much more severe infections as a rule.

TRANSMISSION OF UNDULANT FEVER. Brucellosis is only rarely transmitted from human to human. The organisms from animal sources find portals of entry via the gastrointestinal tract and through cuts and scratches in the skin. On gaining entrance to the body, the organisms travel from the portal of entry by way of the blood and lymph channels. The bacilli tend to localize in lymph nodes in all the various organs. In female farm animals the bacilli tend also to localize in the udder and, in pregnant animals, in the uterus, placenta, and similar locations. The fetus, membranes, and fluids discharged during abortion due to *Brucella* are highly infectious, as is the milk of infected animals, and occasionally of women. The organisms also sometimes appear in the feces and urine both of infected animals and of man, hence their inclusion here among the intestinal infections. In man and male farm animals inflammation of the testis (orchitis) is not uncommon and often results in sterility.

Since the organisms invade the blood, they are present in all the tissues, and for this reason the disease is particularly common among butchers, employees of slaughterhouses, stock raisers, and veterinarians. Persons who take unpasteurized milk or other dairy products from cows or goats which have not been carefully tested to rule out the disease are in danger of contracting the infection, and generally do so sooner or later. It is apparent that human cases of brucellosis have steadily declined in the United States, from the reported (diagnosed) 3510 cases in 1950 to 183 cases in 1971.

SEROLOGIC DIAGNOSIS OF UNDULANT FEVER. In addition to a blood culture (which is the most conclusive test, if positive), an agglutination test, performed almost exactly like the Widal test, is one method of diagnosis. It does not distinguish between species of *Brucella*. The serum of patients and of infected farm animals usually agglutinates the brucellas in significant dilutions, as does the sweet whey from junket made with milk of infected animals. In many confirmed cases of brucellosis, however, agglutinins appear in the serum only in low dilutions or not at all, and they appear sometimes in supposedly normal persons. There is no real "diagnostic titer" of agglutinins, though in practice a positive reaction with serum diluted above 1:320 or 1:640 is generally regarded as indicating infection, either past or present. It is much more significant if there is a rise in titer between two tests done about ten days apart. This is true of all serologic tests and should be remembered by the student (Chapter 19). It shows that the tissues are actively responding to the immunologic stimulus of an infection. The student should compare this rise in titer with, and carefully differentiate it from, the anamnestic reaction and the secondary antigenic stimulus. Antibodies in human sera have also been detected by means of the FA (fluorescent antibody) test.

Sometimes blood or the cream from suspected milk is injected into guinea pigs for diagnostic purposes. These animals are very susceptible to infection with *Brucella* and show characteristic lesions. Cultures inoculated with blood or cream are also often used for diagnostic purposes, with good results. Until the machine age replaced many of the "small time" producers of milk, the "ring test" was widely used and could be easily performed in any barn by practically untrained personnel. To 5 ml of whole unhomogenized milk, 0.2 ml of a heavy suspension of killed, purple-stained *Brucella* cells is added. The two are mixed well and allowed to stand. In the presence of antibodies against *Brucella*, the stained organisms adhere to the fat globules and rise with them to the surface, forming a purple ring of cream, a positive "ring test." This is diagnostic in cows infected with brucellosis, but may also occur in infected cows that have been vaccinated. Milk known to be infectious by any pathogen should not be used. Isolation of specific, causative microorganisms in pure culture is the surest diagnosis in any infection.

PREVENTION OF UNDULANT FEVER.   The disease may be prevented by using only pasteurized dairy products, and by carefully avoiding any infected animals and their flesh or discharges.

Vaccines have been found to be of some value in prevention of loss of calves and other farm animals by abortion, although the infection may occur. There is no good vaccine for human beings.

The patient with undulant fever is not highly infectious unless there are draining lymph nodes or other open lesions. Dressings and clothing soiled with such drainage should be carefully disinfected and not allowed to touch other articles. The organisms are occasionally present in the urine and feces and these should be given the same sort of treatment as stools from typhoid fever patients.

TREATMENT OF UNDULANT FEVER.   Tetracyclines alone are usually adequate; for severe cases chlortetracycline (Aureomycin) and streptomycin are used. Treatment must be continued for at least three weeks; relapses are frequent.

GENUS LEPTOSPIRA

Leptospiras are the smallest and most delicate cell forms of spirochetes. They are tightly coiled, slender, and curved into a hook at one or both ends (Figs. 24–1, 24–2). They may be cultivated in simple mineral solutions (e.g., Stuart's), supplemented with about 10 per cent of rabbit serum and incubated at about 20 to 35 C. In cultures or in infected urine or tissues, they may readily be seen by means of the darkfield microscope, wriggling and twirling with fascinating energy. There are several harmless species of *Leptospira*, which multiply in sewage, stagnant water and feces. These are sometimes grouped as *Leptospira biflexa*. They grow well at temperatures of 5 to 10 C, several degrees below the minimal (13 to 15 C) for pathogenic leptospiras. The pathogens generally exhibit much greater ability to hydrolyze leucyl naphthylamide than the saprophytes. Other differences have been noted.

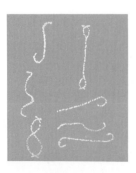

Figure 24–1

Leptospira icterohaemorrhagiae. Appearance of organisms in the darkfield (×1000). (Joklik and Smith: Zinsser Microbiology, 15th Edition, p. 661. 1972, Appleton-Century-Crofts Educational Division, Meridith Corp., N.Y.

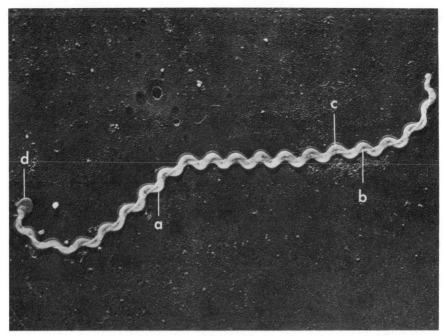

Figure 24-2

L. icterohaemorrhagiae. Spray preparation shadowed with chromium. Note protoplasmic spiral (a), axial filament (b), covering sheath (c), and end bulb (d). 12,500 ×. (From Simpson, C. F., and White, F. H.: *Infect. Dis.*, 1961, *109:*243. Copyright 1961, University of Chicago Press.)

All species, both saprophytes and pathogens, are quite fragile and easily killed by heat, drying, and standard disinfectants; however, all can survive for considerable periods in streams, ponds, and other bodies of fresh water. If pathogenic species happen to be present in such waters, they can (and often do) infect animals or uninformed persons drinking the polluted water, or swimming or wading in it. Like *Brucella,* the leptospiras enter the body via the gastrointestinal tract or cuts or scratches in the skin. Since the pathogenic leptospiras usually damage the kidneys especially, they often occur in the urine as well as in blood and other tissues of infected man and animals. The presence of the spirochetes in bodies of water subject to pollution with human or animal urine or tissues is therefore easily understood. The carcasses of dead infected animals sometimes pollute streams and ponds. Animals likely to be infected (and infectious) include dogs, cattle, swine, mules, rats, and numerous wild mammals.

Leptospirosis

The pathogenic leptospiras, after entry, invade the entire body by way of the blood. Infection with any species of *Leptospira* is properly called *leptospirosis.* Leptospiras are discussed here after our discussion of the enteric group of bacteria because one of their important portals of entry is by way of the mouth and because their important portal of exit is the urinary tract (via urine); hence, like the Enterobacteriaceae they are transmitted by sewage-polluted or urine-fouled water and food. They do not ordinarily occur in the feces.

The several species of *Leptospira* that infect man are so much alike that they can be differentiated only by skilled laboratory workers. The species commonly infecting dogs is called *L. canicola,* that infecting cattle and swine, *L. pomona.* A species causing Weil's disease or infectious hemorrhagic jaundice in man is named *L. icterohaemorrhagiae.* Others causing

357

related conditions are *L. australis* A and B, *L. hebdomadis*, *L. grippotyphosa*, and so on. At the present time 18 serogroups are recognized, with probably over 100 serotypes obtained from all over the world. Clinical manifestations of leptospirosis are varied, ranging from lesions of the eye, to meningitis, hepatitis, jaundice, high fever, "black vomit,"[2] and other symptoms, depending somewhat on the infecting species.

WEIL'S DISEASE.   One of the most familiar forms of leptospirosis in man was originally called Weil's disease, after A. Weil, a physician of Wiesbaden, Germany. It was once confused with yellow fever (a viral disease), partly because of the intense jaundice due to hepatitis and other clinical features (including "black vomit") found in both diseases. This form of leptospirosis is quite widespread in some regions, including the United States. It often occurs in persons who spend much time (especially with bare feet or leaky shoes) in wet, poorly drained places, such as badly constructed mines, trenches during war, rice fields, sewers, and the bilges of boats, where there is human urine and where rats abound. It may also occur in persons living at home, however, and not frequenting any of the situations named, if they come into contact with water or food contaminated with the urine of rats or other infected animals or persons.

Leptospira icterohaemorrhagiae, the cause of Weil's disease, occurs in the blood and urine of the patients and may be cultivated from them in serum media, as previously mentioned. The organisms survive and possibly multiply in polluted water and may easily be cultivated from the water. *Leptospira icterohaemorrhagiae*, is readily transmitted from man to man by polluted water. The disease is often severe and not infrequently fatal, though many mild cases occur. Leptospirosis at the present time is a notifiable disease of low frequency in the United States. In 1971, 62 cases were reported.

RATS AND LEPTOSPIROSIS.   Rats commonly acquire the infection, and in any large number of rats properly examined (kidney examinations by darkfield), a certain proportion (often 50 per cent) will always be found to harbor these organisms. Studies done during 1958 to 1968, and reported in 1971, showed that up to 46 per cent of the brown rat (*Rattus norvegicus*) population is infected with *Leptospira icterohaemorrhagiae*. It is thus evident that rats transmit the disease, polluting sluggish streams, mines, ships, trenches, establishments in which poultry, fish or meat are cleaned, as well as food in kitchens and water in shallow wells. When rats or other infected animals (such as dogs) die in wells, boats, ponds, and streams, their bodies make the water infectious.

OTHER TYPES OF LEPTOSPIROSIS.   The same general sequence of events holds true for other forms of leptospirosis. Leptospirosis due to *L. canicola* causes serious losses in dog kennels; in swine and cattle leptospirosis from *L. pomona* costs farmers many thousands of dollars annually, and carries with it the risk of the farmers themselves becoming infected. Formerly regarded as a rare disease, leptospirosis has been found to be frequent and widespread in both man and animals in many countries other than the United States.

DIAGNOSIS.   Darkfield examination of urine of patients with leptospirosis often reveals the leptospiras. They are not generally found in

---

[2]Black vomit is a lay term for vomitus containing blood blackened by the acid gastric juice. The blood in black vomit comes from hemorrhages in the alimentary tract, which are common in Weil's disease. Damage to the liver causes jaundice, hence the term "hemorrhagic jaundice" for Weil's disease.

blood by this means. Guinea pigs are highly susceptible and inoculation of them with infectious blood or urine usually produces a typical case of leptospirosis. Cultures made with blood or urine also reveal the organisms.

Shortly after the onset of infection with *Leptospira*, agglutinins and cytolytic antibodies begin to appear in the blood. These increase in concentration until the serum of the animal or person is capable of protecting him against large doses of leptospiras. Stable, formolized *Leptospira* serotype suspensions are available and are used satisfactorily in rapid slide agglutination tests for serological diagnosis. Also used is the immune adherence method and the FA (fluorescent antibody) test.

Because of the frequent occurrence of leptospiremia, in taking blood specimens for "blood counts," cultures, and serologic studies, precautions must be taken to see that cotton pledgets, needles, syringes, and so forth, soiled with blood are properly disposed of.

In addition to these precautions, the urine of patients with leptospirosis should be handled as infectious. Such urine, as well as clothing and bedding soiled with it, should be disinfected, with the usual precautions. The patient must avoid contamination of his surroundings with urine. Ordinary cleanliness of hands will usually suffice. Rats should be exterminated. When managing cases of leptospirosis under home or field conditions, water should be boiled or chlorinated before drinking, unless it is from a supply of known purity. Food possibly contaminated with excreta of rats, or from unsanitary sources, should not be eaten.

Supplementary Reading

Alexander, A. D., Wood, G., Yancey, F., Byrne, R. J., and Yager, R. H.: Cross-neutralization of leptospiral hemolysins from different serotypes. Infect. Immun., 1971, *4*:152.

Alexander, A. D., et al.: A new pathogenic *Leptospira*, not readily cultivated. *J. Bact.*, 1962, *83*:754.

Alston, J. M., and Broom, J. C.: Leptospirosis in Man and Animals. 1958, Baltimore, The Williams & Wilkins Co.

Begumnova, F. I.: Epidemiology of nonicteric leptospirosis in the Astrakhan region. Z. H. Mikrobiol. Epideminol. Immunobiol., 1970, *47*:36.

Burton, G., Blenden, D. C., and Goldberg, H. S.: Naphthylamidase activity of *Leptospira. Appl. Microbiol.*, 1970, *19*:586.

Galton, M. M., et al.: Leptospirosis, epidemiology, clinical manifestations in man and animals, and methods in laboratory diagnosis. Public Health Service Pub. No. 951, 1962, Washington, D.C., Government Printing Office.

Hendricks, S. L., et al.: Brucellosis outbreak in an Iowa packing house. *Amer. J. Pub. Health*, 1962, *52*:1166.

Joint FAO/WHO Expert Committee on Brucellosis, 3rd Report. 1958, Geneva, World Health Organization, Technical Report Series, No. 148.

Mazzur, S.: The detection of Australia antigen by immunodiffusion and counterelectrophoresis. Am. J. Med. Tech., 1972, *38*:343.

McKiel, J. A., Rappay, D. E., Cousineau, J. G., Hall, R. R., and McKenna, H. E.: Domestic rats as carriers of leptospires and salmonellas in Eastern Canada. Can. J. Pub. Health, 1971, *61*:336.

National Communicable Disease Center: Epidemiological Notes and Reports, Nosocomial isolations of *Clostridium perfringens*—Oregon. Morbidity and Mortality, 1967, Vol. 16, No. 26, U.S. Department of Health, Education, and Welfare, Public Health Service, Bureau of Disease Prevention and Environment Control.

National Communicable Disease Center: Morbidity and Mortality. 1971, Vol. 20, No. 53, U.S. Department of Health, Education, and Welfare, Public Health Service, Bureau of Disease Prevention and Environmental Control.

Ritchie, A. E., and Ellinghausen, H. C.: Electron microscopy of leptospires. *J. Bact.*, 1965, *59*:223.

Shulman, N. R.: Complement fixation techniques for measuring hepatitis associated antigen and antibody. Am. J. Med. Tech., 1972, *38*:350.

Vedros, N. A., Smith, A. W., Schonewald, J., Migaki, G., and Hubbard, R. C.: Leptospirosis epizootic among California sea lions. Science, 1971, *172*:1250.

WHO Expert Group: Current Problems in leptospirosis research. 1967, Geneva, World Health Organization, Technical Report Series, No. 380.

Enteric Viral Infections

Enteric Viral Infections

25

In addition to various kinds of bacteriophages, many viruses capable of infecting mammalian cells are to be found in the intestinal tract of man and/or animals. One special group of viruses found in the intestine of man is called enteroviruses.

THE ENTEROVIRUSES

These viruses were classified in 1963 as picornaviruses. Picornaviruses are small (*pico* = small), and contain an RNA core (hence *picorna*). Some systems of viral nomenclature have discouraged use of the term picornavirus. However, it continues to be used as the name of a group (genus?) that includes the viruses of foot-and-mouth disease of cattle, and of mouse encephalitis, and three subgroups called, respectively, enteroviruses, rhinoviruses (cause of common colds), and reoviruses (Table 6–2). The enterovirus group includes the viruses of poliomyelitis and those of the Coxsackie and ECHO groups. All the enteroviruses that infect man are distinguished by the facts that: (1) they multiply primarily in cells of the human gastrointestinal tract; (2) when they produce clinically recognizable disease, it usually involves the central nervous system (CNS: brain and spinal cord). ECBO viruses are similar to ECHO viruses but are bovine pathogens. Possibly some of the reoviruses may become eligible for inclusion in the group of enteroviruses since they appear to multiply in the intestine and, like poliovirus, appear in feces or oral secretions and, in animals at least, affect the CNS. Suggested interrelationships of some enteroviruses are indicated in Figure 25–1. For a proposed classification of viruses consult Appendix B. Classification of viruses is still unsettled.

To assist the reader's memory:
ECHO stands for Enteric, Cytopathogenic, Human, Orphan (see page 88).
ECBO stands for Enteric, Cytopathogenic, Bovine, Orphan.
NITA stands for Nuclear Inclusion Type A.

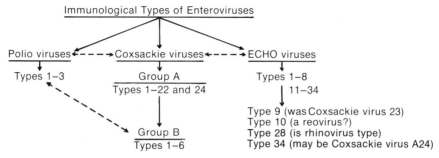

Figure 25-1

Suggested immunologic relationships between some enteroviruses. (Adapted from J. T. Syverton. In *Am. J. Trop. Med. & Hyg.*, Vol. 8.)

REO stands for Respiratory, Enteric, Orphan.
CHINA stands for Chronic Infectious Neuropathic Agents.

These viruses are all members of a large "family" or "spectrum" of viruses. They have certain properties in common but each is different from the others. They can be differentiated from one another by means of immunologic tests and other laboratory procedures and in many cases by the types of clinical conditions and pathologic changes they produce. Currently, at least 64 human enterovirus types are recognized.

Another virus, that of *infectious hepatitis* (*IH*) or *epidemic viral hepatitis*, must also be considered with the intestinal viruses because of its fecal-oral route of transmission. Strictly speaking, it is not one of the group called enteroviruses because it apparently multiplies in the liver, not in the intestine or CNS.

All are among the smallest of viruses and are relatively stable and durable in environments outside the human body. For example, all are resistant to the fermentations, acidities, putrefactions, and other conditions occurring in feces and sewage, and they appear to be more or less regularly transmitted in such materials. All are relatively resistant to certain disinfectants and some (e.g., Coxsackie virus and possibly epidemic hepatitis virus) may survive ordinary pasteurization processes. All are wholly resistant to common antibiotics. Another problem that complicates matters is that enteroviruses are regularly found in sewage even after it has received some treatment.

Any of these viruses, on gaining entrance to a host, may produce little or no obvious disease, or may produce "flulike" or coldlike episodes or gastrointestinal distress of varying severity and symptomatology (especially Coxsackie, ECHO, reoviruses, and polioviruses). Such conditions are rarely specifically diagnosed, and their cause usually remains unknown unless special laboratory investigations are made.

Enteroviruses, although commonly remaining unrecognized in the gastrointestinal or respiratory tracts, sometimes invade the blood (temporarily) and the CNS. They thus manifest one of their outstanding properties, and one that distinguishes them from the hepatitis virus: they are strongly *neurotropic*. Neurotropic viruses have marked affinity for the nervous tissues and characteristically cause diseases of the CNS. The enteroviruses most commonly and distinctively cause anterior poliomyelitis (especially polioviruses), numerous polio-like conditions (especially the Coxsackie viruses) and meningitis or encephalomyelitis (especially the ECHO viruses). The conditions caused by these viruses are frequently not clearly distinguishable from each other by clinical means.

Anterior Poliomyelitis

This disease is sometimes called "infantile paralysis," which is unfortunate since it occurs in persons of all ages and rarely causes permanent paralysis; however, most cases occur in the first 30 years of life and a large proportion before adolescence. More often yet the term "polio" is used by both layman or professional to designate this disease. Poliomyelitis is an acute, febrile disease, and like most viral diseases it is usually sudden in onset, with headache, chills, nausea, and fever. The patients often exhibit extreme irritability, pain when being moved, and characteristically the muscles of the neck are held rigid. If much invasion of the nervous system occurs, especially of the parts called "the bulbar region" (medulla oblongata)—the exception rather than the rule—it results in injury or destruction of the motor cells of the anterior horns of the cord (Fig. 25–2), producing paralysis, or "paralytic polio."

Following the febrile period there sometimes appears a paralysis of the legs and, in some cases, also of the arms and other muscles. These may or may not result in permanent injury, depending on extent of damage to the nerves and the rehabilitation treatment. If the disease extends to the nervous mechanisms controlling respiration, death may quickly ensue from respiratory failure unless some apparatus such as an "iron lung" or a "rocking bed" is used to replace the action of the muscles of respiration. For each case of paralytic poliomyelitis, probably a hundred inapparent or mild, nonparalytic infections occur. These mild cases produce such

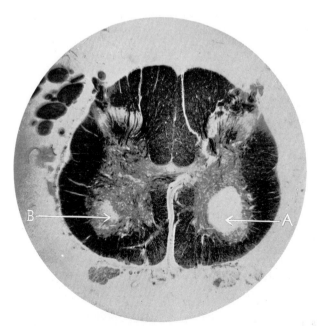

Figure 25–2

The results of acute anterior poliomyelitis. A cross section of the spinal cord in the lumbar region. The gray matter of a large area in the left anterior horn *(A)* has been completely destroyed by the inflammation, leaving a hole. The result of this lesion would be paralysis of the left leg. In the right anterior horn is an area *(B)* of partial degeneration, as evidenced by the light spot. (Wechsler, I. S.: Clinical Neurology. 9th Ed. 1963, Philadelphia, W. B. Saunders Company.)

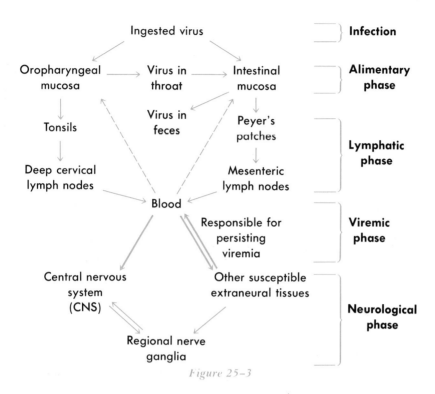

Figure 25-3

A model for the pathogenesis of poliomyelitis based on a synthesis of data obtained in man and chimpanzees. (Modified from Sabin: *Science*, 1956, *123*:1151; and Bodian: *Science*, 1955, *122*:105.)

signs and symptoms as slight fever, malaise, drowsiness, headache, constipation, and sore throat. These are not diagnostic and often pass unnoticed. These conditions range downward in severity from fairly severe "flulike" attacks to the status of healthy carriers. Such infections confer immunity. There are apparently thousands of such unrecognized infections with poliovirus every year. These do no harm in the individual but they disseminate the virus widely.

A model for the pathogenicity of poliomyelitis as postulated from experimental evidence available at present is shown in Figure 25–3.

THE POLIOMYELITIS VIRUS. The virus appears to be quite widespread. Its principal portal of entry appears to be the gastrointestinal tract, via the mouth. In the vast majority of infections it remains in the alimentary tract and is cast off in the feces. It is nearly always demonstrable in municipal sewage, especially during epidemic periods. This proves three things: (1) the virus is not sensitive to life in the outside world; (2) it must occur in relatively large amounts in feces of patients and unrecognized carriers; and (3) it apparently is readily transmitted from person to person by personal and familial contact. It is probably only after the virus invades beyond the alimentary tract that it enters the walls of the nasopharynx and thus becomes transmissible by oral and nasal secretions during the acute phase of the illness. Prevention of spread is therefore doubly difficult since it involves the problems of both enteric and respiratory vectors.

Types of Poliomyelitis Virus. There are three main immunologic types of poliovirus: I, II, and III. Type I, known as the *Brunhilde* strain, has at least three subtypes, *HoF*, Frederick, and Mahoney; type II, the *Lansing* strain, also has three subtypes, known as *MV*, *Yale-SK*, and *MEF₁*; type III, the *Leon* strain, has one antigenic type, known as *Saukett*. Immunity to one type does not confer immunity to another. A large proportion of urban adults have antibodies to all three types in their serum, yet have never had any disease recognizable as polio. They undoubtedly have had subclinical, immunizing *infections.*

Polio Vaccines

In 1949, it was found possible by Enders, Weller, and Robbins (Nobel Prize winners) to cultivate the virus of poliomyelitis in tissue cultures made with various living cells such as those from human kidneys, monkey kidneys, human intestinal tissues, human embryonic tissues, and, most interestingly, human cancer (HeLa) cells. The virus multiplies in and kills the tissue cells.

THE SALK VACCINE. The vaccine developed by Dr. Jonas Salk and first demonstrated by public trial in 1954–55 was prepared by cultivating poliovirus types I, II, and III in cultures of live monkey kidney tissue cells. After several days of incubation the dead tissue cells and other detritus are removed and the fluid, containing the poliovirus, is collected. Formaldehyde is added in about 1 : 4000 concentration to inactivate the virus. After allowing one week at about 37 C for the formaldehyde to act, the excess formaldehyde is removed. Tests are then made to determine that

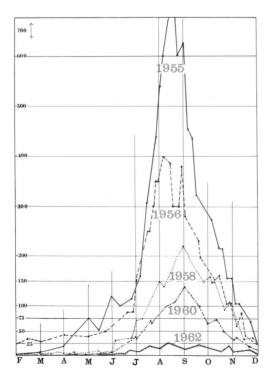

Figure 25–4

Effect of antipoliomyelitis vaccination on incidence of paralytic polio in the United States. Numbers of new cases per week are shown at left; months, beginning with February, along the bottom of the diagram. Salk inactivated vaccine was introduced on a large scale after 1954–55. Sabin active-virus vaccine was introduced for public use after 1961. Note the dramatic decline in incidence of paralytic polio, especially during the summer and autumnal months after 1955. Since 1961–62 not only paralytic but all clinical poliomyelitis has been rapidly disappearing from the American scene. Will measles follow it? (Modification courtesy of Eli Lilly & Company, Indianapolis, Indiana.) See also Figure 25–5.

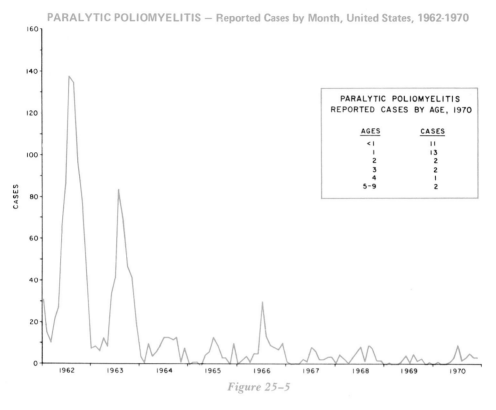

PARALYTIC POLIOMYELITIS — Reported Cases by Month, United States, 1962-1970

PARALYTIC POLIOMYELITIS REPORTED CASES BY AGE, 1970	
AGES	CASES
<1	11
1	13
2	2
3	2
4	1
5-9	2

Figure 25–5

Paralytic poliomyelitis, 1962–1970. Cases by month of onset. (From Morbidity and Mortality Annual Supplement, 1970. U.S. Dept. of Health, Education and Welfare.)

the virus is really inactive and that the material is not contaminated with bacteria. These and other tests being satisfactory, preservative is added, the vaccine is ampouled, and is ready for use.

Use and Effectiveness of Salk Vaccine.   Various schedules of inoculation with polio vaccine are recommended. One commonly used advises four doses: three about four to six weeks apart and a fourth about seven months later. Booster doses are variously recommended at intervals of one of three or more years. Persons of all ages may be vaccinated.

The vaccine does not necessarily prevent *infection* by poliovirus, although incidence of the disease in clinical and severe form rapidly declined to a very low level after Salk vaccine was generally utilized. Gastrointestinal infections by extraneous or "wild," active polio strains frequently occur after vaccination; however, the antibodies in the blood and tissues of vaccinated persons interpose a barrier between the gastrointestinal source of the wild virus in the body and the central nervous system. Thus, the most important effect of the vaccine is to prevent severe *paralytic polio*, especially the crippling and deadly "spinal paralysis" or bulbar polio. The vaccine appears to be at least 90 per cent effective in preventing paralytic polio. The mild infections in vaccinated persons appear to have the beneficial, immunizing effect of booster doses of vaccine (Figs. 25–4, 25–5).

VACCINATION IN PREGNANCY. An important aspect of polio vaccination is the protection of pregnant women as early in pregnancy as possible. Expectant mothers appear to be more susceptible to polio than other adults, and the disease is much more dangerous in pregnancy. Immunization of the mother also probably gives some passive protection to the infant for a few months.

THE SABIN ORAL POLIO VACCINE. Cultivation of the virus in cells in 1949 as noted above, made available on *active,* attenuated-virus vaccine. Large scale experiments with such "living" virus vaccine by the World Health Organization, Sabin, and others led to approval of the "Sabin vaccine" for general use in 1961 and 1962 by the U. S. Public Health Service. It has since been administered to millions of people of all ages. Routinely, the vaccine is given in a small amount of prepared culture fluid in candy, food, or beverage, one dose of each virus separately (to avoid mutual interference of the viruses), at intervals of three to six weeks, to persons over three months of age (to avoid inhibition of the virus by residual maternal antibodies in infants).

Although residual maternal antibodies in newborns may prevent the vaccine virus from multiplying and thus immunizing, good results (about 75 per cent immunized) have been obtained with vaccine administered within the first few hours or days of life. This procedure seems advisable to many workers. It has the advantages that newborns are not yet infected with extraneous enteric viruses that interfere with the vaccine virus and that infants are usually more conveniently "on hand" for the immunization.

Following the oral administration of the Sabin vaccine, multiplication of the virus occurs in the alimentary tract and virus is discharged in the feces. No perceptible symptoms occur. This not only immunizes the recipient, but like ordinary ("wild") virus, soon spreads among the recipient's contacts, thus widening the benefit. In addition to the excellent antibody response, the intestinal infection apparently results in an immunization of the intestinal tract as well, thus preventing subsequent reinfection. With the widespread use of this vaccine, poliomyelitis, previously a dreadful scourge in the world, is rapidly being forgotten, at least in the United States. Nevertheless, in the summer of 1968, an 18-month old infant died of paralytic poliomyelitis in Houston, Texas, and the disease was diagnosed in another child. In laboratory tests the etiologic agents were isolated and confirmed to be poliovirus. It seems that both children had escaped vaccination against poliomyelitis. Other, larger outbreaks were reported in 1972 in unvaccinated children.

"TRIPLE" ACTIVE POLIO VACCINE. In 1963 a second type of oral vaccine (e.g., Orimune) containing all three types of active, attenuated poliovirus was licensed by the U. S. Public Health Service. Because of interference between the three types of virus, not more than two will infect and immunize simultaneously. This type of vaccine, however, yields a high degree of immunity if given in only two doses two months apart instead of in the three or four doses required by other vaccines. It is very effective as a supplement to other immunizing processes: natural in older persons, artificial in infants and children.

The schedule of vaccination employed differs in various countries. In the U.S.S.R., trivalent vaccine is fed more frequently to children than in other countries, supposedly to help eradicate the wild strains of viruses. In the United Kingdom, two doses of trivalent vaccine are given at intervals of 1 to 2 months for primary vaccination, commencing at six months of age, and a third dose is given 6 months later. In the United States, the system resembles the British one and, in addition, children receive trivalent vaccine at one year of age. Sometimes a booster dose is given at entry into school.

It is now abundantly clear that the oral vaccines are among the safest of the live antigens in use.

Because the incidence of poliomyelitis in adults in the United States and Canada is at present negligible, authorities have advised that the vaccine should be given only to those under 18 years of age, except in outbreaks or other circumstances in which adults might be exposed to unusually high risk.

TISSUE CULTURE DIAGNOSIS. The tissue culture technique is widely used to isolate the virus from feces, oral secretions, and similar sources. This permits not only epidemiologic investigations, but also diagnosis by actual demonstration of the virus in specimens from the patient.

Transmission of Poliomyelitis

The possibility of transmission by sewage-polluted water exists, although the spread of epidemics of poliomyelitis is not suggestive of a water-borne disease like typhoid fever. The chief mode of spread suggests, rather, transfer by feces-contaminated hands and objects, in much the same manner as bacillary dysentery is spread. This is almost certainly the principal mode of dissemination. Young children playing together constitute an ideal situation for this type of dissemination, especially in areas of low-grade sanitation and cleanliness. Flies have been shown to harbor virus in their gut for as long as 48 hours. That they are important in its transmission, however, is doubtful.

POLIO AND SURGERY. It has been shown that the virus finds entrance through the tissues around the gums, tonsils, and pharynx very easily, especially if there is injury such as would result from tonsillectomy, adenoidectomy, or tooth extractions. It is therefore recommended that such surgical procedures not be done during seasons of prevalence of poliomyelitis. Many cases have been observed to follow tonsillectomy. The incidence of paralytic cases is definitely higher in persons who have had recent tonsillectomy. Furthermore, paralysis appears more frequently in arms or legs that have recently been the site of injection of materials such as pertussis vaccine, penicillin, or diphtheria toxoid. These injections certainly increase the risk of paralysis, possibly also of infection.

Prevention

The control of the poliomyelitis virus in the care of a diagnosed case is centered around proper disposal of respiratory secretions (as for respiratory infections) during the first two to three weeks from onset, and adequate disposal and disinfection of stools (as done in enteric infections) for four weeks from onset. These are arbitrary figures. There is little basis for exact rules, and the disinfection of feces from the patient who has poliomyelitis is not in practice in some communicable disease units or hospitals. There is every indication, however, that feces and feces-contaminated objects are very important vectors of the infection. Hands, as well as dishes and other objects used by the patient, should therefore be thoroughly disinfected to prevent the spread of the disease. It is known that poliomyelitis virus is inactivated by boiling and by adequate exposure to chlorine (chloride of lime, laundry bleach).

In addition to providing care for patients who have poliomyelitis, the health team has the responsibility of encouraging all people to become vaccinated as recommended by local health officials.

Coxsackie Virus

The first Coxsackie virus was isolated in 1948 by Dalldorf and Sickles from patients ill with a polio-like disease in the town of Coxsackie, N.Y. This virus resembles poliomyelitis virus in size and in resistance to destruction in sewage. Coxsackie virus also resembles poliovirus in being found in feces as well as in nasopharyngeal washings and nervous tissue and in producing disease clinically resembling poliomyelitis. It also produces pleurodynia, a disease of the heart of infants or fetuses; herpangina (febrile disease of children marked by vesicles and ulcers in the throat); and meningitis. As is true of many viruses, Coxsackie virus has been found to include at least two groups, A and B. These are differentiated mainly by their effects on infant mice. There are also, as in other groups of microorganisms, numerous subgroups or types in the major groups (Fig. 25–1). Group A has 23 subgroups (numbered 1 to 22 and 24; type 23 is now considered to be ECHO virus type 9), and group B consists of six prototype strains. Like polioviruses, the Coxsackie viruses are widespread and cause extensive epidemics, often simultaneously with poliomyelitis epidemics. Simultaneous infections with both Coxsackie and poliovirus are not uncommon.

Vaccines can doubtless be prepared against infection by several, if not all, Coxsackie viruses. Because of the considerable number of different antigenic types, however, protection against all Coxsackie virus diseases is not practicable at present.

ENTERIC VIRUSES IN URINE.   As will be pointed out in Chapter 32, at least one virus (mumps) previously thought to be associated only with the respiratory tract, is now known to appear in the urine of patients. Similarly, Coxsackie virus B has been shown to occur in urine, probably due to viral damage to the kidney. This requires that nursing precautions in infections by Coxsackie virus B (possibly in all intestinal viral infections) include handling as infectious materials not only feces and nasal secretions but also urine. In light of these findings, it is conceivable that any virus that injures the kidney may appear in the urine. This phase of the transmission of viruses requires further investigation.

ECHO VIRUSES

Studies of intestinal viruses have led to the discovery that there are many viruses in the bowel, some of which have been mentioned. Attention was drawn to some of these additional viruses not because they caused disease but because, in tissue cultures, these agents caused death and destruction of the tissue culture cells. After several such agents had been described by several workers, they were collectively designated as "enteric" viruses having cytopathic (cell-damaging) effects (Fig. 6–10), of human origin and "orphan" in relationship, i.e., not associated with any particular disease.[1] To shorten this description they were designated ECHO (Enteric, Cytopathogenic, Human, Orphan) viruses.

About 34 different "types" of these ECHO viruses have been described, but undoubtedly more will be found, and some ECHO viruses will be reclassified into other groups. Some of them have been definitely associated with diseases such as aseptic (nonbacterial) meningitis (types 2–6, 9, 14, 16), and summer diarrhea of infants (type 18 and others). The term *reoviruses* was suggested as a new designation for the ECHO type 10 virus and others antigenically related to it, evidence of the close relationship between the two groups.

These viruses are found chiefly in, and cause diseases of, children and young people. The diseases are often influenza-like, frequently with a blotchy, red rash; they are not highly fatal. They often resemble nonparalytic polio, which in turn often resembles "flu."

Prevention in ECHO virus infections centers around control of feces-borne, possibly urine-borne, infection by methods already described, and also around control of respiratory secretion-borne infection, especially if upper respiratory tract symptoms are present. Thus, ECHO viruses, and presumably numerous intestinal-respiratory viruses, present a double, sometimes triple, problem of control.

VIRAL HEPATITIS

The term hepatitis is drawn from pathology and means inflammation of the liver due to any cause, mechanical, chemical, or biologic. Several viruses are known to cause hepatitis in animals (e.g., in dogs, sheep, cattle, horses, swine, mice, ducks, and canaries), but there is no evidence that any of these is etiologically related to viral hepatitis in man. Viral hepatitis occurs in all parts of the world.

Two kinds of human hepatitis virus are known: infectious hepatitis virus or hepatitis virus A, and the virus of homologous serum jaundice or hepatitis virus B. Since both are infectious, virus A is more accurately referred to as the cause of epidemic viral hepatitis; infection with virus B does not occur in truly epidemic form.

EPIDEMIC HEPATITIS VIRUS (INFECTIOUS HEPATITIS OR VIRAL HEPATITIS). The virus of epidemic or *infectious hepatitis* (IH), or *epidemic jaundice*, called hepatitis virus A, once gaining entrance to a host, usually does not remain unnoticed in the gut, but causes overt disease. It invades the blood and liver and often produces prolonged (weeks or months) inflammation in that organ (hepatitis), with resulting fever, regional pain, gastrointestinal distress, and, less commonly, the jaundice that gives the disease one of its older names—*catarrhal jaundice.* Relapses are frequent. Intestinal carriers may occur, but if so they appear to be much less common than carriers of the enteroviruses and related enteric-respiratory viruses. The virus also circulates in the blood. Persons who carry hepatitis virus in their blood (healthy carriers) appear to be fairly common, and such persons are a real menace if selected for blood donations. Immune gamma globulins are of value in prophylaxis of infectious hepatitis (IH) due to virus A. Like poliovirus, virus A is excreted in feces. In 1970, 56,797 cases of infectious hepatitis were reported in the United States,

[1] They were at one time spoken of as "viruses in search of a disease."

VIRAL HEPATITIS — Case Rate by Four-Week Periods, United States, Epidemiologic Years, 1953-1970

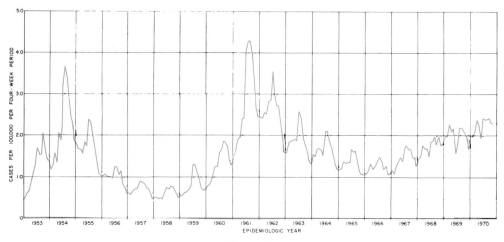

Figure 25–6

Viral hepatitis infections in the United States, epidemiologic years 1953–1970. Note that the disease is on the rise since 1966. Why? (From Morbidity and Mortality, Annual Supplement, 1970. U.S. Dept. of Health, Education and Welfare.)

INFECTIOUS HEPATITIS — Reported Cases Per 100,000 Population, 1970

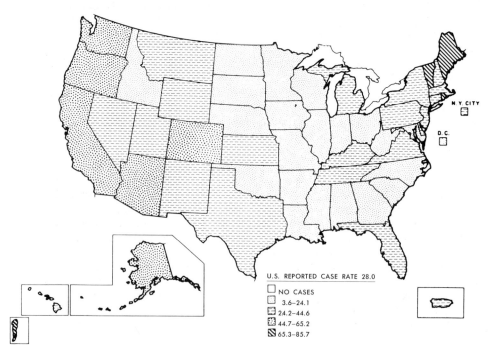

Figure 25–7

Incidence of infectious hepatitis in the United States in 1970. (From Morbidity and Mortality, Annual Supplement, 1970. U.S. Dept. of Health, Education and Welfare.)

with the highest incidence in and around the New England area and California (Figs. 25–6, 25–7).

VIRUS OF HOMOLOGOUS SERUM JAUNDICE (HEPATITIS VIRUS B). We have already described one cause of hepatitis as hepatitis virus A. The second viral agent of hepatitis in man, though closely related to and possibly a variant of virus A, is, nevertheless, antigenically distinct from it and, so far as is known, is not one of the intestinal viruses; therefore, it has not previously been mentioned. It is called the virus of homologous *serum jaundice* (*serum hepatitis*, SH, or *transfusion jaundice*) or hepatitis virus B. The exact relationship between viruses A and B is not known though the two are closely related and similar. Virus B appears to be as yet inseparably associated—in the blood of serum hepatitis patients and carriers —with a very tiny (20–25 nm diameter) particle consisting of two or more proteins. This particle appears not to be an infective agent since it contains no nucleic acid; it may be a separate capsid of the hepatitis B virion. Having been found in association with serum hepatitis in Australia, it is known as the Australia antigen (Au) or hepatitis-associated antigen. For convenience we may briefly discuss hepatitis virus B at this point, even though it is not transmitted in feces or urine.

Virus B appears to occur only in *human* blood or serum, hence, its name of homologous serum hepatitis virus. It differs from virus A mainly in that it does not occur in feces and it does not cause large epidemics. The disease it causes differs in certain clinical details from epidemic hepatitis. Virus B has the distinction of being transmitted (as far as is known) only by artificial means: syringes, needles, dressings, serum, blood, plasma, and so on (see Chapter 38). It is a mystery how, with no natural vector, it has become so widespread in the human race.[2] Like hepatitis virus A, virus B may remain in the blood, apparently for years. Hepatitis due to virus B has a longer incubation period (two to six months) and a mortality rate of 1 to 19 per cent.

VIRAL HEPATITIS.   The term *viral hepatitis* is not directly applicable to IH or to SH, but is an unspecified viral hepatitis. Perhaps this disease is best described as "*post-hepatitis cirrhosis*" of the liver, being a sequel of some other viral diseases (Fig. 25–6). The laboratory diagnosis of viral hepatitis consists chiefly of liver function tests, specifically testing the rise of serum glutamic oxalacetic transaminase (SGOT) levels.

Prevention

With respect to virus A, as mentioned above, precautions applicable to all enteric infections are required. Virus B is not feces-borne.

With respect to both viruses, precautions concerning transmission by blood and certain blood derivatives, syringes, needles, bandages, instruments, and so on, are indicated.

Detection of Au (and presumably of the virus) in the blood is now possible by means of very sensitive serologic methods. This is of enormous importance in prevention of serum hepatitis due to transfusion of Au in the blood of prospective donors.

One additional point must be stressed and borne in mind because it

---

[2]Some imaginative persons have suggested that the common use of bloody swords, daggers, bayonets, and the general quarrelsomeness and bloodthirstiness of our ancient (and not so ancient) ancestors widely disseminated the virus. But how did it originate in the first place?

affects all routines of disinfection and sterilization. Hepatitis viruses are exceptionally resistant to heat. They can resist boiling for ten minutes, probably longer. They are also somewhat resistant to chemical disinfectants.

All health workers will have to keep these viruses constantly in mind when dealing with any materials likely to be contaminated with human blood or blood derivatives. Syringes, needles, instruments, and bloody dressings may transmit the virus via tiny scratches in the hands or because of inadequate sterilization; this is avoided by using disposable syringes and needles. Thermometers, especially rectal thermometers, of patients with infectious hepatitis A are isolated with the patient and discarded after the patient is discharged. Each patient should have his own bedpan. This is true in any infectious disease borne by feces or urine. Disposable plastic thermometers are now available in most modern hospitals.

Supplementary Readings

Burnet, F. M.: Natural History of Infectious Disease. 3rd Ed. 1962, New York, Cambridge University Press.

Carver, D. H., and Seto, D. S. Y.: Production of hemadsorption-negative areas by serums containing Australia antigen. *Science*, 1971, *172*:1265.

Gerin, J. L., Holland, P. V., and Purcell, R. H.: Australia antigen: large-scale purification from human serum and biochemical studies of its proteins. *J. Virol.*, 1971, 7:569.

Goodheart, C. R.: An Introduction to Virology. 1969, Philadelphia, W. B. Saunders Co.

Horsfall, F. L., Jr., and Tamm, I. (Editors): Viral and rickettsial infections of man. 4th Ed. 1965, Philadelphia, J. B. Lippincott & Co.

Luria, S. E., and Darnell, J. E.: General Virology. 2nd Ed. 1967, New York, John Wiley & Sons, Inc.

Lwoff, A., and Tournier, P.: The classification of viruses. *Ann. Rev. Microbiol.*, 1966, *20*:45.

Melnick, J. L., and Wenner, H. A.: Enteroviruses. In: Diagnostic Procedures for Viral and Rickettsial Infections. 4th Ed. 1969, New York, American Public Health Association.

National Communicable Disease Center: Morbidity and Mortality. 1967, Vol. 16, No. 26, U.S. Department of Health, Education and Welfare, Public Health Service.

Pollard, M. (Editor): Perspectives in Virology. 1967, Vol. 5, New York, Academic Press, Inc.

Stanley, W. M., and Valens, E. G.., et al.: Viruses and the Nature of Life. 1961, New York, E. P. Dutton & Co., Inc.

WHO Expert Committee on Hepatitis: Second report. 1964, Geneva, WHO Technical Report Series No. 285.

WHO Scientific Group: Human viral and rickettsial vaccines. 1966, Geneva, *WHO* Technical report series. No. 325.

Intestinal Protozoa and Helminths

26

PROTOZOA

Numerous species of Protozoa inhabit the intestinal tract. Some are ciliates, some are flagellates, others are amebas. Most of these animals are harmless and may be observed by microscopic examination of normal feces or during examination of feces for pathogenic species. Common harmless species of enteric (intestinal) amebas are *Entamoeba coli, Endolimax nana, Iodamoeba bütschlii* and *Dientamoeba fragilis* (Fig. 26–1).

Entamebas, like all typical animal cells, have no rigid cell walls and, in the active, multiplying or trophozoite stage, have no particular or invariable form. Entamebas in the trophozoite stage are continually changing their shapes from round or oval to very irregular forms with protrusions and finger-like processes sticking out from various portions (Fig. 3–2). Their fluid cytoplasm, being constantly in motion (*cytoplasmic streaming*), they can move by "flowing" into any one (or several at once) of these finger-like processes, which are called *pseudopodia*. This kind of motion is called *ameboid movement*. It is seen also in the blood cells called phagocytes. By means of pseudopodia, both phagocytes and amebas can engulf solid particles of food, a type of nourishment called *phagotrophic nutrition* (Chapters 3, 18).

ENTAMOEBA HISTOLYTICA AND AMEBIASIS

Infection by any species of ameba is properly spoken of as *amebiasis*.[1] The most harmful of the species pathogenic in man bears the name *Entamoeba histolytica* (*ent*, inside; *histo*, tissue; *lytic*, dissolving). The organisms, are usually ingested as dormant *cysts* in feces or sewage-polluted food or water. They soon undergo *excystation*, and grow into fragile, actively multi-

---

[1]The term amebiasis includes amebic dysentery and also other disease processes due to invasion of the liver and other organs by the amebas.

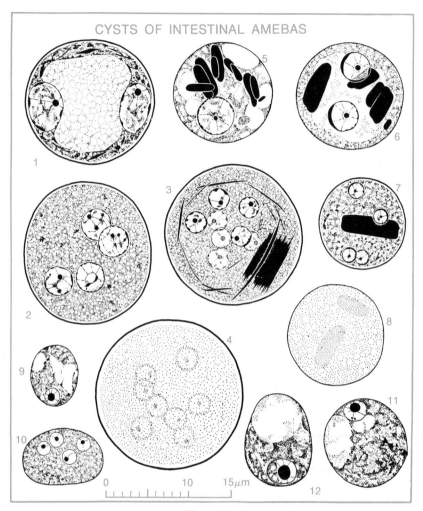

Figure 26–1

(1) Stained* binucleate cyst of *Entamoeba coli.* (2) Stained quadrinucleate cyst of *E. coli.*** (3) Stained mature cyst of *E. coli.* (4) Unstained mature cyst of *E. coli.* (5) Stained uninucleate cyst of *E. histolytica.* (6) Stained binucleate cyst of *E. histolytica.* (7) Stained mature cyst of *E. histolytica.* (8) Unstained cyst of *E. histolytica* showing chromatoid bars. (9) Stained uninucleate cyst of *Endolimax nana.* (10) Stained mature cyst of *E. nana.* (11) and (12) Stained mature cysts of *Iodamoeba bütschlii.* (From Hunter, Frye, and Swartzwelder: A Manual of Tropical Medicine, 4th Ed. 1966, Philadelphia, W. B. Saunders Co.)

*All cysts were stained with iron hematoxylin.

**The student should not confuse *E. coli (Entamoeba coli)* here with *E. coli (Escherichia coli),* the bacterial species.

plying *trophozoites,* which primarily attack the lining (mucosa) of the intestine, usually the large bowel. These entamebas, by means of tissue-destroying enzymes, burrow into, and in places undermine, the intestinal lining and cause ulcers (amebic dysentery).[2] There is little inflammatory reaction unless, as is common, secondary bacterial infection develops.

[2]The student must distinguish between amebic dysentery and dysentery due to other causes, such as *Shigella.*

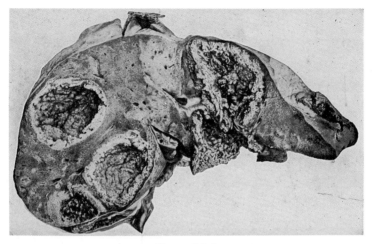

Figure 26–2

Multiple amebic abscesses of liver. (Mense's *Handbuch der Tropenkrankheiten.*)

Entamoeba histolytica in the trophozoite form often burrows through the intestinal lining and deep into the intestinal wall. Occasionally, rupture of the intestine occurs as a result. The patient may then die of peritonitis caused by escape of the bacteria of the feces into the abdominal cavity.

The amebas may also invade the intestinal lymph and blood vessels and then are carried to the liver, lungs, brain, and other organs, where they can become localized and cause the formation of large amebic abscesses (Fig. 26–2).

Like many other infectious diseases, amebiasis is often chronic and may be present with little definite symptomatology for a long time. Carriers of *E. histolytica* are common in some areas of low-grade sanitation. Thus amebic infection is often unknowingly widely disseminated by persons with mild cases or by carriers.

Amebiasis is common in all warm regions and is frequently found in temperate zones around the world.

Entamoeba histolytica is eliminated only in the feces and may appear in one or both of two forms.

CYSTS. The amebas have the property of forming rounded, dormant, thick-walled, drought-resistant cysts (Fig. 26–1), that remain alive and dormant for hours or days in feces or in moist, polluted soil or water. They are slowly killed by drying and exposure to sunlight. They are susceptible to heat and vigorous disinfection. Unless active diarrhea is in progress, which quickly flushes the trophozoites from the bowel before encystment can occur, it is the cyst form that is found in stools. These cysts are transmitted from person to person by the well known (and nauseatingly common!) fecal-oral route of transmission of all types of intestinal infection.

TROPHOZOITES. The actively multiplying, fragile, trophozoite form is excreted only in the watery stools of acute amebic dysentery, is not resistant outside the intestine, and quickly dies when cooled or dried. Trophozoites of *E. histolytica* frequently ingest red blood cells; those of other species rarely or never do. These facts are of diagnostic value.

Transmission of Amebiasis

Anything recently contaminated with infected human feces from a "cyst-passer" (chronic case or carrier) may transmit the cysts. Transmission on fruits and vegetables is said to be a common occurrence in the Orient and other places where human sewage and feces ("night soil") are used

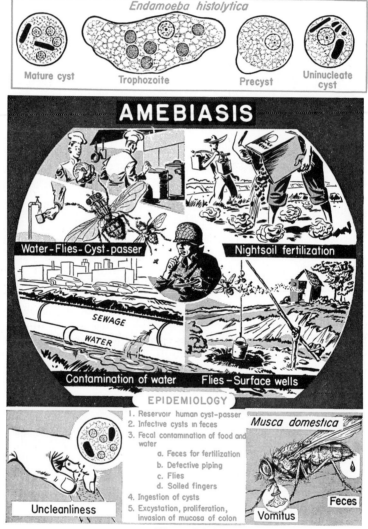

Figure 26–3

Epidemiology of amebiasis and numerous other enteric infections. At the top are shown forms of *Entamoeba histolytica*. At lower right and left are seen two of the main methods of transmission: fingers soiled with excreta, and flies from infected feces. These are avenues of transmission of many intestinal infections. In the central panel are shown means by which various vectors of intestinal diseases (including amebiasis) operate: Carriers or cyst-passers who handle foods contaminate foods and utensils; in the Orient human excreta ("nightsoil") is used to fertilize vegetables eaten raw; water mains become contaminated by leaky sewerage; flies spread feces everywhere. (Hunter, Frye, and Swartzwelder: A Manual of Tropical Medicine, 4th Ed. 1966, Philadelphia, W. B. Saunders Co.)

for fertilizer. Fresh vegetables, lettuce and celery, for instance, may then very readily have live ameba cysts upon them when eaten. Although opinions differ concerning the transmission of amebiasis by fruits and vegetables, it is wisest not to eat uncooked foods in the Orient or tropics (Fig. 26–3). Some serious outbreaks of amebic dysentery in the United States have been caused by sewage-polluted water supplies.

Although amebiasis is more prevalent in areas where unsanitary disposal (or *no* disposal!) of feces is the rule, carriers of *Entamoeba histolytica* exist in all populations and are, of course, dangerous sources of infection. In many areas of the world this infection is present in up to 50 per cent of the people, but even in well sanitized cities 1 to 5 per cent may carry the organism. In the United States, Craig found 11 per cent of 59,336 persons examined to be carriers of *Entamoeba histolytica.* In some groups, as among certain North American Indians, the number of carriers may rise to as much as 25 per cent. Feces-soiled hands and flies appear to be the major vectors. Carriers who handle food may transmit cysts to the food via their soiled hands.

In regions and in countries where modern sanitation in regard to disposal of sewage and feces is effective, little amebic dysentery exists. Unlike *Salmonella* and *Shigella,* the amebas do not multiply in food. It is difficult to cultivate them except on specially prepared media. They usually require bacteria as food.

DIAGNOSIS OF AMEBIC DYSENTERY.   Diagnosis by clinical means is often difficult. The disease may be diagnosed in the laboratory by microscopic examination of the patient's stools. The diagnostically distinctive cysts, and occasionally vegetative forms, may then be found. The cysts are about 12 μm in diameter. When mature, they contain four distinct spherical nuclei in a finely granular cytoplasm. They are readily recognized by those trained to observe them. Complement fixation tests are also valuable in diagnosis. Bars of deeply staining material (chromatoid bars) similarly are diagnostically distinctive in their size and arrangement.

Entamoeba coli.   In making diagnoses by microscopic examination of stool specimens, one must carefully distinguish between *Entamoeba coli*, a harmless species, and the pathogenic *Entamoeba histolytica*. This is usually not difficult, but requires experience, as is seen in Figure 26–1. An important improvement in diagnostic procedure is the use of polyvinyl alcohol fixative and preservative for mounting the protozoa on the microscope slide. In basic principle it is like mounting them in transparent plastic, much as flowers and similar items for ornaments and costume jewelry are mounted. Cysts of *E. coli* differ from those of *E. histolytica* in being about 18 μm in diameter and in containing eight (sometimes 16 or 32) nuclei, larger than those of *E. histolytica.*

Prevention

Although isolation of the patient who has amebic dysentery is not usually required, the potential infectivity of his feces should be recognized. Feces should be disinfected with chlorinated lime (5 per cent) or saponated solution of cresol (5 per cent) for a minimum of one hour unless other, more satisfactory methods of disposal are available. Flies and other insects should be eliminated from the patient's unit so that they may not carry feces from the patient to food. As in the care of all patients who have enteric infections, all attendants should wash their hands carefully so that they do not inadvertently become carriers. The patient should also wash his hands after defecation. It is to be remembered that after the acute diarrheal condition is over, during which it is mainly the fragile trophozoites that are passed, the formed stools often continue to be even more dangerous because of the presence of the durable cysts.

Disinfectant dips for fruits and vegetables have no proved value.

OTHER INTESTINAL PROTOZOA

The student who is interested in more detailed study of other Protozoa which have adopted the human intestinal tract as a place of residence will find the subject a fascinating and profitable one. Because the modes of transmission (fecal-oral) and controlling problems are alike for all, and because of limitations of space and time, we here merely name and briefly describe only two of the common species. Like the entamebas, most of the intestinal flagellates and ciliates occur in both trophozoite and cyst form; the forms of the latter are diagnostically distinctive.

GIARDIA LAMBLIA. In the trophozoite stage, these protozoans (which belong to the group of Mastigophora or flagellates) are fantastic in appearance (Fig. 26–4). They are found in stools of many normal persons in the cyst form. Trophozoites are flushed out only by rapidly moving diarrheic stools. They may at times cause irritations of the gallbladder and upper intestinal tract. Infection with *Giardia* is spoken of as giardiasis. Although annoying, they are not generally regarded as very dangerous pathogens.

TRICHOMONAS HOMINIS. The trophozoites of all common species of *Trichomonas* are egg- or pear-shaped, with three to five free flagella at the rounded anterior end and another forming the edge of an attached, undulating membrane that extends the length of the animal. All have a conspicuous nucleus and a pointed, spike-tipped posterior (Fig. 26–5). *T. hominis* is probably nonpathogenic, but may at times cause mild intestinal irritations. The infection is called trichomoniasis. *T. hominis* does not form cysts as does *E. histolytica* or *G. lamblia*. The other species shown in Figure 26–5 occur elsewhere in the body and are discussed separately.

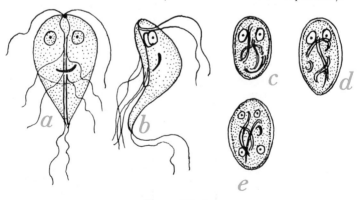

Figure 26–4

Giardia lamblia: a, trophozoite, ventral view; *b,* profile view; *c, d,* immature cysts; *e,* mature cyst (×1600). (Original Faust.) (Faust, Beaver, and Jung: Animal Agents and Vectors of Human Disease, 3rd Ed., 1968, Philadelphia, Lea & Febiger.)

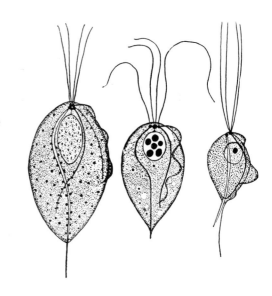

Figure 26–5

Three species of *Trichomonas* found in humans: (left to right) *T. vaginalis*, *T. buccalis* (or *T. tenax?*), and *T. hominis*. The size differences shown are not very constant. *T. buccalis* is not known to be pathogenic, but its continuous presence in the mouth in considerable numbers indicates bad oral hygiene (×2000). *T. hominis* occurs in the intestine where it may cause secondary irritation; *T. vaginalis* causes irritating infections of the genitourinary tract, especially of women (Chapter 35). (Powell.)

HELMINTHS (WORMS)

The term helminth means worm, but it is now generally restricted to pathogenic worms. Many helminths are parasitic in valuable agricultural plants, others in wild and domestic animals and man. The most common intestinal helminths of man are included in two large groups: the phylum Nematoda or roundworms (for example, hookworms), and the phylum Platyhelminthes, containing flatworms in two classes important to man: Trematoda (flukes), and Cestoda or cestodes (tapeworms). Each of these groups contains parasites of blood and tissue of man (Chapter 40).

Figure 26–6

Some common nematode eggs: *A*, Whipworm, *Trichuris trichiura*; *B*, pinworm, *Enterobius vermicularis*; *C*, large roundworm, *Ascaris lumbricoides*, fertilized egg; *D*, hookworm egg. Some cestode eggs: *E*, Human tapeworm, *Taenia sp.* (×750); *F*, dwarf tapeworm, *Hymenolepsis nana* (×750). (Modified from Mackie, Hunter, and Worth: A Manual of Tropical Medicine, 2nd Ed. 1954, W. B. Saunders Co. Philadelphia, Pa.) *A, B, C, D*, courtesy of Dr. R. L. Roudabush, Ward's Natural Science Establishment, Rochester, N.Y. Photos by T. Romaniak. *E* and *F*, courtesy of Photographic Laboratory, AMSGS. Photos by Milt Cheskis.)

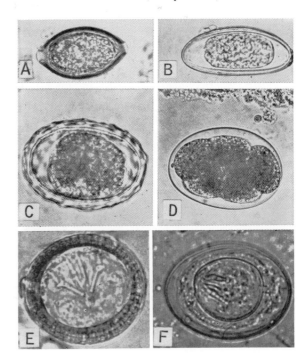

Because adult helminths are far from microscopic and because of limitations of space, they will not be discussed in detail here. As compared with unicellular microorganisms, they have very complex organic structures and life cycles. Some spend a part of their developmental period in the soil, in the sea, in various other hosts such as fish, hogs, rats, snails, and the tissues of man. The student will find the study of such animal parasites both fascinating and profitable. Excellent textbooks are available. Still, do not think that everything is known about these organisms. For example, a new disease (not recognized previously with respect to its etiology) named "intestinal capillariasis" caused by *Capillaria philippinensis*, a roundworm, was first described in 1968. The tremendous protein loss due to this disease of the small bowel leads to death in untreated cases. Yet little is known about its incubation period, transmission, natural reservoir, communicability, susceptibility or resistance.

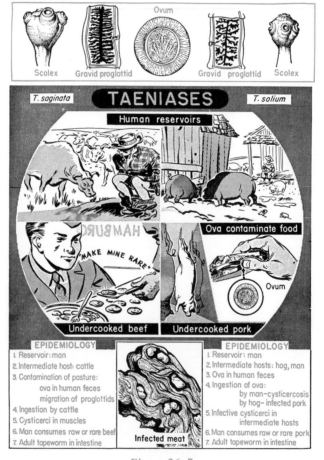

Figure 26–7

Epidemiology of the taeniases (tapeworm infections). *Taenia saginata* is the beef tapeworm; *T. solium*, the pork tapeworm. (Hunter, Frye, and Swartzwelder: A Manual of Tropical Medicine, 4th Ed. 1966, Philadelphia, W. B. Saunders Co.) A scolex is the head of the mature worm, by means of which it fastens itself to the intestinal mucosa; a proglottid is a sexually mature segment of the long "tape" of the worm as passed in the feces. It contains fertile eggs (Fig. 26–6).

COMMON NAME	PRINCIPAL ENDEMIC AREAS	SCIENTIFIC NAME	STAGE USUALLY PRESENT IN FECES	REQUIRES FURTHER DEVELOPMENT IN	PRINCIPAL SOURCE OF INFECTION OF MAN	USUAL PORTAL OF ENTRY TO MAN	IMPORTANT MEANS OF CONTROL	USUAL MEANS OF DIAGNOSIS IN LABORATORY
NEMATODES								
Hookworm	moist tropics and warm temperate zones	*Necator americanus; Ancylostoma duodenale*	immature eggs / immature eggs	warm, moist soil / warm, moist soil	feces-contaminated soil	via skin in contact with soil	avoid skin contact with soil; sanitary disposal of feces; chemotherapy	microscopic examination of stool for eggs
Pinworm (seat worm)	world-wide, especially temperate zones	*Enterobius vermicularis*	adults which lay eggs on skin	none; anus-to-mouth transmission	eggs in perianal area; dust, etc.	mouth	frequent bathing; sanitary disposal of feces; chemotherapy	find eggs on perianal skin
Whipworm	world-wide, except cold and arid areas	*Trichuris trichiura*	immature eggs	warm, moist soil	infected soil, food water	mouth	sanitary disposal of feces; avoid feces-contaminated soil	demonstration of eggs in stool
Giant roundworm	moist warm and temperate zones	*Ascaris lumbricoides*	active, immature larvae	warm, moist soil	as above	mouth	as above	as above
Filaria worms	moist tropics and subtropics	*Loa loa, Onchocerca, Wuchereria bancrofti*	none, transmitted by insects	—	mosquitoes, etc.	mosquito bite	mosquito control; chemotherapy	demonstration of microfilariae in blood
Trichina worm	pork-eating peoples	*Trichinella spiralis*	none; occurs in tissues	hogs, rats	undercooked pork	mouth	adequate cooking of pork; sanitary garbage disposal	microscopic examination of excised muscle
CESTODES								
Dwarf tapeworm	children, world-wide warm areas	*Hymenolepis nana*	mature eggs	none; anus-to-mouth transmission	eggs from feces-soiled clothing, etc.	mouth	cleanliness of perianal region and underwear; chemotherapy	find eggs in feces
Beef tapeworm	beef-eating peoples	*Taenia saginata*	mature eggs in segment of worm	muscles of cattle	undercooked or raw beef	mouth	prevent sewage pollution of pastures; avoid rare beef; chemotherapy	find segments (occasionally eggs) in feces
Pork tapeworm	peoples eating poorly cooked pork	*Taenia solium*	as above	muscles of hogs	undercooked pork	mouth	hogs acquire cysts from sewage, infected meat in garbage, and rats which eat garbage; sanitize hog-raising; avoid undercooked pork	as above
Fish tapeworm	peoples eating raw or poorly cooked fish	*Diphyllobothrium latum*	mature eggs	cool, fresh water; water flea	undercooked or raw fish	mouth	prevent sewage and fecal pollution of fresh waters; avoid undercooked fish	find eggs in feces
Dog tapeworm	areas where man-dog contact is close	*Echinococcus granulosus,* etc.	eggs in dog feces	muscles and tissues of man	eggs in feces of dogs and other canines	mouth	avoid feces of dogs, especially in areas where they are numerous, as arctic, etc.	immunological tests
TREMATODES								
Blood fluke	tropics	*Schistosoma mansoni*	mature eggs (in feces)	fresh water; in snails	sewage-polluted waters where snails abound	skin in contact with polluted water	sanitary sewage disposal; kill snails; do not go into polluted streams, pools, etc.	find eggs in feces
Blood fluke	mainly Africa	*Schistosoma haematobium*	mature eggs (in urine)	as above	as above	as above	as above	find eggs in urine

The fact of chief importance at this point is that the microscopic eggs (Fig. 26–6), or other developmental stages of most of these worms, are eliminated in the feces (or urine). Diagnosis is commonly made by finding the eggs, or parts of worms (e.g., segments of tapeworms), in stools of patients. The portal of entry for most of the intestinal worms is via the mouth or through the skin. For example, beef-tapeworm larvae are ingested in underdone beef, pork-tapeworm larvae in underdone pork (Fig. 26–7); hookworm larvae develop from eggs in feces that have been deposited on moist, warm soil and penetrate the skin of the feet of barefoot persons. For convenience, data pertinent to prevention and control of the more important, more common, or representative types of these worms are given in Table 26–1.

FIVE GENERAL PREVENTIVE RULES

Five general rules may be applied to avoid most of these infections (and many other enteric infections as well); (1) do not come into direct contact (e.g., with bare feet) with feces-contaminated soil, especially in warm, moist areas; (2) do not eat (in *any* area) "rare" or uncooked meats, fish, or shellfish; (3) avoid contact with feces-soiled clothing or persons; (4) avoid eating, drinking, or contact with raw food, vegetables, or water contaminated with feces, urine, or sewage of human or animal origin; and (5) avoid arthropod bites in all areas, especially in warm climates.

Supplementary Reading

Beaver, P. C.: Control of Soil-Transmitted Helminths. WHO Public Health Papers, No. 10, Geneva, World Health Organization.

Faust, E. C., Beaver, P. C., and Jung, R. C.: Animal Agents and Vectors of Human Disease. 3rd Ed. 1968, Philadelphia, Lea & Febiger.

Hunter, G. W., Frye, W. W., and Swartzwelder, J. C.: A Manual of Tropical Medicine. 4th Ed. 1966, Philadelphia, W. B. Saunders Co.

Marcial-Rojas, P. A.: Pathoglogy of Protozoal and Helminthic Diseases. 1970, Baltimore, The Williams and Wilkins Co.

Most, H. (Editor): Health Hints for the Tropics. 6th Ed. Suppl. to *Trop. Med & Hyg. News* (C. L. Gibson, Editor). 1967, Bethesda, Md., National Institutes of Health.

Schliessmann, D. J., Atchley, F. O., Wilcomb, Jr., M. J., and Welch, S. F.: Relation of environmental factors to the occurrence of enteric diseases in areas of Eastern Kentucky. 1958, Washington, D.C., Superintendent of Documents, Government Printing Office, U.S. Public Health Service, Publication No. 591.

WHO Expert Committee on Helminthiases: Soil-transmitted helminths. 1964, Geneva, World Health Organization Technical Report Series No. 277.

Foods as Vectors of Infection and Poisoning; Sanitation in Food Handling

In this chapter we outline the role of foods as vectors of various pathogens and of certain microbial poisons (toxins), differentiating clearly between the terms "food infection" and "food poisoning," i.e., between infection by foods and microbial[1] poisoning by foods. For convenience of the reader the most commonly found food-borne pathogens are outlined in Table 27-1.

---

[1]Many foods (e.g., certain fish, fungi, and so on) are poisonous per se; others may become poisoned accidentally, e.g., mistaking insect poison for flour.

Table 27-1. Most Commonly Found Food-Borne Pathogens

ENTEROVIRUSES and epidemic hepatitis virus (Chapter 25).

FAMILY ENTEROBACTERIACEAE (Chapter 23) — Gram-negative, nonspore-forming, intestinal rods; easily killed by heat and disinfectants.
  ✓ Genus *Salmonella:* Typhoid, paratyphoid, and "food-poisoning" bacilli.
  ✗ Genus *Shigella:* Dysentery bacilli; much like typhoid bacilli.

FAMILY BACILLACEAE (Chapter 36)
  Genus *Clostridium:* Gram-positive, spore-forming, soil-derived rods; resistant to heat and disinfectants. *Cl. botulinum* causes botulism, a dangerous form of food poisoning; *Cl. perfringens causes* acute but transitory gastroenteritis.

FAMILY MICROCOCCACEAE (Chapter 28)
  Genus *Staphylococcus:* Causes one form of food poisoning (enterotoxin).
  Genus *Streptococcus:* Beta type sometimes contaminates milk and other foods.

✓**FAMILY BRUCELLACEAE** (Chapter 24)
  Genus *Brucella:* Gram-negative, nonspore-forming, animal-derived rods easily killed by heat and disinfectants; cause undulant fever or brucellosis in man.

FAMILY MYCOBACTERIACEAE (Chapter 31)
  Genus *Mycobacterium:* Bovine and human tuberculosis via meat and milk.

PROTOZOA, like *Entamoeba histolytica* (Chapter 26).

HELMINTHS, like tapeworms (Chapter 26).

A few of the food-borne microorganisms briefly mentioned in this chapter are discussed in greater detail in other chapters: *Coxiella burnetii* (Chapter 39), *Pasteurella tularensis* (Chapter 38), *Corynebacterium diphtheriae* (Chapter 29), *Entamoeba histolytica* (Chapter 26), and some viruses. Note that of all the organisms listed in Table 27–1, the only distinctively in-testinal ones are the family Enterobacteriaceae, *Entamoeba histolytica*, and some worms and viruses. Others may cause infection or poisoning by foods and may be transmitted in foods, but are not usually, if ever, derived from the intestinal tract in this relationship.

FOOD INFECTION AND FOOD POISONING

Most foods contain living bacteria unless they have just been exposed to radiation or thoroughly heated. Many foods, especially those that are not very acid, salty or syrupy, serve as good culture media for bacteria. Usually bacteria in properly handled and prepared foods are harmless. Many kinds of bacteria can grow rapidly in food if it is not properly refrigerated or cooked. If pathogenic bacteria are present, this may result in (1) *food infection* or (2) *food poisoning*, or both. These two terms mean very different things but are often erroneously used interchangeably. What is actually meant by food infection is *infection* of persons by (active or living) pathogens in food. By food poisoning we mean *poisoning* of persons by toxins already produced in the food by bacterial growth. In true food *poisoning*, infection rarely occurs. Food infection must be dis-tinguished from food poisoning since both the causes and the methods of avoiding these troubles differ completely.

Food Infection

The principal sources of infectious microorganisms in food are in-fected animals and infected persons who handle or inspect foods.

CONTAMINATION BY ANIMALS. Animals may contaminate food in at least two ways. They may pollute it with their excreta (as do flies, roaches, rats, and mice), or flesh used as food may come from infected animals. For example, the meat of tuberculous cattle and dairy products from them may be highly infectious. Flesh and milk of cattle, swine, or other animals with brucellosis often cause human brucellosis if the meat or milk is not intelligently handled. Hunters and market workers often contract "rabbit fever" (*tularemia*, Chapter 38) from infected wild rabbits they handle. Pork, poultry, and eggs are notoriously often infected with *Salmonella* and cause epidemics of salmonellosis.

Salmonella typhi (cause of typhoid fever) is often found in oysters and other seafood if they are taken from sewage-polluted fishing grounds, a practice prohibited by health authorities. Epidemic viral hepatitis is now known to be transmitted in the same way. Another species of *Salmonella, S. typhimurium*, a cause of one form of paratyphoid fever or salmonel-losis or food-borne infection, is a common (though not the only) *Salmonella* parasite of mice and rats. Excreta of these animals can sometimes get into or on food. Rats also transmit in their urine a dangerous disease, lepto-spirosis (or hemorrhagic jaundice), due to spirochetes of the genus *Lepto-spira* (Chapter 24). No vermin should be tolerated around food or elsewhere. Trichina worms (*Trichinella spiralis*) are almost always present in pork, and tapeworms are not uncommon in beef. Raw fish may transmit tapeworms. These foods may all be made safe by *thorough* cooking.

CONTAMINATION OF FOODS BY PERSONS. In addition to the pathogens just mentioned, which are derived from infected animals, directly or indirectly, personnel may contaminate food. The organisms of common colds, influenza, scarlet fever, diphtheria, and tuberculosis are often present in saliva droplets and on the hands of food handlers who are carriers of these pathogens. Toxin-producing staphylococci (see page 387) often are found in respiratory secretions and in pimples and boils on the hands and forearms of food handlers, and thus may gain entrance to food. Shoppers in stores or cafeterias where unwrapped foods are displayed in open cases obviously transmit microorganisms to foods by sneezing, talking, and coughing over them and by handling them with soiled hands. The thumb in the plate, that is handed over to the customer, is the rule and not the exception in some cafeterias.

Intestinal pathogens such as the virus of epidemic hepatitis, *Salmonella, Shigella,* and cysts of *Entamoeba histolytica* may be on the hands of untidy kitchen workers and other food handlers who are carriers.

OTHER FOOD MICROORGANISMS. Also added to the list of food pathogens, or opportunistic pathogens, are certain saprophytic bacteria such as *Proteus* species, *Clostridium perfringens* (Chapter 36) and *Pseudomonas aeruginosa,* certain intestinal cocci (e.g., *Streptococcus faecalis*), and some others that can grow in food and decompose it. Some of the products of decomposition of food by these bacteria may be irritating to the intestine. There is little reason to suppose that ordinarily these organisms or their products cause any but the mildest irritations of the gastrointestinal tract, if any at all. Certain strains of *Escherichia coli,* however, definitely produce enteritis, especially in infants, and can grow in many foods, including unhygienically prepared babies' formulas.

Because spoiled food is esthetically objectionable and unpalatable and may cause gastroenteritis, sour, spoiled, or decomposed food should never be eaten, especially by infants, children, or ill patients. The mere fact that large numbers of bacteria are present in food does not in itself imply that the food is harmful. It is the kind of bacteria that determines the harmfulness of the food. Various foods are prepared by the growth in them of certain bacteria: sauerkraut, buttermilk and cheese are examples.

"PTOMAINE POISONING." Ptomaines are products of protein decomposition that is so extensive that the food is partly liquefied and offensive to sight, taste and olfactory sense. Such putrefied matter is never accepted as food. No human being and especially no dog would eat odoriferous, sulfur-containing ptomaines. The condition that used to be called "ptomaine poisoning" is now known to be, in the vast majority of cases, either infection by *Salmonella* species or poisoning due to enterotoxigenic staphylococci or some strains of *Clostridium perfringens.* The symptom complex of botulism does not ordinarily simulate the acute gastroenteritis popularly associated with "ptomaine poisoning." Ptomaine poisoning, as once commonly thought of, *does not exist.*

Food Poisoning

Food *poisoning* by bacteria results from the growth in the food, not in the patient, of one of at least two organisms: *Clostridium botulinum,* cause of botulism, and *Staphylococcus aureus,* cause of staphylococcal intoxication. Some strains of *Clostridium perfringens* also appear to cause acute but transitory gastroenteritis possibly due to toxin formed by the bacteria in the food.

CLOSTRIDIUM BOTULINUM.   The botulism organism resembles all other clostridia, e.g., *Cl. tetani* and *Cl. perfringens,* in having complex organic nutritional requirements, in being a gram-positive, motile, saprophytic, spore-bearing anaerobic rod, and in being found in the soil. Formation of its large endospore gives it a snowshoe-like form, the basis of the name of the genus (Greek *kloster,* spindle). Like *Cl. tetani,* it cannot invade healthy tissues.[2] How then, does it produce disease?

Clostridium botulinum, an obligate anaerobe, can grow well in such anaerobic places as the center of large sausages (*botulus* is the Latin for sausage) and in canned foods that are not too acid, such as canned spinach, asparagus, beans, meat, or corn. Spores of the organism are enclosed in the cans with soil on improperly washed vegetables or other food. If the spores are not killed by the "processing" or autoclaving at the canning factory or in the home, they may germinate and multiply vigorously inside the container. Some of these spores are among the most heat-resistant organisms known. A related and very similar species is called *Cl. parabotulinum.*

When growing, *Cl. botulinum* and *Cl. parabotulinum* give off extremely potent toxins. Botulinal toxins, when swallowed, frequently prove fatal. The appearance, taste, or odor of the poisoned food may or may not be bad. Food often appears to be normal and gives little or no hint of the presence of toxins that cause the forms of food poisoning called botulism.

BOTULISM.   This disease is due to the effect of botulinal toxin on nerves that activate muscles. Unlike tetanus toxin, which irritates motor nerve cells, producing tetanic convulsions, botulinal toxin blocks nerve terminals (myoneural junctions) so that paralysis occurs. This paralysis progresses downward from eye, to face, throat, speech, swallowing, arms, and so on. Prognosis depends largely on the amount of the toxin swallowed. When the thoracic muscles become fully involved, respiration is impossible and, in the absence of artificial respiration, death supervenes.

Prevention of Botulism.   Protection against botulism is easy because the toxin (not the spores!) is destroyed by ten minutes of boiling. For absolute safety, all home canned foods should be held at boiling, *after* opening the can, for at least ten minutes before eating. Botulism from commercially canned foods is uncommon in the United States. However, every once in a while some isolated case causes public recognition that this danger is still with us. Through the information media we are told what cans are to be withdrawn from sale as being unsafe. The canners themselves take excellent precautions against botulism by clean preparation and thorough autoclaving of all canned goods. Any cans that show even slightly bulging ends (due to gas from bacterial fermentation within) should be discarded, as well as any cans showing other evidences of fermentation, or acid or gas formation or leaks. Never eat, or even taste, sour, spoiled, or discolored food from cans or jars. Unless the food is first thoroughly cooked, it is inadvisable to throw such food to dogs, hogs, or chickens, since they also may die of botulism.

BOTULISM ANTITOXIN.   There is an efficient antitoxic serum, which may be used for the prevention of botulism. Unfortunately, diagnosis of botulism is often delayed. As in tetanus, after definite symptoms have

---

[2] A few cases of botulism resulting from growth of *Cl. botulinum* in soil-contaminated wounds have been reported.

appeared, the patient's chances of recovery are not very good, even with large doses of serum. There are several serologic types of botulinal toxin: A, B, and E are most common, F and C type outbreaks less so. For therapeutic and preventive purposes polyvalent serum, effective against several types, is generally used. In the United States, human botulism is most often due to types A and B, rarely to type E (found principally in improperly processed fish, e.g., as just noted). In 1970, 12 cases of diagnosed botulism were reported in the United States.

In managing cases of botulism, no isolation precautions are indicated and no special attention to infectious disease technique is needed as no infection exists.

STAPHYLOCOCCAL FOOD POISONING.   Another important and common cause of food poisoning is the toxigenic *Staphylococcus*. It has been found that staphylococci grow in many foods, especially precooked hams, milk, custards, cream fillings, salads, and the like. Some strains or species of these staphylococci produce a powerful exotoxin (*enterotoxin*, Chapter 28) when they grow in food. When the food is eaten, food poisoning results, with severe but transitory gastroenteritis, nausea, vomiting, diarrhea, and marked weakness or prostration. Severity depends on the amount of toxin swallowed. No infection occurs. These symptoms come on usually within two to 12 hours after eating the toxin. This permits differentiation from salmonellosis, which produces very similar symptoms, but only after a necessary incubation period, usually of 12 to 24 hours. Staphylococcal food poisoning is rarely or never fatal per se.

The enterotoxigenic species of staphylococci (restricted mainly to phage Groups III and IV) are usually, but not always, of the *aureus* type. They ferment lactose and mannitol, digest gelatin, and in addition to enterotoxin, produce an enzyme called *coagulase*, which causes citrated blood plasma to coagulate. In contrast with the heat-labile botulinal toxin, staphylococcal enterotoxin can resist 100 C for at least 30 minutes and probably longer. Once formed in food, cooking does not necessarily destroy it, though the staphylococci that produced it may easily be killed by heat.

CLOSTRIDIUM PERFRINGENS.   This gram-positive rod resembles *Cl. botulinum* in being distributed in soil, forming heat-resistant spores, and growing well in many foods under anaerobic or partly anaerobic conditions. It is commonly present in feces. It is not as strict an anaerobe as *Cl. botulinum* and is discussed more fully as a cause of wound infection (gas gangrene, Chapter 36). It is mentioned here because some strains appear to be a cause of food poisoning characterized by acute gastroenteritis beginning usually eight to 14 hours after eating and lasting for six to 12 hours.

The toxin, not yet fully studied, is presumably destroyed by heating, in this resembling *Cl. botulinum* toxin. Poisoning by *Cl. perfringens* type A strains (A to F antigenic types are known) may therefore be avoided by clean preparation of foods and by prompt eating or refrigeration of freshly prepared foods. Poisoning by *Cl. perfringens* is often associated with cooked meats. In preparing canned foods the same precautions should be used as for prevention of botulism.

MYCOTOXINS.   These are poisonous by-products of the growth of certain eucaryotic fungi in foods. They have been causes of serious economic losses to stock and poultry growers when the animals have been fed moldy products, mainly vegetables, such as ground peanuts, rice, and corn. The role of mycotoxins in human disease may be more important than is generally known but it is still to be fully evaluated. Among the mycotoxins are the aflatoxins (*Aspergillus flavus*) and the rubratoxins (*Penicillium purpurogenum* and *P. rubrum*).

PREVENTION OF FOOD INFECTION AND FOOD POISONING

COOKING.   Cooking may or may not prevent food infection and food poisoning. This is because of the peculiar heat relationships of the factors involved. Vegetative cells of *Clostridium botulinum*, *Cl. perfringens*, *Staphylococcus aureus*, *Salmonella*, *Shigella*, *Vibrio cholerae* (in the Orient), cysts of *Entamoeba histolytica*, enteroviruses, and toxins of *Cl. botulinum* and (presumably) of *Cl. perfringens* are all inactivated by ten minutes of boiling (100 C). But *spores* of several types of *Cl. botulinum* are among the most heat-resistant organisms known to exist and will survive oven baking and steam pressure cooking (autoclaving), unless prolonged and at high temperature. *Cl. perfringens* spores are also very thermostable. *S. aureus* enterotoxin will resist boiling for an hour or more (Table 27–2). The virus of epidemic hepatitis is also known to be resistant to boiling for up to 30 minutes.

It must be remembered that in solid foods such as roasts, heat penetrates slowly. For example, the outside of a roast or the top of a pudding may be browned, yet the center may never be more than lukewarm. Steaming or boiling is more effective in disinfecting or sterilizing food than is baking or frying. The thrifty housewife thoroughly heats leftover food that cannot be refrigerated and that she is afraid will not "keep" overnight. If it must be kept unrefrigerated longer than overnight, it should be reheated at 100 C for ten minutes in the morning. Food to be eaten uncooked should be selected with care.

Never serve or eat opened or handled (i.e., *potentially contaminated*) food that has remained in a warm place (i.e., incubated) for more than four hours. These precautions apply, of course, to moist, nonacid foods suitable for growth of staphylococci, *Cl. perfringens*, *Salmonella*, and *Shigella*. These organisms will not multiply in such acid foods as stewed tomatoes, rhubarb

Table 27–2.   Relative Heat Resistance of Common Foodborne Microbial Pathogenic Agents

PATHOGENIC AGENT	RESISTANCE TO 100 C OR MORE FOR 30 MINUTES*
Salmonella, *Shigella*, *Vibrio cholerae*, enteroviruses, *Coxiella*, *Mycobacterium*, cysts of *Entamoeba histolytica*	–
Staphylococcus:	
enterotoxin	+
cells	–
Clostridium botulinum and *Cl. perfringens:*	
toxin	–
cells	–
spores	+
Epidemic hepatitis virus	±†

*+ = resistant; – = inactivated.
†A relatively heat-resistant virus but exact limit undetermined.

or pickles, or in dry foods like salted nuts and cookies, but will have a field day in gravies, cheese spaghetti, soups, whipped cream, creamed potatoes, bread or rice pudding, and the like.

REFRIGERATION.   Efficient and prompt refrigeration of foods soon after preparation or possible contamination prevents not only unnecessary and wasteful bacterial spoilage but also goes far to retard excessive growth of any harmful bacteria that may have gained access to the food after it was handled.

Babies' bottles can be prepared for feedings for a 24-hour period and then refrigerated with complete safety, provided that they are sterilized by heat to begin with. Special facilities are usually provided in hospitals and clinics, either for aseptic preparation, using sterilized materials and equipment, or for sterilizing the bottled formulas after preparation (Fig. 27-1). Proper handling and use of commercially prepared products eliminates this problem entirely.

FREEZING.   This is another method of inhibiting growth of microorganisms. Frozen foods are not necessarily sterile, but most will "keep" for months, and many for years, because of the halting of the metabolism of organisms present. Not only foods, but also many medicinal supplies and solutions liable to deterioration or microbial spoilage at room tempera-

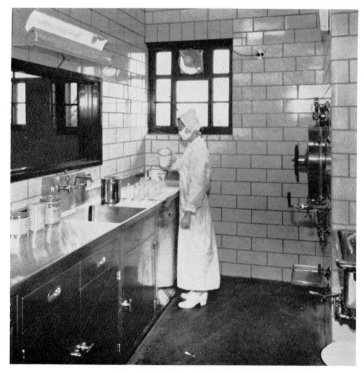

Figure 27-1

Formula preparation room. Note the ultraviolet source above the sink, exhaust fan in the window, tiled walls, built-in autoclave, knee-operated lavatory, and the surgical cleanliness of the process and the environment. (The Manual of Sterilization, Disinfection and Related Surgical Techniques [periodical]. American Sterilizer Co., Erie, Pa.) Smooth walls help to cut down potential contamination. Bricks and rough tiles have hidden crevices and these also contribute to dust. In some hospitals this preparation has been eliminated by using only prepackaged prepared products.

tures are preserved by freezing as well as by refrigeration. (Caution: Aqueous fluids frequently break glass containers on freezing!)

SUPERVISION OF FOOD HANDLERS.   Essential in the prevention of food infection is employment only of noninfectious food handlers. This is not always as easy as it might appear. Many cities require that all applicants for places as food handlers in hotels, restaurants, and institutions be examined for general cleanliness, carrying of enteric infections, the presence of boils or sores due to micrococci, or diphtheria, tuberculosis, or syphilis, and that only those who pass the test be employed. No person harboring infectious disease organisms transmissible by food or fomites should be allowed to work in a kitchen or dining place. The general enforcement of such regulations is difficult.

Clean hands and sanitary habits of food handlers are of prime importance also, since bacteria, either harmful or harmless, enteric or respira-

HAND DISHWASHING PROCEDURES

SANITIZING WITH HOT WATER
REQUIRES 2 STEPS

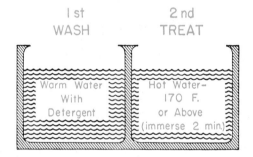

SANITIZING WITH CHEMICALS
REQUIRES 3 STEPS

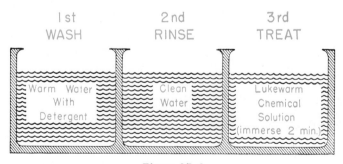

Figure 27–2

Methods of sanitizing dishes washed by hand. The water in the third sink in the chemical method (lower diagram) should contain a commercial disinfectant or at least 50 parts per million of free chlorine, preferably 100–200 ppm. If the water in this sink is too hot, the heat drives off the chlorine. (U.S. Public Health Service, Publication No. 83.)

tory, are commonly transferred from hands to food. Eating of food as it is prepared should be discouraged, especially if the cook sticks his fingers in his mouth in the process, then touches the food others will eat. The hands should always be washed thoroughly before preparing or serving a meal. Hands should always be washed after using the toilet and blowing the nose. The reason is obvious. The problem of clean hands is a pressing and difficult one in institutions such as state mental hospitals, where patients help in kitchens and dining rooms.

PROPER DISHWASHING. The method of dishwashing has great bacteriologic importance and is regarded seriously by health departments and administrators of institutions. Practices in some "soda-lunch" counters and small restaurants are revolting to any educated person. One often notices a stale cigar taste or sees lipstick on his clean (?) glass and not in frequently finds "eggy" saliva adhering to his spoon or fork (not to mention the knife). The mere swishing of tableware through a basin of lukewarm, filthy, saliva-shredded water is obviously of no use from the standpoint of preventive medicine or public health, but it is a too common practice. Also, washing dishes in a pan of lukewarm water with a dirty dishcloth, even with a dash of detergent or soap powder, merely distributes bacteria over them.

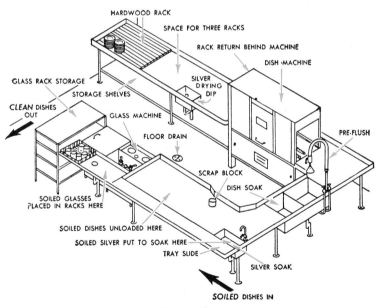

Figure 27–3

One form of modern, sanitary dishwashing equipment. The working bench is of stainless steel. Soiled dishes are piled on the bench in the foreground. They are sorted and scraped, the larger scraps of food dropping into a barrel beneath the counter. Glasses are rinsed over rotating brushes, dipped into disinfectant and placed in trays in a rack (left). Silverware soaks in a pan of special detergent solution (right foreground). The dishes, arranged in baskets, are soaked and then given a preliminary rinse with *hard* streams of *hot* water (right). They then pass through a machine dishwasher (center, background). The silver, after soaking, passes through the same process as the dishes and is self-dried after a dip into a drying agent. Afterward all utensils are stacked and stored in dust-proof cabinets. Eating utensils handled in this way are virtually sterile. (Courtesy of John L. Wilson and Wm. M. Podas, Economics Lab., Inc. In *Modern Sanitation.*)

HAND DISHWASHING. An abundance of tolerably hot water with detergent should be used for initial washing. The proper washing of spoons, forks, cups, and glasses is especially essential. In the absence of a disinfectant, the cleaned dishes should be immersed in almost boiling water (180 F or more) for several minutes to disinfect them. If a chlorine disinfectant is used, the dishes should be rinsed in a basin of cool, clean water containing at least 50 parts per million of free chlorine. Hot water drives off the chlorine. Chlorine content is easily determined by Health Department inspectors (Fig. 27–2). Poorly washed spoons or forks can be the means of transmitting pneumonia, diphtheria, tuberculosis, the organisms associated with Vincent's angina, scarlet fever, septic sore throat, diphtheria, and influenza from one person's mouth to another's.

MACHINE DISHWASHING. This is far more effective than hand methods, and much hotter water can be used (Fig. 27–3). In managing cases of disease transmitted by saliva and sputum, the dishes and eating utensils of the patient should be boiled. Dish towels, if used, should be clean! Since dish towels cannot long stay clean if used, it is better to let glasses or dishes air-dry. Some institutions subject tableware to bactericidal ultraviolet light. One must remember, however, that ultraviolet light does not pass through glass and that it kills bacteria only on those surfaces directly exposed to it for some time.

BACTERIOLOGIC EXAMINATION OF TABLEWARE. It is relatively easy to determine approximate numbers of bacteria on tableware before and after washing, storage, and handling. In one simple procedure a swab, moistened with sterile broth or water, is rubbed over a measured area of the tableware (dish, knife, and so on). The swab is shaken violently in a tube containing a measured volume (5 ml) of broth. An agar plate count is then made of the bacteria that were released from the swab into the broth. There are many modifications of this procedure. In several, a water-soluble, filamentous material (calcium alginate) is substituted for the cotton.

MILK

BACTERIA IN MILK. Bacteria of many kinds grow well in milk. As sold on the market, milk may be processed to be sterile, or it may contain thousands of harmless bacteria per milliliter. Mere numbers of bacteria, however, are not alarming; it is the kind that is important.

Milk as it is drawn from a healthy cow contains a few bacteria, but unless modern, "closed" methods of milking are used (Fig. 27–4), it acquires many more from the cow's body, the dust and dirt in the barn, the hands, the milking machine, and milk cans. Some of this contamination is unavoidable, but it can be greatly reduced by care in the cleanliness of the cows, milkers, barns, cans, and other equipment, which is now routine in all good dairies.

When it has just been drawn, very clean milk may contain as few as 100 bacteria per ml. By the time milk reaches the city consumer from 24 to 48 hours later, the number of bacteria ranges from about 3000 per ml in the very best milk, to millions per ml in unacceptable milk. Good, pasteurized, Grade A milk contains not over 30,000 and should contain as few as 10,000 bacteria per ml. The presence of large numbers of bacteria in milk shows that it has either been produced and handled under unclean conditions, or is stale and has not been kept cool. It may also have

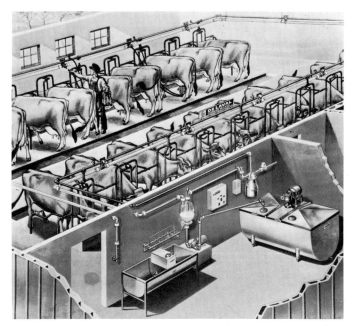

Figure 27–4

A two-unit barn-type combine milker. Milk is conveyed, directly from the cows' udders, in a completely enclosed glass, plastic, or stainless steel pipe, through a filter (glass container, lower center) and into a refrigerated bulk cooler (lower right). The milk is never open to contamination from the air or environment. After milking, the assembled units are connected with a manifold washer in the milk room (attached to wall, lower right). Detergent is placed in a special compartment in the automatic washer. By pressing a button the entire system is prerinsed, washed, and rinsed again automatically. Surely a far cry from the romantic (but unsanitary) "pretty milkmaid"! (Courtesy of DeLaval Separator Company.)

come from infected cows even though it does not contain large numbers of bacteria. Although drawn under good conditions from healthy cows, it may have been inoculated with pathogens by milk handlers who were carriers of enteric or respiratory pathogens, or both (see Table 27–3). Powdered milk is now often used by the consumer and also in institutions where water is added prior to refrigeration and subsequent serving to students, inmates, and so forth. The water must be of acceptable sanitary quality. Evaporated and condensed milks are sterile if properly processed.

PUBLIC HEALTH SUPERVISION OF MILK SUPPLIES.   Good milk is so important that Boards of Health in all states and progressive communities regulate the conditions under which it shall be produced and sold. The farms on which the milk is produced are inspected, and sanitary codes, established in cooperation with State and Federal experts, are enforced in the buildings, among the employees, in the care of the cows and the handling of the milk.

In general, milk from sick animals may not be used, nor may the milk be marketed if there is a case of infectious disease transmissible by milk among the family or employees on the farm. Milk must be kept in the refrigerator in shops and sold only by the bottle or carton. In most states only pasteurized Grade A (see p. 395) milk, powdered, or presterilized bottled milk is permitted to be sold for household use. *Certified milk* ("baby

Table 27–3.   Sources of Pathogens in Cow's Milk

I. Udder of cow is infected *prior* to milking:
    a. *Mycobacterium tuberculosis* (var. *bovis*)
    b. *Brucella* sp.
    c. *Streptococcus pyogenes* (Group A)*
    d. *Coxiella burnetii*
    e. *Staphylococcus aureus**
II. Worker infects milk *after* milking:
    a. *Corynebacterium diphtheriae*
    b. *Salmonella*, sp.
    c. *Shigella* sp.
    d. *Staphylococcus aureus*
    e. *Streptococcus pyogenes* (Group A)*

---

*S. pyogenes (Group A) appears in both upper and lower parts of the table because infected workers can infect both the cow's udder (resulting in mastitis), and contaminate the milk *after* it is drawn. This may be true also of *Staphylococcus.*

milk") is produced by specially licensed and very carefully inspected and controlled dairies.

BACTERIOLOGIC EXAMINATION OF MILK. The bacteria in milk are readily made visible and may be counted if a smear of 0.01 ml of the milk is made over an area exactly 1 cm square, stained with methylene blue, and examined under the microscope. The smear shows whether the predominating species are streptococci (potential pathogens) or other varieties. Pus cells, revealing infected udders, are also easily detected. Since the volume and area of the milk smear are known, it is easy to calculate the numbers per unit volume. This procedure is widely used by creameries and health departments in daily estimations of the quality of the milk. It is known as the "Breed count" (after the famous American bacteriologist, Robert Breed) or the *direct microscopic method*. One drawback of the Breed count is that it does not enable the examiner to distinguish between living and dead bacteria. New or specially cleaned slides must be used. The stained slides may be stored for permanent records.

A widely used method of estimating the number of living bacteria in milk is to dilute the milk appropriately (1:10, 1:100, 1:1000) and mix 1 ml of the diluted sample with about 12 ml of melted nutrient agar of a prescribed composition in a sterile Petri dish. After appropriate incubation (usually 48 hours at 32 C), readily visible colonies will have developed in the plate, each colony presumably having originated from a live bacterium in the milk. To count the colonies and make the required arithmetical calculations is then a simple matter. This method is equally applicable to estimating the number of bacteria in blood, water, or any other fluid if suitable medium is used. The procedure is often called a "plate count."

A peculiarity of this method is that, while each colony theoretically represents a single bacterium, actually many bacteria tend to cling together in clumps of from two to 100 or more, and hence a single colony may represent one of these clumps rather than a single cell. Furthermore, in order to avoid complicated methods, a relatively simple medium is generally used for counting bacteria in milk or water, and many bacteria, especially pathogens and anaerobic species, will not grow in it. For these reasons the Breed count is always higher than the plate count. A combination of the two methods is probably best. It is evident that the enumeration of bacteria in milk or water merely approximates exactness, but the method has given us some of our most useful information about water and milk supplies and means of controlling their quality.

GRADING MILK. Milk is commonly graded or classified according to the conditions under which it has been produced and the number of bacteria which it contains. Standards and regulations may differ somewhat in different communities. Some common standards are the following:

Grade A is produced under very clean conditions from disease-free cattle, and is suitable for infant feeding. It is nearly always required to be pasteurized. It is required that the plate count be lower than 30,000 per ml after pasteurization. The U.S. Public Health Service formulated the Grade A Pasteurized Milk Ordinance in 1965.

Certified milk is produced raw under supervision of the American Association of Medical Milk Commissions. Special licenses are required, and rigid medical and veterinary requirements must be met, all of which tend to safeguard the consumer. A certificate is issued to farms that meet the requirements, and the milk is said to be "Certified."

Grade B milk is produced under ordinarily good conditions, but is usually not sold for public consumption directly. The plate count is less than 1 million before pasteurization and not over 50,000 afterward.

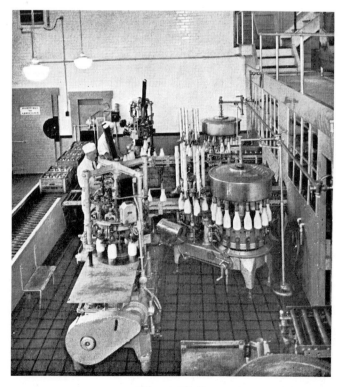

Figure 27–5

Bottling milk in a sanitary dairy. All the piping can be demounted in a few minutes for steam sterilization and for hosing down the floors and walls. In some plants light, transparent, plastic tubing is used. The bottles in this picture have been steam sterilized just before filling. Many large modern milk distributors use paper cartons. Much milk is also distributed in plastic containers. (Dodd's Alderney Dairy, Buffalo, N.Y. Courtesy of Cherry-Burrell Corp.)

CARE OF MILK IN THE HOUSEHOLD.   Milk should be kept covered and cold. The mouth of the bottle or carton should be wiped with a clean cloth before the milk is poured out. One never knows what contaminating influence (e.g., inquisitive dogs or hungry cats) has been at work on the tops of milk bottles standing on porches and doorsteps.

The tops of milk bottles should not be touched with fingers. Milk bottles should never be taken into a sickroom. The use of waxed paper cartons is doing much to eliminate the evils of the glass milk bottle. Their advantages are obvious. A disadvantage is that they sometimes leak and may thus become contaminated.

DISEASES TRANSMITTED BY MILK.   Pathogens transmitted by milk may be listed under two headings, as shown in Table 27–3.

The bacteria causing bovine tuberculosis (*Mycobacterium tuberculosis* var. *bovis*) gain entrance to the milk from infected cows; so also do those causing brucellosis (*Brucella* species) and *Coxiella burnetii*, cause of Q fever. *C. burnetii* may also be transmitted by ticks and dust.

The organisms causing septic sore throat and scarlet fever (*Streptococcus pyogenes*) may get into milk directly from some infected person who handles the milk, or indirectly by means of an infection in the cow's udder, which in turn came from an infected milker. The bacilli of shigellosis, of salmonellosis, and of diphtheria gain entrance to milk only after it is drawn and only from infected human beings, since the udders of cattle are not normally infected by these organisms (Table 27–3).

All these microorganisms, excepting *C. burnetii* and possibly *M. bovis* and *Brucella* sp., grow very well indeed in milk and, if the infectious milk is kept in a warm place, may soon make a milk supply exceedingly dangerous. Milk from an udder heavily infected by *Staphylococcus aureus* (a common cause of bovine mastitis) may contain enough preformed enterotoxin to cause severe poisoning in spite of pasteurization.

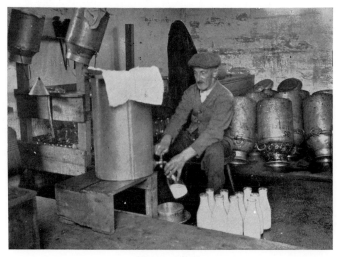

Figure 27–6

Unclean bottling of unpasteurized milk. Suppose the farmer were recovering from "strep throat" and had long been a typhoid carrier! Conditions like these are found occasionally when public health supervision of the milk supply is insufficient or lax. (Photo by Lewis Hine. Courtesy of Cleanliness Institute.)

PASTEURIZATION. As mentioned in a previous chapter, all micro-organisms causing transmissible disease that ordinarily occur in dairy products are killed by the usual commercial processes of pasteurization, i.e., 63 C (145 F) for 30 minutes by the vat or holding process, or 72 C (161 F) for 15 seconds by the "flash" or high-temperature, short-time (H.T.S.T.) process. Many harmless bacteria in milk survive so that pasteurization disinfects but does not sterilize. After pasteurization, the milk must be refrigerated promptly and bottled under hygienic conditions (Fig 27–5), or the pasteurization is futile.

The pasteurized and carefully guarded milk supplies of large cities are rarely the means of spreading infection. Milk consumed in rural districts and in backward areas of the world is sometimes produced under very unsanitary conditions, handled carelessly, and not pasteurized or, worse, ineffectually pasteurized, creating a false sense of security (Fig. 27–6).

Supplementary Reading

Annelis, A., Grecz, N., Huber, D. A., Berkowitz, D., Schneider, M.D., and Simon, M.: Radiation sterilization of bacon for military feeding. *Appl. Microbiol.*, 1965, *13*:37.

Anonymous. The yearly profit on one drug: 25 lives. *The Reader's Digest*, 1968, June:M2

Chesbro, W. R., and Auborn, K.: Enzymatic detection of the growth of *Staphylococcus aureus* in foods. *Appl. Microbiol.*, 1967, *15*:1150.

Cliver, D. O.: Food-associated viruses. *Health Lab. Sci.*, 1967, *4*:213.

Cockburn, W. C., Taylor, J., Anderson, E. S., and Hobbs, B. C.: Food Poisoning. 1962, London, The Royal Society of Health J. (90 Buckingham Palace Road).

Dack, G. M.: Food Poisoning. 3rd Ed. 1956, Chicago, University of Chicago Press.

Food Service Sanitation Manual, 1962. Washington, D.C., Government Printing Office, Public Health Service Publication No. 934.

Foster, E. M., and Sugiyama, H.: Recent developments in botulism research. *Health Lab. Sci.*, 1967, *4*:193.

Frazier, W. C.: Food Microbiology. 2nd Ed. 1967, New York, McGraw-Hill Book Co.

Frobisher, M.: Fundamentals of Microbiology. 8th Ed. 1968, Philadelphia, W. B. Saunders Co.

Hall, H. E., and Lewis, K. H.: *Clostridium perfrigens* and other bacterial species as possible causes of food-borne disease outbreaks of undetermined etiology. *Health Lab. Sci.*, 1967, *4*:229.

Ingram, M., and Roberts, T. A. (Editors): Botulism 1966. 1967, London, Chapman and Hall.

Joint Editorial Committee: Standard Methods for the Examination of Dairy Products. 12th Ed. 1967, New York, American Public Health Association.

Natori, S., Sakaki, S., Udagawa, S. I., Ichinoe, M., Saito, M., Umeda, M., and Ohtsubo, K.: Production of rubratoxin B by *Penicillium purpurogenum* Stoll. *Appl. Microbiol.*, 1970, *19*:613.

Schlinder, A. F., Palmer, J. G., and Eisenberg, W. V.: Aflatoxin production by *Aspergillus flavus* as related to various temperatures. *Appl. Microbiol.*, 1967, *15*:1006.

Strong, D. H., Canada, J. C., and Griffiths, B. B.: Incidence of *Clostridium perfringens* in American foods. *Appl. Microbiol.*, 1963, *11*:42.

Subcommittee on Methods for the Microbiological Examination of Foods: Recommended methods. 2nd Ed. 1966, New York, American Public Health Association.

Thatcher, F. S., and Clark, D. S.: Microorganisms in foods. Their Significance and Methods of Enumeration. 1968, Toronto, University of Toronto Press.

Varga, S., and Anderson, G. W.: Significance of coliforms and enterococci in fish products. *Appl. Microbiol.*, 1968, *16*:193.

Vermilyea, B. L., Walker, H. W., and Ayres, J. C.: Detection of botulinal toxins by immuno-diffusion. *Appl. Microbiol.*, 1968, *16*:21.

Welt, M. A.: When food is irradiated. Letters to the Editor, *Science*, 1968, *160*:483; see also McKinney, M. E., Schweigert, B. S., same source.

White, A., and Hobbs, B. C.: Refrigeration as a preventive measure in food poisoning. *Roy. Soc. Health J.*, 1963, *83*:111.

WHO Expert Committee and F. A. O.: Microbiological aspects of food hygiene. Tech. Report Series, 1968, No. 398, Government Printing Office, Washington, D.C.

Part B
*Pathogens Transmitted
from the Respiratory
Tract*

Staphylococcal, Diplococcal, and Streptococcal Infections

28

Pathogenic microorganisms occurring in the respiratory tract (including sinuses, inner ear, conjunctival sacs, and adjacent tissues) are regularly transmitted via oral and nasal secretions or discharges from infected eyes, or ears, or both. Oral and nasal secretions inevitably contaminate the atmosphere during talking, laughing, sneezing, coughing, and similar actions that produce droplets and droplet nuclei. If we add to the aerial dissemination of saliva and mucus, the spread of oral, nasal, and conjunctival secretions by hands, eating utensils, drinking glasses, and improperly maintained swimming pools (which may be contaminated by feces and urine as well as by respiratory secretions), it is clear that we constantly face a formidable, unceasing, and virtually ubiquitous onslaught of infection.

Pathogens of the respiratory tract, and airborne pathogens in general, are among the most difficult to control. Indeed, except under the most carefully restricted circumstances, such as the use of special breathing apparatus, masks, germicidal vapors in closed rooms, small, irradiated isolation cubicles or rooms, and "life islands" or "bubbles" used for patients being treated with drugs that depress the immunologic responses (e.g., in heart and other organ transplants), we have virtually no control over airborne diseases in ordinary daily human contacts.

INFECTION, NATURAL IMMUNIZATION, AND CARRIERS. On the comforting side, daily experience shows that the majority of normal, healthy persons generally do not suffer serious or even perceptible infectious disease except in times of epidemics. Fortunately, as a result of previous subclinical infections (or vaccinations) and robust health they generally become actively immunized (or *re*immunized) to many of the organisms with which they daily come into contact. Unfortunately, they also often become carriers of pathogenic microorganisms; they remain healthy but transmit their pathogens to others, perhaps to ill or aged persons or young children, who may suffer from being infected with a serious disease as the result.

It is fortunate that none of the common respiratory pathogens forms heat-resistant endospores.[1] All nonspore-formers (except certain viruses) are readily killed by five minutes of boiling and by such standard disinfectants as 2 per cent saponated cresol, household chlorine bleaches (5 per cent NaOCl), and low-surface-tension iodine solutions.

CONTROL OF RESPIRATORY INFECTIONS

There are many effective "road blocks" that may be placed by the health worker in the path of respiratory pathogens. These include the thorough washing (using disinfectant soap) of hands known to be soiled with respiratory tract discharges; adequate sanitization of dishes and eating utensils, most readily accomplished in institutions and homes by machine dishwashers with hot water (185 F or 85 C) as a final rinse; disinfectant laundering of bedding of patients with any infectious disease (i.e., hot water or soaking in disinfectant, hot ironing, and the like); disinfection (not merely "airing") of blankets, mattresses, and so on by autoclaving or sporicidal vapors or gas; use (and proper disposal!) of clean handkerchiefs or paper tissues for sneezing and coughing; use of proper sputum containers for tuberculosis patients (see discussion of tuberculosis); disinfection of air and dust; the use of masks, dust control, and ventilation. Only the last four require discussion here.

MASKS.   These should be sufficiently thick and should cover the nose and mouth completely. They must never be reversed and never reused after dangling about the neck. Masks should be changed when perceptibly moist. When discarded after use they should be placed in a closed container. Washing reusable masks with hot (80 C) water and soap is sufficient routine disinfection. Better yet are sterile, disposable, inexpensive masks, packaged for immediate effective use. Some modern masks are made of molded plastic or metal to which are adapted removable filter units of very fine-pored foam rubber, fibered glass, and like materials (see also Fig. 15–8). Units or entire masks that are completely disposable are highly effective, but each type should be adopted only after actual experimental trial.

Quite noticeable to the traveler in Japan is the number of people who rush through Tokyo, to their daily tasks, wearing a face mask. Either they are concerned about catching a cold, or, more likely, giving a respiratory infection to other people. This is indeed very polite, civilized, and most alert to the ever present danger of the airborne respiratory pathogens around us.

---

[1] Pulmonary anthrax ("wool-sorter's disease") is an exception. This disease is rare, except in the wool and hides industry.

DUST CONTROL.   Since dust (including droplet nuclei) is obviously an important factor in disease transmission by air, methods of suppressing dust have been developed. One consists of treating all floors, window sills, and bedding in barracks, hospital wards, and similar places where infectious dust accumulates, with an imperceptible film of oil. The dust sticks to the oil and is easily removed without being stirred up. The use of oiled "sweeping compounds" in public places, hospitals, and so on, is desirable for this reason.

Modern vacuum cleaning systems are devised to conduct dust taken up by the nozzle, not to a "dust bag," which is often far from efficient in the retention of the dust, but into a built-in vacuum-duct system with intakes in each room that conduct all dust through airtight tubes to an incinerator or dust-tight container.

Devices that combine wet-scrubbing with vacuum cleaning are also excellent means of floor dust control. Probably the perfect dust control system remains to be invented.

VENTILATION.   When ventilation is thorough, it is a very effective means of removing airborne pathogens and of reducing dosage of infectious organisms to a virtual vanishing point.

In cold climates ventilation with outdoor air raises problems of heating costs. Ventilation by recirculation of indoor air raises problems of expensive installations for blowers, dust filters, and incineration; however, these are engineering details with which we need not be concerned in this book.

DISINFECTION.   Air and dust may be disinfected by several means, among which are irradiation with ultraviolet light, surface disinfection, and microbicidal vapors. These methods have been discussed in Chapters 10, 12, and 13. Passage of air through filters and ducts at high temperature (virtual incineration) is also used.

PATHOGENIC COCCI OF THE RESPIRATORY TRACT

CLASSIFICATION AND DESCRIPTION OF COCCI.   Cocci arrange themselves in different ways as they multiply. Those forming predominantly chains are called streptococci; those usually arranging themselves in irregular clusters are called staphylococci if *facultative* aerobes, or micrococci if *strict* aerobes; and those that mainly form pairs are called diplococci (Fig. 4–2). All cocci are gram-positive except the important genus *Neisseria*, containing the gonococci and meningococci. These are discussed further on page 414. The pathogenic gram-positive cocci described in this chapter are:

> *Staphylococcus aureus*
> *Streptococcus pyogenes* and closely related species (often called the hemolytic streptococci, Streptococcus hemolyticus or "hemolytic strep")
> Streptococcus salivarius, *S. faecalis, S. mitis*, and related species (often called Streptococcus viridans)
> *Diplococcus pneumoniae* (often called the pneumococcus; now generally called *Streptococcus pneumoniae*).

The Staphylococci

Staphylococcus aureus is named for its golden yellow pigment.[2] A similar species called *S. epidermidis* (epidermis-inhabiting) produces a chalky white pigment. These pigments are most distinctive in colonies on solid media. Neither produces pigment in broth or when grown anaerobically. *S. aureus* and certain white-pigmented variants of it are distinguished from *S. epidermidis* by producing coagulase. Both species grow well on infusion agar or in peptone broth or milk at temperatures of 25 to 40 C. They are facultative aerobes. Although they form no spores, they are somewhat resistant to drying, and can therefore remain alive for several months under favorable conditions in dust or elsewhere outside the body. One or both species are often present in the normal upper respiratory tract.

Infections by staphylococci commonly cause much pus formation, hence they are said to be *pyogenic* (*pyo*, pus).

STAPHYLOCOCCAL TOXINS.   *Staphylococcus aureus* produces a metabolic product called *leukocidin*, which kills white blood cells. Many strains also produce a poison that is called *enterotoxin* because it causes gastroenteritis. In addition to this, *S. aureus* secretes substances that cause necrosis of skin tissues (dermonecrotic toxins), hemolysis of red blood cells and coagulation of oxalated or citrated[3] plasma (*coagulase*). Coagulase-producing staphylococci, regardless of color, are especially dangerous, and the *coagulase test* is frequently done in the diagnostic laboratory.

A positive coagulase test for either *Staphylococcus aureus* or any similar strain is taken as an indication that the strain being tested is pathogenic. Nonpathogenic strains do not produce coagulase. It should be noted that organisms that cause food poisoning by means of an enterotoxin also usually are coagulase positive. There are several *S. aureus* hemolysins, separable by electrophoresis.

Phosphatase production has also been associated with pathogenicity of staphylococci; however, it does not always agree with coagulase activity. Nontoxic metabolites produced are deoxyribonuclease, hyaluronidase, staphylokinase, lipase, gelatinase, and also protease.

Isolation of Staphylococci

Staphylococcus aureus ferments mannitol, while *S. epidermidis* does not. Also, *S. aureus* can tolerate a high salt concentration of close to 10 per cent. Because of this property, mannitol salt agar is used as a selective medium for the isolation of *S. aureus* from feces and other sources. In 48 hours, salt-tolerant colonies of staphylococci appear, surrounded by a yellow halo on mannitol salt agar. Vogel and Johnson agar permits early detection of coagulase-positive colonies of *S. aureus.* On this red medium, a yellow zone surrounds the black colonies of *Staphylococcus.*

Penicillinase.   One of the dangerous enzymic properties often found in staphylococci (and in some other pathogens, notably *Shigella*) is production of the enzyme *penicillinase,* which *destroys penicillin.* Obviously any organism that can excrete this enzyme can protect itself from penicillin; i.e., it is penicillin-resistant. The power to produce penicillinase often ap-

---

[2]From the Latin word *aurum,* gold. The Greek word *staphyle* means a bunch of grapes.

[3]Sodium oxalate or citrate is usually added to blood specimens for chemical examination to prevent clotting.

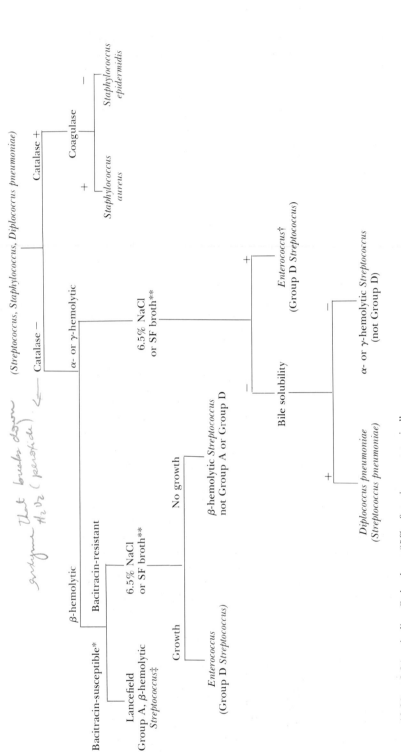

Figure 28–1

Differentiation of pathogenic gram-positive cocci.

*0.02 to 0.04 unit disc. Only about 85% of strains react typically.
**Streptococcus faecalis broth inhibits streptococci and some other organisms which are not enterococci; this includes gram-negative organisms.
†This category may contain some non-catalase-producing strains of Aerococcus. These can be distinguished from Enterococcus by their inability to grow at 45°C.
‡May be confirmed by the Lancefield precipitin test or the direct fluorescent-antibody technique, using group-specific serum.

pears as a result of genetic mutation. Penicillinase is a peptidase and acts on a variety of peptides, of which penicillin is one.

Adaptive or Induced Enzymes.   Sometimes bacteria, notably staphylococci, appear to be stimulated to produce penicillinase by mere contact with the drug, not by genetic mutation. Thus treatment with penicillin may, by itself, induce production of the enzyme. Enzymes ordinarily not produced by an organism but produced *in response to contact* of the organism with a specific substrate are said to be *adaptive* or *induced enzymes.* They represent activation of a latent genetic potentiality. There are many, various sorts in various organisms.

Staphylococcal Infections

Staphylococcus epidermidis, the white, coagulase-negative species, is widely distributed on the bodies of human beings and animals. These cocci are usually harmless residents. If the skin is injured by a cut, a scratch, or in other ways, however, the cocci can get into the underlying tissues and may cause an infection.

Pimples and acne lesions are common forms of infection in which these organisms are found. Infection of stitches following surgical operation (commonly called "stitch abscess") is most frequently caused by these staphylococci. As a rule, infections caused by these organisms are not highly dangerous. However, cocci designated as *S. epidermidis* have been reported in some cases of fatal septicemia. Microorganisms are devious and treacherous!

S. aureus, the dangerous coagulase-producing species, typically produces boils and carbuncles. These cocci can also invade the whole system, causing fatal septicemia, meningitis, endocarditis, puerperal sepsis, pneumonia, destructive abscesses in the internal organs called *multiple abscesses,* and infections of the bones called *osteomyelitis.*

Staphylococcus aureus is of special significance in hospitals, notably in surgical and maternity wards and nurseries, as the cause of epidemics of antibiotic-resistant wound infections, severe abscesses of the lactating breast (mastitis), and distressing ulcers on infants (pemphigus or impetigo neonatorum[4]), as well as other serious infections (nosocomial or "in-the-hospital" infections). As previously mentioned, staphylococci often become antibiotic-resistant and cause hospital epidemics. These outbreaks have received much serious consideration in medical as well as lay literature.

PHAGE TYPES OF STAPHYLOCOCCI.   Specific lytic group types have been established by staphylococcal phage typing. More than 22 of these bacterial strains have been classified into six groups. Of these, for example, Group II, which causes many skin lesions, reacts only with phage 71. The international staphylococcal phage typing system is not yet completely accepted; some laboratories do some additional typing.

DRUG-FAST STAPHYLOCOCCI.   Every hospital is concerned with this problem because of the constant contact of the patients with different visitors and personnel who are unknowingly carriers of *S. aureus.* All hospital personnel should be examined periodically for various pathogenic microorganisms or subclinical infections of any sort, and as far as possible kept from contact with patients. Prevention of the spread of respiratory microorganisms requires rigid precautions as to washing hands, dis-

[4]Greek *neos,* new; *natus,* born.

posing of infectious dressings, disinfecting bedding, dishes, and thermometers, cleanliness of the rooms and wards, wearing gowns and masks, and other details of expert barrier technique. Complete details are given in the report of the American Hospital Association, "Prevention and Control of Staphylococcal Infections in Hospitals; see also Top, F. H., (Ed.) et al.: *Control of Infectious Diseases in General Hospitals.* 1967, New York, American Public Health Association.

In handling staphylococcal infections, the greatest care should be exercised not to let the pus come into contact with anything that will distribute it. Staphylococci, and indeed all organisms, in pus are in a particularly virulent condition. Dressings of boils and other lesions may be dropped into a pot of disinfectant or into boiling water, or wrapped carefully in several thicknesses of newspaper, fastened securely to prevent escape of the infected dressings and burned completely. Probably the most important single factor in the transmission of staphylococcal infections in hospitals is the dissemination of the organisms on lint from bedding and contaminated dust in the environment of infected patients, especially of patients (or personnel) with nasal infections.

STAPHYLOCOCCAL FOOD POISONING. It is obvious that *S. aureus,* though occurring commonly in the respiratory tract, can cause a great variety of pathological conditions and infect almost any part of the body via many portals of entry and exit. It can cause boils of the nose, hands, arms, or face of people, some of whom may work with foods. Its easy transfer to one's lunch can be all too readily envisioned!

As already mentioned, *S. aureus* is the cause of a common variety of food poisoning. The cocci grow readily in many not-too-acid foodstuffs such as "precooked" hams, milk, custards, salads, sandwich fillings, and creamed foods. Many strains give off a potent toxin (*enterotoxin*[5]). This, when swallowed, causes gastroenteritis: nausea, vomiting, cramps, and diarrhea. Thorough cooking destroys the organism but not the toxin. The enterotoxin is very resistant to heat. Ordinary cooking will not destroy it after the staphylococci have produced it in the food. The best safeguard against staphylococcal food poisoning is prompt refrigeration, cooking, or eating of all handled foods and discarding any that are stale or "spoiled." Contaminated food, i.e., any food that has been handled or exposed to people who are coughing, sneezing, or talking, may develop large amounts of the enterotoxin if allowed to stand at kitchen temperatures for more than three to five hours. Staphylococcal food poisoning is rarely fatal, but it has spoiled many a dance date.

The Streptococci

The streptococci comprise a large group of organisms, among which are many useful and harmless species and also some of the most deadly pathogens. Streptococci are catalase negative, do not usually ferment inulin, do not reduce nitrates and are not soluble in bile salts. If a carbohydrate is fermented by streptococci, large amounts of lactic acid are produced, without gas. The pathogenic streptococci grow readily in the laboratory but for best development require blood or serum media and body

---

[5]Note that *enterotoxin* refers to an exotoxin that affects the *enteric* tract (Greek *enteron,* intestine). The word enterotoxin must not be confused with *endotoxin,* which means a toxin that remains inside the bacterial cell (Greek *endon,* inside of).

temperature (37 C). They are facultative aerobes. They are killed by pasteurization, by five minutes of boiling, and by disinfectants such as 1 per cent saponated cresol, 5 per cent sodium hypochlorite, and iodine disinfectants. They may remain alive for some time when dried: for several days or weeks in sputum, in exudate from lesions, or in droplet nuclei. Streptococci may be relatively easily differentiated from other cocci and as to group by the scheme shown in Figure 28–1. Of special value is the growth on blood agar.

BLOOD-AGAR TYPES OF STREPTOCOCCI. All streptococci may be assigned to one of three types, *alpha, beta,* and *gamma,* differentiated by the action of their subsurface colonies on sheep erythrocytes in Petri dishes of blood-agar medium. They are distinguished as follows:

Alpha Type (α-Hemolytic Streptococci). These so-called viridans species of streptococci produce a greenish area around their blood-agar colonies, with or without an outer clear, colorless area of hemolysis. The zones of greening may vary from less than one to several millimeters wide. The outer clear area around the greenish zone may best be seen after the cultures are stored in the refrigerator. Such colonies are said to be of the *alpha type* and the streptococci producing them are called alpha

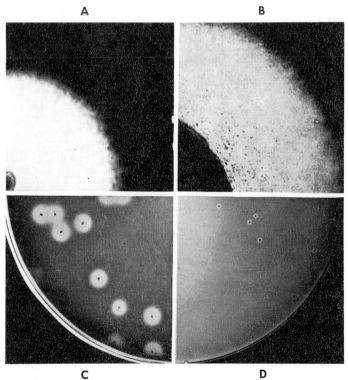

Figure 28–2

Colonies of hemolytic streptococci in blood agar. *A,* One β type colony enlarged to show edge of colony at lower left and absence of erythrocytes in clear hemolyzed zone. *B,* One α type colony enlarged to show edge of colony at lower left, with many intact erythrocytes in hemolyzed zone. *C,* Clear zones of complete hemolysis around colonies of β type (*Streptococcus pyogenes,* Lancefield Group A), natural size. *D,* Small hemolytic zones of α type colony, *S. mitis,* natural size. (Preparations by Dr. Elaine L. Updyke. Photo courtesy of U.S. Public Health Service, Communicable Disease Center, Atlanta, Ga.)

type hemolytic streptococci, viridans streptococci, or Streptococcus viridans (Fig. 28–2).

Several species of alpha type hemolytic streptococci are pathogenic for man or lower animals, or both. Representative species are *S. salivarius*, reputedly harmless, which is commonly found in saliva, and *S. mitis*, also found in saliva. Another is *S. faecalis*, common in feces and sometimes found in saliva. These and several very similar species are often found in abscessed teeth, in growths on heart valves in bacterial endocarditis, and in arthritic joints. In general, they produce less acute infections than do the beta type streptococci, but are nonetheless dangerous because the infections tend to become chronic.

Beta Type (β-Hemolytic Streptococci).   These produce perfectly clear, colorless zones around their subsurface colonies in blood agar. These zones are due to *hemolysin* secreted by the streptococci in the colony. The clear, colorless zone of hemolysis is called *beta type* hemolysis and the streptococci are said to be beta type hemolytic streptococci (Fig. 28–2).

In general, the beta type hemolytic streptococci are *pyogenic* and are pathogenic for man, or animals, or both. The principal human pathogen is *Streptococcus pyogenes*. This and several very similar variants cause scarlet fever, septic sore throat, puerperal[6] sepsis, "blood poisoning" (streptococcemia), and other conditions, many of which are similar to those caused by *Staphylococcus aureus*.

Gamma Type (Nonhemolytic Streptococci).   Some streptococci produce no visible change in the blood agar around their colonies. These are called *gamma type* streptococci, or indifferent or nonhemolytic streptococci. The colonies produced are usually small, gray and translucent.

These streptococci are not commonly pathogenic, some species being found in milk; however, they sometimes are found in the same sorts of lesions as the alpha type streptococci.

Infections by α-Type Hemolytic Streptococci

TOOTH ABSCESSES.   Streptococci of the alpha type are often found in abscesses in the roots of the teeth. These abscesses may cause no definite symptoms and may be found only by the dentist's x-ray picture, and yet the organisms or their toxins may cause serious damage to various organs, especially as the streptococci may localize elsewhere in the body, setting up new foci of infection in vital places such as the heart.

HEART VALVE INJURIES.   Alpha type streptococci may infect injured heart valves and are a frequent cause of *subacute bacterial endocarditis*, which is often fatal. Just how the organisms are transmitted is not known exactly, but they may come via the blood from infected teeth and tonsils or chronic sinus infections, or from the intestines. Infections carried by the blood in this way are said to be *hematogenous* (or *endogenous*).

In endocarditis the streptococci cause an inflammation of the heart valves. This is followed by shrinkage and thickening (scarring) of the valves, causing them to leak (Fig. 28–3). These streptococci may also cause infections of joints, resulting in one type of arthritis.

The care given children's throats and the removal of badly diseased tonsils and teeth in both children and adults probably diminish the number of streptococcal infections of the heart valves.

---

[6]Latin, *puer*, child; *parere*, to bear; give birth to.

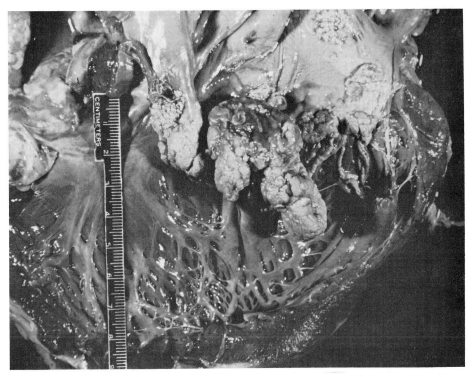

Figure 28–3

Endocarditis due to *Streptococcus faecalis* from the intestine. The heart has been cut open and we look into the left auricle and ventricle. On the leaflets of the mitral valve and the wall of the auricle are irregular, granular clusters of inflammatory tissue called "vegetations." These heal leaving nodules of scar tissue, which causes deformities of the valves that prevent their closure or narrow the opening, with resulting defective circulation. (Robbins, S. L.: Pathology. 3rd Ed. Philadelphia, W. B. Saunders Co., 1967.)

Infections by β-Type Hemolytic Streptococci

CAPSULES OF STREPTOCOCCI. Beta type hemolytic streptococci are frequently encapsulated, especially in infectious material such as pus, exudate, or sputum. These capsules may be stained or they may be demonstrated by mixing the material containing them with a little India ink and observing them under the microscope (Fig. 4–5). As mentioned previously, these capsules contribute to infectivity.

SEROLOGIC GROUPS.[7] The beta type hemolytic streptococci can be divided into several groups (often called Lancefield groups, after their discoverer) on the basis of *carbohydrate* antigenic substances contained in the cell walls of the cocci. For example, the cell walls of all group A streptococci contain a certain complex, group-distinguishing carbohydrate antigen in common; group B streptococci contain another group-distinctive carbohydrate antigen, and so on through groups C, D, E, F, G, to O. It is an easy matter to make these distinctions by means of the pre-

---

[7]Distinguish clearly between the Greek α and β (alpha and beta), which refer to *types as determined on blood-agar plates*, and the Roman capitals A, B, C, and so on, used to designate serologic groups of *beta type* hemolytic streptococci.

cipitin test. It is re-emphasized that, with few exceptions, Lancefield's groupings apply only to beta type streptococci. The term beta type streptococci of group A (or even "group A streptococci") is virtually synonymous with *Streptococcus pyogenes*, the most dangerous of the beta hemolytic streptococci.

The outstanding value of this means of differentiation lies in the fact that group A streptococci cause serious, acute human diseases such as scarlet fever, erysipelas, septicemia, puerperal sepsis, and so on. Most group B streptococci are entirely harmless to man, but they cause mastitis in cattle. Groups C and G cocci cause infections of man such as tonsillitis, sinusitis, and similar conditions, but these are usually not as dangerous as scarlet fever and other group A diseases. Group D streptococci are of minor importance as pathogens, occurring only among the intestinal streptococci or enterococci. The other groups need not concern us here.

Serologic Types of Group A.   Group A streptococci are further divided into some 50 or more *types*, each containing a different *protein* called an M antigen. These M types are differentiated by precipitin tests and may be still further subdivided within the Group A streptococci by T-agglutination.

The terminology seems a little confusing but may be simplified by thinking of a streptococcus as living in a street (blood-agar type), an apartment house (Lancefield group), an apartment (M-protein type), and in a certain room (T and R[1] antigen types). For example:

Streptococcus pyogenes:
Beta type (blood agar)
  Lancefield group A (carbohydrate antigenic substance)
    Serologic type 14 (M protein antigenic substance).
      Slide agglutination T and R antigen types (have not been correlated with virulence, as have the M types)

Regardless of the serologic differentiations of beta type hemolytic streptococci as a matter of professional information, clinical and nursing procedures will be alike for all, differing only as to whether the streptococci are infecting brain, respiratory tract, peritoneum, parturient uterus, or other area.

Group A hemolytic streptococci produce several extracellular toxins and enzymes that explain the pathogenicity of these streptococci. Some of the products are: Streptolysin S and O; diphosphopyridine nucleotidase; erythrogenic toxins A, B, and C; deoxyribonucleases A, B, C, and D; proteinase; hyaluronidase; streptokinases A and B. There are probably others. Most Lancefield group A strains are susceptible to concentrations of the antibiotic bacitracin that do not inhibit most strains of other groups.

Generally, the susceptibility of the Lancefield Group A streptococci to chemotherapeutic agents is as follows: Group A is quite susceptible to sulfonamides but may become resistant, and tetracycline-resistance is about 20 per cent; Groups B and C are moderately susceptible to antibiotics and sulfonamides; Group D, resistant to sulfonamides and tetracyclines, is susceptible to streptomycin and most penicillins.

CELLULITIS.   This is an infection of the skin and underlying tissues and is one of the most dangerous conditions caused by beta type streptococci. The group A cocci give rise to a very severe, rapidly spreading infection, often with much swelling, attended by marked general symptoms

---

[1] R surface antigens are found in M protein types 2, 3, 28 and 48, but not in type 14.

due to potent exotoxins. The infection spreads in subcutaneous and lymphatic tissues. The "red streaks" often seen developing up the arm or leg from a focus of streptococcal infection represent spreading of the infection via lymphatics (lymphangitis). These conditions require immediate medical attention. *Erysipelas* is another form of acute infection of the skin and underlying tissues due to beta type streptococci of group A. It can be rapidly progressive and is frequently fatal unless promptly treated.

The streptococci may enter the tissues through a very tiny break in the skin; for example, when a pathologist pricks his finger through a rubber glove while performing an autopsy on a corpse that harbors a streptococcal infection.

Streptococcal impetigo cannot be distinguished clinically from staphylococcal impetigo. They are inflammatory skin diseases. It is best to remove the crusts that form over the pustular lesions and to keep the skin clean with soap and water to clear up superficial infections.

Beta type hemolytic streptococci of groups A, C, and G may also cause severe *tonsillitis* (*septic sore throat*), and are frequently present in the healthy nose and throat, hence their inclusion in the group of respiratory pathogens. Like staphylococci, they sometimes invade the blood, causing "blood poisoning" (septicemia), and are often found in infections of the lungs (*pneumonia* and *empyema*), *meningitis*, *sinusitis*, and *mastoiditis*.

Fortunately, infections by beta type hemolytic streptococci are efficiently controlled by most of the broad-spectrum antibiotics. Fatalities due to these bacteria are consequently much less common now than before the discoveries of antibiotics.

RHEUMATIC HEART DISEASE.   A very serious and widespread disease called rheumatic fever, with resulting heart disease that often cripples and frequently kills, is related to infection with Group A hemolytic streptococci. Rheumatic heart disease is one of the principal causes of death and disability from infectious disease in the United States. It is probable that allergy toward Group A hemolytic streptococci is the real underlying cause. Relapses (reinfections by the streptococci causing the allergy) in rheumatic fever patients may be, in large part, prevented by special treatment schedules with sulfonamide drugs or antibiotics to prevent repeated reinfections with group A streptococci.

Antistreptolysin in Rheumatic Fever.   The hemolytic toxins (streptolysins) of group A streptococci are of two sorts: streptolysin S, unstable in the presence of heat and acids, and streptolysin O, unstable in oxygen. Streptolysin O is strongly antigenic. In persons infected with group A streptococci, antibodies to streptolysin O are generally found and easily measured. The measurement (titration) of antibodies against streptolysin O, especially when the titer rises sharply over a period of two weeks or so during or after an illness such as sore throat, affords not only a valuable diagnostic test but also a measure of the reaction of the patient. Well over 80 per cent of rheumatic fever patients have a considerable titer of antistreptolysin O.

PUERPERAL INFECTION.   Beta type hemolytic streptococci may be carried into the parturient uterus in one or more of the following ways: from the skin or external parts that have been insufficiently cleansed, on contaminated dressings or instruments, on the hands of the doctor or nurse if hands have not been carefully disinfected, especially if the doctor or nurse is a carrier of hemolytic streptococci, a common situation. Such infections are preventable in practically every case. Formerly the cause of as high as 50 per cent postpartum mortality due to "childbed fever," streptococcal puerperal fever is now very uncommon, thanks to clean obstetric techniques (remember the pioneer work of Ignaz Semmelweis, 1818–1865) and antibiotics; however, infections sometimes develop when labor has been complicated and operative interference is necessary. A woman should, if possible, go to a hospital to have a baby, because there are better facilities for treating any emergencies that may arise, and it is easier to carry out aseptic technique there than in the home.

Puerperal fever and *erysipelas* patients should be isolated to prevent the spread of the infection to other patients. The discharges, packs, and bandages are highly infectious. The recent postpartum patient has an open wound in the uterus and in some instances in the vagina and perineum. These are all very good portals of entry for streptococci, staphylococci, and other microorganisms. Nurses, doctors, and other personnel should not be allowed to care for obstetric or indeed any patients if these staff members have sore noses or throats. Personnel who have infectious lesions anywhere are real hazards to all patients.

BRONCHOPNEUMONIA.   This is a serious complication of other diseases. Often it determines a fatal outcome in patients weakened by other disease. Bronchopneumonia may be caused by one or more of a variety of organisms, common among which are staphylococci and alpha and beta type hemolytic streptococci. Several species of microorganisms that can cause bronchopneumonia are usually in the patient's own mouth and often gain entrance to the lungs by accidental inhalation of saliva and mucus, as during surgical anesthesia.

Organisms that can cause bronchopneumonia are found in large numbers in the droplets of sputum or saliva given off by normal persons talking, sneezing, or coughing. It is evident that patients who are especially likely to develop bronchopneumonia, that is, those having chronic diseases or passing through acute diseases, must be protected from both the bacteria in their own mouths and those from visitors. This involves special efforts to keep the mouth clean, the same nursing precautions in bronchopneumonia as in lobar pneumonia, great care to prevent carrying bacteria from one patient to another, and the exclusion of all but necessary visitors and especially of persons (including medical and hospital personnel) having respiratory infections.

SCARLET FEVER AND SEPTIC SORE THROAT.   Within recent years in the United States, these streptococcal diseases have declined greatly in frequency and severity. This is due, in part, to sanitation of dairy products. These diseases usually occur in epidemics, and formerly were often traceable to unpasteurized milk from cows having mastitis due to Group A streptococci introduced into the cow or her milk by infected milkers. Pasteurization kills the streptococci. Septic sore throat and scarlet fever are really different manifestations of the same infection. Some strains of Group A streptococci form a toxin that produces the rash seen in scarlet fever. Once a person becomes immune to this *erythrogenic* (rash-producing) toxin, he is no longer subject to rash but may still contract infection with Group A streptococci of some other M-antigen type. The infection then develops without rash and therefore is called by different names, a common one being septic sore throat, or "strep throat."

Hence, although scarlet fever is not common in adults, most of whom have some immunity to the erythrogenic toxin, septic sore throat may occur in persons of any age. The desquamation or scaling of scarlet fever is not seen in persons with septic sore throat, since it is due to the erythrogenic toxin. Usually, in an epidemic of septic sore throat, cases of scarlet fever occur; the same streptococci cause both conditions. Not infrequently, in severe cases, the cocci invade the blood. This is usually a sign of waning resistance.

An antitoxin for the scarlet fever rash, analogous in principle to other antitoxins, is sometimes used in the treatment of scarlet fever in the same manner as diphtheria antitoxin is in diphtheria. It neutralizes the erythrogenic toxin but does not kill streptococci. There is also a test (the *Dick test*) that shows who is susceptible to the erythrogenic toxin, and a toxoid for giving active artificial immunity against the erythrogenic toxin. Neither is now very widely used. Similar substances and procedures are used in diphtheria and tetanus, as explained farther on. A diagnostic skin test, based on the Schultz-Charlton reaction, is sometimes made by injecting into the skin of a patient with a rash a small dose of scarlet fever antitoxin. If the rash is due to scarlet fever, it promptly fades or is *blanched*, the "blanching reaction."

Transmission. In mode of transmission from person to person, scarlet fever is an excellent model of most diseases of the upper respiratory tract and may well be discussed in detail. The scarlet fever (and septic sore throat) patient can spread the streptococci from the time of the very first symptoms, and even earlier, and he remains infectious for a considerable but indefinite time after recovery, two to four weeks or months. The vectors are *saliva* and *mucus* from mouth and nose. These are nearly always present on any patient's hands and face to some degree. The dangers of handshaking and of kissing (alas!) are only too obvious.

Convalescents who are released from isolation too soon may transmit the disease since they may remain convalescent carriers for weeks or months. A patient can spread the disease as long as there is any discharge from the nose, ears, or any other part of the body containing the streptococci. Patients with streptococcal infections can be made noninfectious within 24 hours by treatment with penicillin. This is not necessarily a cure and may have to be repeated or a different antibiotic used if the streptococci are penicillin-resistant.

Like many other communicable diseases, scarlet fever and septic sore throat are spread also by healthy carriers and by persons with mild, unrecognized cases, who sometimes exhibit minimal symptoms, e.g., only a slight sore throat or a temperature associated with a faint rash. These infected individuals keep the disease alive in a community and are the starting points of epidemics. The health workers, and especially intelligent and well-informed teachers, are always on the watch for these overlooked cases. A good method of finding such cases, as well as epidemics of many other diseases, is follow-up work by the school nurse in investigating absent pupils. This discloses children with mild cases of a variety of childhood diseases who have not been seen by a physician.

Prevention

As has been indicated, the discharges from any lesion infected with streptococci (or, indeed, with any infectious organisms) are highly dangerous, as the organisms can be transferred to clean wounds, scratches, cuts, the postpartum mother, and possibly to normal mucous membranes such as nose, throat, and eyes. Not only is this so, but pathogens fresh from the body are particularly virulent. Dressings from all septic wounds, including those infected with streptococci, should be adequately wrapped, securely fastened, and burned. Any instruments or objects contaminated by such wounds should be sterilized or at least well disinfected by boiling or with chemicals.

In streptococcal infections such as erysipelas, septic sore throat, scarlet fever, and puerperal fever, the portal of entry and the portal of exit must be remembered and considered. The exudate from erysipelas lesions is very dangerous. The nose and throat secretions of a patient who has septic sore throat or scarlet fever are highly infectious through almost any portal of entry. All these secretions should be received into paper "wipes" or gauze and discarded in a plastic bag at the bedside. The bag should be discarded daily or more frequently, if necessary, by clamping carefully at the top, wrapping in newspaper, securing carefully, and incinerating. Dishes and other objects that have had contact with the mouth or nose should be adequately disinfected.

The Anaerobic Streptococci

These organisms belong to the genus *Peptostreptococcus* and grow only anaerobically or microaerophilically. Many pathogenic conditions affecting the uterus, sinus, ear, etc., are caused by these organisms. They may also produce gangrenous wounds.

Diplococcus pneumoniae

Pneumococci are gram-positive, encapsulated cocci that occur characteristically in pairs. The capsule is a particularly distinctive part of pneumococci and confers on them three important properties: smoothness of colony form (S), antigenic type specificity similar to M-type specificity of streptococci, and virulence. Without the capsule, pneumococci are in the R (rough) phase, have little or no virulence, and have no antigenic type specificity. Pneumococci often grow in chains and are, in fact, a kind of streptococci. They grow best on blood or serum at 37 C under the same conditions as other streptococci and, like streptococci, are quickly killed by boiling and by common disinfectants. In blood-agar plates they produce the alpha type of reaction, often with considerable hemolysis and cause many of the same kinds of infection as do the Group A hemolytic streptococci. They were originally observed in association with pneumonia, hence their name.

Infections by Pneumococci

LOBAR PNEUMONIA. This is an acute infectious disease most frequently caused by *Diplococcus pneumoniae*. (Note for student: Distinguish carefully between bronchopneumonia and lobar pneumonia.) *Bronchopneumonia* localizes in scattered patches throughout the lungs and may be caused by a wide variety of organisms, including not only the staphylococci and streptococci but also *Klebsiella pneumoniae*, a gram-negative short rod. *Lobar pneumonia* derives its name from the fact that one or more entire lobes of the lung become infected. It is most often caused by the pneumo-coccus; however, various streptococci and Friedländer's pneumobacillus (*Klebsiella pneumoniae*) also sometimes cause lobar pneumonia. Formerly one of the leading causes of death, lobar pneumonia now causes fewer deaths, partly because of the use of antibiotics.

The pneumococci cause not only lobar pneumonia, but like group A streptococci, they may also invade: the pleural cavity, causing empyema; the meninges, causing meningitis; and the peritoneal cavity, causing peritonitis; in addition, they sometimes also cause puerperal sepsis, sinusi-tis, and septicemia. *Diplococcus pneumoniae* is found in the saliva and sputum of patients with lobar pneumonia and also occurs in normal persons.

SEROLOGIC TYPES OF PNEUMOCOCCI.   Extensive studies of pneu-mococci have shown that, like group A streptococci, they may be divided into over 80 serologic types, called types I, II, III, and so on.

These types, like those of group A hemolytic streptococci, are differ-entiated by serologic methods, all of which depend on the fact that the capsules of pneumococci contain an antigenic substance (*soluble specific substance*, SSS, or *capsular polysaccharide*, as it is sometimes called) that is chemically different in each type. Each type of capsular polysaccharide calls forth specific antibodies (precipitins and agglutinins) against itself. Formerly an important diagnostic procedure in preparation for type-specific serum therapy, determination of type or "typing" is now rarely done because of reliance on chemotherapy.

IDENTIFICATION OF PNEUMOCOCCI.   Pneumococci are bile-soluble (Fig. 28–1). Optochin (Taxo P Sensi-Disks) disks on blood agar produce a zone of inhibition on a pneumococcus lawn after 8 hours of incubation at 37° C., but no inhibition of streptococci. Most pneumococci typically ferment the carbohydrate inulin with acid (no gas) production. In addition, mice injected with virulent pneumococci die within 24 hours. Finally, the Neufeld quellung reaction is a test for the identification of the pneumo-coccal types; the antiserum used causes "specific" swelling (Ger., *Quellung*) of the capsules, which may easily be seen under the microscope.

TRANSMISSION.   There are three chief sources from which lobar pneumonia is spread: the sputum and saliva of pneumonia patients, of convalescent carriers, and of healthy carriers. Another important vector is infected dust (droplet nuclei, and so on). Pneumococci are quite resistant to drying and have been found in the dust of houses in which cases of pneumonia had occurred. The same remarks apply to streptococcal and staphylococcal infections, diphtheria, and tuberculosis.

Prevention

The care of the patient with lobar pneumonia has changed markedly with the use of sulfonamides and antibiotics because the infectious stage of the disease has been considerably decreased with these drugs. A case of lobar pneumonia caused by a strain of organisms susceptible to these drugs is likely to be noninfectious after 48 hours of adequate antibiotic therapy.

Although lobar pneumonia is probably most frequently transmitted by droplet infection, the use of masks for the protection of medical at-tendants has been almost entirely abandoned. The organisms causing lobar pneumonia are found so frequently in the respiratory secretions of apparently healthy individuals that emphasis is now placed on maintaining good general hygiene (rest, adequate diet, and so on) as offering better overall protection than the doubtful procedure of wearing a mask.

The Respiratory Neisseria

The genus *Neisseria* is named for the German physician Neisser, who in 1879 discovered the gonococcus (*Neisseria gonorrhoeae*), the cause of gonorrhea.[8] The gonococcus is, of course, not associated with the respiratory tract but with the genital tract and the venereal disease gonorrhea. It is unique among *Neisseria* in that it is the only species not characteristically found in the upper respiratory tract; however, it is so much like the respiratory *Neisseria* that the gonococcus and the related respiratory species are distinguishable only by special laboratory tests. We shall therefore describe the gonococcus with the respiratory *Neisseria*, reserving discussion of gonorrhea to Part C of this section.

Among the respiratory *Neisseria* there is only one important pathogen: *N. meningitidis*, cause of epidemic spinal meningitis. It is almost exactly like *N. gonorrhoeae* except for habitat.[9] There are several other respiratory tract species of *Neisseria*, all of which are relatively harmless; however, these "harmless" *Neisseria* species sometimes become important because they can cause a gonorrhea-like vulvovaginitis in preadolescent girls and may be confused with the gonococcus.

DISTINCTIVE MORPHOLOGY OF NEISSERIA.   All species of *Neisseria* have the same characteristic appearance when seen with the microscope. The cocci occur in pairs of hemispheres pressed together, with the flat surfaces apposed. Each pair resembles two coffee beans held together.

---

[8]Greek, *gone*, seed or semen: *rhein*, to flow. It was formerly thought that the copious pus formed in acute male gonorrhea was actually a flow of semen, hence the name.

[9]Some cases of meningitis have been ascribed to the gonococcus and some cases of gonorrhea-like disease to meningococci.

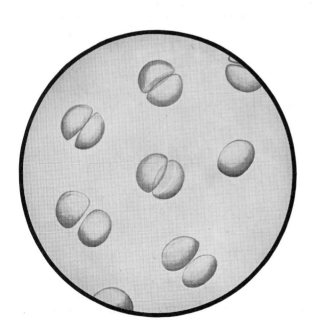

Figure 28–4

Diagrammatic enlargement of *Neisseria gonorrhoeae*. The magnification is in the range of the electron microscope. Note the rounded, hemispheric appearance of each cell of the pairs.

The *Neisseria* species are therefore diplococci (Fig. 28–4). Unlike all other pathogenic cocci they are gram-negative. The pairs are often encapsulated.

PHYSIOLOGIC PROPERTIES. All species of this genus, except *N. gonorrhoeae* and *N. meningitidis,* can grow well on ordinary laboratory media, without blood or serum, at room temperature, and exposed to air. The gonococci and meningococci require a 37 C temperature and special culture media containing heated blood and special nutrients adapted for their growth. Their growth is best in a moist atmosphere containing about 10 per cent carbon dioxide. Thus the two major pathogens are readily distinguished from the lesser ones.

THE OXIDASE REACTION. Colonies of any species of *Neisseria* on "chocolate agar" (blood agar heated at 90 C for ten minutes) are small, watery, and not very distinctive. They may be made quite conspicuous, however, by moistening the growth on the agar with a 1 per cent solution of an *oxidase* indicator, tetramethyl-paraphenylene-diamine. This turns first red, then black, in contact with oxidase-producing colonies, among which *Neisseria* species are outstanding (Fig. 28–5). (Compare with the tetrazolium test for *Corynebacterium diphtheriae,* page 421.

Unlike other species of *Neisseria,* gonococci and meningococci have little resistance to heat, light, drying, or disinfectants, and die quickly outside the body. When kept moist and protected from light, they *may* live on sheets, clothing, or in pus for several hours, but they *rarely* do so. They are easily killed by chemicals containing silver, and hence silver-containing drugs like silver nitrate, Argyrol, or Protargol are often used in gonorrheal infections, especially for the destruction of gonococci in the eye (see gonorrheal ophthalmia). Other ordinary disinfectants are quite effective in disinfecting hands, clothing, and utensils that might be contaminated with either of these organisms. Both, especially the gonococcus, are sensitive to penicillin, although many strains, especially those imported from Vietnam, are now resistant.

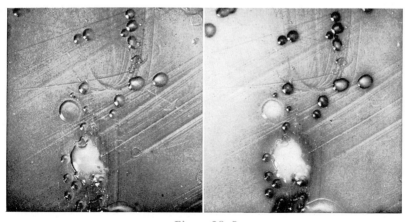

Figure 28–5

The oxidase test for the identification of meningococcus (or any *Neisseria*) colonies. Mixed culture on blood agar. *Left,* colonies of meningococci and contaminants before the application of tetramethyl-*p*-phenylene-diamine solution. *Right,* the same colonies after the application of the reagent. Note that the meningococcus colonies (dark) show the development of color first about the edges, and also a slight discoloration of the medium. (×5). (Burrows: Textbook of Microbiology, 19th Ed. 1968, Philadelphia, W. B. Saunders Co.)

The Meningococcus

The meningococcus, *Neisseria meningitidis*, was previously called *Neisseria intracellularis*. It is the most dangerous pathogen among the upper respiratory *Neisseria*. There are several immunologic groups and types of *N. meningitidis:* type I, type II, type II alpha, and group IV (or types A, B, C, D). Type specificity resides, as in pneumococci, in the chemical nature of the polysaccharide capsular substance. Type I (Group A) type organisms cause the major epidemics.

N. meningitidis causes a very dangerous and often fatal inflammation of the coverings (meninges) of the brain and spinal cord. The disease is called epidemic cerebrospinal meningitis or cerebrospinal fever. *N. meningitidis* is very pyogenic, and in this resembles the gonococcus. The anaerobic organisms in the genus *Veillonella* may also occur in pairs; these parasites occur also in the respiratory tract or genitourinary structures of man, but they are probably nonpathogens.

MENINGOCOCCUS MENINGITIS.   Since this disease, like influenza, is transmitted by respiratory secretions, it usually occurs in epidemics, and is therefore often called *epidemic meningitis.* This form of meningitis should be differentiated from sporadically occurring cases of meningitis, which frequently are caused by blood-borne streptococci, pneumococci, tubercle bacilli, *Salmonella,* and numerous other bacteria, usually secondary to other severe infections. Such cases of meningitis never occur as epidemics.

Epidemic meningitis occurs in persons of all ages and sexes and is spread chiefly by the oral and nasal secretions and droplets of sputum of *carriers.* In many outbreaks the mode of transmission is obscure, but obviously requires fairly close contact (as in very crowded rooms) since the meningococci die quickly outside the body. The carrier rate (i.e., number of persons among each 1000 who carry the cocci) in some population groups, such as military organizations, may be as high as 50 per cent, and yet morbidity (illness) rates may be only 2 to 5 per cent, indicating a high rate of spread but a low degree of susceptibility of persons in general, or low virulence of the meningococci being spread. Virulence, however, apparently may suddenly increase, causing a serious epidemic. The connection between cases is sometimes impossible to trace, as is true of all infections spread by carriers. Persons directly associated with a patient (e.g., doctors, nurses, and the patient's family) contract the disease only infrequently, although they often become carriers.

Meningococcal meningitis is particularly serious in children. Of the 3,000 to 4,000 cases reported in the United States yearly and the 30,000 to 80,000 cases in epidemics, more than 50 per cent of the cases are in children under five years of age.

Since penicillin has not eradicated the carrier state and prevention is preferable to treatment, a vaccine that would give protection against *Neisseria meningitidis* would be a great discovery. Such a vaccine which is reported to have reduced the attack rate in large-scale field trials among military recruits by 87 per cent has been developed. Cell wall polysaccharides of the three major serogroups (A, B, and C) were isolated. Group A and C polysaccharides were found to be antigenic in man. Group C polysaccride was used in the above-mentioned field trials. Should the meningococcal polysaccharides prove effective in the general population

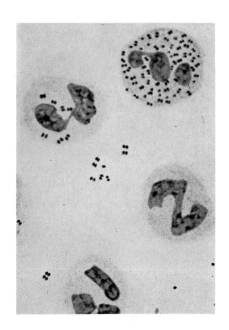

Figure 28–6

Meningococci in spinal fluid stained by Gram's method. The leucocytes have engulfed (phagocytized) large numbers of the diplococci. (Ford: Bacteriology.)

they might serve as models for the future development of vaccines against other infectious diseases.

The meningococcus enters the body via the nasopharynx. In many instances, the meningococci remain localized in the nasopharynx, producing no symptoms whatever, or no more than a rhinitis with purulent discharge. Such cases are regarded as mere "colds," or "catarrh," and probably serve to infect many persons. Once localized in the nasopharynx, the cocci may proceed no further, which appears to be the usual event, or they may invade the blood. The disease is known to be frequently a *septicemia* in its early stages, and blood-broth cultures are often positive for the meningococci. In many instances the organisms invade no farther than the blood. Probably only a small percentage of blood infections result in meningitis.

DIAGNOSIS. In any case in which there is a suspicion of meningitis, it is of extreme importance to make a lumbar puncture very early. The diagnosis is made, or confirmed, usually from a gram-stained smear of the *centrifuged sediment* of the spinal fluid. The organisms are found in the phagocytes and exactly resemble gonococci (Figs. 28–6 and 35–4). Cultures may also be made, in the same manner as for gonococci, using the spinal fluid sediment. The results of cultures are too slow in preparation to be of value for immediate diagnosis and therapy in such rapidly progressive diseases as any form of bacterial meningitis.

THERAPY. Because sulfadiazine was highly effective, both for oral prophylaxis and intravenous therapy in meningococcal meningitis, it was very widely used until most strains of meningococci became resistant to it, necessitating the use of antibiotics like parenteral penicillin or, in penicillin-sensitive patients, broad-spectrum antibiotics like the tetracyclines or chloramphenicol. None of these is as effective as sulfadiazine.

Prevention

The precautions in cerebrospinal meningitis are those observed in dealing with all infections transmitted by the oral and nasal secretions. The same precautions are used as in dealing with pneumonia or scarlet fever.

Supplementary Reading

Andersen, A. A., and Andersen, M. R.: A monitor for airborne bacteria. *Appl. Microbiol.*, 1962, *10:*181.

Blair, J. E., Lennette, E. H., and Truant, J. P.: Manual of Clinical Microbiology. 1970, Bethesda, Md., Williams & Wilkins Co.

Casman, E. P.: Staphylococcal food poisoning. *Health Lab. Sci.*, 1967, *4:*199.

Davis, B. D., Dulbecco, R., Eisen, H. N., Ginsberg, H., and Wood, W. B., Jr.: Microbiology. 1967, New York, Hoeber Medical Division, Harper & Row, Publishers.

Donnely, C. B., Leslie, J. E., and Black, L. A.: Production of enterotoxin in milk. Appl. Microbiol., 1968, *16:*917.

Goldschneider, I.: Vaccination against meningococcal meningitis. *Connecticut Medicine*, 1970, *34:*335.

Guyton, H. G., and Decker, H. M.: Respiratory protection provided by five new contagion masks. *Appl. Microbiol.*, 1963, *11:*66.

Haque, R.: Identification of staphylococcal hemolysins by an electrophoretic localization technique. *J. Bact.*, 1967, *93:*525.

Ivler, D. (Chairman): The staphylococci: ecologic perspectives. *Ann. N. Y. Acad. Sci.*, 1965, *128*(Art. 1):1.

Kirby, W. M. M. (Chairman): Comparative assessment of the broad spectrum penicillins and other antibiotics. *Ann. N. Y., Acad. Sci.*, 1968, *145*(Art. 2):207.

Klarman, E. G.: Surface disinfection and respiratory ills. *Modern Sanitation*, June, 1954.

Krugman, S., and Ward, R.: Air sterilization in an infants' ward. Effect of triethylene glycol vapor and dust suppressive measures on the respiratory cross infection rate. *J.A.M.A.*, 1951, *145:*775.

MacLeod, C. M.: The pneumococci. In: Bacterial and Mycotic Infections of Man. 4th Ed. 1965, Philadelphia, J. B. Lippincott Co.

Morse, J. R.: Pericarditis as a complication of meningococcal meningitis. *Ann. Intern. Med.*, 1971, *74:*212.

Orth, D. S., and Anderson, A. W.: Polymyxin-coagulase-deoxyribonuclease-agar: a selective isolation medium for *Staphylococcus aureus.* Appl. Microbiol., 1970, *20:*508.

Riley, R. L., and O'Grady, F.: Airborne Infection: Transmission and Control. 1962, New York, The Macmillan Co.

Sanborn, W. R.: The relation of surface contamination to the transmission of disease. *Amer. J. Public Health*, 1963, *53:*1278.

Shinefield, H. R., and Ribble, J. C.: Current aspects of infections and diseases related to *Staphylococcus aureus.* Ann. Rev. Med., 1965, *162:*63.

Staphylococcus symposium. *Amer. J. Public Health*, 1962, *52:*1796, 1810, 1818, 1828.

Subcommittee on Taxonomy of Staphylococci and Micrococci. Recommendation. Int. Bull. Bacteriol. Nomencl. Taxon, 1965, *15:*109–110.

Top, F. H., et al. (Eds.): Control of Infectious Diseases in General Hospitals. 1967, New York, American Public Health Association.

Vedros, N. A., and Culver, G.: A new serological troup (E) of *Neisseria meningitidis.* J. Bact., 1968, *95:*1300.

Wentworth, B. B.: Bacteriophage typing of the staphylococci. Bacteriol. Rev., 1963, *27:*253.

Diphtheria

29

[handwritten notes: "review acid fast staining technique" and "stain"]

CORYNEBACTERIUM DIPHTHERIAE

Corynebacterium[1] *diphtheriae*, the bacterium that causes diphtheria,[2] is characteristically confined to the respiratory tract. Unlike streptococci, staphylococci, and pneumococci, which may infect many parts of the body, it is rarely found in any other part of the body.[3] Its mode of transmission is representative of respiratory pathogens in general. Formerly one of the most important causes of death in all parts of the world, diphtheria is now much less significant, especially in the United States. Because diphtheria illustrates many important principles, it will be discussed in some detail. Diphtheria bacilli were discovered in 1883–84 by two German physicians, Klebs and Loeffler, in bacteriologic specimens from the throats of patients. These bacilli are therefore sometimes spoken of as Klebs-Loeffler or K-L bacilli.

PHYSIOLOGIC CHARACTERISTICS. *C. diphtheriae* is nonmotile and does not form spores. As a nonspore-former, it is easily killed by commercial pasteurization (63 C for 30 minutes) or exposure to 60 C or over for ten minutes; however, it survives drying and exposure to light better than many nonspore-bearing pathogenic organisms and can be disseminated in dust.

The bacilli are easily killed by standard disinfectants. A few hours of exposure to direct sunlight kills most *nonspore-forming* pathogenic bacteria, including *C. diphtheriae*.

MORPHOLOGIC CHARACTERISTICS. These gram-positive bacilli have an especially characteristic appearance when stained with slightly alkaline *methylene blue* (Loeffler's stain). When thus stained, the bacilli are

---

[1]Greek, *koryne*, club. Club-shaped rods are one of the numerous distinctive forms of diphtheria bacilli.

[2]Greek, *diphthera*, membrane. This refers to the distinctive, membrane-like film (pseudomembrane) formed in typical cases of diphtheria.

[3]During World War II it caused serious trouble to soldiers in Burma by infecting cutaneous ulcers (cutaneous diphtheria). Vulvovaginal diphtheria may also occur.

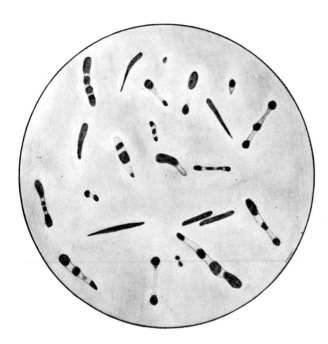

Figure 29–1

Corynebacterium diphtheriae (drawing from pure cultures). These have been stained with Loeffler's alkaline methylene blue solution. Note the great variation in length, the pleomorphism, and the volutin arranged as bars and granules and sometimes filling the entire cell. (× approx. 2500.)

seen to be very pleomorphic, sometimes being slender, pointed, and curved, with deep blue or reddish purple granules of *volutin*[4] at the ends and often several transverse bars. In laboratory cultures four hours old or more, the bacilli usually assume curious shapes, often resembling clubs, hence their generic name. Sometimes, because of volutin granules at the ends, they resemble dumbbells and exclamation points (Fig. 29–1). These morphologic and staining peculiarities are very useful in making bacteriologic diagnoses of diphtheria.

LABORATORY DIAGNOSIS.   The bacilli grow well aerobically in the laboratory at 35 C on Loeffler's medium[5] and on blood or serum agar (or broth) with glucose. In making diagnostic throat cultures on these media, a sterile swab is rubbed gently over tonsils or white patches in the patient's throat and the swab is then rubbed on the surface of Loeffler's medium in culture tubes or on Pai's medium.[6] These cultures are incubated at about 35 C and examined microscopically after about four hours and again after eight, 18, and 24 hours. When smeared on a slide, stained with methylene blue, and examined with a microscope, the diphtheria bacilli in the cultures are usually seen to be mixed with other microorganisms, which also grow on these rich media unless a *selectively inhibitory* substance, potassium tellurite (KTe), is added. Mixed or pure, the distinctive diphtheria bacilli may usually be recognized by a skilled bacteriologist. Hence it is usually possible to tell within four to 24 hours from the time a throat culture is started whether diphtheria-like bacilli are present in a patient's throat.

---

[4]Volutin is a complex metaphosphate, probably stored food reserve. It is commonly associated with nucleic acids and occurs in many species of bacteria. It stains very intensely with basic dyes.

[5]Heat-coagulated serum containing 20 per cent of 5 per cent glucose infusion broth.

[6]Coagulated egg.

PURE CULTURES.   Pure cultures of *C. diphtheriae*, which are necessary for conclusive diagnosis, may be isolated from primary Loeffler cultures or directly from throat swabs by spreading the material on blood or serum agar containing KTe. KTe not only inhibits much contaminating growth but is reduced to a dense black color by colonies of *C. diphtheriae*. The colonies on tellurite medium are greyish-black or metal-grey, without a sheen. On Tinsdale's medium there is a brownish-black halo. In the absence of KTe, the colonies may be recognized by treating them with a solution of a tetrazolium salt, which is reduced first to a distinctive color and then to black. The tetrazolium test is analogous to the oxidase test used in identifying colonies of *Neisseria* in the diagnosis of meningitis or gonorrhea (Chapters 28 and 35). *C. diphtheriae* is catalase positive, reduces nitrate to nitrite and is gelatine and urea negative. Acid is produced from glucose and maltose in 48 hours, but sucrose is rarely fermented.

THROAT CULTURES.   The procedure in preparing diagnostic throat cultures, whether for *C. diphtheriae* or for other microorganisms, is identical. The culture medium, which must be appropriate for the organisms to be cultured, must be moist and fresh and the tube properly labeled with the patient's name, the date, and the hour. If the patient has been on antibiotic therapy or sulfonamides within five days, this information should be sent to the laboratory with the culture, since these drugs may inhibit growth in the cultures.

Pathogenesis of Diphtheria

Typically, diphtheria commences as an acute inflammation of the pharynx caused by the diphtheria bacillus. The organisms are almost entirely lacking in aggressiveness. They usually remain localized in the tonsils,[7] if present, and in the upper respiratory mucous membranes. There the bacilli secrete an exotoxin comparable in deadliness to the exotoxins of *Clostridium botulinum* and *Cl. tetani*, all of which are much more poisonous than cobra venom.

The exotoxin irritates the tissues, which give forth a fibrinous exudate that coagulates into a tough, leathery, greyish white *pseudomembrane*. This is not always present or typical in color or consistency. This membrane, along with swelling due to inflammation, may occlude the air passages, especially if the larynx is invaded (laryngeal diphtheria). Death may be caused mechanically by asphyxiation in a few hours unless the obstructed larynx is bypassed by inserting an air tube into the trachea from the outside (*tracheotomy*). Other serious symptoms, and often death, arise from the effect of the toxin on the heart muscle (myocarditis and sudden "heart failure"), nerves (paralysis), kidneys (nephritis with albuminuria), and adrenal cortex (circulatory failure).

When bacilli grow on the tonsils and walls of the throat (pharynx) of a susceptible person, they cause the usual (pharyngeal) form of diphtheria. The organisms may grow also in the nose, producing *nasal diphtheria*, and in the larynx, causing what used to be known as "membranous croup," but what is now generally called *laryngeal diphtheria*.

In children under five years, diphtheria is likely to be more severe than in older children or in adults. A considerable percentage of deaths

---

[7]Presence of tonsils greatly predisposes to the harboring and carrying of diphtheria bacilli, hemolytic streptococci, and other pathogens.

from the disease occur in children under five years. The number of cases of diphtheria and also of other contagious diseases of children usually rises in the fall because bringing the children together in school increases opportunities for infection, and also because fall and winter are the seasons of various infections of the nose and throat, which may allow diphtheria bacilli to become established. Some cases may occur at any season, although in the United States the disease is now rare, largely due to active artificial immunization with toxoid. In 1971, only 215 cases were reported, of which 106 occurred in the 5 to 9 year old age group.

The disease is not confined to childhood; cases may also occur in older persons of all ages, including doctors, nurses and other members of the health team who have not taken proper precautions.

Transmission of Diphtheria

Diphtheria, typical of diseases of the respiratory tract, is spread by means of the *saliva* and *nasal discharges;* by direct contact, as in kissing; by coughing into another's face; or, as is frequently the case with children, by articles that go directly from the mouth of one child to that of another, such as pencils, "pop" bottles, or drinking cups. Fingers may also carry the bacilli. These methods of transmission convey all sorts of microorganisms of the upper respiratory tract. *C. diphtheriae* may live quite a long time in saliva and mucus deposited on dishes, tableware, and toys. Bits of the fibrinous pseudomembrane that forms in the diphtheria patient's throat may be thrown out in coughing and dry on the furniture or floor. In such fragments of membrane the bacilli may remain alive for weeks and be distributed as dust. Oral and nasal mucus, or exudate from sores in noses or on lips of patients also contain the bacilli.

CARRIERS.   Diphtheria carriers were the first kind discovered, and much of our knowledge of carriers in general has come from the study of diphtheria. There are three kinds of carriers of diphtheria bacilli: (1) convalescents, (2) those who have contact with diphtheria patients, and (3) those who are not known to have had any association with the disease (so-called "casual carriers").

Convalescents.   Convalescents usually get rid of the bacilli in a few days or weeks, but in some cases the bacilli may remain in the throat and nose for a long time after the patient has recovered. In about 5 per cent of the cases they persist for two months, and in about 1 per cent they remain indefinitely. Most health departments require two or three negative cultures (that is, cultures that do not show the diphtheria bacillus) from both the throat and nose, taken at intervals of 24 to 48 hours, before a patient may be released from isolation.

ANTIBIOTICS AND RELEASE CULTURES.   In addition to antitoxin, many physicians administer antibiotics to patients with diphtheria, often before a diagnosis has been made. Although antibiotics do not neutralize diphtheria toxin, they seem to control growth of other bacteria, such as streptococci and pneumococci, in the throats of diphtheria patients, thus decreasing complications.

These antibiotics may continue to be present in oral and nasal secretions for five days to a week after the last dose. They often suppress growth of diphtheria bacilli in diagnostic or quarantine-release cultures. If the laboratory is informed that the patient has received penicillin, the bacteriologist can eliminate it by the use of penicillinase in the cultures. If the patient has received a sulfonamide drug, PABA is added to the culture media. (Explain these devices.)

Even though a convalescent remains a carrier for a long period, he is much less infectious two weeks after the complete healing of all lesions. Experience shows that such carriers may be readmitted to school without any untoward results.

Contact Carriers.   These may be schoolmates of the patient, members of the family, or persons who have taken care of him. These people may be more dangerous than the patient or convalescent because they go about freely. Contact carriers must observe the same precautions as are taken in actual cases of diphtheria to avoid scattering the bacilli by means of the saliva and nasal secretion.

Casual Carriers.   The third class of carriers, those who have had no known contact with diphtheria cases, are discovered accidentally when routine throat cultures are made. Careful studies have shown that it is the person with the clinical case and his family-contact carriers who are most likely to cause the disease. Healthy children found carrying diphtheria bacilli in the schools seldom give rise to epidemics.

If contact or convalescent carriers are wage earners, it is not absolutely necessary to keep them away from work unless it involves some special danger to others, such as the handling of milk and food, nursing, or the care or teaching of children.

SUBCLINICAL INFECTIONS.   The chief sources of diphtherial infections are carriers and subclinical and missed cases. Diphtheria is not always severe. Many children have mild sore throats not recognized as diphtheria and the infection is ignored. Because of their own resistance they do not succumb, but another child whom they infect may die. The carrier state is usually temporary. Removal of tonsils will often cure the carrier state. In children's wards and schools, health personnel should be on the watch for nasal discharges, especially those that irritate the nostrils or are tinged with blood, as these may be due to the diphtheria bacillus (nasal diphtheria). These are often subclinical infections. Hoarse voice, "croupy" cough, or difficulty in swallowing or breathing should also rouse immediate suspicion of diphtheria.

MILK THAT CAUSES INFECTIONS.   *Corynebacterium diphtheriae* does not change the appearance or taste of milk and grows well in it. The milk may be contaminated somewhere in its course from the cow to the consumer by means of a person with subclinical infection or a carrier. Pasteurization kills diphtheria bacilli, but the milk may become contaminated with the bacilli after it has been pasteurized or homogenized. Also, ice cream made from milk containing the bacilli may cause epidemics although this is now rather rare.

The characteristics of a milk-borne epidemic of any disease (e.g., scarlet fever, enteric infections, and diphtheria) are that the cases break out all at once; that they are all on the route of one milkman, or among the customers of one dairy or firm; and that a majority of the patients are children. Dry milk (powder) is rendered noninfectious by the heat-processing to which it is subjected; evaporated and condensed milks are sterile.

VIRULENCE OF DIPHTHERIA BACILLI.   Only those strains of diphtheria bacilli that are *lysogenic*[8] are virulent; i.e., they are toxigenic.

---

[8]Microorganisms are said to be *lysogenic* when they are carriers of a bacteriophage that does not immediately destroy the carrier cells (a so-called *temperate phage*). Temperate phages often confer new genetic properties (e.g., toxigenicity) on the carrier cells (see Transduction, page 109).

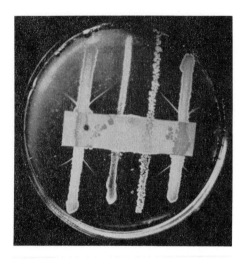

Figure 29–2

The *in vitro* test for toxigenicity. Serum-agar was poured into the dish at about 45 C. Before it hardened, the strip of filter paper, saturated with diphtheria antitoxin, was pressed to the bottom of the agar in the dish. After the agar hardened, it was inoculated on the surface in long streaks at right angles to the paper. As the growth developed, at 37 C, toxin diffused from the culture into the agar. Simultaneously, antitoxin diffused from the paper strip. Where the toxin and antitoxin met in proper concentration for reaction, precipitation occurred. This is seen as thin white lines between the growths of the cultures. This reaction with diphtheria antitoxin is produced only by virulent, i.e., toxigenic, *C. diphtheriae.* (Photo courtesy U.S. Public Health Service, Communicable Disease Center, Atlanta, Ga.)

Virulence may be tested for, in one way, by inoculation of a pure culture of the suspected bacilli into animals. All health departments are prepared to make this test. Guinea pigs, rabbits, and young chicks are often used. Certain characteristic changes are produced that can be recognized by those especially trained in such work.

An alternative method is available that does not utilize animals but is dependent on the production of toxin by the bacilli while growing on a special antitoxin-containing agar. It is called the in vitro toxigenicity test. The presence of diphtheria toxin is made evident by distinct white lines that appear in the agar. The white line is in reality a precipitin reaction between toxin from the growing bacilli and diphtheria antitoxin previously incorporated in the agar (Fig. 29–2).

The Structure of Diphtheria Toxin

Diphtheria toxin consists of two proteins, each with a molecular weight of about 63,000 daltons. One of the proteins consists of intact polypeptide chains, while the other is composed of two fragments (Fragments A and B) linked by at least one disulfide bridge. When treated with low concentration of trypsin, the former (intact toxin) will convert to the latter (nicked toxin) and the toxicity does not change, which indicates that both are toxic. Fragment A alone is not toxic. Linkage to Fragment B is apparently required for toxicity, perhaps to facilitate entry of Fragment A into cells. Treatment of toxin with thiols decreases the toxicity, presumably as a result of dissociation of the nicked fraction into nontoxic Fragments A and B. Toxin is almost devoid of enzymic activity unless treated with thiols. The activity is probably due entirely to Fragment A released upon dissociation of nicked toxin in the presence of thiols. Adsorption of toxin occurs over a wide pH range and does not take place in the absence of salts. Initial binding of toxin to the cell is electrostatic in nature, involving positively charged surface groups No specific receptors are required for the attachment of toxin to cells.

Therapeutic Use of Diphtheria Antitoxin

For therapeutic purposes the dosage of any antitoxin (diphtheria, tetanus, etc.) is determined by the seriousness of the symptoms, the stage of the disease at which treatment is begun, and the age of the patient. The sicker the patient and the later the stage of the disease, the larger the dose must be. It is best given intramuscularly. Only in desperate cases is antitoxin of any kind given intravenously. The antitoxin combines with the toxin circulating in the blood and renders it harmless. It does not repair damage to heart, nerves, and kidneys, once the toxin has combined with the tissues. Severe allergic reactions must be constantly guarded against in administering any serum for any purpose.

THE UNIT OF ANTITOXIN. The potency of diphtheria antitoxin is stated in units. The commercial "unit" of antitoxin is the amount that counteracts slightly over 100 minimal lethal doses (MLD) of diphtheria toxin. An MLD of toxin is the least amount of toxin necessary to kill four of five 250 gram guinea pigs in four to five days. A unit of antitoxin, therefore, neutralizes a little over 100 MLD of toxin. The unit is used for expressing the dosage of antitoxin just as milligrams, cubic centimeters, or milliliters are used for ordinary medicines. Some other units, used mainly in the preparation and testing of commercial diphtheria antitoxin, are shown in Table 29-1. A strong, artificially concentrated diphtheria antitoxin contains from 2000 to 2500 units per ml. The dosage may range from 20,000 to 100,000 units, depending on age, weight, severity of the attack, and time after onset. Similar basic considerations apply in connection with the use of other antitoxins: tetanus, gas gangrene, and so on, though units and dosages may be expressed somewhat differently for each kind of antitoxin.

NECESSITY FOR EARLY DIAGNOSIS AND THERAPY. If sufficient quantities of specific antitoxin are given early in any disease (first day after onset or sooner, if possible), a large percentage of patients with uncomplicated intoxications or infections, including diphtheria, recover (Fig. 29-3). In any infectious or toxic process the effectiveness of serum therapy depends on counteracting the toxin or infectious agent, or both, before the pathogenic agent (toxin or microorganism) has had the opportunity to

Table 29-1.   Units of Diphtheria Toxin and Antitoxin

ALD—The average lethal dose; the same as the LD/50. The dose of toxin that kills *half* of a group of 250-gram guinea pigs in 96 hours.

LoD—The largest amount of toxin that, when mixed with one unit of antitoxin, does not cause symptoms of diphtheria toxication in guinea pigs.

L+D—The least amount of toxin that, when mixed with one unit of antitoxin, kills 250 gram guinea pigs in 96 hours.

MRD—Minimum reaction dose; the highest dilution (i.e., least amount) of toxin that gives a typical skin reaction on intracutaneous injection.

LrD—The highest dilution (i.e., smallest amount) of toxin that, when mixed with one unit of antitoxin, gives a typical skin reaction.

TCID—Tissue culture infective dose.

LfD—The flocculation unit is the amount of toxin that will combine most rapidly with one unit of antitoxin in the in vitro Ramon flocculation test.

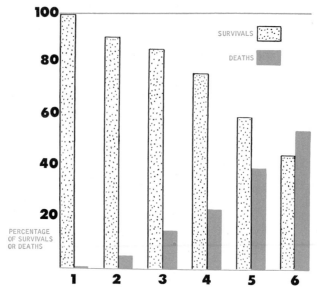

Figure 29–3

Extent to which delay in giving antitoxin decreases chances for survival in diseases due to toxigenic bacteria such as diphtheria bacilli, the food poisoning bacillus *(Clostridium botulinum)*, and the tetanus organism *(Clostridium tetani)*. Prompt diagnosis often depends on proper handling of diagnostic specimens. The percentages given are merely illustrative and may differ greatly in individual instances.

injure the body cells. A few hours lost in beginning treatment may make the difference between life and death. In certain cases of malignant or "bull neck" diphtheria (so called because of the enormously swollen cervical lymph nodes), antitoxin appears to be of no value whatever. The reason for this is not known.

Immunity to Diphtheria

Immunity to diphtheria depends in part on the presence of antitoxin in the blood and in part on the ability of a person to manufacture such antitoxin quickly. This latter ability usually results from previous active immunization by either natural infection or artificial injection of toxoid (primary stimulus). The tissues act as though they have become sensitized (allergic) to diphtheria toxin and bacilli and react very strongly and quickly to any new infection by diphtheria bacilli or to a secondary or "booster" injection of toxoid, thus warding off disease.

NATURAL IMMUNITY. In some urban areas many adults and young children have at least 0.02 unit of antitoxin in their blood as a result of mild or unrecognized (subclinical) infections with *C. diphtheriae* or the action of still obscure natural mechanisms. Such persons are therefore Schick negative (page 428), i.e., immune to the disease, even though exposed to it. In rural areas natural factors of immunization are often much less effective. Infants born of immune mothers usually have maternal antitoxin in their blood for only about three months.

PASSIVE ARTIFICIAL IMMUNITY.   A dose of antitoxin (10,000 units) will usually prevent the development of diphtheria in children below 10 years old and not previously immunized with toxoid, who have been highly exposed to the disease. This is called a prophylactic or preventive dose, but the protection given by it lasts only from two to three weeks. This is a good example of the temporary nature of *passive artificial immunity*. Active immunization with toxoid should be started at the same time.

The use of antitoxin is sometimes followed by serum sickness. This is not due to the antitoxin, but as has been said, is a manifestation of allergy to the proteins in the horse serum containing the antitoxin. The use of horse serum sensitizes the patient, usually for life, to all other antisera derived from horses (for example, to tetanus antitoxin) so that it should not be used prophylactically unless the need is clearly evident.

ACTIVE ARTIFICIAL IMMUNITY.   As previously pointed out, it is possible to stimulate the human body artificially to produce any specific antitoxin by the injection of toxoid made from that toxin. The procedure is commonly used in prophylaxis of diphtheria and also of tetanus (lockjaw).

Fluid Toxoids.   Whether making tetanus toxoid or diphtheria toxoid, these antigens consist primarily of broth culture of the appropriate species of bacteria, filtered to remove the bacteria. The filtrate (filtered broth culture) contains the exotoxin of the bacilli. This is treated with formaldehyde to remove toxicity. Specific antigenicity remains. The product is called "fluid toxoid."

Alum-Precipitated Toxoid.   If alum is added to fluid toxoid it forms a precipitate to which the toxoid is adsorbed and is carried to the bottom of the flask as a white sediment. The supernatant broth is then poured off, leaving the concentrated toxoid in the sediment relatively free from the impurities of the culture broth. The precipitate is resuspended in physiologic saline solution and the milky suspension thus formed is called *alum-precipitated toxoid*, or *toxoid, A.P.*, and is injected after suitable tests for sterility, potency, antigenicity, and nontoxicity.

ACTION OF ALUM-PRECIPITATED TOXOID.   Alum-precipitated toxoid (toxoid, A.P.) is more effective than fluid toxoid because the antigenic stimulus from a deposit of alum toxoid is prolonged. This is because the alum, being insoluble, is not absorbed for some time but remains for days or weeks in the tissues. It slowly and steadily releases the attached toxoid into the blood in a long-continued, antigenic stimulus, simulating actual infection, which is very effective.

Triple Toxoid.   It is now common practice to combine diphtheria and tetanus toxoids (A.P.) and thus accomplish two immunizations with one series of injections. It is also a recommended procedure to include pertussis (whooping cough) vaccine (bacterin) with the two toxoids, in a "triple vaccine" or "triple toxoids." The first injection is given at about three to five months of age, with one or two others after intervals of four to five weeks, another at about one year, and another at entrance to school. Various other injection schedules are also in use; the choice must rest with the physician. The three mixed antigens, tetanus, diphtheria, and pertussis, act better together than any of the three alone. One product has been introduced that also contains Salk (inactivated) poliovirus vaccine. All are very effective.

Primary and Secondary Stimulus. The two or three initial doses of such immunizing agents in infancy constitute a primary stimulus. Even though the antibodies called forth into the blood by such a stimulus may disappear with time, the person who has had such a primary stimulus responds very quickly to a *secondary stimulus.* This second stimulus may consist of actual infection: tetanus, diphtheria, pertussis, or polio, or it may consist of a "booster" dose of toxoid or other specific antigen. The previously immunized person is usually able to respond quickly with the production of specific antibodies (Fig. 20–3).

Immunized persons, especially those who have not had a booster dose at all or not for many years (frequently adults), sometimes get diphtheria, pertussis, tetanus, or polio, but the infection is generally mild or subclinical. Fatality from diphtheria, pertussis, or tetanus in immunized persons is very rare.[9] It is important, therefore, that every child receive at least a primary stimulus with a multiple antigen early in life, a "booster" stimulus a year later, and another usually at the time of entering school.

Infants under two to four months of age are protected from a number of diseases by antibodies derived from their mother's blood. These persist for 3 to 4 months after birth provided the mothers are immune. Diphtheria is one of these diseases. For this and other reasons it is customary not to immunize children to diphtheria until they are about two months of age. After that period their susceptibility increases and artificial immunization is necessary.

The Schick Test. The "Schick test" is named for the Viennese physician who first made practical use of it. It is a test for the presence or absence of significant amounts of diphtheria antitoxin in the blood. The test is performed by injecting into (not under) the skin an extremely small amount of diphtheria toxin ($1/50$ MLD). If the person has no antitoxin in his blood (i.e., is not immune), within 24 hours a small red area appears at the place of injection, which gradually spreads for a centimeter or more. This is caused by the irritating effect of the toxin on the cells of the skin. In five days the area becomes slightly pigmented, and later a few flakes of epidermis may scale off. The test should not be read earlier than the fifth day after the injection because there is often a temporary irritation (pseudoreaction) caused by foreign substances always present in the toxin. The red area due to such impurities is nearly always gone by the end of five days. An area that persists after five days and undergoes the changes described is a positive reaction and means that the person has less than 0.02 unit of diphtheria antitoxin in the blood and may be susceptible to diphtheria, especially for individuals under 15 years of age.

If one has at least 0.02 unit of antitoxin in the blood, this will counteract the toxin injected in the Schick test and the skin remains normal. This is a negative Schick reaction and shows that the person will not contract diphtheria under ordinary conditions of exposure. The test is harmless, painless, and leaves no scar.

IMMUNIZATION. It is scarcely necessary to say that every member of the health team should be protected at the beginning of training, whether their work includes the care of contagious diseases or not. From one half to one fourth of urban adults give a positive Schick test. Most of them were probably once Schick negative, but antitoxin tends to dis-

---

[9]Persons with congenital agammaglobulinemia are exceptions. They usually fail to respond to vaccines, in general, and are likely to have low resistance to infectious diseases.

appear from the blood with passage of time and the Schick reaction reverts to positive; however, diphtheria is relatively uncommon among adults unless they are heavily and constantly exposed. Their resistance depends on the fact that at some time nearly all have received a primary antigenic stimulus: doses of toxoid or mild or unrecognized infection. Reinfection acts as a secondary stimulus. This same principle appears to hold true in many infectious diseases and should be clearly understood and remembered.

It is truly remarkable how this killing disease of small children, once feared by every mother, has been brought under control because of the workers in the field of immunology. In the early years of this century many thousands of cases and deaths from diphtheria occurred annually in the United States. In 1971 only 215 cases were reported in the entire nation, 101 of these occurring in children between the ages of 5 and 15 years. There were very few deaths.

DIPHTHEROIDS

Closely related to *Corynebacterium diphtheriae* are a number of organisms having somewhat similar morphology but incapable, so far as is known, of producing serious disease. Two common species are *Corynebacterium pseudodiphtheriticum* (Hoffman's bacillus) and *Corynebacterium xerosis*. These are frequent in the normal throat and nose. They grow in much the same manner as *C. diphtheriae* and are often mistaken for it in throat cultures by inexperienced diagnosticians, hence, the name diphtheroid, which means "diphtheria-like." They may usually be differentiated by the fact that they are less granular and more uniform in size and shape. In pure culture they exhibit entirely different biochemical and physiologic properties. They give negative reactions in toxigenicity tests. Other related species are *C. ulcerans*, *C. haemolyticum*, *C. equi*, *C. aquaticum*. Some of these are serious pathogens of domestic animals.

THE GENUS LISTERIA

Listeria monocytogenes is the only species in this genus. Formerly classified with the Corynebacteriaceae, it has only a superficial resemblance to them. The species name is derived from the appearance of large numbers of monocytes in the blood of experimentally infected animals. It bears no relation to infectious monocytosis in man, a disease caused by a virus. *Listeria* causes more infections than has previously been suspected. It may be isolated from cerebrospinal fluid, blood, vaginal swabs and other sources, apparently as a contaminant; however, the organism has been definitely established as the etiological agent in certain forms of meningitis, meningoencephalitis and also septicemia. Listeriosis sometimes results as a complication in debilitated patients with alcoholism, diabetes, or neoplastic diseases.

Supplementary Reading

American Public Health Association: Control of Communicable Diseases. 11th Ed. 1970, New York, American Public Health Association.

Blair, J. E., Lennette, E. H., and Truant, J. P.: Manual of Clinical Microbiology. 1970. Baltimore, Williams & Wilkins Co.

Burrows, W.: Textbook of Microbiology. 19th Ed. 1968, Philadelphia, W. B. Saunders Co.

Challoner, D., and Mandelbaum, I.: The protective effect of L-carnitine in experimental intoxication with diphtheria toxin. *J. Lab. Clin. Med.*, 1971, *77*:616.

Craig, J. P.: Diphtheria: prevalence of inapparent infection in a nonepidemic period. *Amer. J. Public Health*, 1962, *52*:1444.

Drazin, R., Kandel, J., and Collier, R. J.: Structure and activity of diphtheria toxin. *J. Biol. Chem.*, 1971, *246*:1504.

Duncan, J., and Groman, N. B.: Activity of diphtheria toxin (intoxication in HeLa cells). *J. Bact.*, 1969, *98*:963.

Gill, D., Pappenheimer, A. M., Jr., Brown, R., and Kurnick, J.: Mode of action of diphtheria toxin. *J. Exper. Med.*, 1969, *129*:1.

Gray, M. L., and Killinger, A. H.: *Listeria monocytogenes* and *Listeria* infections. *Bact. Rev.*, 1966, *30*:309.

Herman, G. J.: Diphtheria. Diagnostic Procedures. 5th Ed. 1970, New York, American Public Health Association.

Karlstrom, A., Barger, R. H., and Brandon, G. R.: Simplification of modified Tinsdale's medium. *Public Health Lab.*, 1962, *20*:44.

Monis, B., and Reback, J. R.: Tetrazolium salts and identification of *Corynebacterium diphtheriae. Proc. Soc. Exp. Biol. Med.*, 1962, *111*:81.

National Communicable Disease Center: Morbidity and Mortality 1967, Vol. 16, No 48. U.S. Department of Health, Education, and Welfare, Public Health Service, Bureau of Disease Prevention and Environmental Control.

Steigman, A. J., and Epting, M. H.: Diphtheria in children. *Amer. J. Nurs.*, 1957, *57*:467.

Laryngotracheitis, Conjunctivitis, Whooping Cough, and "Trench Mouth"

30

THE BRUCELLACEAE

Many species of saprophytic gram-negative rods may occasionally be found in the upper respiratory tract, accidentally carried there by inhaled dust, hands, foods, and other such means. There are three species, however, that are typically respiratory pathogens and are characteristically transmitted only in respiratory secretions. They are the so-called influenza bacillus, the bacillus of "pink-eye" or infectious conjunctivitis,[1] and the bacillus of whooping cough or pertussis.[2] These three organisms all belong to the same family (Brucellaceae[3]) because they have properties of that group in common.

PHYSIOLOGIC PROPERTIES OF THE BRUCELLACEAE. All Brucellaceae are very small, short rods or coccobacilli, ranging in diameter from 0.3 to 0.6 μm and in length from 3 to 8 μm. All are gram-negative, nonmotile, and nonspore-forming. They are fragile and are easily killed by common disinfectants and by pasteurizing or boiling. They grow best at 37 C in atmospheres containing about 10 per cent carbon dioxide and on media containing blood or serum and extracts of flesh. They are highly specialized parasites of the mammalian body, and have special nutritive requirements.

Genus Haemophilus

THE INFLUENZA BACILLUS (HAEMOPHILUS INFLUENZAE). This organism is a typical member of the family Brucellaceae. It is particularly adapted to live and grow in the body. Outside the body it soon dies unless

---

[1]The eyes, being connected with the upper respiratory tract via the tear ducts, can infect the oronasal secretions.

[2]*Per* is from the Latin for much; *tussis* from the Latin for cough. Pertussis is therefore "much cough."

[3]Bruce was a famous British Army surgeon who, in 1887, discovered the cause of Malta fever, *Brucella melitensis*, another member of the Brucellaceae.

provided with media containing whole blood or blood derivatives: *heme* and nicotinamide adenine dinucleotide (NAD). The genus name is derived from its requirement for blood (Greek *haima*, blood; *philus*, loving); its species name is from its formerly supposed causative relationship to influenza, a theory now completely disproven. Note that *H. influenzae* does not cause influenza; a *virus* is the etiologic agent of this disease.

H. influenzae is found in the nose and throat of many normal persons and is transmitted in droplets by sneezing and coughing; hence, it is a typical respiratory tract organism. So are *Haemophilus parainfluenzae* and *Haemophilus parahaemolyticus*, which rarely may cause pharyngitis or subacute bacterial endocarditis. *H. influenzae* is present in and appears to cause many inflammatory conditions of the respiratory tract, such as bronchopneumonia and sinusitis, and has been found in pure culture in the blood of patients dying of other diseases. It may sometimes cause meningitis and endocarditis. It has no causal relation to influenza, but it causes infections of the sinuses and eyes, especially following colds and influenza. Such infections caused by *H. influenzae* are probably secondary, rather than primary.

There are six encapsulated types of influenza bacilli, differentiated by soluble specific capsular substances much as are pneumococci and meningococci. These types are a, b, c, d, e, and f.[4] The type is determined by methods like those used in typing pneumococci; e.g., the quellung reaction and the precipitin test. These organisms resemble pneumococci also in being bile-soluble. Type b influenza bacilli appear to be especially virulent, causing many severe throat infections, especially *laryngotracheitis*, a serious and often fatal disease in infants, causing obstruction of the air passages by severe edema and mucous secretions. A type-specific antiserum as well as sulfonamide drugs and appropriate antibiotics, especially tetracycline, have been used effectively in treating such infections.

Haemophilus influenzae infections of the respiratory tract are treated, as far as nursing precautions and isolation techniques are concerned, like other upper respiratory infections (pneumonia, scarlet fever, and so on).

"**PINK-EYE.**" One of the causes of this disease, more accurately called acute or angular conjunctivitis or inflammation of the lining of the eyelids, is named *Haemophilus aegyptius* (the Koch-Weeks bacillus). This organism has the general characters of *H. influenzae*, which it closely resembles. It requires heme and NAD for growth.

GENUS MORAXELLA. Organisms of this genus occur in the same kinds of infections in which species of *Haemophilus* are found. The genus *Moraxella*, named for a famous French ophthalmologist, includes about eight species of very small, gram-negative, nonspore-forming, aflagellate, aerobic coccobacilli that generally require media containing serum but not heme or NAD. As a group they are not active in attacking carbohydrates, though species differ slightly in this respect (e.g., *M. kingii* ferments glucose). All produce oxidase and several form catalase. Several are actively proteolytic. Among the best known species are *M. lacunata* (the Morax-Axenfeld bacillus) and *M. kingii*.

Acute conjunctivitis due to species of *Haemophilus* and *Moraxella* is very contagious and spreads rapidly in families, institutions, and schools.

---

[4]Other strains are unencapsulated.

Transmission appears to be by means of direct contact with the infected eyes, or by fingers, towels, washcloths, handkerchiefs, and the like, soiled with secretions from the eyes. Dust may also transmit the organisms, but as they are not highly resistant to drying, this is thought not to be important. The disease is easily treated and is usually not serious, although it is extremely annoying, unsightly, and temporarily disabling. It may last for three or four days to two weeks.

Prevention

The eyes of the patient are usually bathed with mild disinfectant or antibiotic solutions to reduce the infection and the inflammation. A child with pink-eye must be kept from contact with other children. The school or institution nurse who has had experience with an outbreak of pink-eye will realize the importance of segregating the child, his bed linen, handkerchiefs, washcloths, towels, and anything that may be soiled with discharge from the eyes, directly or by way of the hands. Conjunctivitis of this origin tends to clear up spontaneously, but while it lasts, the same care should be given as for gonorrheal ophthalmia.

Other causes of acute conjunctivitis are at least one virus, gonococci, pneumococci, streptococci, and staphylococci; also the so-called TRIC agents: *Chlamydia trachomatis* (trachoma) and *C. oculogenitalis* (inclusion conjunctivitis). All these infections are more severe than "pink-eye" and are discussed more fully in connection with the respective etiological agents.

Genus Bordetella

THE BACILLUS OF WHOOPING COUGH (BORDETELLA PERTUSSIS). This organism, for years called *Haemophilus pertussis*, has many of the distinctive properties of *H. influenzae*. It was discovered in 1906 by two Belgian scientists, Bordet and Gengou. It is now called *Bordetella pertussis* in honor of Bordet; it is sometimes also called the Bordet-Gengou bacillus. The bacillus grows slowly and with difficulty outside the body, appearing on the surface of glycerin-potato-blood agar (Bordet-Gengou medium) only after five to ten days' incubation at 37 C. The addition of penicillin to this medium is recommended to inhibit gram-positive organisms that may cause contamination. The tiny colonies of *B. pertussis* are described as being "like droplets of mercury." (Fig. 30–1). They are hemolytic. *B. pertussis* is as delicate and, when first isolated, has the same fastidiousness about its growth requirements as has the influenza bacillus. After growth in artificial media it no longer requires heme or NAD. Both antigenic analysis (encapsulated types I to IV and direct fluorescent antibody staining of smears give promise of more rapid diagnosis.

A related organism, *H. parapertussis*, produces a similar though milder disease, parapertussis. The following discussion of pertussis applies equally to parapertussis.

Another pertussis-like disease is caused by *Bordetella bronchiseptica*, a gram-negative rod grouped with *Bordetella* because of its pathogenic relationship, but so different from all other *Bordetella* that it was formerly classified with the Achromobacteraceae as *Alcaligenes bronchisepticus*. It differs markedly from other *Bordetella* in being actively motile and able

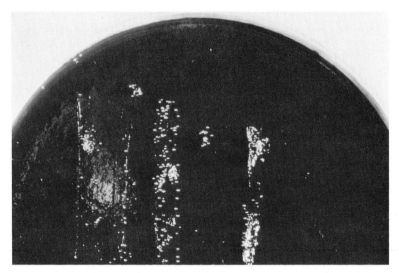

Figure 30–1

This illustration shows typical colonies of *Bordetella pertussis* on Bordet-Gengou medium. Note the colonial growth that resembles "droplets of mercury." (From Schneierson, S. S.: Atlas of Diagnostic Microbiology, Abbott Laboratories, North Chicago, Ill.)

to grow luxuriantly and rapidly at 25 C on plain peptone media. It is most commonly found in respiratory disease of dogs, rabbits, and so forth. Strangely, it shares certain antigens with other species of *Bordetella*.

Pertussis

NATURE AND TRANSMISSION.   Whooping cough, also called pertussis, comes with and without whooping, and whoops come with and without pertussis. Although mass immunization and improvements in care and treatment have reduced the incidence and mortality, this disease still occurs and it still is extremely dangerous, especially during infancy. *B. pertussis* produces an inflammation of the trachea and bronchi, and consequently is found in the sputum, saliva, and nasal discharge. It is transferred directly from person to person by droplet infection during coughing, and by articles freshly soiled with nose and mouth secretions. A spray of sputum and saliva may be thrown out to a distance of four or five feet during the violent attacks of coughing. It is possible to obtain a culture of pertussis bacilli if a Petri plate containing a suitable medium (Bordet-Gengou or substitute) is held before the mouth of a coughing patient. Such plates are called "cough plates" and are useful in bacteriologic confirmation of diagnosis, but they are subject to excessive contamination and difficulties in obtaining a productive cough from infants. The nasopharyngeal swab is simpler.

It is particularly advantageous to add penicillin to the B-G medium. This prevents the growth of most of the unwanted staphylococci and other organisms of the nasal and oral secretions, but permits good growth of colonies of *B. pertussis*. The same principle (selective cultivation) is used in diagnosing other bacterial infections.

Whooping cough begins with the symptoms of an ordinary cold. Like measles, diphtheria, and scarlet fever, it is highly infectious during the first few days of the actual disease when the causative organisms are present in the sputum in enormous numbers and before anything beyond a "cold" is suspected. Health workers should therefore be extremely critical and suspicious of "colds" in children and insist that the patients be kept at home for several days. After six weeks from the onset of whooping cough it is rarely possible to demonstrate *Bordetella pertussis*, even though the child may still cough violently. Carriers of whooping cough are therefore not a problem in prevention of the disease. New cases of whooping cough doubtless arise from mild cases, sometimes in adults, that are not thought to be whooping cough, or from cases in the early, "snuffly" stage before they are diagnosed.

COMPLICATIONS. Whooping cough, like measles, is a serious disease because of the other infections that complicate or follow it. The most important of these are bronchitis, pneumonia, and tuberculosis. Whooping cough is responsible for many fatal cases of bronchitis and pneumonia in young children. About 97 per cent of the fatal cases occur in children under five years of age, and about 70 per cent in those under one year. Care is directed toward preventing exposure of susceptible children, especially those under five years of age, to known cases. The usual general precautions for respiratory diseases are applicable. The organisms are easily killed by standard disinfectants and by drying and sunlight. Before the advent of active artificial immunization it was a common sight to see small children with "nurses" in public parks sitting in the sun. Often the child would start to cough until blood would come up, not a pretty sight to see, and one that is not easily forgotten.

WHOOPING COUGH VACCINE. A vaccine made of killed whooping cough bacilli is widely used for the control of the disease. It has notable value in preventing the disease; if the disease occurs in persons who have had the vaccine, the severity of the infection is usually markedly decreased. The vaccine is not effective as a curative measure, nor if it is used too close to the time of exposure. Time (four to six weeks) must be allowed for immunity to develop after injection. This is true of most methods of active immunization.

Alum-Precipitated and Mixed Vaccines. Pertussis vaccine is prepared by precipitating the killed bacilli, suspended in saline solution, with alum or aluminum hydroxide. The precipitated bacilli, resuspended, constitute "pertussis vaccine, alum-precipitated." It may be used alone, but it is common and approved practice to mix it with diphtheria toxoid, also alum-precipitated, and often also with alum-precipitated tetanus toxoid (triple antigen). The advantages of using alum-precipitated antigens have been pointed out previously. Some preparations also contain Salk polio vaccine. In children, the pertussis vaccine should be started at one month of age of even earlier. Immunization against pertussis is usually not required past six years of age.

The incidence of pertussis in the United States has declined from over 120,000 cases in 1950 to 3036 in 1971; deaths from over 1500 to about 50.

PASSIVE IMMUNITY. Transitory protection may be given highly susceptible children under five years of age by the use of serum or, better, gamma globulin from immune persons. The children who need this type of protection are those who have not received pertussis vaccine and who are debilitated by other disease or malnutrition and who are likely to be exposed to the infection.

PREVENTION.   For as long as four weeks from onset, the child with whooping cough expels large numbers of the organisms from the nose and mouth when coughing and sneezing. A susceptible child is almost certain to contract the disease if he spends any time in a closed room with a person who is discharging the organisms by coughing. Even outdoors, close contact should be avoided for at least four weeks after the onset of the disease and for six weeks if possible. Adults are not commonly victims of pertussis, but unless they are known to be immune they should avoid contact with known cases of the disease. Sometimes people become infected (and infectious) following contact with a case, yet manifest only the symptoms of a cold. All fomites of the patient contaminated with sputum or vomitus, as well as the vomitus itself, should be disinfected. *Bordetella pertussis* is a fragile organism and does not live very long in the outer world; nevertheless, it survives long enough to be effectively transmitted by droplets, saliva, and so on.

Conner reported in 1970 that a pertussis-like syndrome, indistinguishable from pertussis, was caused by adenoviruses types 1, 2, 3, and 5. This viral etiology could be of considerable importance and needs further investigation.

ORAL SPIROCHETES

"TRENCH MOUTH."   *Borrelia vincentii*, a spirochete, is anaerobic and is difficult to cultivate in the laboratory. Although commonly present in the normal mouth in relatively small numbers, it is implicated in a painful, ulcerative disease of the gums, cheeks, and throat often called "trench mouth" (because it was common among troops in the trenches during World War I) or Vincent's angina. Vincent's angina has been thought to be an infectious disease, causing a superficial, gangrenous ulceration or stomatitis, often with an offensive odor (*oral fetor*). It may be that certain vitamin deficiencies are the basic cause of the lesions seen in Vincent's angina and that the spirochetes then multiply in the lesions as secondary invaders or opportunists. The actual relation of the spirochetes to the cause of the disease is not clear. In any event, the spirochetes are always found in enormous numbers in the ulcers, always associated with long, thin, spindle-shaped or cigar-shaped bacilli called *fusiform bacilli* (*Fusobacterium fusiforme*). The organisms may be demonstrated by staining material from the ulcers and examining it microscopically. Both spirochetes and fusiform bacilli stain well and are gram-negative (Fig. 30–2).

The organisms can be transmitted by improperly disinfected drinking glasses and eating utensils, kissing, and articles that pass, undisinfected, from an infected mouth to another; however, other factors, possibly dietary, may also be involved. Vigorous disinfection of the mouth usually cures the infection. The same antispirochetal drugs used for the treatment of the treponematoses also give prompt relief in some cases, and penicillin is most effective. The disease is not very dangerous as a rule, though it can cause great discomfort. The ulcerous lesions are sometimes mistaken for the membrane found in diphtheria.

Other *Borrelia* species, those causing relapsing fever, will be discussed later in Chapter 38.

SYPHILIS.   *Treponema pallidum*, the spirochete that causes syphilis, occurs in the mouth in some cases of primary syphilis and also in later stages

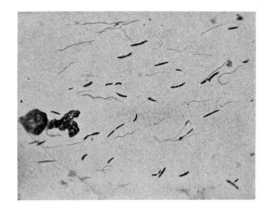

Figure 30–2

Throat smear, Vincent's angina, showing the spirochetes, which stain lightly, and the cigar-shaped bacilli that always accompany them. The darkly stained masses at left are nuclei of leucocytes. (Zinsser and Bayne-Jones: Textbook of Bacteriology. New York, Appleton-Century-Crofts, Inc.)

of untreated syphilis. It may be transmitted by kissing and by objects freshly contaminated with oral secretions. Further discussion of syphilis appears in Chapter 34.

Supplementary Reading

Abbott, J. D., Preston, N. W., and Mackay, R. I.: Agglutinin response to pertussis vaccination in the child. *Brit. Med. J.*, 1971, *1*:86.

Brooks, G. F., and Buchanan, T. M.: Pertussis in U.S.A. *J. Infect. Dis.*, 1970, *122*:123.

Brooksaler, F. S.: The pertussis syndrome. *Texas Med.*, 1971, *67*:56–61.

Burnett, G. W., and Scherp, H. W.: Oral Microbiology and Infectious Diseases. 3rd Ed. 1968, Baltimore, The Williams & Wilkins Co.

Burrows, W.: Textbook of Microbiology. 19th Ed. 1968, Philadelphia, W. B. Saunders Co.

Connor, J. D.: Evidence for an etiologic role of adenoviral infection in pertussis syndrome. *New Eng. J. Med.*, 1970, *283*:390.

Henrickson, S. D., and Bøvre, K.: *Moraxella kingii* sp. nov., a haemolytic, saccharolytic species of the genus *Moraxella J. Gen. Microbiol.*, 1968, *51*:377.

Holwerda, J., Brown, G. C., and Pickett, G.: Symposium on pertussis immunization in honor of Dr. Pearl L. Kendrick. *Health Lab. Science*, 1971, *8*:206.

McGuire, C. D., and Durant, R. C.: The role of flies in the transmission of eye disease in Egypt. *Amer. J. Trop. Med. & Hyg.*, 1957, *6*:569.

National Communicable Disease Center: Pertussis in the United States. *J. Infect. Dis.*, 1970, *122*:123.

Nelson, J. D.: Whooping cough—viral or bacterial disease? *New Eng. J. Med.*, 1970, *283*:428.

Stanfield, J., Bracken, P. M., Waddell, K. M., and Gall, D.: Diphtheria-tetanus-pertussis immunization by intradermal jet injection. *Brit. Med. J.*, 1972, *2*:197.

Top, F. H., et al.: Communicable Diseases. 5th Ed. 1968, St. Louis, The C. V. Mosby Co.

Van Bijsterveld, O. P.: New *Moraxella* strain isolated from angular conjunctivitis. *Appl. Microbiol.*, 1970, *20*:405.

Tuberculosis and Hansen's Disease

31

GENUS MYCOBACTERIUM

The order *Actinomycetales* consists of branching, moldlike bacteria and includes the genus *Mycobacterium*,[1] in which belong the tubercle and leprosy bacilli. Several species of mycobacteria, whose pathogenic status is still not fully clarified, are often found in tuberculosis-like pulmonary conditions, or associated with true tuberculosis. These mycobacteria are often called "atypical acid-fast bacilli" or *unclassified* or *anonymous* mycobacteria. The designation "atypical" is used for mycobacteria other than *M. tuberculosis* and *M. bovis* that also occur in clinical specimens. It is not preferred terminology and the classification of Runyon is to be applied to these organisms instead (Table 31–1). *M. tuberculosis* and *M. bovis* are not assigned to any Runyon group. Others are nonpathogenic, saprophytic mycobacteria that live in the soil and on plants, notably *Mycobacterium phlei*, and on the human skin, *M. smegmatis.*

All mycobacteria are distinguished from virtually all other microorganisms[2] by the property of acid-fastness, which will be explained later in this chapter. Hence, they are often called "acid-fast bacilli." They are all rods, usually slender and curved, often pointed and beaded, but occasionally showing forms more or less branching. This branching character and their bacterium-like size and structure certify their membership in the order of Actinomycetales.

By far the most important members of the genus *Mycobacterium* to humans are *M. tuberculosis*, cause of tuberculosis in man, and *M. leprae*, cause of Hansen's disease (leprosy). They are included here as respiratory tract organisms, since both are commonly transmitted via the respiratory tract, although both often infect other tissues and organs in the body and may appear in feces and urine as well as in respiratory secretions and in tissue and wound drainages.

---

[1]*Myco* is from the Greek *mykes*, fungus or mold.
[2]Except a few species of the closely related *Nocardia*, named for a French microbiologist, Edmund Nocard. (Fig. 1–9.)

438

Table 31-1. Distinctive Properties of Various Mycobacteria*†

SPECIES OR SUBGROUP	NIACIN PRODUCED	NITRATE REDUCTION		CATALASE PRODUCED mm.			TWEEN HYDROLYSIS (DAYS)		TELLURITE REDUCTION IN 3 DAYS	PIGMENT FORMATION		GROWTH ON 5% NaCl	GROWTH IN LESS THAN 7 DAYS AT 37 C	PRODUCE ARYLSULFATASE ENZYME +3 DAYS	GROWTH ON MacConkey AGAR
		>1+	>3	>40	>50	68°+	+5	+10		Dark	Light				
M. tuberculosis●	++	++	++	++	–	–	∓	∓	–	–	–	–	–	–	–
M. bovis	–	++	–	++	–	–	–	∓	–	–	–	–	–	–	–
Runyon Group I (Photochromogenic) (lemon yellow pigment)															
M. kansasii●	–	++	–	–	++	++	++	++	–	–	++	–	∓**	–	–
M. marinum●	–	–	–	±	∓	–	++	++	–	–	++	–	–	–	–
Runyon Group II (Scotochromogenic) (yellow orange to dark red)															
M. sp. scrofulaceum	∓	∓	–	++	++	++	–	–	–	++	++	–	–	–	–
M. sp. aquae	–	–	–	++	++	++	++	++	–	++	++	±	–	–	–
M. flavescens	–	++	+	±	++	++	+	++	–	–	++	±	–	–	–
Runyon Group III (no pigments in light)															
M. avium‡●	–	–	–	++	–	++	–	–	±	–	∓	–	–**	–	∓
M. intracellulare‡●	–	–	–	++	–	++	–	++	+	–	–	–	–	–	+
M. xenopei	–	–	–	++	–	–	–	–	–	∓§	∓§	–	–	±	–
M. gastri	–	–	–	++	–	–	++	++	–	–	–	–	–	–	–
M. terrae complex	–	++	+	++	++	++	++	++	–	–	–	–	–	–	–
"V" (M. triviale)	–	++	+	++	++	++	+	++	–	–	–	++	–	∓	–
Runyon Group IV (rapid growers) (some scotochromogens)															
M. fortuitum	–	±	+	++	++	++	∓	++	++	–	–	++	++	++	±
M. smegmatis	–	++	∓	++	++	++	++	++	++	–	–	++	++	–	–
M. phlei‡	–	++	∓	++	++	++	++	++	+	++	++	++	++	–	–
M. vaccae‡	V	++	+	++	++	++	±	++	+	–	++	++	++	±	+
M. borstelense	–	++	±	++	++	++	–	+	±	++	++	++	++	++	+
(M.) rhodochrous	–	++	±	++	++	–	∓	∓	∓	–	–	∓	++	∓	–

*Modified after Current Item No. 165, Laboratory Program, 1968. National Communicable Disease Center. Courtesy George Kubica, former Chief, Mycobacteriology Unit, NCDC, Atlanta.

†Key to percentage of strains reacting as indicated: ++ = 85 per cent or more; + = 75–84 per cent; ± = 50–74 per cent; ∓ = 15–49 per cent; – = <15 per cent; V = variable.

‡With tests listed the pairs of organisms so indicated cannot be separated; colonial morphology on 7H-10 may be helpful in the case of M. phlei–M. vaccae.

§Pigment increases with age.

**M. ulcerans and M. marinum grow best at about 32 C; M. avium and M. intracellulare at 41 C.

●Mycobacteria that are of clinical significance. The others are rarely or never significant.

THE TUBERCLE BACILLUS

One of the most important discoveries in medicine was that of *Mycobacterium tuberculosis*, first seen and cultivated in the laboratory by Koch in 1882. For hundreds of years previously, however, it had been known that tuberculosis was infectious. In 1865 Jean Villemin, a French pathologist, had produced tuberculosis in animals by inoculating them with material from patients who had died of tuberculosis.

PHYSIOLOGIC PROPERTIES. Tubercle bacilli and, indeed, all mycobacteria are nonspore-forming and nonmotile. They are aerobic and gram-positive. The Gram stain, however, does not give as much information about them as do some other staining methods. Special methods of staining, called the *Ziehl-Neelsen acid-fast stain*, or the *Kinyoun's acid-fast stain*, are generally used.

THE ACID-FAST STAIN (ZIEHL-NEELSEN METHOD)
1. Prepare the smear (e.g., sputum) as usual and dry.
2. Flood with a solution of carbolfuchsin (a red dye).
3. Heat the slide gently so that the solution steams. Do not allow to boil. Do not allow to dry.
4. After three to five minutes, wash off the stain with a gentle stream of water.
5. Apply alcohol containing 5 per cent hydrochloric acid to the slide for one or two minutes. Wash.
6. Counterstain with methylene blue.
7. Wash and blot.

The acid alcohol removes the red fuchsin from everything except the acid-fast bacilli. These retain the red stain in spite of the acid alcohol; everything else appears blue. The Ziehl-Neelsen (or acid-fast) stain is a *differential* stain since it differentiates acid-fast bacilli from other kinds. It is one of the most widely used methods for detecting tubercle bacilli in sputum. The reason for heating the slide is that many workers believe the acid-fast bacteria to have a waxy cell wall. This must be softened so that the stain can soak in rapidly. Once in and cooled, it stays there in spite of the application of acid and alcohol. Tubercle bacilli are more strongly acid-fast than are most other mycobacteria. Note that *Nocardia* species are also somewhat acid-fast, but it is not too difficult to distinguish them from the tubercle bacilli.

MICROSCOPY. Acid-fast bacilli are easily detected with microscopy because of their acid-fastness. Whenever there is bacterial retention of the dye after acid-alcohol treatment, fluorescence staining is as valuable as acid-fastness in the identification of mycobacteria. Auramine and rhodamine stains are excellent for fluorescence microscopy with an ultraviolet light source; even fluorescence microscopy with a blue light source is fully effective and *greatly superior* to the Ziehl-Neelsen technique. The best stain for this method is auramine O. The Truant fluorescence technique permits the observation of mycobacteria and acid-fast *Nocardia* as bright, yellow-orange fluorescent bacilli on a dark background.

CULTIVATION AND DIFFERENTIATION. All mycobacteria (with the exceptions of *M. leprae* and *M. lepraemurium*) grow on appropriate culture media exposed to air. Rate of growth, pigment production and optimal growth temperatures are important primary differential characters (Table 31–1). Among many solid media for mycobacteria are Lowenstein-Jensen's and Middlebrook and Cohn's 7H-10 agar. The latter requires an atmosphere containing 7 per cent carbon dioxide. Glycerin infusion agar or any of several media made with mixtures of eggs, milk, and potato are commonly used for cultivating tubercle bacilli for diagnostic purposes. Most *nonpathogenic* species, especially if exposed to light, generally produce luxuriant, brilliant orange, red, or yellow growth in three to five days at about 25 C.

Human and bovine species of tubercle bacilli grow much more slowly on such media, requiring about two to three weeks or longer to develop perceptible growth. They grow only at about 37 C. The growth is usually very pale yellow or cream colored and is usually rough and granular; experienced microbiologists can recognize it with some assurance. Certain improved methods and media, especially fluid media (e.g., Dubos's medium) containing surface-tension reducers, such as Tween 80, that enable the nutrient fluid to wet the waxy bacilli, speed up the growth of *M. tuberculosis*.

Species of Tubercle Bacilli

There are several species of tubercle bacilli. Some of these grow well at low temperatures and infect cold-blooded (poikilothermic) animals like frogs, snakes, and turtles. There are at least three species that infect mammals: *M. tuberculosis*, which infects man; *M. bovis*, which infects cattle and man; *M. microti*, the so-called vole bacillus, which infects voles (a kind of field mouse) and other rodents. There is also an avian variety (*Mycobacterium avium*), growing best at about 40 C, which infects birds and can be a real problem to poultrymen. Rarely, it infects man; sometimes pigs. The several species are morphologically indistinguishable.

The *bovine* tubercle bacillus (*M. bovis*) affects cattle and some other domestic animals as well as human beings. The two kinds of bacilli, human and bovine, can be differentiated by laboratory tests but are very closely similar in most respects. If a cow has tuberculosis of the udder, the milk will contain the bacilli. Children may be infected by drinking the milk of tuberculous cows. This method of infection accounts for much tuberculosis of the lymph nodes of the neck and abdomen and also of the bones in children, especially in some countries where pasteurization of milk and precautions against tuberculosis in cattle are not as rigorous as in the United States. Tuberculosis of organs other than the lungs (extrapulmonary tuberculosis), however, can also result from infection with human tubercle bacilli.

DIFFERENTIATION OF MYCOBACTERIA. Characteristics that differentiate various mycobacteria are listed in Table 31–1. No single test provides a wholly reliable diagnosis, but tests for virulence in guinea pigs and rabbits are among the most dependable diagnostic procedures for *M. tuberculosis*. *M. bovis* infects both guinea pigs and rabbits; *M. tuberculosis* only guinea pigs. Neither infects fowls, which are susceptible to *M. avium*. *M. tuberculosis* is the only species of *Mycobacterium* known to produce niacin.

It is important for the diagnostician to know the characteristics that differentiate the various kinds of mycobacteria, and especially those differentiating harmless acid-fast saprophytes from tubercle bacilli because the saprophytes are widely distributed in nature in soil, dust, dung of domestic animals, dairy products, hay, and on the surface of the human body. Since they occur in dairy products and dust, their occasional presence in saliva is readily understood. This can cause confusion when sputum is examined microscopically for tubercle bacilli since all mycobacteria closely resemble one another in appearance. Saprophytic mycobacteria may be found also in urine and gastric contents, which are often examined for tubercle bacilli.

TUBERCLE BACILLI AND DISINFECTION. In spite of the fact that tubercle bacilli do not form spores, they are more resistant to some disinfectants and drying than are the previously discussed nonspore-forming pathogens. In dried sputum kept in the dark they may live for several months. In particles of sputum-infected dust, they may remain alive for eight or ten days if not exposed to sunlight. In dried sputum they can withstand temperatures of about 70 C for one hour. Dried organisms are often somewhat more resistant to heat and chemical disinfectants than are the same organisms in a moist or fully hydrated condition. Exposure to direct sunlight kills tubercle bacilli in a few hours (mainly because of the ultraviolet rays). Pasteurization (63 C for 30 minutes or 72 C for 15 to 30 seconds) also kills them in milk.

It is difficult to kill tubercle bacilli in sputum by means of ordinary disinfectants because of their waxy membrane and because they are protected by mucus. Disinfection of sputum with solutions like 5 per cent saponated cresol or full strength chlorine laundry bleach or organic aqueous iodine disinfectant may require from two to five hours. Bichloride of mercury and alcohol are unsatisfactory because they coagulate the sputum around the bacilli and are thereby excluded from contact. Formaldehyde is not reliable for this purpose and is very irritating.

TUBERCULOSIS IN MAN

Clinical Forms

The symptoms produced by tuberculous lesions may be varied and thus simulate many other disease entities. In the diagnosis of any chronic infection, as well as some acute ones, the possibility of tuberculosis must be considered. Thus, tuberculosis may involve practically any organ or tissue of the body, and although about 90% of all tuberculosis infections involve the lung, the rest are tuberculosis of the CNS, the skin, bones and joints, kidney and bladder, genital organs, intestines, liver, middle ear, eye, abdomen, peritoneum, and so forth.

TUBERCLES AND PRIMARY TUBERCULOSIS. By *primary tuberculosis* is meant the disease process resulting directly from the first entry of tubercle bacilli, whether by inhalation, ingestion, or otherwise. Primary infection may occur at any age but is most common in infants, children, and young adults. Man, especially the infant, readily becomes infected with tubercle bacilli, but he is highly resistant to progression of the disease under good living conditions, especially between ages 5 and 15. When the local lymph nodes become involved, the process is called a *primary complex*.

Within a few days after tubercle bacilli first locate in the body of a susceptible person (or animal) they cause a tissue reaction that results in the formation of a distinctive kind of lesion called a *tubercle*. A tubercle consists of one or more tubercle bacilli surrounded by a small mass of pus and phagocytes. They are later enclosed within distinctive, multinucleate tissue cells called *giant cells*, all surrounded by connective tissue cells (fibro-

Figure 31–1

Tuberculous lesion (primary) in apex of left upper lobe (right upper corner) with associated massive involvement of regional lymph nodes (primary complex). Large wedge-shaped lesion in lower half (lateral portion) of left lower lobe. This last lesion (tuberculous pneumonitis) is secondary to bronchial erosion from a tuberculous node. (Courtesy of Drs. Charles Dunlap and James B. Gray in Chapter by High, R. H. In Nelson, W. E., et al. (Eds.): Textbook of Pediatrics. 9th Ed. Philadelphia, W. B. Saunders Co., 1969.)

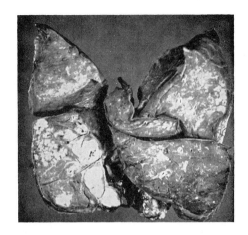

blasts), which form a sort of tough retaining wall or sac with relatively little fluid. This is the *proliferative* type of lesion, a favorable type likely to heal without further progress and without remarkable symptoms of any kind. The disease is called "childhood tuberculosis." The whole lesion is surrounded by a zone of inflammation. The cells and structure of tubercles are so characteristic that a diagnosis of tuberculosis can be made from them alone, even though the bacilli may not be found with the microscope. A single, very early tubercle is a gray mass, the size of a pinhead or smaller, which feels hard to the touch (Fig. 31–1). Numbers or masses of tubercles usually occur together in an organ. Usually the resistance of the healthy childhood patient is sufficient to stop their progress. Tubercle formation is commonly associated with the development of allergy to the tubercle bacilli.

When virulence is high, or dosage large and continuous, or resistance low, as in undernourished children, the bacilli continue to multiply, producing further inflammation and the exudation of fibrinoserous fluid. This is the *exudative* type of lesion, one likely to progress. The bacilli continue to grow, enlarging the tubercles, and killing the tissue at the center. This dead tissue becomes coagulated into a cheesy mass. When the process has extended to this point, *caseation* is said to have occurred. If the process continues, numbers of such caseated abscesses may encounter each other as they expand, finally fusing together to form one large, caseous mass.

If the infection is in a lung, the necrotic process often invades and erodes through the wall of a bronchiole, and then the caseous contents, along with numerous tubercle bacilli, are coughed up with the sputum. This is a very dangerous stage of the disease for other people since the sputum is then highly infectious. Tuberculous sputum and the pus from tuberculous abscesses contain dead tissue, pus, and large numbers of tubercle bacilli. Sputum is often swallowed, especially by young children, and the gastric contents may often reveal tubercle bacilli when sputum examinations are persistently negative or cannot be made. Intestinal or generalized infection may then occur.

If a tuberculous abscess erodes through the wall of a blood vessel, a *hemorrhage* occurs, which may prove fatal.

Tubercles frequently heal, especially in the nonprogressive, primary

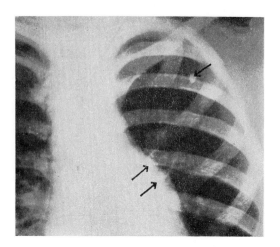

Figure 31–2

Primary infection with the tubercle bacillus. The child, when two years of age, was in contact with a tuberculous mother, who died of the disease. Six years later, at the age of eight years, x-ray of the child shows prominent calcified lesion in the left upper lobe and several calcified hilar lymph nodes. This is a healed primary complex. (Rubin: Diseases of the Chest.)

form of the disease, in which case they become surrounded by thick envelopes of scarlike tissue. Calcium salts may be deposited in them; i.e., they undergo *calcification*. These are readily seen in x-ray pictures. As we shall see later, many of us are carrying healed, calcified tubercles somewhere in our bodies.

Whenever live bacilli in tubercles are present in an organ we say that tuberculosis of that organ exists. Any organ in the body may be attacked by tuberculosis, but in some it is much more frequent than in others. As we have already stated, the lungs and adjacent tissues and lymph nodes are the organs of adults most often affected; in children, however, the lymph nodes (Fig. 31–2), bones, joints, intestines, and the brain and its coverings (tuberculosis meningitis) are also frequently involved. Various types of lesion may occur at almost any age, however.

CLASSIFICATION OF TUBERCULOSIS CASES. There are various classifications of tuberculosis, some based on the extent of the disease, others on bacteriologic findings. Cases of diagnosed tuberculosis may be classified as *active, quiescent,* or *inactive*. In an active case the patient casts off bacilli in the sputum or other excretion. In quiescent and inactive cases bacilli are not given off and lesions are not progressive or are healing. Such cases are not an immediate danger to others. An active case may become inactive if healing takes place; an inactive case may become reactivated and again dangerous to others. The progress of the disease represents a constantly changing balance between the resistance of the patient and the virulence of the organism.

REINFECTION (OR ADULT) TYPE TUBERCULOSIS. This type is said to occur when tubercle bacilli again enter the tissues after a primary infection has healed or partially healed. The bacilli may be reintroduced from an outside source (reinfection or superinfection) or by release internally from a partially healed tubercle (postprimary progression). Most persons are constantly being reinfected from outside sources with no obvious ill effects whatever. If resistance is low, however, reinfection or postprimary progression may result in serious developments. These are associated with allergy to tubercle bacilli.

Allergy in Tuberculosis

In many chronic or prolonged microbial infections such as syphilis, undulant fever, tularemia, relapsing fever, fungal infections, and tuberculosis, the patient develops *an allergic condition,* specific with regard to the particular antigen involved. Generally benign and protective in character, in some individuals this allergy becomes excessive and does great harm. In tuberculosis and in syphilis and some other chronic infections, the ulcerative, softening character of lesions developing late in the disease, or after the lapse of many years in the reinfection type of disease, are believed to be the result of excessive allergy of the tissues. Such lesions tend to break down rather than to heal.

Allergic tissues tend to arrest pathogenic organisms and to prevent their spread throughout the body, although the organisms may severely damage the arresting tissues. Allergy as an arresting agent must, therefore, be regarded as an important defensive mechanism. Whether or not the arrest stops the further progress of the disease depends on the nature of the allergic response and the resistance of the patient. Allergy is probably the chief defensive means of normal adults against repeated reinfection with tubercle bacilli as well as against many other infections.

ALLERGY AND KOCH'S PHENOMENON. The arresting action of allergy in tuberculosis is well illustrated by the *Koch phenomenon.* (Do not confuse with Koch's postulates.) If a normal guinea pig is inoculated (usually in the right groin) with virulent tubercle bacilli, the bacteria form a local abscess, and then proceed almost unopposed from the abscess to the lymph nodes of the abdominal cavity, to the spleen, the liver, the lymph nodes of the thorax, the lungs and kidneys, and the pig finally dies of disseminated tuberculosis in about six to eight weeks. Now, if on the second or third week of this progressive disease a second injection of tubercle bacilli is made into the left groin, there is a strong, local, allergic tissue reaction. The bacilli are held in the site where they are injected and do not progress further, although they may cause a local abscess. The tissues are highly defensive because of the allergy to the first infection. We do not understand why the bacilli of the first infection are not similarly held in check.

Similarly, human beings who have had a mild, unrecognized infection with tubercle bacilli, one perhaps long since healed, are generally much more resistant to tuberculosis than persons who have never had any contact with tubercle bacilli. The first group are moderately allergic (hence resistant) to the bacilli, as shown by the fact that they react not too excessively to the tuberculin test (see following). The second group may readily be made allergic (resistant) to tubercle bacilli by giving them a very mild infection, as is done in BCG[1] vaccination.

THE TUBERCULIN TEST. Intracutaneous injection of diluted antigenic extracts of tubercle bacilli, called *tuberculin,* into the skin of city-living adults commonly evokes a red, indurated, itching wheal in most of them after about 48 hours. It disappears after a few days, and the test is an entirely harmless experiment if small doses of tuberculin are used. The reaction is called a *tuberculin reaction.*

Tuberculins of various types were first developed by Koch (notably "old tuberculin," or O.T.), who thought he had devised a vaccine against

---

[1] Bacille Calmette Guérin. See page 302.

the disease and had great hopes of using tuberculin for the cure of tuberculosis. Modern tuberculins are made from *purified protein derivatives* (PPD) of tubercle bacilli. It has since been found, however, that tuberculin alone will not cure or prevent the disease. In fact, if too much of it is introduced into the body of a person allergic to the protein, a very severe, generalized, and even fatal allergic reaction may occur, instead of merely a local one on the skin. If the patient has live tubercle bacilli in his tissues, the reaction may give the organisms a fresh start, and thus greatly injure him. On this basis it is recommended by some authorities that *tuberculin-positive individuals should not* be vaccinated with BCG.

Healed tuberculous infection in an adult, even though the individual may never have been aware of it, still leaves him in an allergic condition toward tubercle bacillus protein. Thus a positive tuberculin reaction in an older person does not necessarily indicate active or even inactive tuberculosis. Resulting from a healed childhood infection, the tuberculin reaction may remain positive for life or it may revert to negative though the individual may still have resistance. *The tuberculin test is most used to detect early primary tuberculosis in children.*

Among young children and also in adults in nontuberculous environments, many are found who give a negative tuberculin reaction. Allergic sensitivity appears in primary infection at any age within three to ten weeks after infection. Therefore, in children who have only recently developed tuberculin reactivity for the first time, the infection is probably present in a more or less progressive form, since they are not old enough to have recovered completely. The reaction remains positive whenever viable tubercle bacilli are present in the body, whether or not active disease is present.

The presence or sudden appearance of a positive tuberculin reaction does not necessarily mean that the person is going to develop clinical tuberculosis. That depends on his continued reinfection, malnutrition, poor living conditions, and other factors. The tuberculin test merely serves as a warning that proper measures should be taken before it is too late.

METHODS OF PERFORMING THE TUBERCULIN TEST. Tuberculin may be applied in a number of ways, all of which are designed to bring the tubercle bacillus protein into intimate contact with the body cells. Von Pirquet described the method of scratching the tuberculin into the skin, or *scarification.* When the test is done in this way, it is often called the *von Pirquet test.* It is a simple and widely used procedure.

In a popular modification called the *Heaf test,* the tuberculin (PPD) is first spread over a small area of skin. An instrument sometimes called a Ster-needle gun is then pressed against the skin, and a triggered, spring-driven plunger with six short, solid needle points drives the PPD painlessly into the skin. The needle-tipped heads are replaceable for sterilization by heat. In the *Tine Test* the points are precoated with O.T. and dried.

The injection of minute, accurately measured amounts of tuberculin (PPD) *intradermally* was devised by *Mantoux,* and his, quantitatively the most accurate procedure, is designated by his name. *Vollmer* demonstrated the method of applying tuberculin to the surface of the skin on patches of gauze or tape. This is the "*patch test.*" The patch is left on 48 hours, and the test is read 48 hours after its removal. The test is convenient but considered not very accurate.

Diagnosis of Tuberculosis

MICROSCOPIC. A tentative diagnosis of pulmonary tuberculosis is generally made on the basis of x-ray and clinical findings and is confirmed whenever possible by examining the sputum with the microscope. Smears of the material are made on slides and stained by the Ziehl-Neelsen method or Kinyoun's acid-fast stain or fluorescence microscopy (see the following paragraph) by the fluorochrome method to see if acid-fast bacilli are present. It is frequently necessary to make many examinations before the bacilli are finally found; therefore, in suspicious cases one negative report is insufficient.

FLUORESCENCE MICROSCOPY. Fluorescence is a property of numerous substances, as a result which they reflect light waves having a wavelength (color) different from that of the incident rays. A fluorescent object may be invisible when seen by ordinary light, yet glow (or fluoresce) with a bright yellowish luminosity when viewed under ultraviolet ("black" or "invisible") light.

If tubercle bacilli in sputum on a microscope slide are coated with a fluorescent stain (e.g., auramine O), the excess stain washed from the rest of the slide, and the slide then illuminated with ultraviolet light and examined under the microscope, the tubercle bacilli are easily seen as brightly glowing, golden rods in a dark field (see also page 121). An ordinary microscope is readily equipped for fluorescence microscopy by means of a special mirror, appropriate light filters and a good source of ultraviolet light in place of the usual illumination. Do not confuse this application of fluorescence in microscopy with fluorescent-antibody staining, described in Chapters 19 and 34 (see Figs. 19–6 and 34–7).

CULTURAL. Since the bacilli in sputum or other material may be present in such small numbers that they cannot be found by routine examination with the microscope, and since, especially in urine, feces, and gastric contents, it is impossible to differentiate tubercle bacilli from acid-fast saprophytes microscopically, it is absolutely necessary (for first diagnosis, at least) to make cultures from the pathologic material, identify the bacilli by their growth characteristics, and, if in doubt, to prove their pathogenicity by injection of the specimen into animals, usually guinea pigs. Some of the media commonly used in medical laboratories for the diagnosis of tuberculosis have already been mentioned. Many contain a dye such as crystal violet or malachite green. The dye inhibits growth of many microorganisms that often contaminate pathologic material such as sputum in which tubercle bacilli are found. It does not affect the tubercle bacilli. Most of the contaminating bacteria in sputum and other exudates are often killed first by mixing the material with an equal volume of 5 per cent sodium hydroxide and neutralizing after 30 minutes.

To avoid the destruction of a large percentage of tubercle bacilli from sputum and bronchial secretions by strong alkali, a mild decontamination and digestion procedure has been developed. This method uses the mucolytic agent N-acetyl-L-cysteine (NALC) and 2 per cent sodium hydroxide. Another mild method employs trisodium phosphate plus benzalkonium chloride; still another uses dithiothreitol at pH 7.0, followed by 1 per cent NaOH or Zephiran.

It should be noted that besides cultivation from sputum, tubercle bacilli may be isolated from gastric specimens, urine, and cerebrospinal

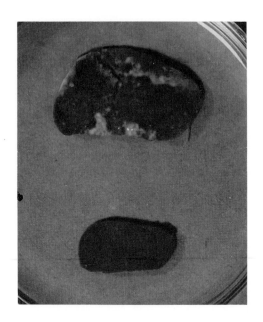

Figure 31–3

Effect of tuberculous infection on spleen of guinea pig. Note great increase in size, inflammation (dark areas), caseation (white areas), and small white specks (tubercles) in tuberculous spleen (upper). The lower picture is of a normal spleen (natural size). (Specimen prepared by Miss Lucille Sommermeyer. Photo courtesy U. S. Public Health Service, Communicable Disease Center, Atlanta, Ga.)

fluid, as well as from other body fluids and tissues removed surgically or at necropsy.

Tubercle bacilli can frequently be cultivated directly from *untreated* sputum if a small amount of penicillin and cycloheximide are placed on the surface of the medium to inhibit growth of extraneous microorganisms.

ANIMAL INOCULATION.   After isolation from pathologic materials pure cultures may be used for confirmatory tests (Table 31–1) and for injection into animals. When only a few tubercle bacilli are present in sputum, urine, pus, or other material, it may be impossible to find them with the microscope or even by means of cultures. Another method of discovering them is to inject a guinea pig with the material. Lesions produced by the bacilli are easily recognized (Fig. 31–3).

URINE SPECIMENS.   In examining urine for tubercle bacilli, the *sediment* is usually collected for staining or injection. In urine, acid-fast bacilli other than tubercle bacilli are sometimes found in stained smears (*Mycobacterium smegmatis, M. phlei*). These bacilli are usually present beneath the prepuce or on the labia as harmless saprophytes. They look exactly like tubercle bacilli but are readily differentiated by tests shown in Table 31–1.

In order to avoid the presence of confusing contaminants in urine specimens to be examined for tuberculosis, it is necessary to draw the urine through sterile catheters into sterile flasks. The important bacteriologic points are to see that the catheters are sterile and that they do not become contaminated with material from the external genitalia, hands, or instruments during the process of catheterization. The specimen is placed in a sterile container, properly labeled with patient's name, the date, and whether the specimen is from the *right* or *left* kidney. The patient's life may depend on this!

X-RAYS.   As noted earlier, diagnosis of tuberculosis of the lungs is commonly made by means of x-rays. Caseous masses, cavities, and calcified tubercles give more or less distinctive appearances, which can be recognized by those trained in x-ray diagnosis; however, so many other diseases cause shadows in x-ray plates of the chest, which may be confused with those due to tuberculosis, that microscopic, cultural, and animal inoculation studies should always be made if x-ray plates are suspicious and clinical data inconclusive. Among the diseases causing confusion in this way are histoplasmosis, coccidioidomycosis, nocardiosis, blastomycosis, cancer, pneumonias due to viral agents, and Q fever. Skin tests with tuberculin, coccidioidin, histoplasmin, and similar antigens from other fungi are of value in differentiating some of these conditions.

Transmission of Tuberculosis

Most of the following discussion is intended to apply in situations in which effective chemotherapy and chemoprophylaxis with drugs like isoniazid (INH) or para-aminosalicylic acid (PAS) are not available. Proper chemotherapy quickly renders most patients non-infective.

It is clear from the foregoing that in tuberculosis of the lungs the sputum is the chief source of infection, although in tuberculosis of the kidneys and bladder (relatively infrequent) the bacilli may also be present in the urine in large numbers. The bacilli are present in the feces in tuberculosis of the intestine (uncommon), and in the pus from tuberculous abscesses. It has been estimated that a single patient who is raising a considerable amount of sputum may discharge, in 24 hours, 500 million to three billion bacilli. A coughing or sneezing tuberculous patient throws out a spray of sputum containing tubercle bacilli, and this may be inhaled directly or in the form of droplet nuclei by other people. Thus, pulmonary tuberculosis is primarily an airborne disease. It means almost certain infection for infants in contact with the patient. In the infant, tuberculosis is very likely to take the form of a generalized, acute, fatal infection, with meningitis.

Unless immediate chemotherapy with isoniazid or other antituberculosis drugs is available, whenever possible, uninfected children should be removed from a home in which there is an active case of tuberculosis, or the patient should be removed as soon as the diagnosis of tuberculosis is made. The community health worker is often an important personal factor in explaining to families the need for such separations. The difficulties are often financial or stem from lack of proper institutions for the care of the tuberculous patient.

Tuberculous infection can occur through the mouth, especially in children. For example, a careless or ignorant person with active pulmonary tuberculosis kisses the children or contaminates the floor or furniture with sputum, or expectorates into the street or other public places. Children, creeping on the floor, or playing around the room or in the street, get the bacilli on their hands and thus into their mouths. Oral infection probably accounts for much of the nonpulmonary tuberculous infections of childhood. As previously noted, children may also be infected orally by drinking unpasteurized milk from tuberculous cows.

While probably a vector of only secondary importance, food may be contaminated by handling it with fingers soiled with sputum, or by flies that have crawled over tuberculous sputum. The tuberculous food handler may cough or sneeze over it. The common drinking cup or imperfectly

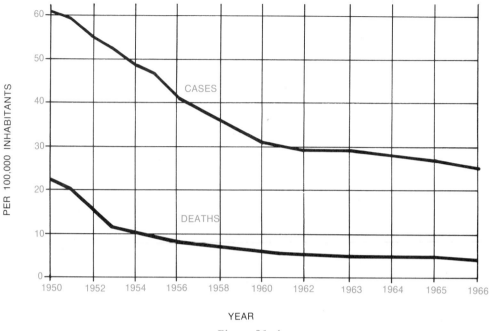

Figure 31–4

Tuberculosis morbidity and mortality in the United States 1950–66. (International Work in Tuberculosis. 1949–1964 WHO, Geneva, 1965 and Nelson, Vaughan, and McKay: Textbook of Pediatrics. 9th Ed. 1969, Philadelphia, W. B. Saunders Co.)

washed spoon or fork may also carry the bacilli. One of the great difficulties in preventing the spread of a constantly present disease like tuberculosis is the ignorance and indifference of the public. In 1966 there were about 60 times as many deaths from tuberculosis per 100,000 population as from poliomyelitis in spite of the fact that the tuberculosis death rate per 100,000 had dropped from about 225 in 1911 to about 4 in 1966. Figure 31–4 shows the decrease in deaths due to tuberculosis from 1950 to 1966. Note, however, that the number of active cases is still too high, considering what is known about this disease. In 1970, 37,137 new active cases occurred in the United States (Fig. 31–5).

Tuberculosis Infections

Tubercle bacilli are so widespread, especially in city streets, public transportation, theaters, and other places where people congregate, that no one in an urban community escapes eventual contact with the organisms. It is well known that 50 to 80 per cent of city-dwelling adults have at some time been slightly infected with the tubercle bacillus (probably in childhood). The healed lesions are found in the lungs in a large proportion of adults upon whom autopsies are performed following death due to wholly unrelated causes. Probably most of these persons never showed any recognized evidence of tuberculous infection. In 1958 it was estimated

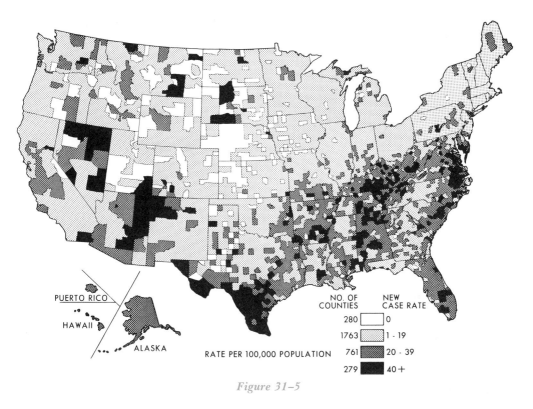

NO. OF COUNTIES	NEW CASE RATE
280	0
1763	1 - 19
761	20 - 39
279	40 +

RATE PER 100,000 POPULATION

Figure 31–5

New active cases of tuberculosis per 100,000 population. (From Morbidity and Mortality, Vol. 19, 1970. U.S. Dept. of Health, Education and Welfare.)

that over 8000 persons in New York City had active, open tuberculosis, unknown to anyone, and the situation has improved little since then.

There appears to be a very delicate balance between health and disease in tuberculosis. In most people the balance is heavily weighted in their favor by robust health (both physical and mental), a well balanced diet, rest, exercise, and recreation. In others, the balance in favor of health may be insufficient, rest and food inadequate, and the scales thus tipped in favor of the tubercle bacillus. Treatment, aside from the use of chemotherapy and surgery, is aimed largely at tipping the balance of health in favor of the patient. Resistance is kept at a high level by everything leading to a normal life: good food, fresh air, sufficient rest, and recreation—everything, in short, that keeps one in good condition. It is diminished by anything that decreases bodily vigor. Among these influences are: other infections, such as measles, whooping cough, and influenza; frequent childbearing; continuous overstrain and fatigue; poor living conditions of all kinds; the use of drugs; tobacco; alcoholism; and malnutrition.

Socioeconomic Conditions

Tuberculosis is closely connected with social and economic conditions in a community. It is much more frequent among the poor than among the well-to-do. Low standards of living mean lack of isolation, rest, sunlight, fresh air, cleanliness, medical care, and also insufficient food. The death rate from tuberculosis in any community clearly indicates what the social conditions are. During and after World War II conditions in war-torn countries in Europe created an enormous increase in tuberculosis. This has also been true for almost any other war.

Prevention and BCG

As mentioned in the section on active artificial immunization, a vaccine against tuberculosis was prepared in 1923, in France, by Calmette and Guérin, from an attenuated strain of *M. bovis*. It is called *BCG* (bacille Calmette Guérin). Its value has been and still is disputed by some health workers. Outstanding authorities have confirmed its effectiveness as an antigen. The United Nations (UNICEF) has given it to 226 million children, both tuberculin positive and tuberculin negative, in 95 countries, with gratifying results.

The physical examination of candidates for a school of medicine or nursing should include an intradermal tuberculin test and a chest plate if the tuberculin test is positive. Such a study results in diverting into less arduous occupations persons who would be unusually likely to develop the disease. It also detects tuberculous infection, previously unsuspected, and allows the infected persons to begin a modified way of living at a very favorable period and long before the disease would have been detected otherwise.

In using BCG, it must be remembered that this vaccine induces tuberculin hypersensitivity (i.e., a positive tuberculin reaction), thus eliminating the diagnostic significance of the positive reaction in persons vaccinated with BCG.

The importance of maintaining complete vigilance for tuberculous infection in patients, who are sources of disease in persons who care for them, unless the patient is under a regimen of treatment with INH or PAS (which renders the patient non-infective within a few days), becomes obvious. It is especially important to examine, by x-ray, sputum smear, tuberculin test, and physical examination, patients who will be in an institution for long periods, such as psychiatric patients and those with chronic disease. Hospital employees, especially orderlies, maids, and cooks, should be similarly examined.

The majority of hospitalized patients with tuberculosis have the pulmonary form. If they are in active stages of the disease, the sputum coughed up from the lungs must be destroyed. Unless the patient has copious pulmonary secretion, he is instructed to cough into disposable paper wipes and place these wipes in a disposable plastic or paper bag pinned to the bed or fastened to the bedside stand. When the bag is approximately three-quarters full of wipes, it is removed, and carefully closed at the top to prevent spilling of the wipes, wrapped in plastic bags and burned. If an incinerator is not readily available, the packages should be placed in marked trash cans. The personnel who are responsible for emptying these cans must be instructed in the importance of complete incineration of this material. Sputum cups are used only when absolutely necessary because they are difficult to disinfect completely and special care must be used in incineration to guarantee complete destruction of all the material in a closed incinerator system. All patients with excessive pulmonary secretions should be considered as possible cases of pulmonary tuberculosis until proven otherwise. Disregarding this simple precaution is probably the single most important cause of the incidence of pulmonary tuberculosis among nurses and others responsible for caring for patients with chronic respiratory conditions.

With the advent of chemotherapy and chemoprophylaxes, hospitals are not used as much as previously to *keep* the patients. The principal role of the hospital now is to care for the *acutely* ill and release the ambulatory patient who *cooperates* in *regular* chemotherapy.

Unless continually receiving INH or PAS or other effective chemotherapy, every patient with an active case of tuberculosis must be taught to live so as to avoid being a danger to others, and should be isolated like a person with an acute infectious disease, whenever possible. If he is not isolated, he must take proper precautions to protect others. He should not cough or expectorate openly. When away from home he should carry a pocket sputum flask. He should have a separate set of dishes, which should be boiled after use. He should sleep alone. He should take special pains not to soil his hands with sputum, and to wash them if he does. He should adequately cover his nose and mouth while coughing or sneezing. He should avoid contact with children under five years of age and elderly persons.

Every tuberculous patient must be trained to avoid exposing others. This teaching is an important function of the health team, and it can also be carried out successfully at home.

HANSEN'S DISEASE

The disease "leprosy" has an historical stigma attached to it. Modern knowledge has repudiated this and shown it to be completely unjustified. Therefore, it is now preferable to call it by its more modern name, "Hansen's disease."[4] The microbiologist and other knowledgeable professional people should lead the way to enlightenment and progress in this as well as other respects.

Although Hansen's disease is not primarily a respiratory disease, it is included here because it is commonly transmitted from extensive open lesions that develop in the upper respiratory tract, especially in the nasal septum, and because it is caused by *Mycobacterium leprae.*

Hansen's disease is one of the "historical diseases," ranking in importance with bubonic plague, cholera, typhus, yellow fever, and some others. That is, it has been known for centuries and has played a role in the history of mankind. In ancient and medieval times Hansen's disease had definite effects on religious activities, architecture, politics, science, literature and many other aspects of human life. Although not now common in the United States, it is nevertheless present. It exists almost unknown among our more than 200 million people, many of whose medieval ancestors' lives were haunted by fear, loathing, and hatred of the leper.

The disease is caused by an acid-fast bacillus (*Mycobacterium leprae*), first observed in significant relationship to the disease by Hansen in 1874. Both bacillus and disease are often called by his name. *M. leprae* can be seen

---

[4]Gerhard Armauer Hansen (1841–1912), a Norwegian physician, was first to recognize leprosy as a clinical entity.

in histologic sections of infected tissues from lepers. It is acid-fast and morphologically indistinguishable from other mycobacteria. Many workers have cultivated species of mycobacteria from leprous tissues and called them "*M. leprae;*" however, these have all the characteristics of the saprophytic mycobacteria. Experimental transmission of Hansen's disease, even with fresh leprous tissues, is very difficult. Shepard, in 1960, was able to grow *M. leprae* in the foot pads of mice. It produced infections and could be transferred for many passages without loss of virulence. In World War II, two American marines developed Hansen's disease in areas of the skin that had been previously tattooed while they had been on leave in Australia. Thus, without having proved Koch's postulates for *M. leprae*, even the skeptic now accepts it as the causative agent of Hansen's disease.

Contrary to centuries-old notions, Hansen's disease is *not* highly contagious. The natural method of transmission of Hansen's disease is obscure. Although lesions and discharges, including nasal discharges when the nasal tissues are involved, contain the bacilli in large numbers, prolonged, close contact appears to be necessary. Persons under 25 are more likely to contract the disease than are older people. As in tuberculosis, children are very susceptible to infection from leprous parents. The incubation period appears to range from a few months to as long as 20 years. In certain regions of the world Hansen's disease is endemic, that is, always present. Among these regions are tropical and subtropical Asia and Africa, Polynesia, and South America.

It is estimated that there are approximately 3 million leprous persons in the world, with about 30,000 in Central and South America and virtually none in Europe. In 1959 there were about 500 known cases of Hansen's disease in the United States, most residing in the National Leprosarium at Carville, Louisiana, and possibly 1000 unknown cases. In this country the disease spreads only in certain restricted areas along the Gulf Coast. In 1969, only 98 new cases were reported in the United States, and in 1970, only 129.

Hansen's disease is most distinctive in its so-called lepromatous phase. Nodules and gross deformities and ulcerations occur in the skin, with thickening, discolorations, and wrinkling. Nerves are often affected so that wounds go unnoticed; the individual has no pain sensations, and revolting and terrifying (to the ignorant and superstitious) disfigurations occur (Fig. 31–6). It was largely because of the disfiguring that the ancient world so feared lepers. Many disfiguring nonleprous diseases (various fungal and protozoal infections, yaws, and bejel) were doubtless confused with Hansen's disease. Modern surgery and chemotherapy with sulfones, such as DDS (dapsone) and 4,4'-diacetyldiaminodiphenyl-sulfone (DADDS), a repository or long-acting drug, are working wonders to combat this scourge of the Dark Ages.

HANSEN'S DISEASE AND TUBERCULOSIS. There are several striking similarities between Hansen's disease and tuberculosis. The causative agent of each is a species of *Mycobacterium;* both tend to be slowly progressive and chronic in many patients and to be most readily acquired in early childhood; progress of both diseases in patients appears to be related to personal resistance and to factors involving allergy. With respect to allergy, the *lepromin test* is analogous to the tuberculin test; the results of the tests have similar significance. Most significantly, BCG can induce lepromin sensitivity, and there is encouraging evidence that BCG vaccination can be of great value in immunization against this historic spectre.

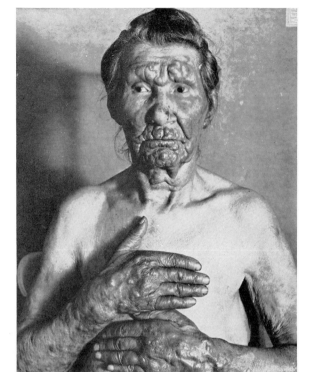

Figure 31-6

An advanced lepromatous case with leonine face, both furrowed and nodulate, and with marked involvement of the forearm and hands, less of the upper arms, and still less of the body. (Hunter, Frye, and Swartzwelder: Manual of Tropical Medicine, 4th Ed. 1966, Philadelphia, W. B. Saunders Co.)

From the standpoint of community health today in the United States, Hansen's disease is not a serious problem. To those concerned with the treatment and control of lepers, however, it is a dedication for life.

ACTINOMYCOSIS

ACTINOMYCES. This is a genus of bacteria in the order Actinomycetales that resemble molds in forming branched, filamentous structures. The organisms are much smaller than true molds, having diameters of 0.5 to 3 μm, like true bacteria. Also like bacteria, the *Actinomyces* are procaryotic in structure. No other bacteria normally exhibit branching to the extent that it occurs among the Actinomycetales. The degree of branching varies greatly in different species, being almost negligible in the previously discussed genus *Mycobacterium*, to which the tubercle bacillus belong. *Actinomyces* are characterized by having definitely a greater degree of branching than *M. tuberculosis*.

ACTINOMYCES ISRAELI. This organism is part of the normal flora of the human mouth. It may, however, cause disease in man. It is rigidly anaerobic and gram-positive but not acid-fast. Under unusual conditions, such as trauma following the extraction of a carious tooth, it becomes a pathogen when imbedded deep in the tissues. Swellings and abscesses form and are filled with pus. Sinus tracts may drain to the surface of the face. The surrounding tissue becomes hard. Colonies of the organism occur in the pus as yellowish granules (called "sulfur granules" because of their color), ranging up to a millimeter or more in diameter. Each granule con-

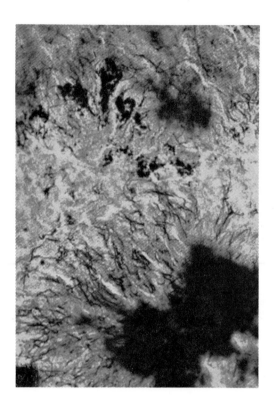

Figure 31-7

A mass (sulfur granule) of *Actinomyces bovis* from pus in an abscess. This organism causes a disease called lumpy jaw in cows. It grows around the jaw bone in pus and sulfur-like granules. The granule has been crushed and shows the central mass of mycelia and the radially arranged filaments. (Courtesy of L. A. Weed and A. D. Boggenstass: *Amer. J. Clin. Path.*)

sists of a central mass of very fine, branching, tightly interlaced and tangled, moldlike filaments (Fig. 31-7). The tips of the branches project radially at the periphery of the mass, like spines on a sea urchin or chesnut burr. This radial arrangement of the filaments in the granule gave rise to the name *Actino* (radial) *myces* (moldlike). These radial structures are not formed when the organism is grown in culture. *A. israeli* may also cause sulfur granules in lung abscesses. The reader should note that the condition called actinomycosis, associated with "lumpy jaw" in cattle, is due to *A. bovis* and is not identical to the human disease, caused by. *A. israeli;* nevertheless, the two conditions and the causative organisms are similar.

Actinomycosis is not contagious, though infections following human bites are known. This is, therefore, one of several reasons for keeping saliva out of a deep, penetrating wound. Actinomycosis is considered here not because it is a respiratory disease but because it is transmitted through saliva, as are the truly respiratory diseases.

RESPIRATORY FUNGOUS DISEASES

Several important and widespread infections of the respiratory tract are caused by fungi, notably histoplasmosis and coccidioidomycosis. As these and some other fungus infections are rarely transmitted from person to person by oronasal secretions, but arise mainly from soil, they are discussed more fully in Chapter 37 on fungous pathogens of the soil.

One important and widely distributed fungous disease that is not transmitted from soil but presumably often from the mouth or intestinal or vaginal tract is *candidiasis*, due to *Candida albicans*. This too for convenience is discussed with other fungi in Chapter 37.

Supplementary Reading

Almeida, J. O., and Bechelli, L. M.: Immunological problems in leprosy research. *Bull. WHO*, 1970, *43*(6):870.

Alvarez, W. C.: Tuberculosis often a geriatric disease. *Geriatrics*, 1971, *26*:82.

Becker, B.: Leprosy vaccines. *J.A.M.A.*, 1971, *216*(6):1038.

Bullock, W. E.: Studies of immune mechanisms in leprosy. *New Eng. J. Med.*, 1968, *278*:298.

Gruft, H., Gaafar, H. A., and Kaufmann, W.: Identification of mycobacteria—what constitutes adequate examination? *Am. J. Pub. Health*, 1970, *60*:2055.

Murohashi, T., and Yoskida, K.: Cultivation of *Mycobacterium leprae* in cell-free, semi-synthetic soft agar media. *Jap. J. Bacteriol.*, 1969, *24*:202.

Mushlin, I., and Amberson, J. B.: Tracking down tuberculosis. *Amer. J. Nurs.*, 1965, *65*:91.

Newman, R., Doster, B., Murray, F. J., and Ferebee, S.: Rifampin in initial treatment of pulmonary tuberculosis. A U.S. Public Service tuberculosis therapy trial. *Amer. Rev. Resp. Dis.*, 1971, *103*:461.

Runyon, E. H., Kubica, G. P., Morse, W. C., Smith, C. R., and Wayne, L. G.: Mycobacterium. In: Manual of Clinical Microbiology. 1970, Bethesda, Md., American Society for Microbiology.

Russell, D. A., Shepard, C. C., McRae, D. H., Scott, G. C., and Vincin, D. R.: Treatment with 4,4'-diacetyldiaminodiphenylsulfone (DADDS) of leprosy patients in the Karimui, New Guinea. *Amer. J. Trop. Med. Hyg.*, 1971, *20*:495.

Silcox, V. A., and David, H. L.: Differential identification of *Mycobacterium kansasii* and *Mycobacterium marinum*. *Appl. Microb.*, 1971, *21*:327.

Smith, D. T.: Which children in the United States should receive BCG vaccination. *Clin. Pediat.*, 1970, *9*:632.

UNICEF News: The fight against leprosy. 1968, 52(April):12.

Weg, J. G.: Tuberculosis and the generation gap. *Amer. J. Nurs.*, 1971, *71*:495.

WHO Chronicle: Therapy on leprosy. 1970, *24*:374.

WHO Chronicle: Leprosy: Progress and problems. 1971, *25*:178.

Young, W. D., Jr., Maslansky, A., Lefar, M. S., and Kronish, D. P.: Development of a paper strip test for detection of niacin produced by mycobacteria. *Appl. Microb.*, 1970, *20*:939.

Respiratory Viral, Mycoplasmal, and Chlamydial Infections

virus caracteristics – page 75.

VIRAL INFECTIONS

In considering any group of viruses the reader will no doubt wonder at the wide assortment of clinical entities that are associated with a given group of viruses, such as the "respiratory viruses," and the occurrence of any given virus in more than one group of clinical entities. Poliomyelitis is but one example of this problem of viral classification. This agent has been described as a *neurotropic* virus because of its frequent and striking affinity for nervous tissue; however, the presence of the virus in secretions of the respiratory tract warrants its mention in this chapter. Yet, the initial site of poliovirus multiplication is in the alimentary tract and therefore the poliovirus is now classified as one of the intestinal viruses or *enteroviruses*. It is most widely and frequently disseminated in feces (Chapter 25).

The classification of viruses and viral diseases changes frequently, primarily because of our rapidly increasing knowledge of the chemical, physical, and biologic properties of viruses. Such important taxonomic features as genetic storage of information in DNA or RNA, protein coat composition, enzymes produced, particle size, natural and experimental host range, susceptibility to chemicals, and serologic properties, to mention but a few, are being intensively studied in an attempt to resolve this problem. Therefore, in dealing with respiratory diseases of viral etiology, the student will note that a disease may be included in this chapter for a particular purpose related to control measures and further considered in other chapters for equally valid reasons (e.g., site of primary infection, epidemiology, or tissue affinity).

For recent concepts of viral classification and relationships the reader is referred to Appendix B.

SMALLPOX (VARIOLA)

It is hard to realize today that smallpox was once one of the most prevalent and most dreaded diseases in the world. Before the days of vac-

458

cination 95 persons of every 100 contracted it, and about one fourth of those died. Many who recovered were blinded or disfigured. Smallpox is readily transmitted by contact with patients or their fomites, as is measles, and both rank among the most contagious of human diseases. In both diseases the causative virus is present in oral and nasal secretions. In smallpox it is also present in the pox fluid and in the scales and crusts that form later. It is quite resistant to drying and may persist for some days in scales, dust, and so on.

Smallpox has been widespread in China and other Eastern countries from antiquity, and has repeatedly swept over Europe in great epidemics. It is still frequent in some countries, especially those of the East, but owing to vaccination and the rigid enforcement of quarantine laws, it has decreased in, and virtually disappeared from, more developed countries. Two clinically and epidemiologically distinct forms of smallpox are recognized. These are the mild form of the disease characterized by a less than 1 per cent mortality rate and termed *"variola minor"* or "alastrim" and the classical, severe form—*"variola major"*—which results in an overall mortality of 15 to 30 per cent. There are still backward communities that do not require general vaccination and some religious cults that actively object to it. In an epidemic in Tipera, East Pakistan (now Bangladesh), in 1957, smallpox killed 1061 persons in only 38 days of survey. Surprisingly enough, smallpox broke out in a small epidemic in Heidelberg, Germany, in 1959; it was said to be due to a virus brought from India.

Figure 32–1 shows the number of smallpox cases that occurred in Bombay, India, between 1966–1967. Of 840 cases, 346 died. One person who left Bombay via air on February 21, 1967, imported smallpox into Regensburg, Germany; another similarly imported the disease into Prague on March 4. Others transmitted smallpox still later from Bombay to Hanover and elsewhere. The imported cases did not cause epidemics in their home cities because the local populations were largely protected by vaccination.

Until 1971 everyone entering the United States had to be vaccinated or show proof of recent vaccination. This protective regulation has been relaxed by governmental agencies. Let us hope we will not regret it! Perhaps the measures applicable to international travelers, as specified in International Health Regulations of the World Health Organization (WHO), in force since January 1, 1971, will take its place.

IMMUNITY TO SMALLPOX. Smallpox was the first disease to which immunity was intentionally obtained by artificial means. The method was developed on the basis of practical experience and was carried on more or less successfully for centuries before there was any knowledge of the scientific principles on which it is based or of the etiologic agent involved. Even before the Christian Era, it was the custom in India and China to introduce under the skin of a healthy person a bit of pus from the eruption of a person with a mild case of the disease in the hope of producing a light attack. This procedure was called *variolation* or *inoculation*. Its disadvantages were that the disease thus produced was contagious, and the attack sometimes proved to be severe or fatal. Nevertheless, it continued to be practiced until *vaccination* took its place (see Chapter 20).

MODERN METHOD OF VACCINATION. The skin is washed with soap and water and then with alcohol, which is allowed to evaporate. Disinfectant such as iodine should not be used on the skin as it will inactivate the virus in the vaccine. The fluid or lymph containing the virus is expelled

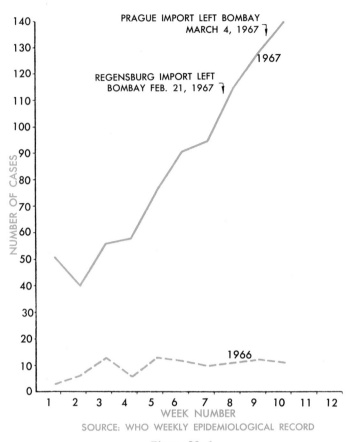

PRAGUE IMPORT LEFT BOMBAY
MARCH 4, 1967

1967

REGENSBURG IMPORT LEFT
BOMBAY FEB. 21, 1967

1966

WEEK NUMBER

SOURCE: WHO WEEKLY EPIDEMIOLOGICAL RECORD

Figure 32-1

Smallpox cases by week of report—Bombay, India—1966 and 1967 (see text). (From National Communicable Disease Center: Morbidity and Mortality. 1967, Vol. 16, No. 12. U. S. Department of Health, Education, and Welfare, Public Health Service, Bureau of Disease Prevention and Environmental Control.)

from the tube onto the skin, and with a sterile needle, two shallow punctures or slight scratches are made through the drop of virus and into the vascular layer of the skin. Vaccination is a small surgical operation and should be done only by a person who understands surgical cleanliness. The wound may become infected like any other wound. The occasional complications of vaccination are often due to this.

VACCINIA. After vaccination of a previously unvaccinated person there is an incubation period of three or four days, during which there are no noticeable changes. Then, if the vaccination "takes," the mild, immunizing infection called *vaccinia* occurs. An eruption appears at the place of inoculation and goes through a series of characteristic stages, during a period of about two weeks (papule, vesicle, pustule, scab, and finally healing), leaving a distinctive scar. About the seventh day there is often a reaction on the part of the whole body, lasting several days, and often shown by fever, loss of appetite, general discomfort, and headache. During this time specific antibodies are formed in the body.

REACTIONS IN IMMUNE PERSONS. (See Fig. 20–2.) If the vaccinated person is completely immune, a small red papule, sometimes with a tiny vesicle or blister, appears within ten to 72 hours and heals within five to seven days. This is spoken of as an "immune (or immediate) reaction." If the person is only partly immune, what looks like a small and rapidly evolving "take" with pustule and scab develops, beginning within one to five days lasting about a week or ten days. This is spoken of as an "accelerated or vaccinoid reaction" or reaction of partial immunity. If no reaction of any kind occurs, it is likely that the vaccine virus was inactive, the person vaccinated was not allergic to it, disinfectants on the skin inactivated the virus, or some other error occurred and the vaccination should be repeated.

Protection Given by Vaccination.   This is complete for some time and then it gradually wanes. It usually begins to disappear in two years and is almost completely gone in ten years. In endemic areas or specially exposed populations every child should be vaccinated between the ages of six months and two years and again when about 12 years old. Much disfigurement, sickness, and death could be prevented by a reasonably intelligent view of vaccination on the part of those in control (Fig. 32–2).

Medical personnel may never see a case of smallpox in the United States; however, they may see the disease during foreign service. Applicants to most schools of medicine, nursing, or other health professions are required to have a recent vaccination against smallpox before being accepted. It is most important to impress people with the importance of vaccination against smallpox.

Compulsory Vaccination.   During a sudden outbreak of smallpox in Tabriz, Iran, in 1957, 123 cases of smallpox and 17 deaths had occurred by the time the outbreak was recognized, and the disease was spreading rapidly when the epidemic was reported. By prompt action of the authorities 92 per cent of the population were vaccinated in three weeks, and the epidemic was promptly stopped. Thus smallpox can be absolutely prevented by the organized, compulsory vaccination of a whole population. There are many other illustrations of this.

Figure 32–2

Children of one family who were brought to the Municipal Hospital of Philadelphia with the mother and father, who had smallpox. The child in the center had been considered too young to be vaccinated. The other children had been vaccinated a year before; they remained free from the disease, although for several weeks they lived in the wards of patients with smallpox. (Schamberg and Kolmer: Acute Infectious Diseases. Philadelphia, Lea & Febiger.)

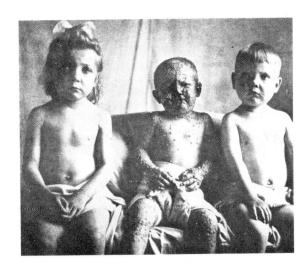

It seems obvious that it is far less dangerous to have a case of small-pox accidentally introduced into an immune community than into a susceptible one. In addition to long range preventive measures, all contacts of known cases should be vaccinated as soon as possible after the diagnosis has been made. A great deal of detective work often has to be done to identify these contacts, particularly if the patient had traveled extensively.

The pustules and the oral and nasal exudates of smallpox patients are infective in the eruptive stage, and bedding, fomites, and similar items are highly infective and must be handled with appropriate precautions to avoid spread of lint and dust. Because the discharges may have a very disagreeable odor, it is usually advisable to use a disinfectant such as saponated solution of cresol or chlorine laundry bleach, both of which have deodorant, or at least "counter-odorant," properties.

MEASLES (RUBEOLA)

Measles is one of the most common and perhaps the most infectious of human diseases caused by viral agents. True measles, also known as rubeola, may be confused by the layman with rubella (German measles, "three-day" measles), or with roseola, which is another related disease. To resolve this confusion (or to compound it even more), a suggestion has been made to use the Latin term morbilli instead of rubeola for the true measles, also called the "red measles."

Like smallpox, measles is extremely contagious. A person who has not had measles, exposed at any age, is almost certain to contract the disease. The reason that rubeola is chiefly confined to children is that most persons have had it before reaching adult life. When rubeola was a common disease, its clinical features, especially the rash, were well recognized by physicians and parents. Since the incidence of measles has been remarkably decreased by vaccination (Fig. 32–3), it becomes more and more important to confirm the diagnosis with laboratory tests. In the United States about 300,000 cases of measles were reported in 1964; 75,290 in 1971; 27,300 in the first nine months of 1972.

TRANSMISSION OF MEASLES. The measles virus does not appear to survive long outside the body. It is presumably transmitted by direct contact, by droplet infection during coughing and sneezing, and by articles freshly soiled with the nose and mouth secretions. A very important fact is that the organism is present in the nasal secretion and saliva before the rash breaks out and for about five days after the rash appears. The first symptoms of the disease resemble those of an ordinary cold, and the rash does not appear until three or four days later. A number of other diseases may begin in the same way—for example, whooping cough and scarlet fever. Rubeola may be easily diagnosed during the pre-skin eruption period by 104–105 F fever, and Koplik's spots, which appear on the mucous membranes in the mouth. These spots are bright red, but have bluish white center specks. As in mumps, urine is infectious.

Measles is most infectious during this early stage and during the rash; there is little danger of the patient's spreading the disease after the temperature has returned to normal.

COMPLICATIONS ATTENDING MEASLES. Measles itself, although it may make a patient very ill, seldom causes death. Complications, however, may be very serious or even fatal unless properly treated. The most common of these are bronchopneumonia and abscess in the ear, caused

MEASLES — Reported Cases by Month, United States, 1963-1970

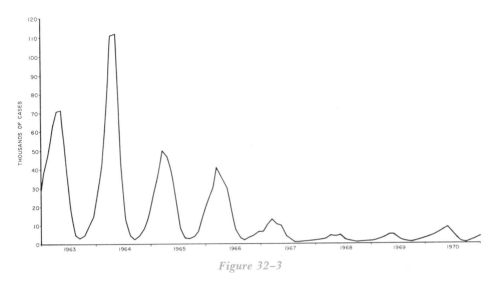

Figure 32-3

Measles incidence in United States, 1963–1970. (From Morbidity and Mortality, Annual Supplement, 1970. U.S. Dept. of Health, Education and Welfare.)

by pneumococci or streptococci. Measles is sometimes regarded lightly, but it is potentially a serious disease because of the infections that often accompany or follow it. As with many other infections, the younger the child, the more serious the disease. Less than half of the cases occur in children under five years, but about 75 per cent of the deaths are in children of five years and under. Since the introduction of antibiotics, the death rate from bacterial complications in measles has been reduced to a very low level.

PREVENTION OF MEASLES. The best means of prevention is by vaccination with measles vaccine. However, if vaccination of children has not been done, when a case of measles has appeared in a school or an institution, the greatest hope of limiting the spread of the disease lies in isolating all persons having symptoms of a cold, or known to have been in contact with the patient while he had the early or later symptoms. Although it is very difficult to diminish the number of cases, a great deal can be done to decrease the number of deaths due to the disease by preventing the complications, through good nursing and antibiotics, and by protecting very young children from infection. Many children are being immunized by vaccination against measles, just as they are against smallpox, so that (hopefully) in a very few years measles, too, will be one of the "conquered" diseases.

In the hospital, complete isolation of measles cases is desirable. In an open ward it is practically impossible to prevent the spread of measles, even with the most painstaking technique. Rigid terminal disinfection is not necessary for the short-lived measles organisms, but streptococci that often accompany them are vigorous and long-lived. It is best, therefore, to disinfect the bedding and clothing, and to give the room a thorough cleaning with soap and water and disinfectant.

prophylactic

GAMMA GLOBULIN.   Until recently, gamma globulin (obtained from the serum of measles-immune persons) was commonly used to protect children under four years of age when exposed to the disease. This protection, like all passive immunity, is temporary but is valuable in protecting young children, in whom complications are apt to be severe. To avert the attack, the gamma globulin must be given within three days after exposure.

Therapeutic

If the material is injected in small doses between the fourth and sixth days after exposure, it does not prevent the disease but modifies its course, making it very mild. This mild attack, however, probably gives permanent protection. Children under nine months of age contain maternal antibodies if the mother has had measles. In spite of the maternal antibodies, gamma globulin may be administered as a precautionary measure. Vaccination against measles, where done, makes this practice obsolete except in special situations (see below).

ACTIVE IMMUNIZATION.   With the isolation and propagation of the measles virus in tissue culture, dramatic progress has been made in the preparation of vaccines for mass immunization. The adaptation of the Edmonston virus (named after the patient from whom this strain was originally isolated) to grow in chick embryo–tissue cultures has decreased its pathogenicity for man while still retaining its antigenicity (i.e., capacity to stimulate the production of antibodies).

Active Virus Vaccine.   This virus, developed by Dr. John F. Enders and his coworkers, provides a vaccine analogous to the Sabin oral, active-virus polio vaccine. The active measles vaccine differs from the Sabin active polio vaccine in that the measles vaccine must be injected instead of being given orally, and the infection produced by it is not transmissible. One dose of measles vaccine (0.2 to 0.25 ml in a single subcutaneous injection) may be given to susceptible young persons and children not younger than nine months, especially to those most likely to be exposed and to be adversely affected by measles, but not to pregnant women or to those with leukemia and other malignancies or certain other conditions. Use of the live attenuated virus vaccine is frequently accompanied by such clinical reactions as the fever and rash characteristic of the disease; however, field trials have shown that the simultaneous injection of measles-immune gamma globulin has significantly reduced the incidence of these undesired clinical manifestations. More recent preparations of vaccine contain measles virus of very low pathogenicity. The immunity induced by the vaccine appears to be durable, prompt and very effective.

Inactivated (killed) virus measles vaccine has been tested but is not recommended because of severe, atypical forms of measles that resulted from later exposure to the disease.

The importance of controlling or eliminating measles is further emphasized by findings in studies made in 1972 suggesting that there may be a causal relationship between infection with measles virus and multiple sclerosis.

Contraindication to the Use of
Active Virus Vaccine

Children with debilitating disease, leukemia, or on drugs affecting immune responses should not be vaccinated; however, *immune human gamma globulin* should be given to such children within three days after exposure to measles.

GERMAN MEASLES (RUBELLA)

This viral disease is fairly common, but is in itself rarely serious. It may be called the "three day measles" because, although the duration of the disease is from one to five days, the rash usually evolves over a three day period. Rubella is probably transmitted in much the same way as measles. The incubation period is about ten days to three weeks. It not infrequently occurs in adults. When it occurs in an expectant mother during the first three months of pregnancy, it often causes severe damage to the fetus since it appears to have a special affinity for the embryonic tissues. Deformities or defects are particularly likely to occur in heart, ears, brain, and eyes.

Because an attack of German measles in childhood is rarely harmful and probably confers lifelong immunity, it was recommended by some that girls be purposely exposed to the disease between the ages of six and eight years in order to avoid contracting it during pregnancy later in life. Vaccination of all children is now the preferred procedure.

Passive immunization of nonimmune women during the first three months of pregnancy to protect the unborn child has been recommended. Gamma globulin (antibodies) from the blood of immune persons is used.

RUBELLA VACCINE. An extremely important advance toward the control and elimination of rubella was made in 1962 when a "rubella associated agent," the virus of rubella, was isolated from rubella patients and cultivated in tissue culture. The step from this to the preparation of a rubella vaccine was not unlike the ones exemplified by the preparation of vaccines against yellow fever, polio, influenza, measles, and several other viral diseases. A single dose of active attenuated rubella virus vaccine was found to protect between 90 and 95 per cent of susceptible children when exposed to the German measles. In the United States vaccination of all children between one year of age and puberty will assure protection against rubella in pregnant women. This will eliminate the need for therapeutic abortions (now legal in some states) to avoid *congenital rubella* in some 20 to 25 per cent of infants born to women who had German measles during the first trimester of pregnancy. *Under no circumstances* should a pregnant female be vaccinated. Women of childbearing age should not be vaccinated unless shown to be susceptible and unless they promise to prevent pregnancy for at least two months following vaccination.

EXANTHEMA SUBITUM (ROSEOLA INFANTUM)

This acute viral disease is often confused with rubella because it, too, sometimes causes a three day rash. Roseola typically occurs in infants about 12 months old. The high temperature and the sudden onset are frequently accompanied by convulsions. The fever remains high for three or four days. After the fever, the rash appears and lasts for one to two days. Allergies may confuse the diagnosis. Many infections remain subclinical.

CHICKENPOX (VARICELLA)

The virus of this annoying malady is contained in the early-stage "pock," or eruption, and is probably transmissible by this; however, the respiratory secretions are probably the most important vector. Chickenpox is extremely contagious. The disease is usually mild, although severe, and—rarely—fatal cases occur, more often in adults than in children. Pustules develop in successive lots. Complications are usually not serious. No prophylaxis is available as in measles. Infected individuals may be isolated, especially if very young children are in a family. The expectant mother should also avoid contact with chickenpox. Congenital varicella is usually fatal to the infant; however, infection of the small infant contracted after birth is likely to be very mild.

HERPES ZOSTER ("SHINGLES")

This painful disease is due to a virus identical to the chickenpox virus. The agent is therefore called the varicella-zoster (V-Z) virus. The dermal lesions are often very similar. Patients with herpes zoster, commonly persons over 40, usually have a history of clinical childhood varicella.

Herpes zoster affects the dorsal nerve roots and areas of skin to which the corresponding sensory nerves extend. There seems to be a tendency for the skin lesions to occur where there exists continuous irritation, such as caused by restricting clothing. It is usually, but not always, confined to one side. The pain and lesions may occur in successive patches and crops, as in chickenpox, anywhere from neck to lumbar region, or even legs and arms. Itching and pain are often intense. Brownish spots may remain after healing. The disease is rarely fatal, but can cause much intense discomfort.

The mode of transmission appears to be like that of measles and chickenpox. An adult with herpes zoster can infect children, who usually develop chickenpox. Children with chickenpox can infect adults, who may develop herpes zoster. The two occasionally occur together in children. Zoster-immune gamma globulins prevent the disease.

HERPES SIMPLEX (FEVER BLISTERS)

The herpes simplex virus, *Herpesvirus hominis*, causes local eruption of "fever blisters" or "cold sores" around the mouth, face, and mucous membranes. This disease is mentioned here because of its name, which may be confused with the previously described herpes zoster. Clinical conditions more severe than fever blisters have been attributed to the virus, such as conjunctivitis, invasions of the central nervous system, asymptomatic conditions in the neonatal infant, and, as will be discussed in Chapter 35, acute vulvovaginitis. It is then transmissible by coitus and other forms of sexual contact.

It is probable that the herpes simplex virus is continually present as a latent infection in the facial tissues of some people. Eruptions occur when extreme changes in temperature, either hot or cold, or fever from whatever cause are encountered that favor its active reproduction. Exposure to ultraviolet irradiation, menstruation, or emotional stress also may cause fever blisters to form.

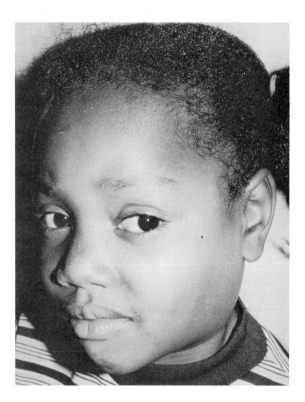

Figure 32–4

Mumps (epidemic parotitis). Firm, elastic swelling of the parotid slightly elevating the ear. (Courtesy of L. R. Regattieri and J. P. Thomas *in* Finn: Clinical Pedodontics, 4th Ed., W. B. Saunders, Philadelphia, 1973).

MUMPS (CONTAGIOUS PAROTITIS[1])

This disease, due to one of the small viruses, is characterized by sudden onset, with swelling and pain in the salivary glands, usually only the parotids; however, the sublingual and submaxillary glands and numerous other glandular tissues may also be involved. In many cases of mumps these glandular involvements do not occur or are so slight as to pass unnoticed. Thus mild, unrecognized cases of mumps (i.e., inapparent infections) occur, which actively immunize the patient but also serve to spread the disease.

The virus may also seriously affect the ovaries or, more commonly, the testes in sexually mature persons, resulting in sterilization; it not infrequently invades the central nervous system, causing meningoencephalitis, which may cause permanent damage to the brain.

SKIN SENSITIVITY. As in many other viral infections, a degree of skin sensitivity follows infection with the mumps virus. This sensitivity may be detected by the intradermal inoculation of persons who have previously been infected by mumps virus, with an extremely minute quantity of the heat-inactivated virus, and by then observing the wide zone of erythema resulting at the site of inoculation within 20 to 24 hours. Unfortunately the dermal test cannot be depended on as an indicator of immune status.

---

[1] Avoid the error of the red-faced student who confused parotitis with parrot fever!

TRANSMISSION. The virus is transmitted in saliva and by objects recently contaminated with saliva. The virus may be present in the saliva from seven days before the onset of symptoms until nine days after glandular swelling subsides.

Transmission by Urine. Mumps virus has been repeatedly demonstrated in the urine of mumps patients within two weeks from onset and often longer. This necessarily alters the older concept of mumps as a disease requiring only those preventive precautions applicable to respiratory secretion-borne pathogens. Urine of mumps patients, as well as their respiratory secretions, must be dealt with as infectious. Is it possible that other viruses infecting the respiratory tract may also appear in the urine?

Prevention

Persons of any age with mumps should be isolated, as should any patient with communicable respiratory disease. There is no effective specific treatment. Patients virtually always recover promptly and without serious complications, except when the ovaries, testes, or central nervous system are involved. Hyperimmune mumps gamma globulin has been tested, but may even increase the incident of the disease. A vaccine is available and may be included in routine immunization programs with a revaccination schedule required. Its full value is still under investigation.

RABIES (HYDROPHOBIA)

Although caused by a distinctively neurotropic virus, and apparently not at all a disease of any part of the respiratory tract, rabies is transmitted, like mumps, with respiratory secretions in saliva. Man can also be infected by way of the respiratory tract by dusty guano in bat caves. Hence, for convenience, it is included in this section.

Rabies is primarily a disease of mammals (an encephalitis), which is transmitted to man usually as a consequence of the saliva of rabid animals gaining entrance to wounds caused by bites or scratches. The disease may be transmitted to and by a great many species of biting mammals: dogs, cats, skunks, rodents of all sorts, foxes, horses, cattle, swine, and so on. Vampire and other species of bats are important vectors in certain parts of Europe, South America, and in the United States.

Rabies is caused by a virus that particularly affects the central nervous system, to which it is conveyed from the wound chiefly by the path of the nerve trunks. The disease in man is very terrible: the patient, usually with clear consciousness, passes through periods of depression and excitement, attended by painful spasms, to a stage of paralysis and death. The name hydrophobia means fear of water. Human beings, as well as other mammals with the disease, have this symptom. The muscles involved in swallowing develop such painful spasms upon attempts to swallow food or drink that the patient comes to fear even the sight or suggestion of them. If symptoms have once appeared, death has seemed inevitable. However, in the case of one boy bitten by a supposedly rabid bat, recovery occurred after a series of treatments designed to anticipate separate disease stages the patient encountered and his body had to combat. The attack was clinically atypical.

Figure 32–5

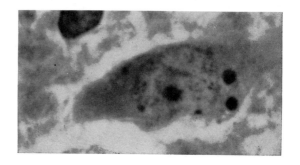

Negri bodies in a nerve cell in a section of the brain of a rabid cat. The three dark, spherical bodies within the cytoplasm of the cell are Negri bodies. A mixture of dyes like Sellers' stain (see footnote on Seller's stain, in text) has been applied to improve visibility. (Schleifstein.)

DIAGNOSIS OF RABIES. The brain cells of mammals whose death is due to rabies contain certain cytoplasmic inclusions called *Negri bodies* after the Italian investigator who discovered them in 1903 (Fig. 32–5). These inclusions contain viral particles and rabies antigens. The examination of the brains of rabies-suspected animals for the presence of Negri bodies is an extremely important method of diagnosis; further, it takes only an hour or so to complete the examination. A small bit of the portion of brain called the hippocampus major, or Ammon's horn, is smeared thinly on a slide, stained, preferably with Seller's stain,[2] and examined for the characteristic intracytoplasmic inclusion bodies.

Failure to find Negri bodies does not necessarily exclude the possibility of rabies. If there is any doubt, injection of the brain into other animals is highly advisable because mice, rabbits, and guinea pigs are very susceptible to the disease. Inoculation of the brains of suspect animals into the brains of such rodents is a much more reliable means of diagnosis than is microscopic examination, but it requires several days or weeks for observation of the test animals. Antigen in infected brain cells is readily demonstrable by means of fluorescent antibody staining.

IMMUNITY TO RABIES. Formerly fairly common, rabies is now infrequent among human beings in civilized countries for three reasons. First, there is much better control (though still very imperfect control in the United States) of stray cats and dogs and wild animals, who disseminate the disease.

Avianized Vaccine. Second, it is now possible, and indeed a common practice in intelligent communities, to vaccinate all pet dogs and cats. This is harmless and very effective. A single subcutaneous injection of an active virus attenuated by cultivation in living avian embryos is often used. It is called "avianized vaccine." This prophylactic treatment with active virus is not yet permissible in man.

Pasteur Treatment. Third, a course of immunizing injections with the avianized vaccine (inactivated by chemicals, ultraviolet irradiations, or heat) is given to all persons who might have been infected by bites. The method, based on principles established (1881–1886) by Pasteur, results in active immunity. It is not a cure. It must be begun as soon after the bite as possible in order that the patient may develop antibodies before the disease has time to establish itself. Fourteen injections of Semple vaccine are the treatment used.

---

[2]Seller's stain: *a*, Basic fuchsin (1 per cent solution in methyl alcohol) — 5 ml. *b*, Methylene blue (1 per cent solution in methyl alcohol) — 10 ml. Mix *a* and *b*; keeps well in tightly stoppered bottle. Stain smear five to ten seconds; wash with water; blot dry. Examine with oil-immersion lens.

The Duck Embryo (Avianized) Vaccine.   Semple vaccine (virus in rabbit brain inactivated by phenol) may cause encephalomyelitis because of the brain tissue it contains. For this reason, the duck embryo vaccine is an excellent prophylactic treatment. Three injections, followed by a booster dose after one month and again several months later, then followed by single injections every few years give perfect protection to veterinarians and animal handlers. (See also the section on artificial active immunization.) After a bite, the duck vaccine is administered subcutaneously once a day for 14 days, or if the bite was on the face or if very severe injuries resulted, for 21 days.

Antirabies Serum.   In case of very severe bites and almost certain infection, antirabies serum, usually horse serum, is sometimes injected into the tissues about the bite wounds at the time of beginning the injections of vaccine. It has proved to be of striking value when so used. Allergic reactions to the equine proteins must be anticipated.

PRACTICAL PROCEDURE.   The bite of a rabid animal does not necessarily mean that rabies will develop, since the virus may not be in the saliva at the time of the bite, or if present, it may not be so in effective concentrations. Also, the presence of thick clothing worn at the site of the bite may prevent the inoculation of virus into the tissues. It is important, however, that bites of animals suspected of being rabid, or bites of unknown, "bite and run" animals, be immediately and thoroughly cleansed with soap and water. A soft syringe may be used to force soapy water to the depths of the wound. When the disease is still in incipient stages in dogs or cats, the saliva is infectious and may infect if transferred by any means to cut or scratches on the hands. Bites or infections on hands, arms, or face are more dangerous than those on the legs and feet because the virus is then inoculated closer to the brain. The incubation period of the disease is variable: from two to six weeks or longer in human beings, in dogs from one to eight weeks. If it seems reasonably probable that the biting animal was rabid, the treatment should be started without delay. Many very painful Pasteur treatments have been given on the basis of hysteria and in the absence of real danger of rabies.

Do not kill the animal unless it is diagnosed rabid by a competent veterinarian. If it is caught, hold it (well caged!) for observation for ten days. Rabid dogs rarely survive ten days after development of symptoms. If the dog has rabies, it will show unmistakable symptoms before this time and may then be killed. Rabies can then be definitely established by examination of the dog's brain for Negri bodies and by mouse inoculation, or by means of fluorescent antibody staining of brain tissues. If the dog shows absolutely no symptoms at the end of ten days, it may be released, and the victim may then discontinue the treatment. His mind will be much more at ease to know that the animal is free from rabies than if it had been killed with the suspicion still upon it. If the animal has already been killed, send the head, packed in ice, immediately to the laboratory of the State or City Department of Health, or a competent veterinarian, for examination. Wild animals suspected of having rabies should be killed immediately and examined for the disease.

RABIES IN DOGS AND CATS.   It is important to be able to recognize rabies in a dog or cat. The first sign of rabies in a dog is usually an alteration of its disposition: it develops a nervous, furtive manner, becomes restless, and seems afraid. Because of its vague apprehensions it may seek human company and appear unusually affectionate. Later it acts in a definitely abnormal manner, develops a peculiar wolflike bark or howl and becomes snappish and even more restless, sometimes running away for days at a time, during which it may bite animals or persons. This is "furious rabies." In "dumb rabies" the furious phase is much less evident. In any case, difficulty in eating develops, and drooling ("foaming at the mouth") occurs because swallowing is difficult. The dog may bite any animal or person and often chews sticks and stones and may swallow them. Paralysis eventually ensues and death supervenes.

In cats, rabies is usually less difficult to recognize than in dogs because cats do not attempt to maintain their favored position in the affections of their owners, in spite of the disease, as do dogs. The early symptoms are much like those in dogs, being manifested as irritability and restlessness, but the disease soon develops into the furious stage as a rule, and the cat becomes entirely wild and ferocious, with dilated pupils, salivating, open mouth, and extended claws. Cats are especially dangerous because of their claws, which become contaminated with saliva, and because cats give allegiance to no one.

Transmission of rabies from one human being to another is very rare. Since the virus is present in the saliva of human patients, precautions must be taken to prevent its entrance into cuts and scratches on the nurse's or physician's hands or face, or from reaching wounds or scratches on other persons. The use of face masks in caring for human beings who have rabies is probably indicated. The disease may also be transmitted by affectionate licking by rabid animals.

ANTERIOR POLIOMYELITIS (INFANTILE PARALYSIS)

Mention has already been made of the dramatic and frequently fatal paralytic effects resulting from invasion of the CNS (central nervous system) by the poliomyelitis virus. Because of this, the disease has for years been regarded as intimately related to nervous tissues. Although this is true, we now know that poliomyelitis may be considered primarily an infection of the gastrointestinal tract (caused by one of the *enteroviruses*) and that, like other enteric infections, it is transmitted partly in and by feces, and is discussed more fully in Chapter 24, with other diseases of the intestinal tract.

In this section on respiratory viruses it suffices to say that the poliovirus is also present in the respiratory (pharyngeal) secretions of many patients, probably for several days before onset of symptoms and for some days (up to two weeks?) afterward. The respiratory (pharyngeal) secretions of patients in early stages, and objects contaminated with them, must therefore be treated as though highly infectious. Whether feces or respiratory tract secretions are the more important vectors of the virus (a debated question), both are acknowledged to be effective and frequent vectors.

Precautions must be in part based on the modes of transmission. With respect to proper handling of respiratory secretions, in poliomyelitis the precautions already described for diseases of the respiratory tract apply fully. With regard to fecal transmission, consult the section on enteric diseases. The same remarks apply to the reoviruses and some ECHO viruses.

INFLUENZA

In 1918–1919 a terrible epidemic of influenza swept over the entire world, causing more than ten million deaths; in the United States alone at least 450,000 died. There is relatively little direct evidence of the true nature of this disease. It is often referred to as pandemic influenza. We do not know with certainty whether this epidemic was the same as the infection now called influenza. Serologic studies indicate that it was due to the virus of swine influenza.

TRANSMISSION.   The mode of transmission of influenza is like that of other respiratory infections. Probably crowded indoor (low humidity) conditions, with droplet infection, favor epidemics.

INFLUENZA VIRUS TYPES.   There are at least three main types of human influenza virus, all causing epidemics of the same (clinical) disease. The first types to be differentiated were called types A (1933) and B (1940). Later type C was discovered. There are numerous subtypes, which are distinguishable mainly on the basis of antigenic and immunologic properties. A whole set or family of such variants of type A was found in 1957 in the world-wide epidemic commonly called Asian influenza ("Asiatic flu"). These viruses are termed variants of Far East (FE), or Asian, influenza (A). During the Christmas–New Year's season of 1968–1969, Asian influenza virus, "Hong Kong flu" (A2) variant, was widespread in the United States, though fatality rates were relatively low. In 1972 the "London flu epidemic," due to influenzavirus A/England/42/72, spread widely and rapidly all over the world by air travel.

COMPLICATIONS.   When uncomplicated, influenza is usually not a fatal disease; however, there is a special tendency to bronchopneumonia, which is responsible for most of the deaths associated with the disease. The bronchopneumonia may be caused by pneumococci, streptococci, the influenza bacillus, or other organisms, alone or in combinations. Thousands of deaths in the army camps in 1918 were due to the bronchopneumonia accompanying influenza. Apparently, the virus of the pandemic of 1918 so lowered the local resistance of the lungs that almost any bacterium could invade the lung tissues and cause pneumonia. Chemotherapy is very effective in controlling these bacterial complications of influenza, as well as of measles, but is of no value in curing or preventing the viral infection in either disease.

ACTIVE IMMUNIZATION.   It is possible to prevent influenza by means of vaccines. These are made of virus propagated in chick embryos, purified, and inactivated with formalin (Figs. 5–3 and 5–4). In preparing influenza vaccine it is important to use a mixture of viruses representing all the antigens of the various groups, since vaccine for only one type offers little or no protection against the others. The immunity is short-lived, lasting for from two to 12 months, and vaccinated persons may get influenza unless vaccination is repeated frequently. The infecting virus strains tend to vary continually so that a vaccine effective today may be ineffective next month.

Treatment

If influenza develops, it is possible in the great majority of cases to avoid the complicating pneumonia by proper care: first, by keeping the patient in bed from onset and during convalescence; and second, by giving protection from the bacteria that are known to be the cause of pneumonia. This is done by means of chemotherapy and by carrying out the same precautions as are prescribed for bronchopneumonia. Care must be taken to keep susceptible persons from contact with the patient. Fomites should be disinfected as in any respiratory disease, viral, bacterial, or other. Careful washing of the hands and proper wearing of a gauze mask may protect health workers. Opinions differ on this point.

THE "COMMON COLD"

The term "common cold" has been used for many years to designate infectious diseases of the upper respiratory tract characterized by various all-too-familiar signs and symptoms in multiple combinations, including adenopathy, inflammation of the mucous membranes of nose, pharynx, and bronchial tree, fever, headache, copious watery nasal exudate, muscular pains, sinusitis, lacrimation, conjunctivitis, general malaise, sneezing, and coughing. As previously mentioned, many of these appear also in early stages of measles and several other diseases so that there is nothing very distinctive about them. Probably most subclinical viral infections are quickly diagnosed as "flu" or the common cold, and if the immune response overcomes the infection, nobody is any the wiser.

The whole, rather vague, clinical picture of the "common cold" had been for many decades confused with the somewhat similar picture of influenza. Clinically, the two are often distinguishable with difficulty. It is now clear from virological studies that in this situation we have to deal with several viruses, which may be found in several fairly distinct but related groups.

"COLD" VIRUSES.   As a result of advances in laboratory procedure and our increasing knowledge of the serologic properties of viruses, rapid progress is currently being made in the isolation and identification of agents implicated in the syndrome designated as "coldlike" illness. Among these agents are members of the *myxovirus* group, including classic influenza and mumps, and the parainfluenza group, of which at least four distinct types have been isolated.

Others are the *respiratory syncytial (RS) virus,* which is apparently responsible for some of the severe respiratory illnesses that occur in infants and small children; *Mycoplasma pneumoniae,* the cause of primary atypical pneumonia; and the *2060-JH virus* (now ECHO 28), isolated from a number of cases of the so-called common cold. Names of other differentiated groups of viruses associated with coldlike diseases of the respiratory tract are rhinoviruses, coryzaviruses, reoviruses, ECHO viruses, and adenoviruses.[3] We may use the last to exemplify respiratory viruses in general.

ADENOVIRUSES.   These viruses cause conditions variously called "acute respiratory disease" (ARD), "respiratory illness" (RI), and so on. An inexact term commonly used is "common cold" or "virus cold." By 1967, 45 or more types of adenoviruses (based on serologic studies and designated by numbers) had been distinguished. The number known is now 55, although some authorities only recognize 31 that were recovered from human sources. Several corona viruses and other myxoviruses and picornaviruses were also found to cause colds under varying conditions.

---

[3]The names are derived as follows: *rhino,* Greek for nose; *coryza,* Greek *koryza* for catarrh; *reo* and *ECHO,* see page 360; *adeno,* Greek *aden* for gland (adenoid tissues or lymph nodes).

"**Cold" Vaccines.**   A vaccine against one virus type does not necessarily give good protection against "colds" or "flu" due to other viruses in the group. It may give some protection or none. Several polyvalent (active against several types) vaccines have been found effective in preventing some of these infections. Their usefulness is greatest in large, closed groups of persons such as troops in barracks, ships' crews, and the like.

Although often neglected, infections with respiratory viruses can lead to serious difficulties. The inflammation of the nose and throat that accompanies such infections prepares a favorable place for pneumococci, streptococci, influenza bacilli, and other organisms to lodge and set up more serious disease. Furthermore, if a person who is carrying streptococci, pneumococci, diphtheria bacilli, or other disease organisms in his throat has a respiratory virus infection, his sneezing and coughing will distribute not only the organisms causing the virus infection, but the other organisms as well.

Transmission of Respiratory Viruses.   The nasal discharges and saliva carry the organisms, and the ways in which these infections are spread are many: coughing, sneezing, kissing, carelessness about handkerchiefs, hands soiled with nasal secretion, imperfectly washed dishes and eating utensils, and the use of common towels and drinking cups. These are methods of transmission common to all infectious diseases of the respiratory tract. The health worker may therefore disregard the virological complexities of serologic grouping and nomenclature since all of the respiratory viruses and bacteria are transmitted and controlled in the same way (see Chapter 28).

Aside from vaccines that, although effective, are somewhat limited in scope of usefulness, as previously noted, there are no known specific measures for curing or preventing these respiratory diseases. Specific immune globulins are useful in some situations: measles, rubella, herpes zoster, rabies, polio.

Antihistaminics do not cure diseases due to adenoviruses, although some of them alleviate some of the symptoms. Different people respond to some of these drugs in entirely distinct ways. One type of antihistaminic may help one person but be toxic to another; thus, medical supervision is essential.

PNEUMONIA CAUSED BY PLEUROPNEUMONIA-LIKE ORGANISMS (PPLO)

Mycoplasma, or PPLO, has been discussed in general in Chapter 4. Some PPLO occur normally in the mouth and other parts of the body. Although many of these organisms infect animals, and mammalian cells in tissue cultures, only those PPLO that are known to produce respiratory infections in man are discussed here.

Atypical Pneumonia in Man.   Many cases of pneumonia that defy clinical diagnosis are too easily dismissed as "virus pneumonia." In fact, PPLO often cause these infections, which are truly pneumonia-like diseases. With fluorescent antibody staining and improved cultural methods, this type of pneumonia is being recognized more frequently. The disease caused by *Mycoplasma pneumoniae* responds, somewhat, to treatment with streptomycin and tetracycline, although the true viral pneumonias do not. Penicillin is of no value in mycoplasmal infectious. Why?

Transmission is as in other infectious diseases of the respiratory tract. The disease is self-limiting and fatality rare.

PSITTACOSIS (PARROT FEVER)

INTRODUCTION.   The causative agent of psittacosis[4] is *Miyagawanella psittaci.* Pneumonitis of cats and pneumonitis of birds are other respiratory infections due to related species of *Miyagawanella.*

Psittacosis attacks parrots and related species of birds, as well as pigeons, chickens, and others, causing diarrhea, sneezing, a generally sick appearance, and often a high (and costly!) mortality rate. This condition in birds other than psittacines is usually called *ornithosis.* Psittacosis was probably first brought to the United States by infected lovebirds, and it has also appeared in European countries. It is readily transmitted to human beings by the dust from dried feces, feathers, and exudate from the nostrils and mouths of the sick birds.

In man it causes a generalized reaction with chills, fever, headache, and vomiting. It especially attacks the lungs, causing a form of bronchopneumonia. The disease in man is frequently fatal, and several microbiologists have lost their lives as a result of studying this pathogenic agent. Commercial handling of psittacine birds is very apt to transmit the organism to the persons engaged in the work. Purchasers of these birds not infrequently contract the disease.

TRANSMISSION AND CONTROL OF PSITTACOSIS.   The nose and mouth secretions of infected human beings can transmit the causative organisms; however, most cases in man result from contact with sick birds. The preventive precautions applicable in influenza and pneumonia are also applicable in human cases of psittacosis.

All parrots or other birds suspected of having the disease should be killed and incinerated, and their cages either burned or soaked in saponated solution of cresol or some other disinfectant solution.

A practical application of our knowledge of the susceptibility of *Miyagawanella* to antibiotics is the feeding of appropriate antibiotics (e.g., tetracyclines) to flocks of psittacine birds to eradicate psittacosis. This is said to be very effective and is important to both the industry and the purchasers.

---

[4]Psittacidae is the scientific name of the zoologic group containing parrots, lovebirds, and similar species. The name of the virus is derived from the fact that it causes a disease of psittacine birds ("parrot fever") that is transmissible to man.

Supplementary Reading

Anthony, R. L., Taylor, D. L., Daniel, R. W., Cole, J. L., and McCrumb, F. R.: Studies of variola virus and immunity in smallpox. *J. Infect. Dis.,* 1970, *121*:295.

Baker, J. A.: Measles vaccine for protection of dogs against distemper. *J. Amer. Vet. Med. Ass.,* 1971, *156*:1743.

Baretta, R. O.: Measles in vaccinated communities. *Lancet,* 1971, *2*:910.

Benenson, A. S.: Control of Communicable Diseases of Man. 11th Ed. 1970, New York, The American Public Health Association.

Burk, R. F., Schaffner, W., and Koenig, M. G.: Severe influenza virus pneumonia in the pandemic of 1968–1969. *Arch. Int. Med.,* 1971, *127*:1122.

Dawson, C., and Darrell, R.: Infections due to adenovirus type 8 in the United States. I. An outbreak of epidemic keratoconjunctivitis originating in a physician's office. *New Eng. J. Med.*, 1963, *268*:1031.

Debre, R., and Celers, J.: Clinical Virology, The Evaluation and Management of Human Viral Infections. 1970, Philadelphia, W. B. Saunders Co.

Dixon, C. W.: Smallpox. 1962, Boston, Little, Brown & Co.

Enright, J. B.: Geographical distribution of bat rabies in the United States, 1953–1960. *Amer. J. Public Health*, 1962, *52*:482.

Fredericksen, H., and Motamedi, S. T.: The 1954–1955 epidemic of smallpox in Tabriz. *Amer. J. Trop. Med.*, 1957, *6*:853.

Gibbs, R. C.: Possible mechanisms for maintaining immunity to varicella-zoster virus. *Amer. J. Dis. Child.*, 1970, *120*:456.

Haire, M., and Hadden, D. S. M.: Rapid diagnosis of rubella by demonstrating rubella-specific IgM antibodies in the serum by direct immunofluorescence. *J. Med. Microbiol.*, 1971, *5*:237.

Jacobs, J. W., Peacock, D. B., Corner, B. D., Caul, E. O., and Clarke, S. K. R.: Respiratory syncytial and other viruses associated with respiratory diseases in infants. *Lancet*, 1971, *1*:871.

Kenny, M. T., Albright, K. L., and Sanders, R. P.: Microneutralization test for determination of mumps antibody in vero cells. *Appl. Microbiol.*, 1970, *20*:371.

Koechli, B., Martin du Pan, R., and Douath, A.: Protection of nonimmune volunteers against rubella by intravenous administration of normal human gamma globulin. *J. Infect. Dis.*, 1972, *126*:341.

Krugman, S., Muriel, G., and Fontana, V. J.: Combined live measles, mumps, and rubella vaccine. *Amer. J. Dis. Child.*, 1971, *121*:380.

Lennette, E. H., and Schmidt, N. J. (Editors): Diagnostic Procedures for Viral and Rickettsial Infections. 4th Ed. 1969, New York, American Public Health Association.

National Communicable Disease Center: Smallpox imported into Germany from India. Morbidity and mortality. 1967, Vol. 16, No. 12, U.S. Department of Health, Education, and Welfare, Public Health Service, Bureau of Disease Prevention and Environmental Control.

Notes on the prophylaxis of rabies in man. *Monthly Bull. Minist. Health*, 1962, *21*:88.

Oxford, J. S., Potter, C. W., McLaren, C., and Hardy, W.: Inactivation of influenza and other viruses by a mixture of virucidal compounds. *Appl. Microb.*, 1971, *21*:606.

Parkman, P. D., Meyer, H. M., and Hopps, H. E.: Production and laboratory testing of experimental live rubella virus vaccine. *Canad. J. Public Health*, 1971, *62*:30.

Prineas, J.: Paramyxovirus-like particles associated with acute demyelization in chronic relapsing multiple sclerosis. Science, 1972, *178*:760.

Quick rabies test. *Medical World News*, 1971 (November 12):15.

Recommendations of the Public Health Service Advisory Committee on Immunization Practices. Morbidity and Mortality, 1972, *21*(No. 25):1–34.

Ruben, F. L., and Jackson, George G.: A new subunit influenza vaccine: acceptability compared with standard vaccines and effect of dose on antigenicity. *J. Infect. Dis.*, 1972, *125*:656.

Schmidt, N. J., Lennette, E. H., and Magoffin, R. L.: Immunological relationship between herpes simplex and varicella-zoster viruses demonstrated by complement fixation, neutralization and fluorescent antibody test. *J. Gen. Virol.*, 1969, *4*:321.

Skehel, J. J., and Schild, G. C.: The polypeptide composition of influenza A viruses. *Virology*, 1971, *44*:396.

Steele, J. H.: Rabies and rabies control. *Amer. J. Nurs.*, 1958, *58*:531.

Some Pathogens Transmitted from the Genital Tract

Trachoma, Inclusion Conjunctivitis, the Venereal Granulomatoses

The Chlamydiaceae have been described in Chapter 5. *Some species* can be cultivated in embryonated eggs, some cannot. The Chlamydiaceae are sometimes called Chlamydozoaceae or Bedsonia. More than 30 different species or varieties have been distinguished on the basis of differing antigenic composition, animal hosts, and diseases caused. There still is not complete agreement on their taxonomy. All are closely related and much alike. At least two groups or genera cause diseases in man: *Chlamydia* and *Miyagawanella*.

Chlamydia (or Chlamydozoon) causes diseases of the eye (trachoma and inclusion conjunctivitis) that occur in man only. These so-called TRIC agents[1] are *not cultivable* in embryonated eggs. Species of *Miyagawanella* (*cultivable* in embryonated eggs) cause various diseases in man, in other vertebrates, or in both: lymphogranuloma venereum (a venereal disease) in man only, psittacosis or ornithosis in man and various species of birds. Other species of *Miyagawanella* cause infections only in vertebrates other than man.

TRACHOMA

This disease, known since antiquity, is caused by *Chlamydia trachomatis* and has been estimated by the World Health Organization to affect about 400 million persons at the present time, of whom nearly 20 million have been made blind by trachoma. The infection is contracted in childhood and progresses toward inflammatory chronic keratoconjunctivitis, with secondary bacterial infections, and, finally, scarring of the cornea with blindness. It is spread by contact with excretions of infected eyes, dust, and so on, and probably also by houseflies (*Musca sorbens*), but it is not highly contagious. No immunity to trachoma seems to develop as the result of infection, although specific antibodies have been found in eye secretions of patients. The disease is most prevalent in countries of the Mediterranean region, especially Egypt. Anyone who has ever seen the inward curvature of the eyelid and the deformation and discharges of

---

[1] TRIC agents applies to the agents of trachoma (TR) and inclusion conjunctivitis (IC). See page 73.

A   B

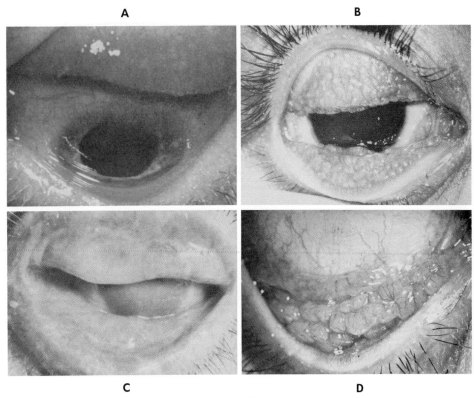

C   D

Figure 33–1

A — Early trachoma with follicular and papillary hypertrophy of upper tarsal conjunctiva and
  beginning pannus at upper limbus.
B — Established trachoma, State IIa MacCallan. Note predominant follicular hypertrophy in absence
  of scars.
C — Stage IV (healed) trachoma with conjunctival and corneal scars and loss of useful vision.
D — Inclusion conjunctivitis in young adult. Note massive follicular hypertrophy of conjunctiva of
  lower fornix. There was an associated urethritis.
(Thygeson, P. and Hanna, L., *in* Diagnostic Procedures for Viral and Rickettsial Infections, 4th Ed.,
1969. Edited by Edwin H. Lennette and Natalie J. Schmidt, Am. Public Health Association, New
York, N.Y. 10019.)

advanced stages of this disease does not easily forget it. Control is mainly
dependent on avoidance of contact, personal cleanliness, and education
of the public. Topical applications of tetracyclines or sulfonamides are
useful in *early* cases.

INCLUSION CONJUNCTIVITIS

Inclusion conjunctivitis (IC), or blennorrhea, the result of an infection
by *Chlamydia oculogenitalis*, is, like trachoma under natural conditions, a
disease of man only. Like the gonococcus, *C. oculogenitalis* is an inhabitant
of the genital tract that can also infect the eyes. It is transmitted during
coitus and also by contaminated hands and fomites. Unlike the gonococcus
and *Chlamydia trachomatis*, *C. oculogenitalis* does not produce scars. It usually

develops and reproduces in the newborn's eyes, unlike trachoma, which rarely occurs in neonates. Eye-to-eye infections have not been reported; however, adults may contract the ocular disease, usually from swimming pools contaminated by genital secretions.

The disease in the baby resembles gonococcal ophthalmia (see Chapter 35), and it is contracted in the same way, during the birth process. Infections of the adult cervix do not cause any symptoms; in the male, the organism may be found associated with urethritis but does not cause discomfort of any consequence.

In the newborn who has been infected, a few days after birth the conjunctivae become inflamed and there is copious mucopurulent discharge, but, even without therapy, the infection is self-limiting. The incubation period (five to seven days) is longer than that of gonococcal ophthalmia (two to three days). No scar or blindness develops, although the disease may take a year or longer to clear up. Diagnosis may be made by microscopic examination of stained scrapings from inflamed conjunctivae. Epithelial (not pus) cells contain diagnostically distinctive *inclusions* (organisms).

THE VENEREAL GRANULOMATOSES

Lymphogranuloma Venereum[2]

Granuloma is a pathologist's term for an abnormal, swollen tissue made up of fleshy granules, generally of an inflammatory or ulcerative character and often seen in healing tissues, especially if infected. It is sometimes colloquially called "proud flesh." Granulomas may be caused by, or associated with, injuries due to mechanical, chemical, or infectious agents.

Lymphogranuloma venereum (LGV) is a painful and destructive disease caused by *Miyagawanella lymphogranulomatosis*. This LGV agent is closely related immunologically to the TRIC agent of trachoma. No immunity seems to develop toward this agent either. The disease is transmitted generally by sexual contact and is common in the tropics and among promiscuous persons. It begins one to 12 weeks after exposure as a small, transitory, local sore on the genitalia, which, in males, is followed by development of swollen, inguinal "glands" (lymph nodes), and, perhaps weeks later, of swellings in adjacent parts. These swellings (buboes) ulcerate and discharge seropurulent fluid. In females the pelvic organs are involved, with lesions in the lower bowel. Discharges from active lesions are highly infectious and may persist for years.

Various other organs and tissues may eventually become involved and large swellings occur. Stricture of the rectum is a common complication, especially in females, and is very painful and troublesome; however, many cases pass unnoticed and serve to disseminate the disease. Many cases give positive reactions in syphilis serology with cardiolipid antigens. For diagnosis, tests for allergy to the organism (like the Frei test) are made. These are analogous in principle to the tuberculin test but are less reliable.

---

[2]This disease has several names: lymphogranuloma inguinale, venereal lymphogranuloma, and so on. Do not confuse with granuloma inguinale, a different disease, which also has several names.

The tetracycline antibiotics are useful therapeutically in early and older cases, but they cannot repair damage done by infections of long standing.

Granuloma Inguinale (Granuloma Venereum)

This supposedly venereal disease (it is only mildly communicable) is due to diagnostically distinctive microorganisms (*Calymmatobacterium granulomatis* or *Donovania granulomatis;* so-called Donovan bodies), which are gram-negative, encapsulated rod-shaped bacteria. These are readily seen within phagocytic cells in stained smears made with exudate from the lesions of the disease. It is now thought that the Donovan bodies closely resemble heavily encapsulated *Klebsiella pneumoniae*. Most likely, *Donovania granulomatis* is identical with *Klebsiella*.

The disease occurs principally in the tropics. It is also not uncommon in the southern United States. Because of similarity in names, it is sometimes confused with lymphogranuloma venereum, and it is mentioned here partly for this reason. The two diseases are similar in epidemiology and modes of transmission. They both exhibit extensive gross superficial lesions, which are painful and progressive, with destruction of tissues.

Prevention of Venereal Granulomatoses

Since the causative microorganisms occur in the discharges, these, as well as dressings, clothing, or rubber gloves contaminated with them, should be handled with care and sterilized or disinfected with appropriate measures. There is little other danger of infection. The same precautions should be used in chancroid (see Chapter 35). The organisms are easily killed by the usual disinfectants.

Supplementary Reading

Jawetz, E.: Agents of trachoma and inclusion conjunctivitis. *Ann. Rev. Microbiol.*,1964, *18*:301.
Lymphogranuloma venereum. *Pfizer Spectrum*, 1958, *6*:484.
McComb, D. E., and Nichols, R. L.: Antibody type specificity to trachoma in eye secretions of Saudi Arab children. *Infect. and Immun.*, 1970, *2*:65.
McDaniel, W. E.: Four lesser venereal diseases *J. Kentucky Med. Assn.*, 1964, *62*:281.
Thygeson, P. and Hanna, L.: TRIC agents. *In* Diagnostic Procedures for Viral and Rickettsial Infections, 4th Ed. 1969, New York, American Public Health Association, Inc.
Vedros, N. A.: Species-specific antigen from trachoma and inclusion-conjunctivitis (chlamydial) agents. *J. Immunol.*, 1967, *99*:1183.

The Treponematoses

34

THE SPIROCHAETALES

The term spirochete is commonly applied to helically coiled, flexible bacteria (Fig. 4–3). These have been described in page 54.

SUBDIVISIONS. In the seventh edition of *Bergey's Manual of Determinative Bacteriology* the order Spirochaetales is divided into two families, the Spirochaetaceae and the Treponemataceae. The family Spirochaetaceae (genera *Spirochaeta, Cristispira,* and *Saprospira*) includes only saprophytic organisms of no medical significance and will not be discussed here. Some changes in their arrangement are projected for the eighth edition of Bergey's Manual.

The family Treponemataceae includes three genera of great medical importance: the genus *Borrelia,* species of which (e.g., *B. recurrentis, B. novyi*) cause relapsing fever; the genus *Treponema* (of which important species are *T. pallidum,* the cause of syphilis, *T. pertenue,* cause of the tropical scourge, yaws, and *T. carateum,* cause of pinta, a tropical skin disease); and the genus *Leptospira,* of which the species *L. icterohaemorrhagiae* is well known as the cause of Weil's disease or infectious hemorrhagic jaundice. It was discussed with urinary enteric pathogens (Chapter 24) because it is excreted in, and transmitted by, urine.

THE TREPONEMATOSES. All treponemal diseases are collectively referred to as treponematoses. Generally, they are extremely destructive to tissues (Fig. 34–1). An exception is pinta, in which there is no ulceration, as in other treponemal diseases. Pinta lesions are flat, spreading, erythematous areas which are at first hyperpigmented. There is little generalized reaction. The lesions, on healing after months or years, become completely depigmented, wide and patterned areas, sometimes showing remarkable bilateral symmetry. Transmission is by personal contact, not necessarily venereal. Serologic tests for syphilis become positive.

In the United States the most important species of spirochetes is *Treponema pallidum,* cause of syphilis. In certain tropical areas, identical

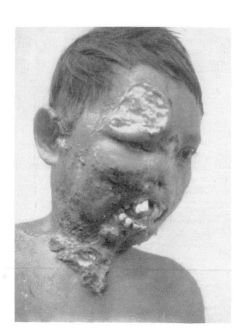

Figure 34–1

Disfigurement due to yaws *(Treponema pertenue)* characteristically restricted to skin, bones, and cartilage. Analagous destruction of tissue, both internally and externally, characterizes syphilis and bejel. These treponematoses yield readily to combined sanitation and penicillin. In old times these and similar diseases were confused with Hansen's disease (leprosy). It is easy to understand the medieval horror of lepers (and *supposed* lepers). (Courtesy of Dr. H. van Zile Hyde, Division of International Health, U. S. Public Health Service.)

or very closely related species of *Treponema* cause at least two other important diseases: *yaws*, caused by *T. pertenue* and common in native tropical peoples around the world; and *bejel* or *nonvenereal syphilis*, caused by *T. pallidum* and found among some less advanced peoples in Southeastern Mediterranean and adjacent areas.

Syphilis is venereally transmitted. Yaws and bejel are transmitted in tropical and sub-tropical regions principally by nonvenereal personal or household contact, especially among children and between mothers and babies, and probably by flies, fomites, and so forth. Although sometimes probably also transmitted by sexual contact, yaws and bejel, like pinta, are not regarded as primarily venereal diseases.

SYPHILIS

Treponema pallidum was discovered in 1905 by Schaudinn (1871–1906), a German scientist, in the primary sores (*chancres*, pronounced *shank'ers*) of persons infected with syphilis. *T. pallidum* has never been successfully cultivated in a virulent state in an artificial (nonliving) medium, although several cultures of nonvirulent spirochetes closely resembling *T. pallidum* (and probably variants of it) exist. One now widely used as a source of antigen in serologic diagnostic tests for syphilis is the Reiter; another is the Nichols treponeme. *T. pallidum* may be kept alive for some time in artificial media, but it does not multiply significantly, if at all. It may also be frozen with CO_2 and 15 per cent glycerol and thus remain alive for years.

All species of *Treponema* are morphologically alike. All are relatively small, thin, tightly coiled spirochetes (Fig. 34–2). Their eight to 14 spirals are close and regular unless the protoplasmic contractions change them. The ends of the organisms are drawn out into extremely fine fibrils, which have been mistaken for flagella. Progressive motion depends presumably on the propeller-like action of the spirals when the treponemes rotate. They move slowly and flex slightly.

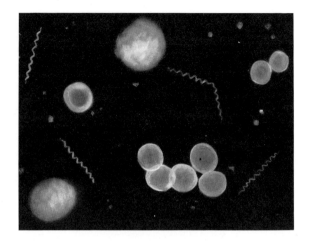

Figure 34-2

Scrapings from a syphilitic chancre as seen in the microscope with darkfield illumination. The spirochetes are *Treponema pallidum.* The eight small, rounded objects are erythrocytes; the two larger, rounded objects are tissue cells or pus cells; the smallest irregular objects are salt crystals, cell detritus, and other bacteria (approximately ×1000). Courtesy of Chas. Pfizer and Co., Inc., Brooklyn, N. Y. In *J.A.M.A.*, Vol. 157.)

DEMONSTRATION OF TREPONEMA. The recognized species of *Treponema* are not easily stained, and consequently other methods are generally used to observe them microscopically. The following are outlines of some methods:

Negative Staining. This is not really a method of staining. Appropriate material, e.g., exudate from pathologic conditions such as syphilitic ulcers, is mixed with a little India ink or nigrosin (a dense, black dye), spread thinly on a slide, and allowed to dry. The ink or nigrosin forms a dark background and the organisms, unstained by the ink or nigrosin, appear as transparent, wavy lines since the ink and nigrosin fail to penetrate them. Many other microorganisms may also be demonstrated in this way (Fig. 9–10).

Silver Impregnation Method. In this method ammoniacal solutions of silver salts are first allowed to penetrate the inside of the cells. Metallic silver is then precipitated on the surface of the spirochetes by means of a reducing solution. The organisms appear thick and black against a yellowish background (Fig. 34–3).

Darkfield Method. Probably the quickest and easiest method of demonstrating treponemes, and indeed any bacteria in fluid material, is by means of the darkfield microscope technique. The ordinary compound

Figure 34-3

Congenital syphilis in lung. *Treponema pallidum* demonstrated by Levaditi silver impregnation method (approximately ×1600). (Smith, L. W., and Gault, E. S.: Essentials of Pathology, 2nd Ed. New York, Appleton-Century-Crofts, Inc.)

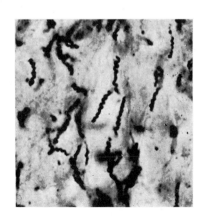

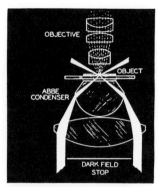

Abbé Condenser with
Darkfield   Stop

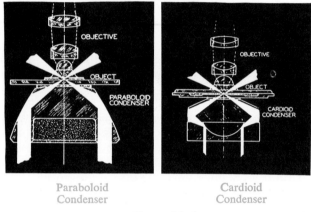

Paraboloid
Condenser

Cardioid
Condenser

Figure 34–4

Various forms of condensers for oblique illumination of the darkfield. In the upper picture an object on the slide is reflecting light up through the objective lens. In each arrangement note that only peripheral light rays pass the condenser. (Courtesy of Bausch & Lomb Optical Co.)

microscope may be easily equipped for this work. A special substage dark-field condenser with an opaque stop in the central part is used in place of the usual type of substage condenser. This darkfield condenser is designed to prevent the entrance of any rays of light from the light source straight upward into the tube of the microscope. By means of the darkfield condenser all rays from the light source emerge from the upper surface of the slide at such an angle that they do not enter the objective lens (Fig. 34–4). The field therefore appears dark when examined with the objective lens of the microscope, hence the term *darkfield*. When a fluid containing any particles, such as dust, bacteria, or spirochetes, is placed on the slide at the focal point of these oblique rays, the oblique light rays are reflected from the surfaces of the spirochetes or other objects upward through the lenses to the eye of the observer. Each particle on the slide becomes visible as a brightly illuminated speck owing to the light reflected from its surface. The remainder of the field remains black. The principle is the same as that which makes the moon and planets visible as bright objects in a dark sky, or dust particles visible in a dark room into which a single ray of sunlight falls.

Only outward form and motility are demonstrable by means of the darkfield, but as these are two of the chief means by which treponemes and other spirochetes are distinguished, the method is very valuable.

The Phase Contrast Microscope.   The use of the phase contrast condenser (especially anoptral phase) permits better contrast without having to resort to the darkfield technique.

The Fluorescence Microscope Method.   This method (see Chapter 19) is often used to demonstrate microorganisms in tissue sections and other materials. Its use in demonstrating pathogenic treponemes for the Fluorescent Antibody Technique is discussed farther on in this chapter.

PROPERTIES OF TREPONEMA PALLIDUM.   The syphilis organism dies quickly outside the body because it is very sensitive to drying, cooling, and standard disinfectants. Soap and other detergents quickly destroy it. Material that has dried will not carry the disease-causing organism, but objects very recently soiled and still warm and moist with secretions containing the spirochete are possible sources of infection, especially to health personnel and laboratory workers who handle syphilitic materials and patients. The survival time of the spirochetes on ordinary objects is very short. Except as noted, the disease is very rarely (some say never) transmitted by fomites, virtually all cases being acquired by direct contact with an infected person.

The Course of Untreated Syphilis

PRIMARY SYPHILIS.   *Treponema pallidum* gains entrance to the body through the skin or mucous membranes. Most often it infects the genitalia during coitus, occasionally the lips during kissing. Not infrequently it is homosexually acquired. Close contact between an infected lesion and a break in the skin on the genitalia, the mouth, lips, anus, face or even the finger or other part of the body is required to contract the spirochete, though usually it is coitus that spreads the disease.

The organisms begin to multiply locally in the tissue almost immediately, producing an initial lesion or *chancre* (Fig. 34–5) that appears two to four weeks after exposure. The chancre is typically a rather flat, indurated or "hard" ulcer (the so-called "hard chancre"). It is often absent or unrecognizable, or inconspicuous, and usually heals over temporarily with a "scab" and finally may heal completely without treatment; however,

Figure 34–5

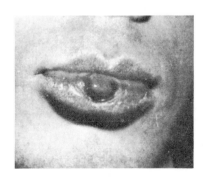

Chancre of lip. (From Domonkos: Andrews' Diseases of the Skin, 6th Ed. 1971, Philadelphia, W. B. Saunders Co.)

this does not mean the disease is cured. It simply means that the organisms have long since left the initial portal of entry and invaded the body. Within a short time, varying probably from a few hours to several days after infection, the spirochetes appear in the local lymph nodes, producing a swelling (bubo). Thence they enter the blood and are carried to every organ in the body. Within two to four weeks after infection, specific antibodies called *reagin* may be demonstrated in the serum. Although *T. pallidum* may be present in the blood during the incubation period of syphilis, there is little danger that the disease is transmitted through blood transfusions. The spirochete does not remain viable in drawn refrigerated blood longer than 2 to 3 days, thus three day old blood from blood banks may be safe, though any blood giving a positive serologic reaction (STS)[1] should be rejected.

SECONDARY SYPHILIS. As a general rule, although not always, a rash appears following the general invasion of the body. This seems to be of an allergic nature and indicates that the body is responding to the infection immunologically. There is nothing especially distinctive in the form or appearance of the rash. It may resemble almost any known type of rash. This is one of the reasons why syphilis, which in later stages produces such a great variety of lesions in so many organs and tissues, is often spoken of, from a diagnostic point of view, as "The Great Imitator." The rash may occur as late as several months after the appearance of the chancre but usually earlier. At about this time, sores may appear on the genitalia or in the oral cavity (mucocutaneous lesions), or both, accompanied by sore throat, slight fever, and headache. This is called the *secondary stage*. It is rarely disabling at this stage and is often ignored by the uninformed as trifling. Syphilis in this stage is, however, a highly infectious disease. The rash, ulcers, and sores swarm with spirochetes, and the disease may be spread at this stage by contact with the patient or by articles still moist with secretions.

TERTIARY SYPHILIS. After a number of weeks or months these secondary symptoms also tend to recede without treatment, probably due to the development of some degree of immunity. But the patient is not cured; the living spirochetes are still boring from within, and the disease enters a *chronic stage*, called the *third* or *tertiary stage*.

LATE SYPHILIS. Like the tubercle bacillus, *Treponema pallidum* may remain alive in the body for many years without causing any definite or acute symptoms, but it is always doing great damage during this time, and new lesions eventually appear in various parts of the body. It may attack almost any organ in the body. The lesions are called *gummas* and may be on external surfaces and be ulcerous, or internal and abscess-like. These gummas tend to extend and also to heal at the same time, thus causing much distortion due to the contractile scar tissue. They rarely contain spirochetes, but exudates may be infectious. In the later stages of the disease there are long periods during which damage progresses slowly, symptoms are indefinite, and the ignorant patient may believe himself cured. The disease then breaks out again. In older days, the long time interval between the original infection and the late manifestations of syphilis caused many of the symptoms and lesions of the later stages to be regarded as entirely different diseases, and to be named as such until their syphilitic

---

[1]STS stands for "serologic test for syphilis" and there are many different ones (see page 489).

nature was fully understood through the demonstration of the spirochetes in the tissues.

The late symptoms of syphilis depend on the organ that is attacked by the spirochetes. The most frequent, serious, and disabling results of syphilitic infection are diseases of the *heart, arteries,* and *nervous system.* These are frequent causes of early death in syphilitic patients.

The spirochetes lodge particularly in the walls of the arteries, causing a chronic inflammation and destroying tissue. Consequently, the vessel walls are weakened and may bulge, causing saclike dilatations called *aneurysms.* These not infrequently burst and the patient may suddenly die of the hemorrhage. Syphilis is one of the principal (but not the only) causes of *aneurysm of the aorta,* of *diseases of the aortic valves,* and it is among the several recognized causes of *arteriosclerosis* and *cerebral hemorrhage* in comparatively young persons.

Unless treatment is given early the spirochetes lodge also in the central nervous system (brain and spinal cord), where they cause a chronic inflammation and destroy the nerve tissue. Various forms of insanity result. These lesions result in *paresis* (general paralysis, or dementia paralytica) and *locomotor ataxia,* or tabes. In paresis, spirochetes are present in the tissues of the brain; in tabes, in the spinal cord.

CONGENITAL SYPHILIS.   Syphilis is sometimes incorrectly said to be inherited. This implies transmission of the spirochete by the sperm or ovum, which probably occurs very rarely, if at all. A woman may transmit syphilis to her child if she has the disease at the time of conception or acquires it during pregnancy. The spirochetes pass from the mother through the placenta into the blood of the fetus; they are one of the few organisms that can pass the placenta. The baby is thus infected before birth and comes into the world with living spirochetes in its body. This is called "congenital syphilis." Syphilitic babies with rashes and sores (rhagades) around the mouth and anus or with "snuffles" (chronic discharge from syphilitic lesions in the nose) are infectious. There is practically no danger, however, from older congenitally syphilitic children, or from the advanced stages of syphilis in adults, if there are no open sores. "Late congenital syphilis" refers to clinical manifestations which appear only after infancy. In fact, congenital syphilis is often not suspected, or is misdiagnosed, and may not be recognized until the child is 10 years old or older. Congenital syphilis generally responds very well to a full treatment with aqueous procaine penicillin (called APP).

Since congenital syphilis is acquired in utero, it cannot be called a venereal disease.

SYPHILIS AND FETAL DEATH.   Many pregnancies in syphilitic women, unless energetically treated, end in miscarriages or stillbirths. Syphilis is a very frequent cause of death of the fetus unless adequate treatment is given. The child may be born alive with signs of syphilis and die very early, or these signs may develop later, depending on the status of immunity in the mother. Syphilis has been a cause of much infant mortality.

LATENT SYPHILIS.   As in the case of adults, the spirochetes may remain alive in the child's body for a number of years without causing symptoms (*latent syphilis*) and then become active. After infancy, the most serious consequences of congenital syphilis are stunting of growth, diseases of the eye, deafness, epilepsy, and feeblemindedness, but these conditions are not by any means always due to syphilis.

Diagnosis of Syphilis

A very satisfactory method of diagnosis in the first stage of the disease is the demonstration of the spirochetes with the darkfield microscope technique (see page 484) in fresh, unstained material obtained from the chancre or sores in the mouth or elsewhere. These contain the organisms in great numbers. The complement fixation and precipitin reactions and other manifestations of immunity, such as antibodies that kill and immobilize the spirochetes, become positive only in the second or third week after the appearance of the chancre. They cannot, therefore, as a rule be used for diagnosis in the very earliest stages, although later they are reliable tests. It is very important to make the diagnosis early.

COMPLEMENT FIXATION TESTS. Application of the complement fixation reaction to the diagnosis of syphilis was first described by a scientist named Wassermann and usually bears his name or the name of some person who has modified the technique, such as Kolmer. Serum of the patient is required. Blood for the test is drawn from a vein at the bend of the elbow, at least 10 ml usually being required.

A strongly positive complement fixation test with cardiolipin antigen is usually designated by the symbol of four pluses (++++); weaker reactions are designated by three pluses (+++), two pluses (++), one plus (+), plus-minus or doubtful (±) and negative (−). There are various other notation systems designed to indicate the amount of antibody in the patient's serum. These tests require several hours or overnight to perform. Other, improved specific diagnostic complement fixation tests for syphilis will be mentioned farther on.

PRECIPITIN TESTS. Various forms of the precipitin reaction (which is closely allied to the complement fixation reaction and, in syphilis, probably dependent on the same antibody or reagin) bear names of the persons who devised them, as Kahn, Eagle, Hinton, Kline, VDRL,[2] and Mazzini. Since performance of any of the precipitin tests requires only the patient's serum and the antigen, they are simpler, quicker, and less expensive than the complement fixation tests and are thought by many investigators to be more reliable.

The precipitin tests depend on the fact that when a concentrated alcohol-ether extract of antigen, similar to that used in the complement fixation test, is mixed in certain proportions and in a certain way with the serum of a syphilitic patient, visible particles are formed that cloud the mixture and eventually clump together into flakes or *flocs* and precipitate to the bottom of the tube (Fig. 34–6).

BIOLOGIC FALSE-POSITIVE (BFP) REACTIONS. None of the reactions obtained in the complement fixation or precipitin tests as just described is specific because the "antigen" used in them is not of syphilitic origin. The lipid (fatlike) substance used as antigen is extracted from normal, bovine heart muscle with an alcohol-ether mixture; hence, they are called *cardiolipid* antigens. These have no relation to *T. pallidum* whatever, though for little understood reasons they react especially with serum of syphilitic patients.

Because the antigens are not specific, falsely positive reactions not infrequently occur in normal persons or in patients with diseases other than syphilis. A positive reaction to tests made with such antigens does not, by itself, necessarily prove that a person has syphilis. Persistently

---

[2]Venereal Disease Research Laboratories of the National Communicable Disease Center.

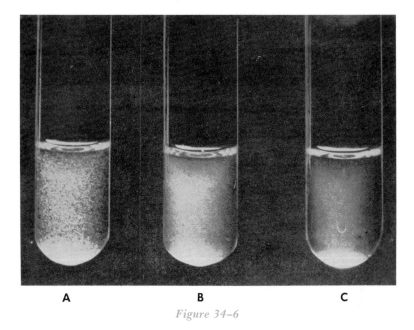

A   B   C

Figure 34–6

The Kahn reaction, a precipitin reaction test for syphilis. *A*, Strongly positive. Definitely visible particles are suspended in the transparent liquid. *B*, A weaker reaction. Fine particles are suspended in a somewhat turbid liquid. *C*, Negative reaction. The liquid is transparent and free from particles. (The light areas at the bottoms of the tubes are caused by reflections of light.) (Kahn: The Kahn Test. Williams & Wilkins Co.)

positive reactions with these antigens in healthy persons are called BFP reactions. They have no significance in relation to syphilis. BFP reactions may also be encountered with people who have malaria, relapsing fever, leprosy, yaws, or some 18 other known diseases. BFP reactions may even occur in pregnancy. This nonspecificity, unless carefully investigated, can introduce error into the tests, sometimes with tragic results; however, in general, these serologic tests are usefully accurate in diagnosing syphilis and evaluating the effect of treatment when intelligently used. When there is doubt concerning the result of these tests recourse may be had to tests depending on specific antibodies. As mentioned previously, serologic tests for syphilis are usually designated STS. Those made with cardiolipid antigens are sometimes designated as standard serologic tests (SST).

Specific Diagnostic Tests

TREPONEMA PALLIDUM IMMOBILIZATION (TPI) TEST. As the disease progresses, specific antibodies appear in the serum which immobilize and kill *T. pallidum*. These antibodies act only in the presence of complement. They are entirely distinct from the nonspecific complement-fixing and precipitin reagins previously discussed. They are highly specific, react only with *T. pallidum*,[3] and persist in the patient longer than the non-specific complement-fixing and precipitin reagins.

---

[3] The antibodies also react with a few very closely related species like *T. pertenue*, cause of yaws and *T. carateum*, cause of pinta.

The *Treponema pallidum* immobilization test is an exceedingly valuable supplement to the nonspecific complement fixation and precipitin tests in diagnostic syphilis serology. The TPI test is used mainly in large diagnostic laboratories, with excellent results when the nonspecific tests are in doubt. It is technically difficult and too expensive for routine use by the smaller laboratories. The spirochetes used in these tests are derived from the testes of rabbits artificially infected for the purpose.

THE SPECIFIC COMPLEMENT FIXATION (TPCF) TEST. Equally specific are complement fixation tests using antigens extracted from *Treponema pallidum* with a mixture of sodium desoxycholate and sodium citrate followed by acetone-ether. These tests are valuable, but preparation of such antigens is difficult and expensive.

THE REITER PROTEIN COMPLEMENT FIXATION (RPCF) TEST. As previously noted, although *T. pallidum* in a virulent state has not been cultivated in artificial media, very similar but avirulent spirochetes (possibly variants of *T. pallidum*) have been artificially cultivated—for example, the strain known as the Reiter spirochetes. These cultured spirochetes contain antigens much like those of *T. pallidum* and are used as sources of antigen in CF tests for syphilis. These tests are thought by some to be not as specific as tests made with *T. pallidum* antigens, but they are valuable diagnostic adjuncts. Experience with them indicates that whereas cardiolipid antigens tend to give some falsely positive BFP reactions, Reiter treponeme antigens tend to err in being not excessively sensitive.

FLUORESCENT ANTIBODY TECHNIQUE. Among the most promising new developments in diagnostic techniques for infectious diseases of all kinds, including the treponematoses, are procedures based on fluorescent antibodies. The Fluorescent Treponemal Antibody Absorption (FTA-ABS) test is done by what is called the indirect method (Fig. 34–7). Details are given in the literature cited. In brief, it may be said that syphilis antibodies in the patient's serum (human) are brought into contact with

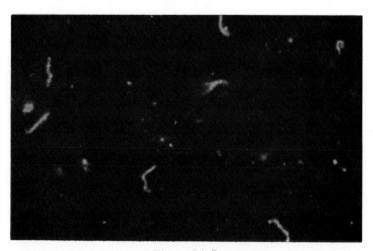

Figure 34–7

Treponema pallidum stained by the fluorescent-antibody technique (approximately ×1200). (Courtesy of Baltimore Biological Laboratory, Inc.)

Treponema pallidum (antigen). The two combine. The specific antigen-antibody complex is then made visible by coating it with anti-human-serum antibodies conjugated with a fluorescent dye. Viewed in the microscope by ultraviolet light the antibody-coated treponemes glow with a yellow fluorescence. The same principle applies to any specific antigen-antibody combination and is being widely used in diagnosis.

OTHER SEROLOGICAL TESTS.   Other serological tests are the FTA-200 (which was later modified to become the previously mentioned FTA-ABS) and the "*Treponema pallidum* immune adherence" test known as TPIA. Some of the tests are now automated.

Other nontreponemal antigen tests are the "Unheated Serum Reagin" test (USR) and the "Rapid Plasma Reagin (RPR) (circle) Card" test. Both of these are rapid reagin tests that use a modified VDRL antigen suspension with enhanced reactivity.

SEROLOGY AND CLINICAL PROGRESS.   A patient in the first (chancre) stage of syphilis may have a negative reaction to all serologic tests because in the very early periods of syphilis, as in most diseases, not enough antibody has appeared to give a positive reaction. The reaction usually becomes positive ten days to two weeks after the appearance of the chancre, sometimes earlier. When treatment is instituted, the reactions usually get progressively weaker and may finally become negative. This is a favorable sign, and repeated tests are therefore made to find out how the treatment is progressing. Congenitally syphilitic children usually have a positive reaction.

If the brain or spinal cord is affected by syphilis, a positive serologic test is usually obtained with the *cerebrospinal fluid*. The reactions are practically always positive in paresis and frequently positive in locomotor ataxia.

Treatment

PENICILLIN IN SYPHILIS.   A single treatment with 2.4 million to 4.8 million units of benzathine penicillin G will render a patient noninfectious in primary syphilis, and probably in early secondary syphilis although the latter may require additional treatments. The same treatment will also cure early gonorrhea unless the strains of *N. gonorrhoeae* are penicillin-resistant. For patients sensitive to penicillin other very effective drugs are available: tetracycline, doxycyclin (Vibramycin), and so forth. Any of these drugs can have undesirable and even dangerous side effects and are to be administered only under medical supervision. It is worth noting also that other treponematoses, especially yaws, bejel, and pinta, respond equally promptly to penicillin therapy.

Unfortunately, new cases of both syphilis and gonorrhea still occur in enormous numbers annually (Fig. 34–8, Table 34–1). The high rate of occurrence is not due to failure of the drugs or of the medical profession but to ignorance, fear, indifference, and prudery of the public. Tragically, the greatest increase is among teenagers, much of it homosexually acquired. Nevertheless, the mortality from venereal disease has declined. For example, the death rate per 100,000 population from syphilis was 11.0 in 1911, 4.1 in 1950, and only about 2.0 in 1961. Yet we cannot be proud of the fact that in 1971 96,000 cases of syphilis (all stages) were reported in the United States. Of these 23,783 were primary and secondary syphilis. Incidence increased by 4% in early 1972.

Like other communicable diseases that are a menace to public health,

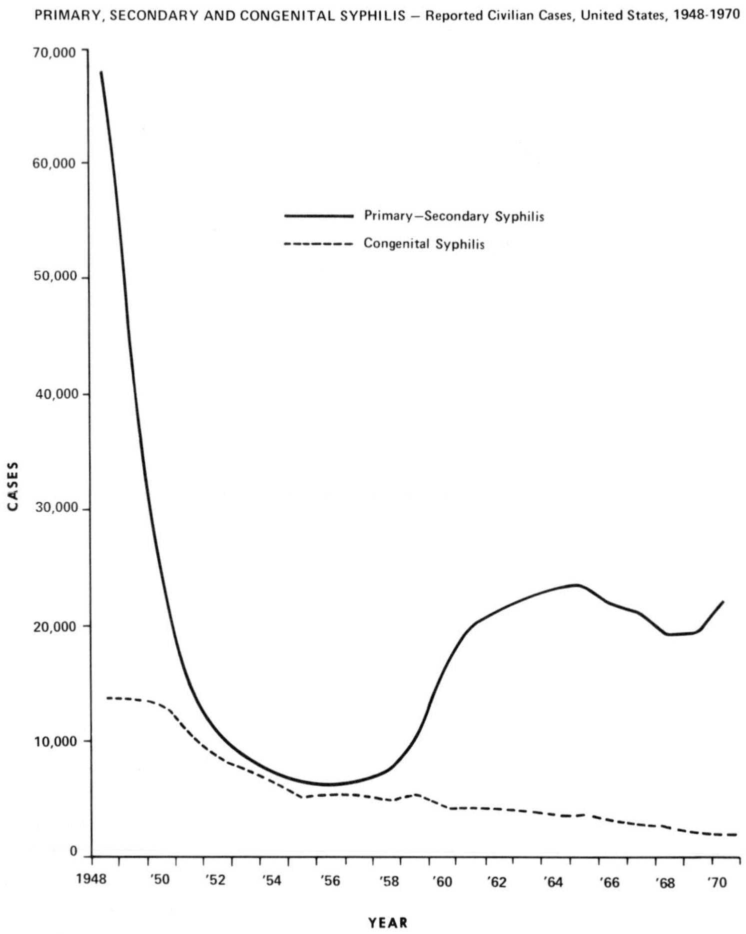

PRIMARY, SECONDARY AND CONGENITAL SYPHILIS — Reported Civilian Cases, United States, 1948-1970

Figure 34–8

Reported cases of primary, secondary and congenital syphilis in the United States, 1948–1970. (From *Morbidity and Mortality.* 1970. Vol. 19, No. 53, U.S. Department of Health, Education, and Welfare.)

venereal diseases are reportable to the health department, but many infections go unreported and untreated. The decline in death rate does not represent a decline in new infections. Many infections occur, but modern methods of treatment lower the death rates. The number of new cases of syphilis increases annually.

IMPORTANCE OF PROMPT AND THOROUGH TREATMENT. Unless all the spirochetes in the body are reached by whatever drug is used, the patient is not cured. If the drug is then discontinued, the disease will again make progress and reaction to the diagnostic serologic tests will again become positive. Drugs can arrest but not repair damage done by the spirochetes. Much depends on how soon after infection treatment is started. If the spirochetes are located in some deep, obscure, well-protected lesion in the body, drugs may not reach them for a time and repeated injections may be necessary.

The chances of permanent cure diminish in proportion to the length

Table 34–1.   Reported Cases of Venereal Disease by Age
Group, United States, 1956–1970

AGE GROUPS	1956	1960	1965	1970	PERCENTAGE INCREASE 1956–1970
PRIMARY AND SECONDARY SYPHILIS					
0–9	11	20 ⎱	281 ⎱	296	+344.2
10–14	75	139 ⎰	⎰		
15–19	1,093	2,577	4,039	3,933	+359.7
0–19	1,179	2,736	4,320	4,229	+358.7
All Ages	6,399	16,144	23,338	21,983	+343.5
GONORRHEA					
0–9	1,222	1,619 ⎱	⎱	7,015	+192.3
10–14	2,425	3,261 ⎰	⎰		
15–19	44,264	53,649		144,805	+327.2
0–19	47,911	58,529		151,820	+316.9
All Ages	224,687	258,933		600,926	+267.5

*Adapted from a report of the U.S. Public Health Service Task Force on Eradication of Syphilis, L. Baumgartner, M.D., Chairman 1962; and National Communicable Disease Center: *Morbidity and Mortality*, 1967, Vol. 16, No. 23, U.S. Department of Health, Education, and Welfare and updated to 1970.

of time that elapses between the time of infection and the beginning of treatment. It is of the utmost importance to place every syphilitic patient under treatment as early as possible, both for his own sake and that of the persons with whom he comes into contact.

TREATMENT AND COMMUNITY HEALTH.   There are two views about the desirability of starting treatment during the primary stage. From the standpoint of preventive medicine, an infectious patient with an open lesion at any stage may be made noninfectious quite promptly by treatment. The patient should, on this basis, be treated immediately in order to prevent spread of the disease. Mere suppression of the infectious state, however, does not imply a cure.

This patient may actually be cured before he has time to develop any immunity, and he may promptly become infected again and be just as infectious until he is treated all over again. From the standpoint of the patient and the physician, it is considered by some to be useful to allow time for the disease to progress until the patient develops a good concentration of antibodies and tissue resistance, but the patient should be warned about his infectious condition and his cooperation enlisted until the time is suitable to begin treatment. Much depends on the intelligence and cooperativeness of the patient.

SYPHILIS AS A FAMILY DISEASE.   Syphilis is a family disease quite as much as tuberculosis. In the lower social levels, if the husband has the disease, it is quite probable that the wife and children have also been infected. A single ignorant or irresponsible syphilitic person can originate many new cases (Fig. 34–9).

If one person in a family is found to have syphilis, it is of the greatest importance to have the other members examined. By placing the infected members under treatment early, the late results of the disease may be avoided.

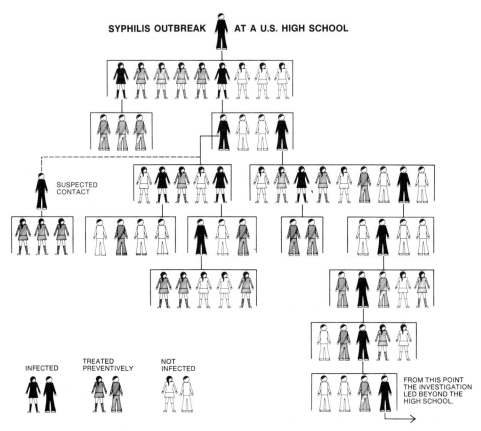

Figure 34–9

Persons involved in a high school syphilis epidemic. (From Today's VD Control Problem – 1971. Courtesy of American Social Health Association, Committee on the Joint Statement – 1970. W. L. Fleming, M. D. Chairman.)

Prevention

Adequate treatment with penicillin quickly renders the syphilitic patient noninfectious so that no special preventive procedures are necessary in contacts with persons who have been so treated. In dealing with untreated cases of syphilis, the clothing, bed linen, towels, and washcloths must be regarded as potentially infectious and should be separately handled and disinfected. In the cases of persons with primary or secondary lesions of skin, genitalia, or mouth, such things as handkerchiefs, eating utensils, and toothbrushes are also potentially infectious. Dressings of any open lesions must of course be burned or otherwise hygienically disposed of. The person faced with the problem must be guided by the nature and location of lesions, as no general rule may be laid down.

After the primary and secondary lesions have healed, and as long as no gummas or other lesions are draining to the exterior, the syphilitic patient is no longer infectious in the ordinary relations of life, although unknown numbers of spirochetes remain alive in the body. This is an important point to remember, as members of the health professions are often unnecessarily afraid of patients in the later stages of the disease.

Rashes, mouth ulcers, and possibly cutaneous gummas, however, are infectious at any stage.

YAWS

As previously mentioned, yaws is not primarily a venereal disease, though its clinical progress has parallels to the venereal disease syphilis. Like syphilis, it begins with an initial lesion called a "mother yaw," accompanied by mild general symptoms. After weeks or months, very characteristic and diagnostically distinctive secondary, raspberry-like excrescences occur over the body. These are especially painful on the feet ("crab yaws"). The name frambesia, commonly given to yaws, is from the French word *framboise*, raspberry. As in syphilis, healing tends to occur but new lesions recur intermittently after long "latent" periods. There are progressive and widely destructive and frequently revolting lesions of skin, cartilages and bones (Fig. 34–1). Unlike syphilis, there is no involvement of the CNS, eyes, aorta or viscera. Fatality rates are low. All serological tests for syphilis are positive in yaws. One treatment with slowly-absorbed penicillin is promptly curative. The United Nations World Health Organization (WHO) has treated millions of patients, with brilliant and dramatic cures.

Supplementary Reading

Annotated Bibliography on Venereal Diseases for Nurses. Current edition. Washington, D.C., U.S. Department of Health, Education, and Welfare.

Caldwell, J. G.: Congenital syphilis: a nonvenereal disease. *Amer. J. Nurs.*, 1971, *71:*1768.

Coffey, E. M., Naritomi, L. S., Ulfeldt, M. V., Bradford, L. L., and Wood, R. M.: Further evaluation of the automated fluorescent treponemal antibody test for syphilis. *Appl. Microbiol.*, 1971, *21:*820.

Fleming, W. L. (Chairman): Today's VD Control Problem—1971. American Social Health Association. Committee on the Joint Statement—1970.

Manual of Tests for Syphilis. Public Health Service Publication No. 411. 1969, Washington, D.C., Government Printing Office.

Reed, E. L.: The rapid plasma reagin (circle) card test for syphilis as a routine screening procedure. *Pub. Health Lab.*, 1965, *23:*96.

Gonorrhea, Chancroid, Trichomoniasis, Venereal Herpes, Prevention of Venereal Diseases

35

GONORRHEA

Gonorrhea[1] is an infection primarily of the glandular tissues of the cervix (in the female) and urethra (in the male) and of adjacent reproductive organs in both male and female, and is caused by the gonococcus (*Neisseria gonorrhoeae;* see Chapter 28). It begins four to ten days (rarely longer) after exposure as an acute inflammation that later (four months and longer) becomes chronic. A great deal of pus is formed in the early stages. Gonorrhea is one of the most frequent of all the serious infectious diseases. Although accurate statistics are not available, recent reliable studies indicate that in this country over 1,200,000 cases of gonorrhea are constantly under medical care. In addition, there are great numbers of cases, possibly another million, that remain unreported, neglected, and untreated. New cases are constantly occurring (Fig. 35-1). In 1971, 670,268 new cases of gonorrhea were reported in the United States. Of these roughly 71 per cent were males. Diagnosis in females is frequently difficult. The disease is transmitted, in the great majority of cases, by sexual intercourse, although gonococcal infections of other parts of the body are acquired in other ways. These will be described later.

Newsweek (Jan. 24, 1972) has stated:

Though the VD epidemic is worldwide, the gonorrhea rate in the U.S., according to latest figures, is markedly higher than in such Western European nations as Britain (118 per 100,000) and France (30 per 100,000). But in the comparatively more permissive Scandinavia, the national average is much higher than in the United States. Denmark, for instance, reports a rate of 319 per 100,000 and in Sweden the rate is an astonishing 514 per 100,000 — higher even than it is in California. Only in Communist China is the VD rate down appreciably. There, thanks perhaps in some measure to Chairman Mao Tse-tung's puritanical thoughts on promiscuity and prostitution, VD seems to have been all but eliminated.

---

[1]Gonorrhea is also known as "clap" or "GC."

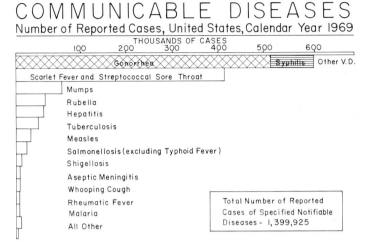

Figure 35–1

Reported cases and specified notifiable diseases. (From Today's VD Control Problem — 1971. American Social Health Association, after United States Public Health Service.)

IN THE FEMALE.   The gonococcus causes an inflammation of the cervix uteri, vulva, various local glands in the genitalia, and of the uterus, fallopian tubes (salpingitis; Greek *salpinx*, tube), and ovaries. Involvement of the tubes and ovaries is quite common and makes necessary many gynecologic operations. Pelvic peritonitis can cause great pain. In most gynecologic clinics it is the custom to examine routinely the cervical secretion of every female patient for the gonococcus. The infection tends to chronicity especially in females.

The adult vaginal wall does not readily become infected with gonococci, but the vagina of preadolescent girls can easily be infected, not only with gonococci but with other *Neisseria* (see Chapter 28), because the membrane lining the vagina and covering the vulva of immature girls is thin and delicate, whereas that of the sexually mature female is thicker and more resistant to infection.

Proctitis, an involvement of the rectum, has been shown to be a secondary infection in about 50 per cent of females with urogenital gonorrhea. An additional 5 to 10 per cent occurs at the rectal site only.

IN THE MALE.   The gonococcus causes inflammation of varying intensity, especially of the urethra. This often spreads to adjacent portions of the genitourinary system; the epididymis, seminal vesicles, prostate, and bladder may be affected, with painful and disabling illness, even death. The urethra may become so scarred (often due to self-medication with caustic disinfectants, or as a result of the infection) that urine cannot pass. This condition is commonly called *stricture* and requires surgical treatment.

Untreated gonorrhea is a frequent cause of childless marriages because it destroys parts of the genital organs. In the female the fallopian tubes become closed by scar tissue, which replaces tissues destroyed by the intense local inflammation set up by the gonococci. In the male a similar process results in the occlusion of the vas deferens. The former condition

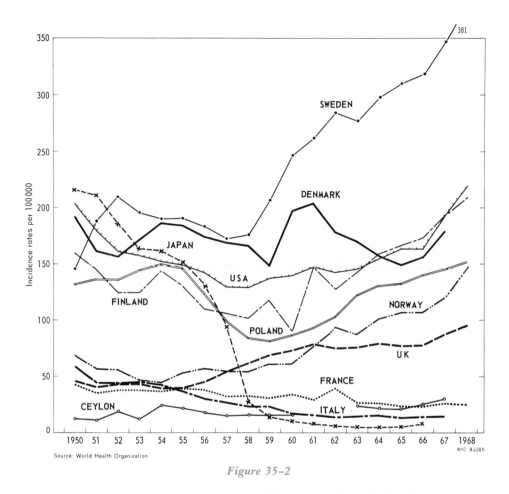

Figure 35–2

Reported gonorrhea in 9 countries 1950–1968. (From World Health Organization.)

prevents the ova of the female, and the latter prevents the sperm cells of the male, from reaching the uterus. This results in sterility.

The infection of children with gonococci also often takes place in families in which there is an adult case of gonorrhea. Such infection in female children may result from sleeping in the same bed with the patient or from the common use of washcloths, towels, bathtubs, and toilets. In adults, on the contrary, extracoital transmission of gonorrhea is rare.

Ophthalmia

Ophthalmia is severe inflammation of the eye or conjunctivae or both. It may be due to physical or chemical causes or to infection. Infectious ophthalmia may be due to several microorganisms, including staphylococci, streptococci, pneumococci, *Haemophilus* species, viruses, rickettsias, and gonococci. The diagnosis should be confirmed by laboratory studies.

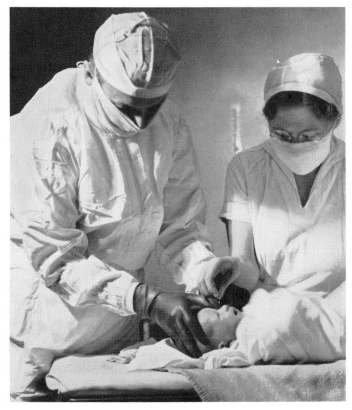

Figure 35–3

Physician and nurse placing silver nitrate solution in eyes of infant shortly after birth to prevent gonorrheal ophthalmia. The solution is contained in a wax ampule to be crushed between the fingers of the nurse. Note the caps, gowns, gloves, and other evidences of surgical asepsis so necessary at the puerperium. (Courtesy of National Society for the Prevention of Blindness.)

GONOCOCCAL OPHTHALMIA.   Ophthalmia caused by the gonococcus occurs both in adults and in newborn babies. An adult patient with gonorrhea may infect his (or someone else's) eyes by means of his hands or fomites. Conversely, a child or adult with gonorrheal ophthalmia may infect his own genitalia. The organisms occur inside *pus* cells. Doctors, nurses, and medical students, if they become careless, may contract gonorrheal ophthalmia through caring for patients.

If a woman who has gonorrhea gives birth to a child, the baby's eyes may become infected during the process of birth; unless the condition is treated promptly and vigorously, the child's eyes may be destroyed within a few days. Gonorrheal ophthalmia neonatorum was formerly the most frequent cause of blindness in infancy.

Blindness due to the gonococcus is diminishing in civilized countries because of the general practice of putting a drop of a silver nitrate or other prescribed antiseptic into each eye immediately after birth (Fig. 35–3). If done properly, this is an almost sure preventive of gonococcal ophthalmia. In a certain maternity hospital in New York City there were 4,660 births during a period of six years in which this method was carried out without a single case of ophthalmia neonatorum. The disease is so easily prevented that its continued existence is criminal, and yet only by eternal vigilance can protection from it be assured to every newborn child. Inclusion blennorrhea (or inclusion conjunctivitis, see Chapter 33), however, is not prevented by this means.

In all enlightened states the use of a silver preparation (silver nitrate 1 per cent) or other legally prescribed drug (antibiotics or sulfonamides or combinations) in the eyes at birth is required by law, and in most states a report must be given to the health department within 24 hours of any inflammation of the eyes of a newborn baby. Devices for treating the eyes at birth are furnished free by most health departments. They usually consist of small wax ampules, which are crushed between the fingers so that the contents drop into the eye of the infant.

Diagnosis of Gonococcal Infections

In the acute stages of a gonococcal infection in a person admitting exposure, the diagnosis is usually made by finding the distinctive gram-negative diplococci with the microscope in gram-stained specimens of the pus. The cocci are characteristically enclosed within the leucocytes (Fig. 35–4). In the chronic stages gonococci are very scarce, and cultural procedures may be necessary to make the diagnosis.

In female children, in persons with ophthalmia, or in adults, especially females, who effectively deny exposure, microscopic evidence is insufficient to prove that organisms resembling *Neisseria* are actually gonococci. In such instances it is necessary to inoculate "chocolate" blood-agar (blood-agar heated at 90 C for ten minutes) containing antibiotic supplements, either Vancomycin-colistin-nystatin or polymyxin-ristocetin. This medium,

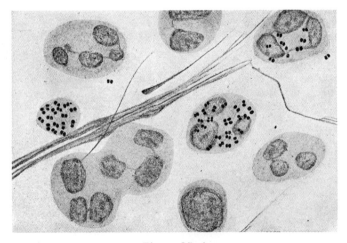

Figure 35–4

Gonococci in leucocytes in smear of pus from case of gonorrhea, stained with methylene blue. (Compare with Figure 28–6.) The long, fibrous objects are shreds of fibrin and mucus in the pus. Note that the pairs of gonococci are nearly all within the leucocytes. (Ford, W. W.: Bacteriology, New York, Paul B. Hoeber, 1939.)

called Thayer-Martin medium, is prepared in Petri plates and after inoculation is incubated at 35 C in an atmosphere containing 5 to 10 per cent CO_2 to isolate the organisms in pure culture, and make complete biochemical and serologic identifications. *Neisseria gonorrhoeae* typically ferments only glucose but without gas, and colonies of the gonococcus are catalase and oxidase positive. A specific FA[2] staining test is also very useful in making rapid tentative identification of the organism. Error in diagnosis can be particularly embarrassing and costly for both patient and medical personnel. (See next paragraph.)

Vaginitis or Vulvovaginitis

This condition in preadolescent girls is often due to *Neisseria* from the upper respiratory tract. The causative *Neisseria*, which are morphologically identical with gonococci, are introduced into the vagina by dirty hands, clothing, towels, and so on. These organisms are easily distinguished from the gonococcus by cultural methods. By such means it has been found that, especially in children's wards and institutions, may cases of suspected gonorrheal vaginitis are in reality innocent self-infections or fomite-borne infections with respiratory *Neisseria*. *Neisseria* common in the nose and throat and found in vaginitis are *N. sicca, N. flava* and *N. meningitidis* (the meningococcus; see Chapter 28). *N. catarrhalis, Trichomonas vaginalis* (discussed later in this chapter), and *Candida albicans* (Chapter 37) are also causes of vulvovaginitis in both children and adults. It is sometimes difficult either to cure the condition in the individual child or to prevent its transmission to other children. It is the custom in many hospitals to delay the admission of girls to the general children's ward until vaginal smears or cultures have been examined and found negative for *Neisseria*. Gonococcal infection of preadolescent children can occasionally occur.

Antibiotics and Neisserian Infections

Appropriate antibiotic therapy is generally effective in dealing with *Neisseria*. A single intramuscular dose of 2.4 million (male) or 4.8 million (female) units of aqueous procaine penicillin G cures about 95 per cent of cases of gonorrhea, especially in the acute stage. So-called resistant infections, estimated to be caused by up to 60 per cent of the gonococcal strains in the United States, still respond to greatly escalated doses of penicillin. Tetracycline and related drugs are also effective. The application of creams containing estrogenic hormones to "mature" the preadolescent vulvovaginal epithelium is reported to be a valuable prophylactic.

CHANCROID

Haemophilus ducreyi was named for Ducrey, a famous Italian physician. It causes a severe ulcerative and *necrotic* (Gr. *nekros,* dead; tissue-destructive) disease of the external genitalia and adjacent parts, called *chancroid* or *soft chancre* (in contrast with the syphilitic chancre, which is hard).

---

[2]Fluorescent antibody.

Chancroid is common, especially among unclean peoples. The disease is more common and severe in men than in women. It is transmitted primarily by sexual intercourse and very rarely by contact of the genitalia with articles (clothing, bedding, towels, toilets) freshly contaminated with the pus and serum from lesions. The causative organism is much like the influenza bacillus but is even more fragile and difficult to cultivate (Chapter 30).

After an incubation period of three days or less a macule, and then a soft, necrotic, spreading ulcer, develop. The lesion spreads over the surfaces and into the deeper structures and erodes the tissues of the genitalia and adnexa. It produces painful inguinal buboes or adenitis ("swollen inguinal glands"). Diagnosis is by microscopic examination of exudate, and by cultural studies of the organism. The disease may often be prevented in exposed persons by vigorous disinfection of the affected parts and by attention to personal hygiene. Tetracycline antibiotics and sulfonamides appear to be of value in treating soft chancre.

TRICHOMONIASIS

TRICHOMONAS VAGINALIS. Although differing in some morphologic details, such as number and length of flagella, size, and length of posterior spike, the protozoan *T. vaginalis* is very much like *T. hominis* (Chapter 26). As its name implies, however, *T. vaginalis* is commonly found in the normal human vagina. It is also found in the normal human prostate and adnexa and in the urine of male or female.

Transmission is generally by sexual contact, but may possibly be also by common toilet seats, freshly soiled (damp) washcloths, clothing, or common vaginal douches. The protozoans are killed by a few hours of drying.

GENITOURINARY TRICHOMONIASIS. Protozoa of the genus *Trichomonas* that inhabit the human genital tract ordinarily live unnoticed as parasites of humans. Under some conditions, however—including, probably, infections by other microorganisms—they can multiply enormously in either male or female, and they can set up, especially in females, a local irritation, with itching and burning that may range from slight and transitory to prolonged and very distressing.

Diagnosis is made by finding the organisms, through microscopic examination, in prostatic secretions or scrapings from the vagina, or in urine. The organism may be cultured in trypticase-liver-serum medium.

The infection may readily be cured in males by chemotherapy; in females it is difficult. If one partner of a married couple is found infected, it is advisable to examine the other and treat the infected person or both as required.

VENEREAL HERPES

In numerous cases the herpes simplex virus has been demonstrated in venereally (also manually) transmitted vesicular and ulcerative lesions of both male and female genitalia. Venereal herpes may be unexpectedly common. The reader is referred to Chapter 32 where the herpes simplex virus is discussed in more detail. "Genital herpes" in women may become quite painful and extensive; in men the lesions remain discrete. In both sexes the disease recurs frequently and provides a portal of entry for other venereal infections.

THE PREVENTION OF VENEREAL DISEASES

The most obvious means of preventing venereal disease is, of course, to prevent contact of uninfected persons with persons of promiscuous sexual behavior or persons known to be infected. Because this so often fails, prevention of venereal disease is one of the most urgent public health questions. One of the great difficulties is *finding* persons who are sources of infection. Patients sometimes reveal information to health personnel about contacts with persons who have venereal infections.

Unfortunately, persons in the most infectious stages of venereal disease are usually not incapacitated and are sometimes secretive and uncooperative through fear or stupid irresponsibility. Some are indifferent, partly because of reliance on effectiveness of treatment. For example, a man may become infected with *N. gonorrhoeae* by a prostitute on Sunday, infect his wife on Tuesday and appear at the clinic for treatment on Thursday morning. Receiving a complete course of antibiotic, he returns home cured in the evening, but comes to the clinic again on Monday morning with a new acute infection contracted on Friday from his wife, whom he had infected on Tuesday. It is the practice, in some clinics, to give treatment to a person only if his sexual partner also agrees to receive treatment simultaneously, in order to avoid a sequence such as that just described.

TREATMENT. Syphilitic, gonorrheal, chancroid, and lymphogranuloma venereum patients can be made noninfectious in the ordinary relations of social and business life by adequate treatment with appropriate chemotherapy (see Chapter 14). This is one of the most practical ways of diminishing chancroid, syphilis, and gonorrhea, and a less practical way of diminishing lymphogranuloma venereum and granuloma inguinale. Incomplete treatment, sufficient only to achieve temporary abatement of clinical symptoms, frequently results in relapse with greater damage than ever. This is what occurs when a patient, contracting syphilis and gonorrhea at one exposure, is treated (or treats himself) for a day or two with antibiotic sufficient to cure gonorrhea but only enough to mask the early stages of syphilis, which later appears in generalized form.

Most state and many city health departments now conduct clinics where proper treatment may be obtained free of charge. Many hospitals cooperate in the campaign.

PERSONAL AND HOUSEHOLD PRECAUTIONS. Until the patient is adequately treated and shown to be noninfectious the principal precautions in handling a case of any venereal disease revolve around preventing transfer of urethral or other discharges to other persons. Although gonococci and syphilis spirochetes cannot survive more than a few minutes of drying or an hour or so of exposure to sunlight or moist room temperature, other microorganisms are much more resistant. Therefore all towels, toilet articles, personal washcloths, underclothing and bed linen should be kept apart from those belonging to others, and disinfected by heat or chemicals. Bandages and dressings should be incinerated. The patient should sleep alone and no one else should get into that bed at any time. The patient should not fondle children. Systematic washing of the hands after each voiding by the patient and by health personnel after handling infectious linens and other articles must be insisted on. Bathtubs and toilet seats must be disinfected in families in which there is a still-infectious patient. The use of public toilet seats is always undesirable. Paper seat covers are available in most department stores or can be improvised from a sheet of newspaper.

GONORRHEAL AND OTHER OPHTHALMIAS. In cases of infectious ophthalmia due to any organism, the exudate or pus is highly dangerous. Dressings soiled with exudates should be carefully handled, discarded, and later incinerated. Precautions as to bed linens and other cloths are as described above. The hands are dangerous vectors of infectious material from the eyes. If only one eye is infected, the noninfected eye should be protected with adequate bandages and the infected eye irrigated or cleaned by washing or wiping away from, instead of toward the good eye. This may prevent transfer of the infection from one eye to the other.

CASE-FINDING. Finding as many of the infected persons as possible and getting them under treatment is a most important part of the program for the prevention of venereal diseases. The public health team is of great assistance here. A blood test (or other appropriate diagnostic test) should be made on every hospital, dispensary, and institutional patient because unrecognized and far-advanced cases of syphilis are found in every large group of the general population. Most states require that all applicants for a marriage license submit to a blood test for syphilis. Surprising results are sometimes found.

ELIMINATION OF CONGENITAL SYPHILIS. The treatment and prevention of congenital syphilis is one of the most important parts of the program against syphilis. Every pregnant woman should have a blood test, and all those with a positive reaction should have thorough treatment. The earlier in pregnancy the mother comes under treatment, the better the chance that the child will escape injury or death due to damage by the spirochetes during embryonic or fetal life. Infection of the fetus rarely occurs before the fourth month.

The children of parents known to be syphilitic should be kept under medical observation even though they show no signs or symptoms of the disease. Congenital syphilis yields to treatment much more readily in infancy than in later childhood. If congenital syphilitic patients always received good treatment in infancy, the number of children showing the late and irreparable consequences of congenital syphilis would be much reduced.

PROPHYLAXIS. Transmission of syphilis and gonorrhea during coitus may usually be prevented by the use of intact rubber sheaths, but this does not necessarily prevent transmission of chancroid or lymphogranuloma venereum, or of syphilis or gonorrhea if lesions are outside the protective coverage of the sheath.

Prophylaxis with penicillin is reportedly effective against both syphilis and gonorrhea for some days following 2.4 to 4.8 million units of aqueous procaine penicillin G. Allergic complications must be guarded against.

The educational, legal, and social methods of attack on venereal diseases rank in importance with the medical, but it is not within the province of this book to do more than mention them.

The educational campaign is being conducted continuously by means of literature, notices, talks, lectures, and motion pictures. The aim is always to acquaint the public with the method of spread, diagnosis, and treatment of these diseases and their results, using accurate, clear, and simple language, and presenting the subject in an unsensational and unsentimental way. The gradual sex teaching given to children and young people in the home and school would be included here.

The legal attack centers around blood and other diagnostic tests for persons intending marriage, breaking up prostitution as a business, and the protection of young people from sex racketeers, drug addiction, and the like.

Supplementary Readings

Brown, W. J.: Acquired syphilis: Drugs and blood tests. *Am. J. Nurs.*, 1971, *71:*713.

Burch, T. A., Rees, C. W., and Reardon, L. V.: Epidemiological studies of human trichomoniasis. *Amer. J. Trop. Med.*, 1959, *8:*312.

Gray, L. A., Kotcher, E., and Giesel, L. O., Jr.: Evaluation of a systemic drug, a nitro-imidazole ("Flagyl"), in the treatment of trichomoniasis. *J. Kentucky Med. Assn.*, 1961, *59:*672.

Greenberg, M., and Vandow, J. E.: Ophthalmia neonatorum: Evaluation of different methods of prophylaxis in New York City. *Amer. J. Public Health*, 1961, *51:*836.

Guthe, T., and Willcox, R. R.: The international incidence of venereal disease. *Royal Soc. Health Jour.*, 1971, *91:*122.

Hodges, J. R., and Lawrence, J. V.: A comparative study of the laboratory diagnosis of gonorrhea. *Health Lab. Sci.*, 1971, *8:*17.

Kotcher, E., Keller, K., and Gray, L. A.: A microbiological study of pediatric vaginitis. *J. Pediatrics*, 1958, *53:*210.

Lassus, A.: Doxycycline treatment of gonorrhea in cases with decreased penicillin susceptibility of gonococci. *Chemotherapy*, 1970, *15:*125.

Lenz, P. E.: Women, the unwitting carriers of gonorrhea. *Amer. J. Nurs.* 1971, *71:*717.

Mathews, R.: TLC with the penicillin. *Amer. J. Nurs.*, 1971, *71:*720.

Nicol, C. S.: Venereal disease in women. II. *Brit. Med. J.*, 1971, *2:*383.

Schwartz, W. F.: VD: Communities strike back. *Amer. J. Nurs.*, 1971, *71:*724.

Shapiro, L. H., and Lentz, J. W.: Therapy of female gonorrhea with Cephaloridine. *Amer. J. Obstet. Gynec.*, 1971, *108:*471.

Thayer, J. D.: Current diagnostic methods in gonorrhea. *Public Health Lab.*, 1968, *26:*85.

Vandermeer, D. C.: Meet the VD epidemiologist. *Amer. J. Nurs.*, 1971, *71:*722.

Wax, L.: The identity of *Neisseria* other than the gonococcus isolated from the genitourinary tract. *J. Ven. Dis. Inform.*, 1950, *31:*208.

Winsser, J., and Altieri, R. H.: Herpes simplex virus infection as a venereal disease. *Public Health Lab.*, 1963, *21:*134.

Bacterial Pathogens of the Soil: Gas Gangrene, Tetanus, Anthrax, and Melioidosis

36

Many species of pathogenic microorganisms occur in the soil: bacteria, viruses, fungi, protozoa, and helminths. Some injure agricultural crops or other plant life; some infect lower animals, some, man. Many occur only occasionally or accidentally in soil, as when infected animal matter transitorily pollutes the soil. Most *bacterial* pathogens of man that are indigenous to fertile soil are species of the genus *Clostridium*. One, *Clostridium botulinum*, causes a form of food poisoning that was discussed in Chapter 27. Two others (occurring also in feces) are: *Cl. tetani*, cause of lockjaw or tetanus, and *Cl. perfringens*, cause of gas gangrene and one form of food poisoning. Figure 36–1 shows a simplified scheme used to classify some of the clostridia.

Bacillus anthracis, the cause of anthrax, is included in this chapter as a soil-borne pathogen although it is transmitted also by fomites and by the blood, fluids, and tissues of infected animals that contaminate soil. It is included here also because, like all species of the genus *Clostridium*, it forms highly heat-resistant spores. Species of the genera *Clostridium* and *Bacillus* are the only known pathogenic microorganisms that form such highly heat-resistant spores.

GAS GANGRENE

All species of *Clostridium* (of which there are nearly 100), including those involved in gas gangrene, are strict anaerobes and form very heat-resistant spores. Autoclaving for at least 20 minutes at 121 C or oven baking for two hours at 165 C is necessary to kill these spores for purposes of surgical asepsis. Neither boiling nor ordinary chemical disinfectants (except certain sporicidal gases such as ethylene oxide and beta-propiolactone) can be relied on to kill them. Any object open to the air and dust is likely to be contaminated with these spores because the organisms are found in all fertile soils. Many of them are also common inhabitants of the intestinal tract and feces of man and animals.

Most species of *Clostridium* are harmless and several species can produce fermentations of great industrial value. Only a few need be considered here: the species that are involved in gas gangrene, *Clostridium perfringens*, also called Clostridium welchii or Welch's gas bacillus, *Clostridium histolyticum*, *Clostridium paraputrificum*, and several others; and the cause of tetanus or lockjaw, *Clostridium tetani*.

506

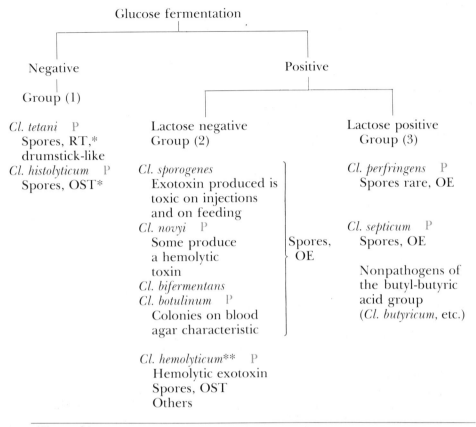

Glucose fermentation

Negative — Group (1)

Cl. tetani P
Spores, RT,*
drumstick-like
Cl. histolyticum P
Spores, OST*

Positive

Lactose negative
Group (2)

Cl. sporogenes
Exotoxin produced is
toxic on injections
and on feeding
Cl. novyi P
Some produce
a hemolytic
toxin
Cl. bifermentans
Cl. botulinum P
Colonies on blood
agar characteristic

Spores, OE

*Cl. hemolyticum*** P
Hemolytic exotoxin
Spores, OST
Others

Lactose positive
Group (3)

Cl. perfringens P
Spores rare, OE

Cl. septicum P
Spores, OE

Nonpathogens of
the butyl-butyric
acid group
(*Cl. butyricum*, etc.)

*Types of Spores:
R = Round
O = Oval
ST = Subterminal
T = Terminal
E = Eccentric
**Also named *Cl. haemolyticum*
 P Indicates pathogenic organisms

Figure 36–1

Classification scheme of *Clostridium* species. (Modified after Bayley and Scott: Diagnostic Microbiology, 3rd Ed. 1970, St. Louis, The C. V. Mosby Co.)

Some types of *Cl. perfringens* have been implicated in outbreaks of food-poisoning, especially associated with cooked meats. *Cl. botulinum* is notorious as a cause of food poisoning (see Chapter 27).

For growth, all clostridia require rich organic media such as blood, serum, dead meat or vegetables, and complete exclusion of atmospheric oxygen. Special media and methods designed to exclude oxygen are used to cultivate them. One simple but effective apparatus is shown in Figure 8–4. When free oxygen (air) is present, growth stops and the vegetative cells (but not the spores) die.

CLOSTRIDIUM PERFRINGENS.   This organism is the most important member of the group that causes the condition called *gas gangrene*.

Clostridium perfringens is a short, gram-positive, nonmotile bacillus with rounded ends. The spore is formed near the center, and since spores resist penetration of stains as well as of disinfectants, the spore appears like a hole in the stained bacillus unless stained by special stains that penetrate the spore wall. When cultivated in milk, *Cl. perfringens* ferments the lactose and produces acid, which clots the milk. Gas is then formed, the clot is torn to shreds and the plug may be blown from the tube. This process, called "stormy fermentation," is a characteristic (though not unique) cultural appearance of *Cl. perfringens,* which is often spoken of as the "gas bacillus." Since *Cl. perfringens* is always found in the normal intestinal tract of man and animals, it is easy to understand why its spores should be widely scattered in the soil. Deep, anaerobic wounds that become contaminated with soil, especially manured soil, may readily become infected with *Cl. perfringens* and the related gas gangrene clostridia, which are similarly distributed. War wounds, especially if received on manured farmland, tragically illustrated this fact during World War I and previous wars.

The organisms of gas gangrene are vigorous growers under proper conditions. They thrive in a medium made with ground meat and broth. This is often spoken of as "cooked-meat medium," and in fact it closely resembles the necrotic tissues in a deep, contused, soil-contaminated wound likely to develop gas gangrene.

GAS GANGRENE. The spores of *Clostridium perfringens* and the other clostridia of gas gangrene find in a deep, dirty wound ideal conditions for germination and growth. It is warm and moist, there is dead tissue for food, and because the wound is deep, air is excluded and strict anaerobes can grow. Gas is formed. The bubbles press on blood vessels and the tissue dies, partly for lack of blood. *Cl. perfringens* produces, among several other toxins, alpha, beta, epsilon and iota toxins, and an enzyme (collagenase or kappa toxin) that helps to destroy the tissue. Other species of *Clostridium* that commonly accompany *Cl. perfringens* in soil contribute to death and destruction of the tissues.

The tissue soon becomes gangrenous and distended (*crepitant* or "bubbly") with gas, and the bacilli multiply in the newly killed tissue and secrete more toxins. There is much foul-smelling fluid exudate. The condition spreads rapidly and may destroy a whole limb in a comparatively short time. Proteolytic species of *Clostridium,* such as *Cl. paraputrificum, Cl. histolyticum,* and others, all saprophytes in the soil, contribute to the septic process by liquefying the dead tissue. There are others, more invasive, such as *Cl. septicum* and *Cl. novyi,* that cause septicemia and toxemia. Several of these organisms, including *Cl. perfringens,* produce very dangerous hemolytic exotoxins. The entire syndrome is often spoken of as a *histotoxic clostridial infection.*

Gas gangrene is not, properly speaking, a contagious disease, since it is not commonly transmitted from one person to another by close contact, as are diseases like smallpox and scarlet fever. It is *transmissible,* however. In a surgical ward or operating room, or in circumstances such as emergency field dressing stations under war or disaster conditions, in which the organisms or spores from one patient's wound may be transferred to another by dirt, soiled dressings, bedding, unsterile instruments, or hands, gas gangrene may be considered a communicable or transmissible disease, and controlled accordingly. It was a particular horror of old-time battlefields.

PREVENTION.   Gas gangrene can be prevented to a great extent by proper and prompt treatment of wounds. Preliminary surgical cleaning (débridement) is essential to prevention by any means. Deep, dirty wounds are to be carefully cleaned, opened as much as practicable, drained, irrigated and made to heal from the inside out. All dead tissue should be cut away. Exposure of the depths of the wound to air, as far as possible, discourages growth of the anaerobes. Polyvalent antitoxins and broad-spectrum antibiotics are lifesaving. Because of the prompt and early treatment of wounds in World War II and the Korean and Vietnam conflicts, far fewer cases of gas gangrene occurred than in World War I. Several *Clostridium* antisera can be obtained commercially, suitable for animal protection. Some of these are:

C. perfringens types A, B, C, D and E
C. novyi types A and B
C. chauvoei
C. tetani
C. botulinum types A, B, C, D, E and F.

Typing of the bacterial strains may be done by protecting mice with known antitoxins prior to injecting the culture.

Because gas gangrene is caused by spore-forming organisms, autoclaving or oven sterilization of infected objects, or treatment with sporicidal gases, are the only safe methods of preventing transmission by fomites. Disposable substances, such as dressings, may be burned. The nurse's or surgeon's hands should be protected with sterile gloves when changing the dressings. The gloves, if not disposable, can be washed, wrapped, and autoclaved. It is largely because bacterial and mold spores are everywhere that autoclaves are closely associated with operating rooms.

TETANUS

CLOSTRIDIUM TETANI.   Like *Clostridium perfringens*, this bacterium is often found in the normal intestinal tract of man and other mammals. Here it does no harm. It is very widely distributed in the soil, especially in manured farmlands. Like *Cl. perfringens*, it is dangerous to man and livestock only when it gains entrance to some deep, dirty wound where there is dead tissue. In farm accidents and war wounds, *Cl. tetani* and the gas gangrene group are often found together. Culturally, they have similar requirements. They can be differentiated in the laboratory by their microscopic appearance, specific serologic tests, and their effects on different carbohydrates, proteins, and other substances.

There are also deaths of newborn infants due to tetanus (*tetanus neonatorum*). This results from infection of the stump of the umbilical cord with soil or feces (usually both). High tetanus neonatorum mortality (50 per cent or more) commonly occurs among primitive peoples who live in filth and who have no knowledge of or interest in cleanliness or sanitation, much less aseptic midwifery. This is readily understood, but tetanus neonatorum has also occurred in these United States of America. In fact, careless illegal abortion is known to produce lethal tetanus and other infections in the aborted woman as well; this, too, in the United States. This happens much too frequently.

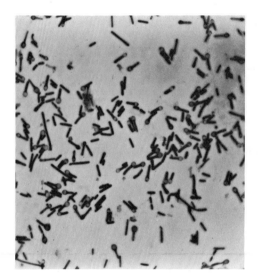

Figure 36–2

Clostridium tetani, a gram-stained smear showing terminal spores that swell the rods and produce the typical drumstick appearance. Cells of *Cl. tetani* are about 0.5 to 1.0 μm in diameter and range from 2.0 to 10.0 μm in length (approximately $\times$ 1000). (Courtesy of General Biological Supply House, Chicago, Ill.)

The tetanus bacillus is a gram-positive, motile, spore-forming rod. The spore, situated at the end of the bacillus, gives the organism a "drumstick" appearance (Fig. 36–2). The spores, like those of other clostridia, may remain alive and virulent in soil and dust for many years.

When the bacilli grow in a wound, they produce the deadly tetanus toxin, which causes the disease tetanus. If, however, they are taken into the intestinal tract, they are entirely harmless, a striking demonstration of the fact that many bacteria can cause an infection only when they enter through an appropriate route. Like *Cl. perfringens, Cl. tetani* cannot invade living tissue and thus lacks aggressiveness.

TETANUS TOXIN. Tetanus toxin is one of the most deadly biologic poisons known; the *injection* of 0.0008 ml of a suitable broth culture of the bacillus would probably kill a man. However, he could drink 100 times this dose with impunity, because the toxin is promptly digested in the stomach. The harmful action of tetanus toxin is due to its action on the nerves that activate muscles. This action is shown by the tetanic convulsions to which death from the disease is in part due.

TETANUS ANTITOXIN. This is obtained in the same way as diphtheria antitoxin, that is, by drawing blood from horses that have received repeated injections of broth in which tetanus bacilli have grown, and that contains their toxin or toxoid. Serum is separated from the blood, the antitoxin-containing gamma globulins are extracted from the serum and concentrated, and the purified concentrate is then dispensed in syringe packages for use, after proper tests for potency and sterility. The curative power of this antitoxin is limited, but it has immense value in preventing the development of tetanus. It has been, therefore, a not uncommon practice to give a prophylactic or passively immunizing dose of 500 to 1500 units to patients who have wounds in which tetanus bacilli are likely to develop, especially if they have not previously had immunizing toxoid "shots." Severe allergic reactions, however, may occur, and the patient is made permanently allergic to all therapeutic sera from horses. The necessity for serum should therefore be clearly evident in the wound situation before it is given to the patient.

After tetanus toxin has affected nerve tissue, the antitoxin cannot effectively neutralize it, hence the great importance of giving the antitoxin as soon after the injury as possible. Poor results obtained with antitoxin given after symptoms of the disease are far advanced are largely due to this fact. When symptoms of the disease are present, the antitoxin is given in larger doses both intravenously and intraspinally, but not as much is to be expected of it under these circumstances. The same ideas underlie the use of any antiserum (Fig. 29–3).

TETANUS TOXOID.   Persons can (and should) be actively immunized against tetanus by giving them a series of injections of tetanus toxoid. When a wound likely to cause tetanus occurs in a toxoid-immunized person, that person receives an immediate injection of a "booster dose" of toxoid at the time of treating the wound. In response, his tissues promptly form antitoxin. A prophylactic dose of antitoxin may also be given as an additional protection, but only if conditions seem to the physician to warrant it.

PREVENTION.   Unless the patient with tetanus has an open, draining wound, he need not be on isolation precautions. With a draining wound, the patient should be managed with the same isolation technique as for gas gangrene. Tetanus is usually prevented entirely by the proper early surgical treatment of wounds, toxoid and chemotherapy.

ANTHRAX; THE GENUS BACILLUS

Spore-forming bacteria of the genus *Bacillus* are, typically, gram-positive rods that in many ways resemble those in the genus *Clostridium.* In contrast to the strictly anaerobic *Clostridium*, most species of the genus *Bacillus* require access to air at all times and will not grow in its absence; i.e., these species of *Bacillus* are strict aerobes. A few species are facultative.

The genus includes some 20 or more common, harmless, and useful species found in soil and dust virtually everywhere. Frequent among these harmless species are *Bacillus subtilis* (source of the antibiotic bacitracin), *B. polymyxa* (which produces the antibiotic polymyxin), and *B. cereus* (var. *mycoides*). The last forms very distinctive colonies (Fig. 36–3). These various

Figure 36–3

Colony of *Bacillus cereus* (var. *mycoides*) growing on nutrient agar. The curiously curled growth is distinctive of this organism. It is interesting to note that the growth is very frequently counter-clockwise in direction. (Courtesy of Dr. F. E. Clark, U.S. Agricultural Research Service, Beltsville, Md.)

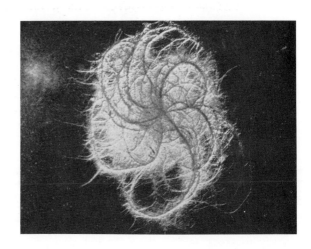

species are found in "hay infusions" (hay soaked for a day or two in water) and were called "hay bacilli." They are of no particular medical importance, except that their spores are very heat-resistant and often appear as embarrassing witnesses to careless sterilization by growing as accusing contaminants in supposedly sterile situations. Occasionally they can cause serious infections of wounds. Most of the species grow readily on simple organic media at room temperatures. They are as active in fermentations and putrefactions as *Clostridium* species. They are valuable scavengers, and many produce industrially valuable products by their growth.

BACILLUS ANTHRACIS.   The only species that regularly causes serious infection is *Bacillus anthracis* (Fig. 36–4). It causes a disease, anthrax (Greek for *carbuncle*; malignant boil or pustule), of farm animals and man. The organism forms highly resistant spores that can remain alive many years. They occur in soil, and are often found in the hair of domestic animals, where they are a menace to workers in the wool, hair, hides, and leather industries. Government regulations require the proper disinfecting of hides and wool before they may be handled in the industries. This is the reason why brushes made from animal hair or bristles must be sterilized and so marked. Some cattle and sheep fields in France and other parts of Europe have come to be called "anthrax pastures," so permeated are they with anthrax spores.

ANTHRAX.   Three forms of anthrax may be recognized in man: cutaneous, usually appearing on hands or forearms; pulmonary, which is very severe and often fatal; and gastrointestinal, which is rare and almost invariably fatal. Cutaneous anthrax, untreated, has a fatality rate of from 5 to 20 per cent. The death rate is very low if antibiotic therapy is promptly and properly administered. *Bacillus anthracis* gains entrance to the animal or human body chiefly through cuts and scratches in the skin. The bacilli multiply at the portal of entry very rapidly, forming a large, angry, black pustule called "malignant pustule." From this site they may invade the blood, where in a few hours they become exceedingly numerous. Toxins are produced by the bacilli and appear to be the principal pathogenic

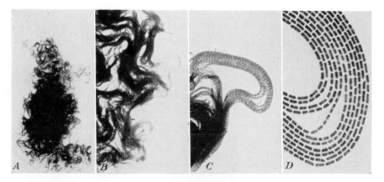

Figure 36–4

Bacillus anthracis. Photomicrograph of a colony on agar, stained with methylene blue. *A* shows the entire colony at an original magnification of × 45. Distinctive curled strands or "ropes" of bacilli are seen. *B*, *C*, and *D* show one portion of a strand at increasing magnifications (×95, ×400, and ×1600). Note the square-ended (cigarette-shaped) bacilli in *D*. Some notion of the astronomic numbers of cells in a single small colony of bacteria may be gained from this picture. (Courtesy of Dr. C. D. Stein, Agricultural Research Service, U.S. Dept. of Agriculture, Washington, D.C.)

agent in the infection. Death may be due to septicemia and usually ensues quickly. Pulmonary anthrax is associated with the wool industry and is called "wool-sorters disease"; it is due to inhalation of the spores from wool dust.

All body fluids (with the possible exception of urine) teem with the organisms; therefore the patient or animal with anthrax is a real source of danger because the bacilli sporulate as soon as the exudates, tissues, or blood are exposed to air. The fluids and carcass of an animal dead of anthrax are clearly sources of permanent contamination of the premises and a menace to careless handlers.

PREVENTION. The care of a patient with anthrax requires extreme precautions and can be dangerous. It requires safe disposal of any objects or dressings contaminated with purulent materials or, in fatal cases, fluids exuding from wounds, eyes, nose, and mouth. If feasible, these materials should be burned promptly to prevent sporulation or spread of spores whenever possible. Once dried, spores may be scattered far and wide by wind and dust. It is best to use surgical gloves and a rubber or plastic apron in handling such material. Only autoclaving, exposure to hot air oven at sterilizing temperature, or exposure to sporicidal gases for a sufficient time can be relied on to disinfect articles not burned, since the spores are highly resistant to heat and ordinary disinfectants and will remain alive in dust for many years.

A precipitin test, called the *Ascoli test,* is used to diagnose anthrax in dead animals. This is done to determine if hides removed for industrial use are safe to process.

Pulmonary anthrax requires the same care as other respiratory infections, with the added precautions necessitated by the presence of disinfection-resistant spores in the exudates.

When growing in infected tissues or when cultivated in organic media containing serum and bicarbonate ions, *B. anthracis* produces a potent exotoxin, and production of capsules is greatly enhanced. Virulence is related to the presence of both toxin and capsules. Antibodies are engendered against both. The exotoxin can be used to induce artificial immunity and is available for certain persons who are heavily exposed to anthrax.

MELIOIDOSIS

Melioidosis, a disease first described by Whitmore in 1912, occurs in man and some other mammals and is caused by *Pseudomonas pseudomallei.* The disease is endemic in many Southeast Asian areas and islands, but scattered cases have occurred around the globe. The disease caused frequently fatal infections in the U.S. Armed Forces in Vietnam.

Clinically, melioidosis in man resembles glanders in horses. Typically it is a generalized infection spreading from an initial cutaneous lesion or by way of the oral or respiratory tract. It is marked by high fever, muscular pains, nodular abscesses and pustules, especially in nose, mouth, and respiratory tract, with copious mucopurulent discharges. Symptoms vary, depending on what organs are affected (e.g., meningitis and pneumonia). Like many other diseases, melioidosis varies in severity from subacute, to (commonly) rapidly fatal (in two to four days), to chronic. In the acute cases septicemia and generalized invasions occur. General symptoms are probably due to endotoxins, exotoxins, or both.

Infection appears to be commonly derived from soil, vegetation, or water polluted by discharges from infected animals or persons, or by direct contact with discharges, blood, or tissues, all of which are highly infectious. Personnel attending cases of melioidosis must exercise the utmost care in handling patients and in disposing of fomites and all materials contaminated with discharges, and so on. Portals of entry appear not to be specific and may be via cuts and scratches, mucous membranes, inhalation of infectious dust or contact with contaminated water, clothing, and so on. Rodents are common vectors.

Pseudomonas pseudomallei is a small, gram-negative, nonspore-forming rod with bipolar flagella and polar granules that are conspicuous when stained by Wayson's stain.[1] The organism grows well at 37 C on selective medium (EMB) used for Enterobacteriaceae, or on Saboraud's medium with antibiotics at pH 5.6, or on infusion agar on which it forms smooth, viscous, honey-colored colonies. It forms acid, but no gas, from glucose, lactose, and sucrose and several other carbohydrates, as well as from several alcohols. It reduces nitrates and gives a positive cytochrome oxidase reaction. It has also been called *Actinobacillus pseudomallei* and is easily confused with *Bacillus mallei* and with *Malleomyces mallei,* the cause of glanders in horses. Malleus is the Latin word for glanders.

---

[1] Wayson's stain:
    Solution A

Basic fuchsin	0.20 g
Methylene blue	0.75 g
Ethyl alcohol (absolute)	20.00 ml

    Solution B

5% phenol in distilled H_2O	200.00 ml

Add solution A to solution B. Stain for ten to 30 seconds; wash with water.

Supplementary Reading

Angelety, L. H., and Wright, G. G.: Agar diffusion method for the differentiation of *Bacillus anthracis. Appl. Microbiol.,* 1971, *21:*157.

Berggren, W. L., and Berggren, G. M.: Changing incidence of fatal tetanus of the newborn. *Amer. J. Trop. Med. & Hyg.,* 1971, *20:*491.

Brundage, W. G., Thuss, C. J., Jr., and Walden, D. C.: Four fatal cases of melioidosis in U.S. soldiers in Vietnam. *Amer. J. Trop. Med & Hyg.,* 1968, *17:*183.

Bryan, F. L., and Kilpatrick, E. G.: *Clostridium perfringens* related to roast beef cooking, storage, and contamination in a fast food service restaurant. *Amer. J. Pub. Health,* 1971, *61:*1869.

Perlstein, M. A., Stein, M. D., and Elam, H.: Routine treatment of tetanus. *J.A.M.A.,* 1960, *173:*1536.

Redfearn, M. S., Palleroni, N. J., and Stanier, R. Y.: A comparative study of *Pseudomonas pseudomallei* and *Bacillus mallei. J. Gen. Microbiol.,* 1966, *43:*293.

Smith, L., and Holdeman, L. V.: The Pathogenic Anaerobic Bacteria. 1968, Charles C Thomas, Springfield, Ill.

Stein, C. D.: Anthrax (1955 revision). Washington, D. C., U.S. Department of Agriculture, Farmers' Bulletin No. 1763.

Sterne, M., and van Heyningen, W. E.: The clostridia. *In* Dubos, R. J., and Hirsch, J. G.: Bacterial and mycotic infection of man. 4th Ed. 1965, Philadelphia, J. B. Lippincott Co.

van Heyningen, W. E.: Tetanus. *Sci. Amer.,* 1968, *218:*69.

Weaver, R. E.: Laboratory identification of *Pseudomonas pseudomallei.* Public Health Lab., 1967, *25:*202.

Wright, G. G., Angelety, L. H., and Swanson, B.: Studies on immunity in anthrax. XII. Requirements for phosphate for elaboration of protective antigen and its partial replacement by charcoal. *Infect. and Immun.,* 1970, *2:*772.

The Mycoses

37

Diseases caused by yeasts and molds are referred to as mycotic diseases or *mycoses*. These diseases may be classified into two main groups: superficial or *cutaneous* mycoses, involving the skin, hair, and nails; and *systemic* or *deep* mycoses, invading subcutaneous tissues and internal organs. Most fungi that cause *systemic* mycoses of man live primarily in the soil as saprophytes. Most fungi that cause *cutaneous* mycoses of man are not indigenous to the soil, but are included in this chapter for convenience in discussing fungal infections in general. We shall discuss the cutaneous mycoses first.

THE CUTANEOUS MYCOSES

Most fungi invading skin, hair, and nails grow as branching filaments or hyphae (Fig. 37–1). They invade only the dead outer layer of these tissues; the hyphae cannot grow significantly into the deeper or living layers. The fungi that cause superficial mycoses are spoken of collectively as *dermatophytes*, literally, "skin plants." The diseases they cause are called dermatomycoses (singular: dermatomycosis). The dermatophytes can attack and utilize *keratin*, a tough insoluble protein, principal component of hair, nails, horn and epidermis.

When the *skin* is infected, metabolites[1] of the fungi diffuse down into

---

[1] As the term is used in this book, a metabolite is a product of the metabolism of any microorganism.

Figure 37–1

A mold (*Trichophyton*) causing "ringworm" of feet or "athlete's foot," sometimes contracted in swimming pools and gymnasiums. This slide shows material scraped from superficial lesions on the foot and treated with 10 per cent KOH (× 350). (Courtesy of Miss Rhoda W. Benham.)

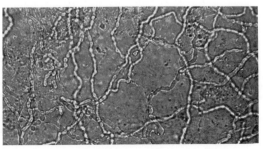

the living layer of dermal cells. Most people are sensitive to these materials, and their skin responds with a reddened (erythematous) area, which itches. Little blisters soon appear within the erythematous area. The infecting fungus spreads radially into adjacent skin. The lay term "ringworm" for some of these conditions arose because when the center of the lesion eventually becomes scaly and heals, it leaves an enlarging, red, outer ring covered with blisters.

When *hair* is infected, infection of the hair shaft takes place within the hair follicle just above the area where the shaft is being formed by living cells. As these cells continue to form the hair shaft, the infected portion of the shaft is brought upward. Hyphae of some fungi may invade the internal structure of the hair shaft, which causes the hair to break readily, often within the hair follicle. This causes the infected area of the scalp to appear bald. When only the surface of the hair shaft is infected by the fungal hyphae, the hair is not as fragile. It will often break, however, giving the scalp a moth-eaten appearance. Children are much more susceptible to fungal infections of the hair than are adults.

Infected *nails* become yellow and then start crumbling. Such infections are almost always secondary to fungal infection elsewhere on the body.

"Ringworm"; The Tineas

Superficial fungal infections ("ringworm") of the skin, hair, and nails are known by the medical term *tinea*. When tinea occurs on the scalp and involves the hair, the infection is called *tinea capitis*. When fungal infections occur on the foot, a condition commonly called "athlete's foot," the infection is designated as *tinea pedis* (Fig. 37–2). Infections on other parts of the body by various dermatophytes are also given specific names (nail, *tinea unguium;* groin, *tinea cruris*).

These infections are collectively called *dermatophytoses* or *dermato-*

Table 37–1.   Three Genera of Dermatophytes, with Common Species of Each and Some of the Conditions They Often Cause[1]

1. *Microsporum* (invades hair and skin; rarely nails)
   M. canis (dermatomycosis in animals; ringworm; tinea capitis[2] in children)
   M. audouini (epidemic tinea capitis in children)
   M. gypseum (ringworm; tinea capitis)
2. *Trichophyton* (invades skin, hair, and nails)
   T. mentagrophytes (athlete's foot; various infections of skin and nails)
   T. rubrum (athlete's foot; tinea cruris[3]; nail infections; sycosis[4])
   T. tonsurans (tinea capitis)
   T. schoenleini (favus[5])
3. *Epidermophyton* (invades the skin and nails but not hair)
   E. floccosum (athlete's foot; tinea cruris; nail infections)

[1]With a few exceptions, almost any species may cause any of the conditions mentioned, subject to the restrictions listed for each genus regarding hair or nails; clinical differentiation is often difficult.
[2]"Ringworm" (dermatomycosis) of the scalp.
[3]"Ringworm" (dermatomycosis) of the groin.
[4]*Sycosis*—pustular inflammation of the hair follicles, especially on the face, due to dermatophytes ("barbers' itch").
[5]*Favus*—a dermatomycosis distinguished by honeycomb-like, itching, yellow crusts over the hair follicles, usually in the scalp.

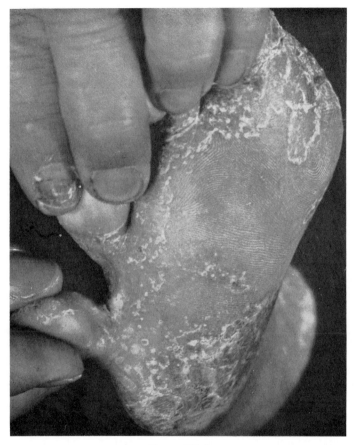

Figure 37–2

Chronic intertriginous type of tinea pedis, showing maceration and fissure between fourth and fifth toes. (Conant et al.: Manual of Clinical Mycology, 3rd Ed. 1971, Philadelphia, W. B. Saunders Co.)

mycoses, from the group name *dermatophyte.* The dermatophytes are closely related fungi comprising three genera and about 20 species. Some are listed in Table 37–1. Almost any species of dermatophyte may cause any form of superficial mycosis, the clinical appearance depending largely on the location of the infection.

A few of the dermatophytes live in soil.[2] Infection takes place when the fungus from the soil is rubbed onto the skin. The fungi grow as hyphae in soil or in cultures, but they also produce conidiospores. Other species occur only on the skin and hair of man and animals. Infections by such fungi are not spread by soil but directly from one individual to another. As the infecting hyphae age in the tissues the fungus cells may develop directly into chains of spores.

Dermatomycoses are spread easily. It is important to remember that each scale from a ringworm lesion, or each stub of infected hair, contains hyphae and spores. These begin growth readily if they become lodged on

[2]Notably *Keratinomyces ajelloi.*

the skin or scalp of another susceptible individual, especially a child. The hyphae promptly grow out from the infected skin scale into the skin of the new host. Dogs, cats, cattle, and other animals are often the source of a ringworm infection. Close inspection of the suspected animal will (if it is infected) show scaly patches with a loss of hair. Remember, too, that an infected child can transmit his infection to the family cat or puppy as well as to his human playmates.

Treatment of Superficial Mycoses

As has been mentioned in Chapter 14, injections of griseofulvin are quite effective if the infection is superficial; also therapeutically useful is nystatin or fungicidin (Mycostatin) for candidiasis and monilial infections. Ringworm has been treated with various topical antifungal agents, Whitefield's Ointment or Tinactin, with ultraviolet irradiation and, in small girls, with estrogens, which cause the child to mature prematurely and cures the tinea infection. For some tineas, selenium sulfide (Selsun) is excellent.

THE SYSTEMIC MYCOSES

Fungi causing systemic mycoses occur naturally in soil as saprophytes. Man and animals become infected with certain of these fungi via the air, i.e., when they inhale dust containing spores or small fragments of hyphae. When lodged in the lung, these begin to grow. If the host's defenses, such as the macrophages, are not capable of destroying these organisms, they multiply and soon a lesion forms in the lung. From these the fungi may (depending on species) enter the lymph or blood and be carried to all parts of the body, where they may produce more lesions. In most people, however, infection is limited to a small area of the lung, and these infections soon heal.

The portal of entry of some soil fungi is via wounds of hands or feet. Millions of people are infected by pathogenic fungi every year, but only a few develop obvious disease.

Coccidioidomycosis

Coccidioidomycosis is a deep (systemic) mycosis that begins as a respiratory infection. In this stage it resembles influenza.

This disease was first recognized as occurring commonly in the San Joaquin Valley of California, and consequently the name San Joaquin Valley fever became popular. We know now that the responsible dimorphic fungus, *Coccidioides immitis,* grows as a saprophyte in the soil in many areas of the arid southwestern United States and in several similar environmental zones elsewhere in the world. People living in these areas become infected by inhaling fungus-laden dust. About 60 per cent of these people experience no symptoms. Their infections are recognized only in retrospect when they are skin-tested and found to react to *coccidioidin*. This is a material derived from *C. immitis* cultures, similar to tuberculin, and the skin test, called the *coccidioidin* test, is analogous in application and significance to the tuberculin test. Following injection of a small quantity of

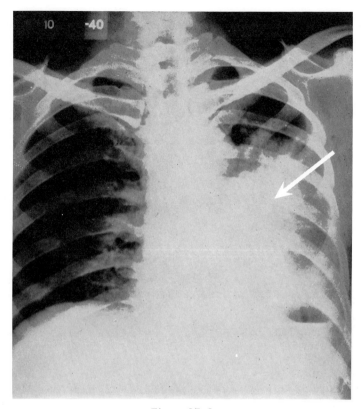

Figure 37–3

Chest x-ray of patient with progressive coccidioidomycosis of the lungs. The light area at the right of the picture, nearly filling the patient's left chest (arrow), represents the x-ray shadows cast by the lesions in the lung. This was a fatal case. (Courtesy of Dr. C. E., Smith *in*: Conant et al.: Manual of Clinical Mycology, 3rd Ed. 1971, Philadelphia, W. B. Saunders Co.)

coccidioidin into the skin, a hard, red area develops in those persons who have coccidioidomycosis or who have had infections by *C. immitis* in the past. A person does not lose the ability to react to this antigen once he has recovered from the infection.

About 40 per cent of people infected experience symptoms. Most of these have only a mild, influenza-like syndrome with fever. A few patients also have painful red bumps on their legs called *erythema nodosum*. In some, pulmonary symptoms are more severe, appearing as pneumonia (Fig. 37–3). In others, symptoms suggestive of tuberculosis occur. In less than 1 per cent of those infected, the fungus is disseminated to all parts of the body. Skin and bone lesions may develop, meningitis is common, and the patient is seriously ill. In a few patients there may be no dissemination, but the lung lesions may progress and giant cavities may form in the lung. Lesions of pulmonary coccidioidomycosis cast x-ray shadows that often cannot be distinguished from those of tuberculosis. The coccidioidin test is then of special value.

The fungus in infected tissue grows as a large, thick-walled, spherical cell called a *spherule,* with little spores forming inside. When the spherule

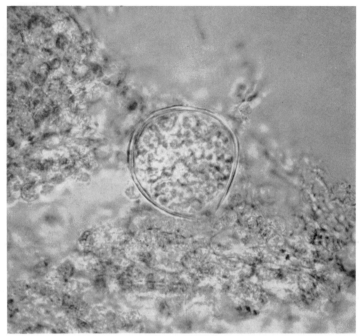

Figure 37–4

Coccidioides immitis in sputum. Spherical, thick-walled cell (*spherule*) containing spores (×700). (Conant et al.: Manual of Clinical Mycology, 3rd Ed. 1971, Philadelphia, W. B. Saunders Co.)

ruptures, these spores are released into the tissue, and each repeats the cycle (Fig. 37–4). If pus or sputum containing these cells is placed on culture media at room temperature, the fungus grows, forming no spherules. It develops a moldlike growth identical to its growth in soil. Because of its ability either to form spherules or to grow as mold it is said to be a *diphasic* or dimorphic fungus. In the soil the hyphae form chains of lightweight arthrospores (Fig. 37–5), which break free and are readily blown about by the wind. Most infections occur during dust storms or when soil is disturbed, as when a tractor plows a field. Cattle, dogs, and many other animals also acquire coccidioidomycosis by inhalation of *Coccidioides* spores in the dust. Direct transmission from person to person is very rare.

Figure 37–5

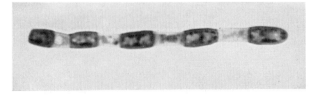

Arthrospores of *Coccidioides immitis.* These are formed from mycelial cells by enlargement and by thickening of the cell wall (approximately ×1000). (Photo courtesy of U.S. Public Health Service, Communicable Disease Center, Atlanta, Ga.)

Primary infections of coccidioidomycosis are extremely common in endemic areas in the United States but the disease is usually not reported to the U.S. Public Health Service. Still, in 1970, optionally reported to this agency were 542 cases in Arizona, 456 in California and 10 in the rest of the states. That these figures do not present a true picture is evidenced by the fact that in epidemic areas 46 to 90 per cent of the population will give a positive coccidioidin test.

The specific treatment of benefit in disseminated infections is amphotericin B (Fungizone), at a near toxic level.

Histoplasmosis

Histoplasmosis is a disease caused by *Histoplasma capsulatum*.[3] This fungus grows in moist, fertile soil in many parts of the world. In the United States it has been found in soil throughout the Middle West and in the eastern half of the country. It is unusually common in soils that have been enriched by fecal material from chickens and other birds, especially starlings. As in coccidioidomycosis, infection takes place by inhalation of spores or fragments of hyphae in dust. Transmission from person to person is very rare.

Skin-testing surveys with *histoplasmin* (a material similar in principle and use to tuberculin and coccidioidin) indicate that millions of people have been infected by *H. capsulatum*. Most of them, however, do not recall having had any recognizable symptoms. Apparently, the healthy body is able to destroy the fungus before much lung tissue is involved.

X-rays made on some healthy people living in the areas where histoplasmosis is endemic often show calcified nodules resembling somewhat those of healed tuberculosis. These people react to histoplasmin skin tests but not to tuberculin unless they have had a tuberculous infection. Most of them are unaware that they have had pulmonary histoplasmosis.

In some infected individuals, large areas of the lung become involved, and these persons experience symptoms that may resemble influenza or pneumonia. Sometimes histoplasmosis may present many symptoms similar to tuberculosis, so much so that laboratory tests are necessary to distinguish which infection is present. When pulmonary symptoms are mild, the patient recovers quickly. When pulmonary disease is severe, the prognosis (outlook for recovery) may be serious.

H. capsulatum, like *C. immitis*, is a diphasic fungus. In the body *H. capsulatum* grows as a small, budding, yeast-like cell. These yeast-like organisms are quickly engulfed by cells of the reticuloendothelial system. The phagocytic cells usually are very active in destroying invading microorganisms, but in the serious forms of histoplasmosis this is not so. The fungus grows actively within these cells. Budding rapidly, the parasites quickly fill the phagocytes.

In symptomless or mild infections the growth of budding *Histoplasma* is controlled, but in serious infections the fungi are carried by the blood to all parts of the body and continue to invade reticuloendothelial cells. Organs such as the liver and spleen, containing large numbers of these cells, become greatly enlarged. These patients are seriously ill.

---

[3]The disease discussed here is clinically entirely different from African histoplasmosis (often confusingly just called histoplasmosis), caused by *Histoplasma duboisii*.

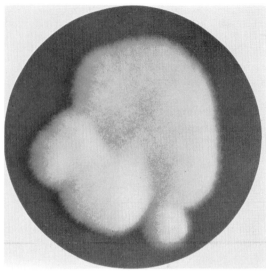

Figure 37–6

A relatively young colony of *Histoplasma capsulatum* on agar, showing the woolly, moldlike growth characteristic of this organism in aerobic cultures. (Courtesy of Dr. J. M. Kurung.)

Figure 37–7

Histoplasma capsulatum. Moldlike phase found in cultures in the laboratory and in soil. The round bodies with projections are called tuberculate chlamydospores and are distinctive of *H. capsulatum* (approximately ×900). (Courtesy of Dr. J. M. Kurung, Ray Brook State Tuberculosis Hospital, Ray Brook, N. Y. In *Amer. Rev. Tuberc.,* Vol. 66.)

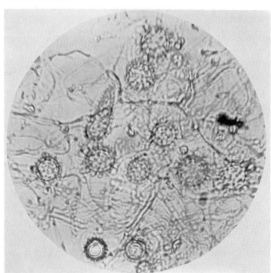

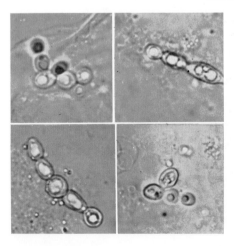

Figure 37–8

Yeast-like cells of *Histoplasma capsulatum* found in the sputum of a patient with pulmonary histoplasmosis (approximately ×1000). (Courtesy of Dr. J. M. Kurung.)

H. capsulatum grows in soil and on culture media at *room* temperature (about 23 C) as a mold producing characteristic conidiospores (Figs. 37–6 and 37–7). If the fungus is cultivated on special media at *body* temperature (37 C), it will grow as small, budding cells identical to those seen in infected tissue or sputum (Fig. 37–8).

Histoplasmosis also occurs in dogs, cats, rats and other animals. For chronic pulmonary cases, amphotericin B is used with caution because of its side effects; large doses of sulfonamides may also be beneficial.

Blastomycosis (North American)

North American blastomycosis and South American blastomycosis are different diseases and are caused by distinctly different dimorphic fungi.

Blastomyces dermatitidis, the cause of North American blastomycosis, is another mold indigenous to the soil. It becomes yeast-like when it grows as a pathogen in the body.

Infection is believed to begin in the lung following inhalation of a spore or hyphal fragment. Dissemination in the tissues is common and

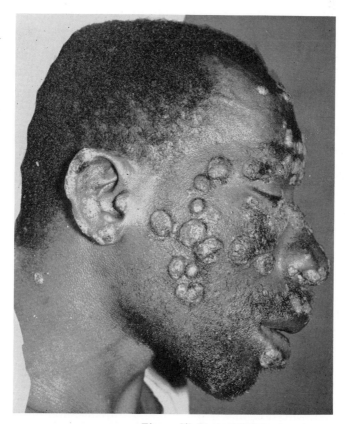

Figure 37–9

North American blastomycosis of the skin, showing multiple, discrete, elevated, granulomatous lesions. (Conant et al.: Manual of Clinical Mycology, 3rd Ed. 1971, Philadelphia, W. B. Saunders Co.)

may be to all parts of the body. Lesions on the skin and in the bones are especially common (Fig. 37–9). Direct transmission from person to person is rare.

Very few people other than patients with blastomycosis react to *blastomycin* (see histoplasmin) when skin-tested. This leads to the belief that subclinical infections are rare and that blastomycosis is not as common as coccidioidomycosis or histoplasmosis. Blastomycosis cases due to *B. dermatitidis* have been found only in the Middle West and eastern half of the United States and Canada; hence this disease is often called North American blastomycosis. All infections with this fungus reported elsewhere in the world have been in people coming from this area.

No preventive measures or immunization regimens for blastomycosis are known. The treatments are amphotericin B or hydroxystilbamidine isethionate as an effective alternative.

Blastomycosis (South American)

South American blastomycosis, also called paracoccidioidomycosis, is a serious, often fatal, chronic mycosis with lung involvement and ulcerative lesions of the skin and mucosa in the oral, nasal or rectal areas. All viscera may be affected, especially the adrenal gland. The fungus causing this disease is *Paracoccidioides brasiliensis*, previously called *Blastomyces brasiliensis*.

The disease is endemic in South America, especially in Brazil, in rural areas. It affects adults rather than children and is perhaps ten times as common in males as in females.

Intravenous use of amphotericin B promptly arrests the spread of lesions, although prolonged treatment with combinations of sulfonamides is also indicated to prevent relapse.

OPPORTUNISTIC MYCOSES

There are a large number of fungi living in soil that are capable of producing infection in man under unusual conditions. The diseases they cause may be considered in the following two categories.

PRIMARY PATHOGENS.   In one category fall the diseases *sporotrichosis* (due to *Sporotrichum schenkii*, Fig. 37–10), *chromoblastomycosis*, and *maduromycosis* (the last due to various fungi). In these mycoses infection takes place only when the fungus is introduced into the skin and subcutaneous tissues by some form of trauma. A localized lesion develops, and the fungus can be found growing in the damaged tissue. Usually there is no dissemination of the organisms in the body beyond enlargement of the lesion, or infection of the lymphatics draining the area. The patient does not develop widespread disease that endangers his life. In each of these diseases caused by a specific *opportunistic fungus*, a more or less characteristic clinical appearance is imparted to the infected area.

SECONDARY PATHOGENS.   There is another category of opportunistic fungal infection that is increasing greatly in importance. This is infection by species of saprophytic soil fungi not ordinarily pathogenic to man. In these cases infection takes place only in patients who are debilitated by other diseases. For instance, a patient with leukemia or lymphoma is more susceptible to *cryptococcosis* (infection by *Cryptococcus neoformans*, a yeast-like fungus somewhat similar to *Blastomyces dermatitidis*) or to *aspergillosis* (infection by *Aspergillus fumigatus;* Chapter 3) than is someone

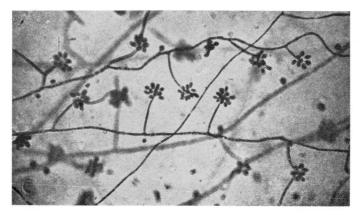

Figure 37–10

Growth of *Sporotrichum schenkii*, on Sabouraud's agar, from a case of sporotrichosis. Note the distinctive arrangement of the bunches of conidia. (Starrs and Klotz: *Arch. Int. Med.*, Vol. 82.)

in good health. A patient who is receiving antibiotics or cortisone for some other condition is also more likely to develop a secondary fungal infection. Most often these begin in the lung and spread to other organs of the body. In *Cryptococcus* infection, meningitis often results.

With an increasing population of older, chronically ill patients, many of whom are receiving antibiotics and steroid therapy, there will be an increasing number of opportunistic infections by fungi. The healthy individual appears to be nonsusceptible to infection, but debilitated patients cannot cope with these ordinarily harmless but potentially pathogenic fungi. Dung and dust of pigeons, starlings, etc., can be infectious.

In general the systemic mycoses are believed to be noncontagious. Care must be given, however, to the proper disposal of sputum, pus, dressings, and other materials that might contain organisms from the patient. These materials present a health hazard.

Other Opportunistic Mycoses

Of the more than 70 species of *Aspergillus* some may become associated with infections in man. This is especially true for *Aspergillus fumigatus*, a pathogen for birds and occasionally for man. Penicilliosis is a very rare disease; only a few of the more than 140 species of *Penicillium* have been isolated from cases with this disease. Just as rare are mucormycosis and infections that may be caused by *Rhizopus*.

Candidiasis[4]

Candida albicans (previously known as *Monilia albicans*) is a yeast-like organism that is common to the mouth and gastrointestinal tract of many normal people. It is *not* indigenous to the soil. Ordinarily it is present in normal persons only in small numbers and produces no disease. Whenever conditions become favorable for its proliferation, this organism multiplies greatly and may even change its growth form. When it is actively invading

[4]The disease is also known as candidosis or moniliasis.

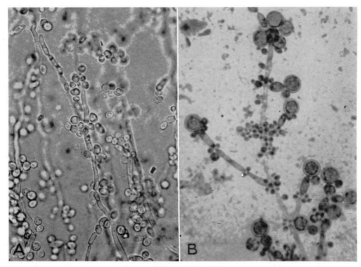

Figure 37–11

Candida albicans. A, Pseudohyphae and clusters of blastospores on Sabouraud's glucose agar (×650). *B*, Typical chlamydospores on corn meal agar (×750). (Conant et al.: Manual of Clinical Mycology, 3rd Ed. 1971, Philadelphia, W. B. Saunders Co.)

tissue, it grows as long filaments as well as in the form of budding, yeast-like cells (Fig. 37–11).

Some conditions that may promote *candidiasis* (infection by *Candida albicans* and occasionally other species of *Candida*) are diabetes, general debilitation, steroid therapy, and the prolonged administration of antibiotics. Pregnant women are also prone to develop *Candida* vaginitis. Some people may develop skin lesions of the interdigital webs or of the finger-nails, especially if their hands are wet for long periods of time. This is another reason why the electric dishwasher is preferred to hand dishwashing.

Treatments often are not necessary if antibiotic therapy, for other diseases, is discontinued. In gastrointestinal infections with *Candida*, nystatin (Mycostatin) is useful; amphotericin B is helpful in generalized disease; and for topical applications, nystatin or gentian violet is used on lesions of the skin and mucous membranes.

THRUSH.   Most *Candida* infections are associated with the mouth and gastrointestinal tract, where this organism is part of the normal flora. When it invades tissues, it causes them to be inflamed, and a white *pseudomembrane* (see Diphtheria) appears on the surface. On the lips and in the mouth this condition is called *thrush*. It is also known as oral moniliasis. Thrush is common in newborn infants whose mothers have a *Candida* vaginitis. The infants acquire their infections during birth. This infection is self-limiting, but to avoid its spread, topical application of 1 per cent aqueous gentian violet is recommended.

Thrush is especially common in patients who have been on antibiotic therapy for a long time. Because of the prolonged antibiotic treatment, there is a tremendous decrease in the kinds and numbers of bacteria in the gastrointestinal tract, which ordinarily suppress growth of *C. albicans*. Under these conditions *C. albicans*, whose growth is not inhibited by most antibiotics, proliferates greatly and may cause diarrhea and other distressing symptoms. Perianal rashes or itching may also result.

Candida is also a common secondary or opportunistic invader, especially in the lungs. When lung tissue has been damaged by cancer, tuberculosis, or other infectious agents, this yeast can grow abundantly in the necrotic tissue and may obscure the diagnostic laboratory findings. Rarely, C. albicans enters the blood. When this happens it may cause vegetations on the heart valves or lesions in the kidneys, always dangerous developments.

Candida albicans is readily transmissible by fluids and excretions from infected areas and tissues: skin, vagina, oral mucosa, urine, feces and so on. Personal contact with lesions should be avoided. Fomites should be disinfected; dressings and bandages must be burned.

MYCOTOXINS

Not all fungal diseases are infections. Some are due to ingestion of toxic metabolites of fungi, collectively called *mycotoxins*. Among the best known of these at present is the group of aflatoxins, metabolites of *Aspergillus flavus*, though a dozen or more are known. Aflatoxins and several other mycotoxins are produced when the molds grow in "spoiled" vegetable products such as hay, peanuts, grains, and so forth, commonly used as stock and poultry feeds. The role of mycotoxins in human disease has yet to be fully evaluated. Recognized cases of acute human mycotoxicosis are rare, presumably because humans do not commonly eat "moldy" or "spoiled" foods; though certain cheeses might be cited as popular exceptions.

Supplementary Reading

Ajello, L.: Comparative ecology of respiratory mycotic disease agents. *Bact. Rev.*, 1967, *31*:6.
Beneke, E. S.: Medical Mycology: Laboratory Manual, 2nd Ed. 1966, Minneapolis, Burgess Publishing Co.
Burnett, J. H.: Fundamentals of Mycology. 1968, New York, St. Martin's.
Conant, N. F., Smith, D. T., Baker, R. D., and Callaway, J. L.: Manual of Clinical Mycology, 3rd Ed. 1971, Philadelphia, W. B. Saunders Co.
Emmons, C. W., Binford, C. H., and Utz, J. P.: Medical Mycology. 1963, Philadelphia, Lea & Febiger.
Fiese, M. J.: Coccidioidomycosis. 1958, Springfield, Ill., Charles C Thomas.
Furcolow, M. L.: Histoplasmosis. *Amer. J. Nurs.*, 1959, *59*:79.
Gilardi, G. L.: Nutrition of systemic and subcutaneous pathogenic fungi. *Bact. Rev.*, 1965, *29*:406.
Goldblatt, L. A. (ed.): Aflatoxin. 1969, New York, Academic Press.
Gordon, M. A., and Devine, J.: Filamentation and endogenous sporulation in *Cryptococcus neoformans. Sabouraudia*, 1970, *8*:227.
Louria, D. B.: Experiences with and diagnosis of diseases due to opportunistic fungi. *Ann. N.Y. Acad. Sci.*, 1962, *98* (Art. 3):617.
Loverman, A. B., and Kotcher, E.: Favus in Kentucky: Diagnosis, treatment and epidemiology. *J. Kentucky State Med. Assn.*, 1962, *60*:No. 7.
Martinson, F. D.: Chronic phycomycosis of the upper respiratory tract. *Amer. J. Trop. Med. & Hyg.*, 1971, *20*:449.
Rakich, J. H.: Nursing aspects of histoplasmosis. *Amer. J. Nurs.*, 1959, *59*:81.
Rebell, G., and Taplin, D.: Dermatophytes: Their recognition and Identification. 1970, University of Miami Press, Coral Gables, Fla.
Skinner, C. E., and Fletcher, D. W.: A review of the genus *Candida. Bact. Rev.*, 1960, *24*:397.
Spensley, P. C.: Mycotoxins. *Roy. Soc. Health Jour.*, 1970, *5*:248.
Walter, J. E., and Atchison, R. W.: Epidemiological and immunological studies of *Cryptococcus neoformans. J. Bact*, 1966, *92*:82.

Pathogens Transmitted
in Blood

Secondary and Accidental
Infections; Arthropod-Borne
Bacterial Infections

38

INTRODUCTION

There are at least three ways in which microorganisms may gain entrance
into blood: either as the result of other infections, or through cuts and
wounds, or by way of natural vectors, such as arthropods that transmit
disease-causing organisms. These ways are listed in Table 38–1. In addition, do not forget blood transfusions!

INVASION OF BLOOD AS SEQUELAE TO PRIMARY INFECTION. As
previously stated, many pathogenic organisms commonly invade the blood
secondarily after they have established a primarily localized infection at
the initial portal of entry (e.g., *Salmonella typhi* via the alimentary tract,
Treponema pallidum via the genital tract, streptococci from abscessed teeth,
and so on). Infections of various parts of the body by microorganisms
transmitted in blood from initial or other local sites are often called *hematogenous* infections.

Artificial or Accidental Infection
of Blood

Many pathogenic agents in infected blood may be transmitted by any
vector that can transfer the infectious blood into the body of another person. The vector in such infections may be artificial: unsterile hypodermic

Table 38–1. Blood Infections and Their Vectors

I. Sequelae to infections acquired via other portals of entry (secondary, endogenous infections).
II. Artificial or accidental vectors, such as cuts, pricks, scratches with infecting instruments;
injection of infected serum or blood; careless handling of infectious blood, instruments,
or dressings; careless tattooing: may transmit any pathogen present in the blood at the
time, including viruses of epidemic hepatitis (hepatitis A) and serum hepatitis (hepatitis
B), and those listed below.
III. Natural vectors (sanguivorous arthropods) may transmit:
    1. Bacteria (e.g., plague, tularemia, relapsing fever)
    2. Rickettsias (e.g., typhus and typhus-like fevers)[1]
    3. Viruses (e.g., yellow and dengue fevers, various encephalitides)
    4. Protozoa (e.g., malaria, African sleeping sickness, kala-azar)
    5. Helminths (e.g., various types of filariasis).

---

[1]We are not so well informed about the means of transmission of chlamydial diseases.

syringes, bloody dressings, any cutting or piercing instrument, unprocessed serum, plasma, and so on. Such infections are usually accidental, or are irregular occurrences due to carelessness or ignorance. For example, in one dramatic instance a group of drug addicts, one of whom was malarious, all used the same needle and syringe at one sitting and all contracted malaria. In another, fatal, instance a pathologist pricked his finger with a knife during an autopsy on a person who had died of plague. Others have similarly acquired "blood poisoning" from human tissues carrying streptococcal or staphylococcal infection. A nurse handling bloody dressings, contaminated with *Pasteurella tularensis*, became careless or negligent. She had a tiny scratch on her hand and the microorganisms entered her blood.

SERUM HEPATITIS. The *homologous serum jaundice* (or hepatitis B) virus is found, so far as is known, only in human blood. It is transferred only by artificial procedures that transmit blood (or certain blood derivatives) from one person to another. These procedures include accidents, as just noted, and also blood transfusions and serum injections and the use, without vigorous and adequate sterilization, of any skin-piercing instrument on a succession of persons. These instruments include surgical instruments, hypodermic needles and syringes (before disposable ones became generally available), needles used to obtain blood specimens, and so on. These modes of transmission are entirely artificial and man-made. How such a virus comes to be widely present in people all over the world is not clear. Apparently, chronic carriers of the virus are fairly common, and many very mild or latent infections occur. In 1971, 9556 cases of serum hepatitis (SH) were reported in the United States. Note that infectious hepatitis (IH), i.e., infection by hepatitis virus A, was much more common; during the same period 59,606 cases were observed. For a discussion of both SH and IH, see pages 369–372.

The virus is one of the small-sized ones and is not affected by any known chemotherapeutic drugs. It differs from other known viruses (except that of infectious or *epidemic* hepatitis which it most closely resembles) in that it is unusually resistant to heat. Ordinary ten minute boiling cannot be relied upon to inactivate it on syringes, needles, and instruments. The only safe sterilizing procedures are autoclaving and the use of the hot air oven. Disinfectant handwashing and use of sterile needles when collecting blood specimens or injecting successive persons and handling of bloody cotton or dressings or blood during specimen-taking or surgery should be done with scrupulous care. The now almost universal use of disposable needles, syringes, and lancets (used for small blood samples) helps greatly in avoiding the transmission of this infection. Homologous serum hepatitis characteristically has a long incubation period of weeks or months. The overt disease is an acute febrile one, with general constitutional symptoms of varying severity. Hepatitis and jaundice are common but not invariable. Children are especially susceptible. Fatality rates can be high.

Australia Antigen. A distinctive, antigenic protein particle, variously called Australia antigen (Au ag), hepatitis antigen (HA), hepatitis B antigen (HB ag), serum hepatitis antigen (SH ag), and hepatitis-associated antigen (HAA), is so regularly found in the serum of patients, convalescents and carriers of hepatitis B (or SH) that it is generally accepted as serologically equivalent to the virus itself. Diagnostic demonstration of this antigen by serologic means is now possible and is of great importance in the selection of blood donors. Unlike hepatitis A, immune serum globulins are of no prophylactic value against hepatitis B infection.

Natural Vectors (Sanguivorous Arthropods)

Numerous infectious agents are transmitted under natural conditions directly into the blood, mainly by sanguivorous arthropods such as malaria-transmitting mosquitoes.

In the remainder of this chapter we shall discuss arthropods as disease vectors and some arthropod-borne *bacterial* diseases.

ARTHROPODS AS DISEASE VECTORS

Man-biting and animal-biting arthropods constitute one of the most important classes of disease vectors. Arthropods may conveniently be divided into two groups with respect to the means by which they transmit disease.

MECHANICAL MEANS.   When flies walk on feces, boils, or sores, soiling their bodies, feet, and legs, and then walk on food, on plates or glasses, on the lips of a sleeping infant or on the ulcers of a sick person, the implications are obvious and need no elaboration.

TRANSMISSION BY FECES AND VOMITUS.   Flies, ants, roaches, and other coprophagic (feces-eating) arthropods may harbor in their gut intestinal pathogens taken in with the feces they eat. These vermin also feed on vomitus, infectious blood, open sores, and so on. Such arthropods deposit the disease agents with their fecal droppings on food and about the house, as well as on the wounds, eyes, lips, and skin of waking or sleeping human beings. Many species also regurgitate (vomit) contents of their gut when they bite. This also needs no further discussion.

BIOLOGIC MEANS.   This generally implies passage of the pathogenic agent from the gut of the insect into the tissues and body fluids of the arthropod vector, especially into the saliva. One of the best known of this type of disease is malaria. Others are various forms of viral encephalitis, yellow fever, bubonic plague, and elephantiasis (filariasis). Some important diseases carried by sanguivorous arthropods, as well as the general nature of the disease agents, may be tabulated as shown in Table 38–2. The lowly bedbug has not been convicted as a disease vector, although it is often suspected of being one, and probably is.

Arthropod-borne diseases prevail especially in warm regions where numerous species of sanguivorous flies, mosquitoes, and ticks abound; they occur also in temperate climates under conditions of uncleanliness and crowding in which vermin such as lice, fleas, and flies flourish, and in swampy and woodland areas where mosquitoes and ticks breed.

ZOONOSES

A number of diseases can be transmitted to man from wild animals in forest or field, "far from the madding crowd's ignoble strife." Infectious diseases of animals transmissible to man by any means are called *zoonoses*.

The name "zoonoses" was first applied by Rudolph Virchow to the infectious diseases that man acquires from domestic animals. The Second Report of the Joint World Health Organization Food and Agriculture

Table 38–2. Some Common Arthropod-Borne Diseases and Their Vectors

Mosquitoes:
    Malaria (protozoa)
    Yellow fever (virus)
    Dengue (virus)
    Encephalitis (virus)
    Filariasis (helminths)
Ticks:
    Relapsing fever (spirochetes)
    Rocky Mountain spotted fever or tick typhus (rickettsias)
    Texas fever of cattle (protozoa)
    Tularemia or "rabbit fever" (bacteria)
Fleas of rats and other rodents:
    Endemic typhus or flea typhus (rickettsias)
    Bubonic plague (bacteria)
    Tularemia (bacteria)
Lice, ticks, fleas, and "red spider" ("chigger") larvae of mites:
    Typhus fever, tsutsugamushi or mite typhus, and related diseases (rickettsias)

Organization Expert Group on Zoonoses (1959) redefined zoonoses as, "those diseases and infections which are naturally transmitted between vertebrate animals and man." Experimental infections from laboratory animals, not normally harboring the infectious agents, are not considered zoonoses. Over a hundred zoonoses are known today, a great increase since the turn of the century when only a few zoonotic diseases like anthrax, cowpox, glanders, rabies, and a few zooparasitic infections were recognized.

Salmonelloses are common in fowls, pigs, dogs, cattle, rats, mice, primates, cats, goats, sheep, pigeons, hares, rabbits, foxes, mink, and guinea pigs, as well as other mammals and birds, and reptiles and arthropods.

Two distinct etiologic agents have been recognized as causing what had previously been considered a single pathologic entity, rat-bite fever. The organism causing one form of the disease called sodoku is *Spirillum minus*. Sodoku in humans usually results from the bite of an infected rodent. Haverhill fever is another form of rat-bite fever, the result of infection with the bacterium, *Streptobacillus moniliformis.*

The causative agent of pseudotuberculosis in laboratory animals is *Pasteurella pseudotuberculosis rodentium*. It attacks the guinea pig chiefly but can also infect mice, rabbits and man, but not rats.

Leptospirosis is not a serious disease among laboratory animals but may become so in the wild counterparts of experimental animals. One causative agent in rodents is *Leptospira icterohaemorrhagiae*. Other serotypes of *Leptospira* implicated in rodent disease include *L. saxkoebing* and *L. ballum*. In many, symptomatology and pathology are varied.

Arthropod-Borne Bacterial Diseases

Not all infections common to man and animals are of bacterial origin. For example, lymphocytic choriomeningitis is a viral disease that affects the brain of monkeys but also causes aseptic meningitis in humans, as well as meningoencephalitis. Transmissions of the virus to guinea pigs by infected woodtick nymphs and by *Aedes aegypti* mosquitoes have been described.[1]

Some other zoonoses will be discussed here.

Genus Pasteurella and Related Organisms

The genus *Pasteurella* contains two species that cause serious disease in man (*P. pestis*, bubonic plague; *P. tularensis*, tularemia). A third species, *P. multocida*, is mentioned here as representative of the remaining six species, all of which cause disease in lower warm-blooded animals, rarely in man. *Pasteurella pestis* is now commonly called *Yersinia pestis* in honor of A. E. J. Yersin (1863–1943), a colleague of Pasteur and discoverer of the bacillus of bubonic plague; *P. tularensis* is now commonly called *Francisella tularensis* in honor of Thomas Francis, Jr., American microbiologist who demonstrated the role of rodents in the transmission of tularemia.

Pasteurella multocida ("killer of many") is so named because it causes frequently fatal hemorrhagic septicemia (or hemorrhagic fever) in many species of lower vertebrates: cattle, sheep, birds, and so on, often resulting in great commercial losses.

Francisella tularensis is given the name *tularensis* for the Tulare areas near San Francisco where it was first observed causing "rabbit fever."

Yersinia pestis is the cause of bubonic plague. Since all of these diseases are primarily infections of animals transmissible to man, they are properly classed as zoonoses.

All species of *Pasteurella* (including *Yersinia* and *Francisella*) are small, gram-negative, nonspore-forming rods. When observed microscopically

---

[1] Most of the above data on zoonoses are taken from *Charles River Digest*, Vol. IV, No. II, April, 1967.

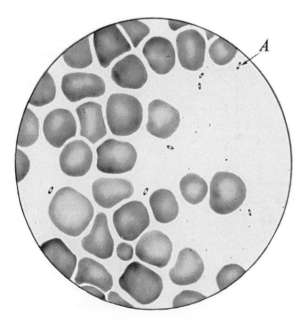

Figure 38–1

Drawing made from a microphotograph of blood of a mouse that died of hemorrhagic septicemia, a plague-like disease of animals. At *A* are seen *Pasteurella multocida*, morphologically like *Y. pestis*, cause of bubonic plague. Note the rounded ends and bipolar staining distinctive of *Pasteurella*. The large, rounded objects are erythrocytes distorted by shrinkage due to drying of the smear. (Courtesy of Dr. C. D. Stein, Bureau of Animal Industry. U. S. Dept. of Agriculture.)

in smears of blood, pus, or other pathologic material, they are characterized by staining (with special stains like Wayson's) more intensely at the
tips than in the center (bipolar staining) (Fig. 38–1). They are easily recognized, and, with pertinent corroboratory data, the infection can be diagnosed by this appearance. Cultures and animal inoculations are also useful.

These species produce bacteriemias and generalized infections, which
tend to localize especially in the lymph nodes. In man, these nodes swell
up and then are spoken of as *buboes*, especially when in the groins, axillae,
or neck. The buboes are filled with pus and bacilli. They often rupture
and the draining pus is highly infectious. Attendants have to consider this
in handling patients with any infection due to these organisms.

Hemorrhagic Fever.   Since this form of bacteremia is primarily a
disease of animals, it need not be discussed in detail here. The organisms
(*P. multocida*) occur in blood and body discharges. They persist in the dust
and dirt of animal cars and pens and are inhaled and swallowed or gain
entrance through cuts and scratches in the skin. The occasional human case
may be handled as described for tularemia (see next paragraph). Arthropod transmission of this disease is probably not important, but the organisms occur in the mouths of rats, whose bites probably infect animals and
occasionally man.

Tularemia.   This disease, often called "rabbit fever," is caused by
Francisella tularensis, a species very similar to *Y. pestis* and *P. multocida* in
many respects. It causes a similar disease among wild rodents, notably
rabbits and ground squirrels.

TRANSMISSION.   Ticks, fleas, deer flies, and probably other sanguivorous arthropods found on rabbits and other rodents transmit tularemia
from animal to animal and to man. A pustule forms at the site of the initial
infection and the pus is highly infectious. Tularemia often occurs in persons (hunters, market men, housewives) handling wild rabbits. Tularemia
has a wide range of hosts, including man; over 50 species of mammals,
birds and reptiles are susceptible to it. Why then implicate only the poor
rabbit?

Infected wild animals occasionally die on the banks of streams, infecting the water and causing serious outbreaks of tularemia among persons drinking the untreated water — another reason for boiling or chlorinat-
ing water from unknown sources, if it must be used.

Blood, pustular sites of primary infection, and draining secondary
buboes in man are infectious. Biting arthropods must be kept away from
patients as well as from other persons. Tularemia is much less fatal than
plague but it is very protracted, very debilitating, and sometimes in-
capacitating for long periods. In a 1971 outbreak of tularemia in Sweden
the epidemiological, bacteriological and clinical data indicated that the
infection was generally transmitted through inhalation of dust from hay
contaminated with animal feces.

Some tularemia-specific skin-test antigens have been tested and found
to give a positive reaction very early in the illness (Foshay's test). In 1971,
187 cases of tularemia in man were recorded in the United States.

Bubonic Plague.   This is one of the so-called "classic" diseases, a scourge
of the ancient and medieval worlds and still a dangerous menace in many
parts of the Eastern and Southern Hemispheres. The presence of buboes
gave plague its name: bubonic. The arthropods most commonly responsible for transmission of bubonic plague to man are fleas from infected rats
and ground squirrels. The disease is maintained constantly among the

rodents by these arthropods. An infectious disease that is regularly transmitted among lower animals is said to be *enzootic*. If it becomes unusually prevalent among them, it is said to be *epizootic* (compare *endemic* and *epidemic*). Plague among prairie and forest animals is called "sylvatic" or "campestral" plague (*sylvatic*, in the forest; *campestral*, in the fields). Occasional cases of plague occur in persons who handle carcasses of such animals.

Bubonic plague is primarily a disease of rats and other rodents. When these become very numerous in contact with humans, bites of fleas (*Xenopsylla cheopsis*, the oriental rat flea) from infected rodents, especially rats, are apt to be numerous. Under such conditions plague becomes epidemic. When this happens, great and devastating outbreaks are apt to occur. The *Black Death*, famous in history and legend, was bubonic plague in acute epidemic form. The term "black death" was derived from the fact that in such epidemics the disease was marked by intense septicemia and subcutaneous hemorrhages that occurred over the whole body, giving it a dark appearance. In the United States such epidemics are now unknown because we now know that rats and ground squirrels harbor the disease and that their fleas transmit it, and we take appropriate measures to control both rodents and fleas. However, sporadic cases sometimes occur, especially in southwestern United States.

Rats and ground squirrels are controlled by the United States Public Health Service in cooperation with local and private agencies. This involves poisoning, trapping, elimination of rats from ships (rats in ships from plague areas are exceedingly clever at getting ashore in spite of immigration and other officials), rat-proof building, the destruction of shelter places, and the elimination of garbage dumps, open feed bins, and similar places where rats can feed. The use of residual DDT powder in homes and in rat runways has been very effective in ridding the rats of their fleas, although it does not eliminate the rats. When dead rats cool off, their fleas leave them and go to other warm-blooded animals. Therefore, avoid dead rats (Fig. 38–2).

The rat control bill passed in 1967 by Congress should help in diminishing these animals that are always potential carriers of bubonic plague. Since January 1, 1971, measures applicable to any transport, land, sea or air, arriving from plague areas are specified in International Health Regulations, WHO, Geneva. Medical personnel in North America will seldom see a case of plague unless it is on foreign service to the Orient, Mediterranean, or certain South American countries.

PLAGUE VACCINE. A vaccine (Haffkine's vaccine), much like antisalmonellosis vaccine, is used to immunize persons going to plague districts, e.g., military and health personnel, and doctors and nurses working in plague areas. The immunity conferred is not absolute, and is of short duration, probably not over six months. All contacts of a person having plague should be immunized. Persons remaining in endemic areas should receive semiannual booster doses. Early use of broad-spectrum antibiotics, especially streptomycin, is extremely valuable in therapy.

PNEUMONIC PLAGUE. This is really a respiratory tract disease, but it may be considered here as a development from bubonic plague. Occasionally, in a patient with flea-borne plague of the bubonic type, the organisms may invade the lungs, causing a plague pneumonia (pneumonic plague). This disease, like other diseases of the respiratory tract, is exceedingly difficult to control. It is highly contagious by means of respira-

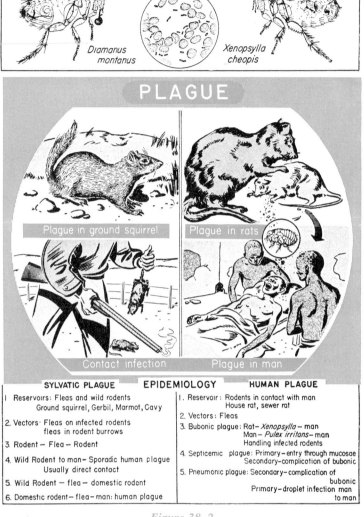

Figure 38–2

Epidemiology of plague. (Hunter, Frye, and Swartzwelder: A Manual of Tropical Medicine, 4th Ed. 1966, Philadelphia, W. B. Saunders Co.)

tory secretions and droplets thereof, and is highly fatal (up to 90 per cent or higher). Outbreaks of pneumonic plague, unless controlled expertly and promptly by state and federal health authorities, are apt to become devastating scourges. Any severe case of bubonic plague may become pneumonic.

PREVENTION. The area surrounding the bite of an infected arthropod, in both plague and tularemia, is usually marked by a pustule containing highly infectious pus. In both diseases drainage and dressings from the initial lesion, as well as all other exudates, must be carefully handled and immediately disinfected, preferably burned. The clothing of the

HUMAN PLAGUE — Reported Cases by Age and Sex, United States, 1950-1970

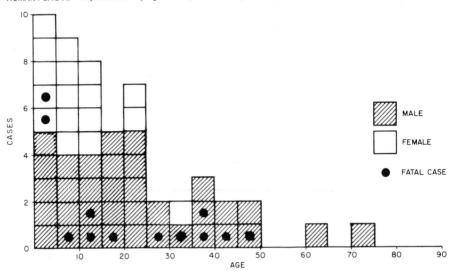

Human Plague by Five-Year Periods, United States, 1926-1970

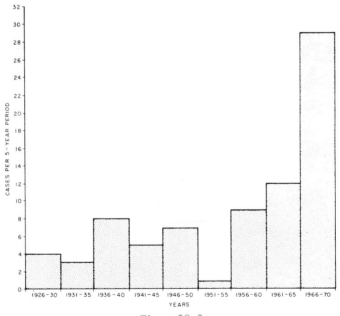

Figure 38–3

Epidemiology of human bubonic plague. (From Morbidity and Mortality, Annual Supplement, 1970. U.S. Dept. of Health, Education, and Welfare.)

patient admitted with bubonic plague should be put into a tight bag immediately and treated to kill fleas. The patient must be absolutely isolated. Nurse, attendants, and physician must wear complete gowns, and in pneumonic plague, head coverings with celluloid masks, as well as rubber gloves. The utmost precautions must be taken with any fomites. Nothing should leave the room that has not been disinfected or enclosed. Droplet and dust infection must be most carefully prevented in pneumonic patients. Bodies are autopsied or buried only under special license and precautions. Rats or fleas on the premises must be eliminated. A good insect spray that really kills fleas, used daily for three successive days and repeated weekly for five or six weeks throughout the infested premises, will often eliminate fleas.

However, it is erroneous to conclude that plague simply does not occur any more in the United States. Statistics show that between the years 1965 to 1968, one person died each year in this country from this disease. In 1970, 13 cases were reported; this, and the data shown in Figure 38–3 indicate that the plague is still with us.

Genus Borrelia

BORRELIA AND RELAPSING FEVER.[2] *Borrelia*[3] is the name of a genus of spirochetes that infect the blood and tissues of man and other animals

---

[2] Distinguish between *relapsing* fever, due to spirochetes of the genus *Borrelia*, and *undulant* fever, due to *Brucella abortus*, etc.

[3] Named for A. Borrel (1867–1936), a famous French microbiologist who made pioneering studies of these organisms.

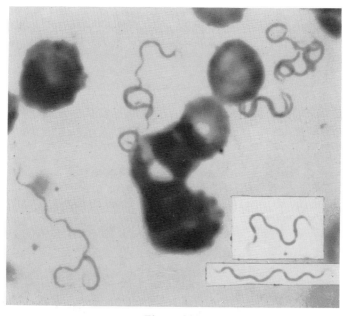

Figure 38–4

Borrelia recurrentis in a droplet of blood (the large, rounded, dark objects are blood cells). This is one of the species of *Borrelia* that cause relapsing fever (×2700). (Courtesy of Dr. A. Packchanian, The University of Texas Medical Branch at Galveston.)

(Fig. 38–4), and that are transmitted by two types of arthropod: lice and ticks. The spirochetes cause relapsing fever in man. Diseases caused by *Borrelia* are often spoken of collectively as borrelioses. The borrelias are somewhat thicker and less regularly curved than treponemes, but the two have often been confused with one another. Tick-borne and louse-borne borrelias, though morphologically identical, are of different species: *B. duttoni* (and several differently named but very similar varieties) in ticks; *B. recurrentis* (also with several differently named but very similar varieties) in lice.

Spirochetal relapsing fever is found in the western United States, in the northwest part of South America, in all of Africa, and in Asia and the Pacific Islands, as well as in Central Europe.

LOUSE-BORNE RELAPSING FEVER. Relapsing fever due to *B. recurrentis* occurs chiefly in limited areas of Europe, North and South Africa, and Central America. The common vector is the body louse (*Pediculus humanus*). Louse-borne diseases, including typhus fever and louse-borne relapsing fever, are rare or nonexistent in the United States (why?). Since relapsing fever can occur in louse-infested populations, it often appears as an epidemic. The same populations also suffer from epidemics of typhus fever, since this also is louse-borne. Such populations are generally those who wear clothes, i.e., they are not tropical natives who go mostly naked.

TICK-BORNE RELAPSING FEVER. Cases of relapsing fever due to *B. duttoni*, seen in some of our western states, are transmitted from wild animals, especially rodents, to man by bites of various species of soft (*Ornithodorus*) ticks. Such infectious tick bites, unlike the constantly present bites of lice, are rather uncommon and accidental, not epidemic, and sometimes occur during picnics.

Relapsing fever due to either species of *Borrelia* gets its name from the frequent and regular recurrences of the fever in the patient. Relapses of fever, chills and pain recur at intervals of five to 15 days and last for several days. Usually five to eight relapses of diminishing severity occur. The spirochetes circulate in the blood during the febrile relapses and may readily be seen with the microscope in stained smears or darkfield preparations. Thompson reported in 1969 that the largest outbreak of tick-borne relapsing fever in the Western hemisphere occurred in 1968 in Washington state. It was thought that the chipmunks and pine squirrels were the reservoirs for this outbreak.

PREVENTION. There are only two problems important to the prevention of transmission of either louse-borne or tick-borne relapsing fever. One consists in taking suitable precautions to prevent the arthropod vectors from biting either patients or well persons. In military action this may be a difficult problem. Blood-engorged ticks, lice, and other man-biting arthropods, regardless of when or where found, should be handled with forceps and immediately incinerated.

A second set of precautions is based on the fact that the blood of patients in the febrile stage will infect through cuts or scratches on the hands or possibly through the unbroken skin. This is important to know when collecting blood specimens or giving intravenous injections.

Supplementary Reading

Buchanan, T. M., Brooks, G. F., and Brachman, P. S.: The tularemia skin test. 325 skin tests in 210 persons: serologic correlation and review of literature. *Ann. Intern. Med.*, 1971, *74:*336.

Burrows, W.: Textbook of Microbiology, 19th Ed. 1968, Philadelphia, W. B. Saunders Co.

Cavanaugh, D. C., et al.: Some observations on the current plague outbreak in the Republic of Viet Nam. *Amer. J. Pub. Health*, 1968, *58:*742.

Dahlstrand, S., Ringertz, O., and Zetterberg, B.: Airborne tularemia in Sweden. *Scand. J. Infect. Dis.*, 1971, *3*(1):7.

Emmons, R. W., Woodie, J. D., Taylor, M. S., and Nygood, G. S.: Tularemia in a pet squirrel monkey (*Saimiri sciureus*). *Lab. Anim. Care*, 1971, *20:*1149.

Faust, E. C., Beaver, P. C., and Jung, R. C.: Animal Agents and Vectors of Disease, 3rd Ed. 1968, Philadelphia, Lea & Febiger.

Felsenfeld, O.: Borrelia, Borreliosis and Relapsing Fever. 1970, St. Louis, Warren H. Green, Inc.

Frobisher, M.: Fundamentals of Microbiology, 8th Ed. 1968, Philadelphia, W. B. Saunders Co.

Goldenberg, M. I.: Laboratory diagnosis of plague infection. *Health Lab. Sci.*, 1968, *5:*38.

Goodman, R. L., Arndt, K. A., and Steigbigel, N. L.: *Borrelia* in Boston. *J.A.M.A.*, 1969, *210:* 722.

Horsfall, W. R.: Medical Entomology. 1962, New York, The Ronald Press Co.

Hubbert, W. T., and Rosen, M. N.: *Pasteurella multocida* infection: 1. Due to animal bite; 2. unrelated to animal bite. *Amer. J. Pub. Health*, 1970, *60:*1103, 1109.

Human bubonic plague – New Mexico. *Morbidity and Mortality*, 1971: *20:*283.

Hunter, G. W., III, Frye, W. W., and Swartzwelder, J. C.: A Manual of Tropical Medicine, 4th Ed. 1966, Philadelphia, W. B. Saunders Co.

Mullett, C. F.: The Bubonic Plague and England: An Essay in the History of Preventive Medicine. 1956, Lexington, The University of Kentucky Press.

Nutter, J. E.: Antigens of *Pasteurella tularensis*: Preparative procedures. *Appl. Microbiol.*, 1971, *22*(1):44.

Thompson, R. S., Burdorfer, W., Russell, R., and Francis, B. J.: Outbreak of tick-borne relapsing fever in Spokane County, Washington. *J.A.M.A.*, 1969, *210:*1045.

Arthropod-Borne Rickettsial and Viral Infections

39

RICKETTSIOSES

An infection with any of the rickettsias is properly spoken of as *rickettsiosis.* Several names of long standing, however, are commonly used to differentiate various rickettsioses transmitted by different arthropods and in different geographical areas. There are perhaps 20 such diseases, which have been placed into major groups as outlined in Table 39–1 and represented, respectively, by *typhus-like fevers, spotted fever, scrub typhus, Q fever,* and others. Of these, only two are of major importance in the United States: typhus, especially murine or rat-borne typhus, and Rocky Mountain spotted fever. Q fever is probably more widespread than is generally supposed.

THE TYPHUS-LIKE FEVERS

The typhus fever-like diseases are often differentiated according to their arthropod vectors, as follows:

LOUSE TYPHUS. The so-called classic or epidemic disease, louse-borne typhus, is transmitted through the feces of body lice deposited when the louse bites. The feces may then be scratched into the wound made by the bite. Epidemic typhus has been known to decimate armies and various populations since antiquity. In more recent times, it was probably in large part responsible for the eventual downfall of Napoleon's armies in Russia and possibly that of the German armies in Italy and the defeat at Stalingrad in World War II.

FLEA TYPHUS. This disease is transmitted from rats to man by the feces of infected rat fleas. This disease is also called murine or endemic typhus. Although sometimes less fatal than louse-borne typhus, it is essentially the same disease. Due to anti-rat campaigns, it has decreased in the United States (Fig. 39–1). Chemotherapy has reduced the death rate to zero.

TICK TYPHUS. This typhus occurs in several forms and is best known to North Americans as Rocky Mountain spotted fever. It is transmitted

540

mainly by wood ticks (*Dermacentor andersoni*) in the West, and mainly by dog ticks (*Dermacentor variabilis*) in the eastern part of the United States. São Paulo typhus in Brazil, transmitted by ticks (*Amblyomma cajennense*), and Boutonneuse fever (fièvre boutonneuse) in Africa are closely related forms of this disease.

MITE TYPHUS. Prevalent in Japan, the Malay peninsula, and the South Pacific Islands generally, mite typhus has many names, such as scrub typhus, tsutsugamushi, river fever, swamp fever, and so on. It is caused by *Rickettsia tsutsugamushi*, and is transmitted from rodents such as field rats and field mice to man by the bite of the larval stage of a "chigger"-like mite known as *Leptotrombidium akamushi* or *Trombicula akamushi*.

These typhus-like rickettsial diseases differ from each other in some clinical and immunologic details, but they are basically so similar that it is convenient to think of them as a group differing chiefly in geographic distribution and vectors.

Louse-borne Typhus Fever

The word "typhus," freely translated (from the Greek *typhos*), means stupor and refers to the stuporous, confused mental state of typhus patients. This disease, caused by *Rickettsia prowazekii,* has been known since very ancient times. *Typhoid* fever (due to *Salmonella typhi*) received its name because some typhoid patients are stuporous and to this extent resemble typhus patients, but the two diseases are otherwise totally unrelated.

Epidemic or louse-borne typhus occurs in Central and Eastern Europe and also in South and Central America, Asia, Africa, Russia, and (only rarely) in the United States and Canada. It becomes epidemic whenever conditions are suitable for populations to become thoroughly infected with lice. Troops in trenches, sailors in old-time ships, and crowded, poverty-stricken peoples during times of war or famine are thus especially likely to be visited by the disease. The course of history has been turned time and again by devastating epidemics of typhus fever; hence, it is a "classic" disease of antiquity.

Typhus fever is characterized by an onset of about two days during which there are nausea, headache, dizziness, and high fever. There then appears a rash, which may cover the whole trunk. It lasts for a week or more and disappears slowly. The patient is lethargic and delirious. The mortality in some epidemics is high. The blood of patients is infectious for lice, man, and animals, although the organisms have not been demonstrated microscopically in the blood.

WEIL-FELIX REACTION. A peculiar immunologic phenomenon, known by the name of its discoverers as the Weil-Felix reaction, occurs during typhus fever, and in some of the other typhus-like diseases such as Rocky Mountain spotted fever and mite typhus or tsutsugamushi. It is sometimes used for diagnostic purposes. Agglutinins appear in high concentration in the blood during the first week of the diseases and later. Curiously, they are active not only against the infecting species of rickettsias but also against certain strains of *Proteus vulgaris*.[1] *Proteus* apparently has no other relationship to the rickettsial diseases.

---

[1]These are gram-negative, nonspore-forming, motile rods classified with the Enterobacteriaceae. See Chapter 23.

Table 39-1.   Human Rickettsial Diseases*

RICKETTSIOSIS GROUP	DISEASE NAMES	INFECTIOUS AGENT	GEOGRAPHIC REGIONS	VERTEBRATE HOSTS	ARTHROPOD TRANSMITTING AGENTS
Typhus fever group	Epidemic typhus fever, epidemic louse-borne typhus, typhus fever (classical type), typhus exanthematicus	*Rickettsia prowazekii*	In colder areas worldwide	Man	Body louse, *Pediculus humanus*
	Brill's disease, a recrudescence of typhus (not a new infection)	*Rickettsia prowazekii*	As typhus	Man	None
	Endemic typhus fever, endemic flea-borne typhus, murine typhus	*Rickettsia typhi* or *Rickettsia mooseri*	Worldwide	Rat, *Rattus rattus, Rattus norvegicus*	Fleas, *Xenopsylla cheopsis*
Spotted fever group	Rocky Mountain spotted fever, New World spotted fever, tick-borne typhus fever	*Rickettsia rickettsii*	(1) Eastern U.S., Southern U.S. (2) Northwestern U.S., (3) Southwestern U.S., Brazil, Columbia	Rodents and other animals, dog, opossum, etc.	(1) Dog tick, *Dermacentor variabilis* (2) Wood tick, *Dermacentor andersoni* (3) Lone Star tick, *Amblyomma americanum*
	Boutonneuse fever, Marseilles fever, Mediterranean fever, African tick fever, Kenya tick fever	*Rickettsia conori*	(4) Mediterranean area (5) South Africa, India, Asia	Rodents and other animals	(4) Dog tick (5) Various other ticks

		Organism	Geographic distribution	Host	Vector
	Queensland tick typhus (Note: this is not Q fever)	*Rickettsia australis*	Australia	Marsupials and rodents	Tick, *Ixodes holocyclus*
	North Asian rickettsiosis, Siberian tick typhus	*Rickettsia siberia*	USSR, Mongolia	Rodents	Ticks of genera *Dermacentor* and *Haemaphysalis*
	Rickettsial pox	*Rickettsia akari*	Cities U.S. and U.S.S.R., Equatorial and South Africa	House mouse, *Mus musculus*	Rodent mite, *Allodermanyssus sanguineus*
Scrub typhus	Scrub typhus, tsutsugamushi, rural typhus, Japanese river fever, mite typhus	*Rickettsia tsutsugamushi* (*Rickettsia orientalis*, *Rickettsia akamushi*)	Japan, Korea, China, South East Asia, Philippines, Indonesia, Australia	Rodents	Larval stage of mites *Leptotrombidium akamushi* or *Trombicula akamushi*, *Leptotrombidium deliensis* or *Trombicula deliensis*
Q fever	Q fever	*Coxiella burneti* (*Rickettsia burneti*)	Worldwide, Western U.S.	Sheep, cattle, goats, birds	Various ticks
Trench fever	Trench fever, five-day fever	*Rickettsia quintana* (*Rickettsia pediculi*)	Europe during World War I and II	Man	Human louse, *Pediculus humanus*

*This table is compiled from numerous sources. No attempt is made to name *all* synonyms of organisms or all rickettsial diseases.

TYPHUS FEVER, FLEA-BORNE (ENDEMIC, MURINE)— United States, 1933-1970

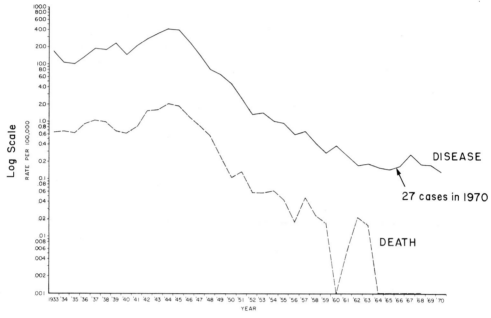

Figure 39–1

Incidence of flea-borne typhus fever. (From Morbidity and Mortality, Annual Supplement, 1970. U.S. Dept. of Health, Education, and Welfare.)

The *Proteus* bacilli and the rickettsias both possess similar antigens, which give rise to antibodies that react with either organism. Thus, *Proteus vulgaris,* the nonspecific organism, contains certain proteins that are also present in certain rickettsial strains, the specific organisms.

Some strains of *Proteus* in the nonmotile or O phase, designated OX-2, OX-19 and OX-K, are especially likely to be agglutinated by sera from persons convalescent from certain of the typhus-like rickettsial diseases (Table 39–2). These tests are useful but, like many biologic tests, not wholly reliable. For example, they are often strongly positive in persons not infected with rickettsias but with strains of *Proteus.*

COMPLEMENT FIXATION REACTION. A more accurate method for diagnosing rickettsial infections is based on the complement fixation

Table 39–2.   Representative Weil-Felix Reactions of Patient's Serum

(ANTIGEN) *Proteus* STRAINS	LOUSE AND FLEA TYPHUS (CLASSIC TYPHUS) (*R. prowazekii*)	TICK TYPHUS (ROCKY MOUNTAIN SPOTTED FEVER, ETC.) (*R. rickettsii*)	MITE TYPHUS (TSUTSUGAMUSHI OR SCRUB TYPHUS) (*R. tsutsugamuski*)
OX–19	++++*	+	–
OX–2	+	+	±
OX–K	–	±	++++

*++++ = strong agglutination in relatively high dilutions of serum; +++, ++, +, and ±, lesser degrees of agglutination; — = no agglutination.

reaction. The antigens used in this test are *specific*, being derived from rickettsias cultivated in the yolk sacs of living embryonated eggs. Similar material is also made into vaccines.

PREVENTION OF TYPHUS FEVER.   For the prevention of louse-borne typhus fever a vaccine is prepared from killed *R. prowazekii* cultivated in embryonated eggs. This has considerable value in modifying the disease but is not an absolute preventive. The use of DDT insecticide to combat lice, along with measures of general cleanliness, was an important factor in helping the United States and British troops win the Italian campaign in World War II.

Flea-borne typhus (murine typhus) is prevented by rat-control measures and also by dusting rat runways and burrows with DDT and other insecticides to kill the fleas on the rats. These measures, practiced by the U.S. Public Health Service in several areas of the United States where murine typhus was formerly rampant, have virtually eliminated the disease from those areas. Fleas remain infectious during their lifetime. The rash caused by the infection is milder and may not occur at all in contrast to the much more severe and extensive distribution of rash in louse-borne typhus.

Rocky Mountain Spotted Fever

This disease, caused by *Rickettsia rickettsii*, is like typhus fever in several respects. The sheep ticks or wood ticks that transmit it occur infected in nature, probably maintaining the disease among rabbits and other rodents by bites. The ticks maintain the rickettsias among themselves by transmission of the infectious agent from males to females and from females to their progeny through the eggs (i.e., transovarially) (Fig. 39–2). In patients with the disease the rash is typically confined to arms and legs but may cover the entire body.

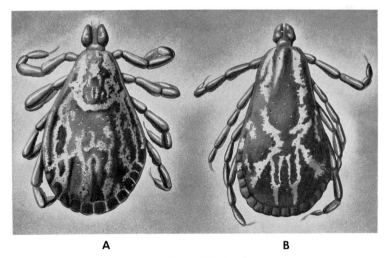

A   **B**

Figure 39–2

Spotted fever ticks. *A, Dermacentor andersoni,* major vector of spotted fever in the West. *B, Dermacentor variabilis,* common eastern dog tick, a vector of spotted fever in the East. (Sharp & Dohme Seminar, Vol. 4, No. 2.)

An effective preventive vaccine is prepared from cultures of the rickettsias grown in chick embryos, in much the same manner as typhus vaccine. Hyperimmune rabbit or goat serum is also available for treatment and is probably of value if given early, but is not much used.

To avoid tick-borne diseases, stay out of woods or meadows where the ticks are known to be present. If forced to go into such areas, wear white clothing, preferably long trousers, and examine the whole body for ticks at three-hour intervals. Do not handle dogs with ticks on them, nor re-move or crush engorged ticks with bare hands. Use insect repellents. Still, 432 cases of Rocky Mountain spotted fever were reported in 1971 in the United States; most of these occurred in the South Atlantic area.

Broad-spectrum antibiotics, like chlortetracycline and chloramphenicol, are very valuable in treatment of rickettsial infections, especially Rocky Mountain spotted and typhus fevers.

Q Fever

This disease, caused by a *Rickettsia* (*Coxiella burneti*,[2] also known as *Rickettsia burneti*), clinically resembles influenza or pneumonitis and in this respect differs from other known rickettsial diseases. Q fever is not one of the typhus-like rickettsioses. The disease was first observed in 1935 by Derrick and by Burnet in Australia. The designation "Q" stands for "Query," since the first observers were puzzled by the nature of the disease. It is true that this disease was discovered first in Queensland, but this did not give it the name Q fever, as is often assumed.

Q fever has since been observed in all continents, and is probably quite widespread, even in areas where it has not yet been recognized. Diagnosis is based primarily on complement fixation tests and secondarily on isolation of the rickettsias, which is readily done by inoculation of animals.

The exact mode of transmission in nature is not entirely clear. Probably there are several modes. Persons working with cattle, goats, and sheep, especially during birth of young animals, as well as in stockyards, abattoirs and dairies, and in contact with infected animal materials seem to be especially likely to contract it. Cattle carry the infection, and the organisms occur in milk. Drinking raw, infectious milk commonly transmits the disease. Person to person transmission is rare.

Many species of ticks, some of which feed on cattle, others on sheep, are known to harbor the rickettsias. Various wild animals also harbor the organisms. Their role as vectors to man has not yet been fully evaluated.

Q FEVER AND PASTEURIZATION. Pasteurization of milk for 30 minutes at 145 F (62.8 C) or for 15 seconds at 161 F (71.7 C) is required to kill the rickettsias. They may survive for weeks in infectious butter.

PREVENTION. The urine in Q fever has been shown to contain the organisms and should be disinfected. In addition, during the febrile stages of the typhus-like fevers the blood is often highly infectious and due care to avoid infection should be taken in drawing samples of blood for any purpose. The best method makes use of disposable needles and plastic syringes, which are subsequently incinerated in the proper manner.

Care should be taken to eliminate arthropods of all kinds, as well as

---

[2]Named for its discoverers, H. R. Cox and F. M. Burnet.

rats, from the premises. In epidemic typhus areas and in Oriental areas where mite typhus occurs this may prove a problem of major difficulty and importance.

A vaccine of killed rickettsias is available for specially exposed workers but may cause severe reactions.

ARTHROPOD-BORNE VIRAL INFECTIONS

Viruses causing diseases in human beings and other vertebrates and that *are transmitted by*, and *multiply* in, sanguivorous arthropods are called arboviruses; *arbo* is an abbreviation of arthropod-borne.

These viruses are generally transmitted among infected birds (herons, sparrows, blackbirds, pheasants, pigeons, and many others) and among horses, monkeys, pigs, and other mammals, and from them to man, by mosquitoes, ticks, and sandflies, the vector and animal reservoir depending on geographical location and kind of virus. At least 300 different arthropod-borne viruses are recognized to cause diseases in man, and the number is growing rapidly.

There are three major groups of arboviruses, differentiated on the basis of antigenic properties and serologic cross-reactions (complement fixation, hemagglutination-inhibition [HI], and so on). Most arboviruses are named for the place of their discovery, the animal principally infected, or the clinical effect. For example, in Group A we find Chickungunya, Semliki Forest, and Eastern and Western equine encephalitis viruses (the last two designated EEE and WEE, respectively); in Group B, dengue fever, yellow fever, St. Louis, West Nile, and Russian spring-summer encephalitis; in Group C, Marituba and Oriboca. There is also California encephalitis, Colorado tick fever, Bunwamyera, the Sandfly fever group (*Phlebotomus* fever) with five different identified viruses, and others. The student need not remember these groupings beyond the fact that they exist and that some have the mosquito as vector, some the sandfly, or the tick, or a yet unknown infective source.

Prevalence of these diseases in man implies: a large reservoir of infected birds or mammals, numerous transmitting arthropods, and fairly close proximity of man to reservoirs and vectors. Transmission by sanguivorous arthropods implies viremia in animals during early stages of infection. Man-to-man transmission by the arthropods can occur, resulting in large epidemics, as of yellow fever.

Yellow Fever

This disease has been known for centuries as a scourge of tropical Africa and tropical America and even in North Atlantic and European shipping ports, where it was introduced in the days of sailing ships, in the summertime, by ships carrying infected tropical mosquitoes. It was introduced to the Western Hemisphere from Africa as early as 1500 by slave traders, probably to Central America. In 1898–1900 it nearly caused the defeat of American troops in Cuba, and along with malaria and dysentery had earlier discouraged the French Government from completing a Panama canal. About 1900, a United States Army Commission under Major Walter Reed demonstrated that the disease is caused by a virus and

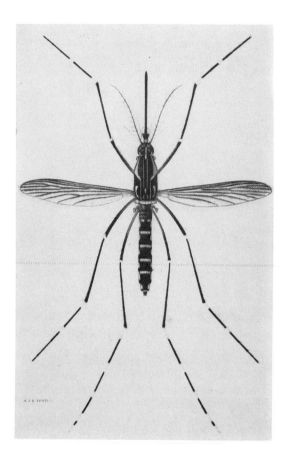

Figure 39–3

Aedes aegypti, the classic urban vector of yellow fever (and some other viral diseases). Note the lyre-shaped markings on the back of the thorax and the silvery bands on the legs. These handsome yellow fever-carrying mosquitoes have been common in the southeastern and U. S. Gulf states, but fortunately there is not (at present!) any virus there for them to transmit. (Smart: Insects of Medical Importance. After Edwards.)

that it is transmitted in populous areas principally by the bite of a mosquito called *Aedes aegypti* (Fig. 39–3), common in tropics and subtropics such as U. S. Gulf states. The virus circulates in the blood during the first four or five days of the initial febrile stage. Mosquitoes can then become infectious if they bite the patient. After about the fifth day the virus is found mainly in the viscera. Here it does extensive damage to the liver, kidneys, and blood vessels, causing jaundice, albuminuria, and hemorrhages into the gastrointestinal tract. Because it damages the viscera it is (for convenience) often spoken of as a viscerotropic virus. The jaundice gives the disease its name. The vomitus, blackened by the blood in the stomach, gives rise to the well known old term "black vomit," so effectively used by Captain Ahab in *Moby Dick*.

VECTORS.   The *Aedes aegypti* mosquito is a household pest, breeding mostly in artificial water deposits such as cisterns, rain gutters, flower vases, and water jars. It is not an extensive outdoor breeder. Control in urban and suburban areas therefore centers mainly around the elimination or covering of these man-made water containers. When such mosquito control has been effective in cities, the disease has disappeared almost entirely.

RECENT OUTBREAKS.   In Africa, only a few sporadic cases of yellow fever were reported in 1970 in contrast to the series of outbreaks which occurred in several African countries in 1969. At that time, a total of 322

Table 39–3. Jungle Yellow Fever—Reported
Numbers of Cases and Deaths in South America,
1969–70*

COUNTRY	1969		1970	
	Cases	*Deaths*	*Cases*	*Deaths*
Bolivia	8	—	2	—
Brazil	4	4	2	—
Colombia	7	7	7	7
Peru	28	24	75	57
Surinam	1	1	—	—
Total	48	36	86	64

*Morbidity and Mortality. 1971, 20:37.

cases and 119 deaths were reported in Ghana, Mali, Nigeria, Togo, and Upper Volta. In 1970, however, 21 cases with 11 deaths were recorded in Cameroon, Equatorial Guinea, Ghana, Nigeria, and Togo.

JUNGLE YELLOW FEVER.   Yellow fever has not disappeared absolutely because, as discovered in 1931, certain jungle-inhabiting mosquitoes (and possibly other arthropods) can also transmit the disease, and certain wild animals (mainly monkeys) can act as an animal reservoir of the virus. Complete suppression of these jungle mosquitoes and monkeys is impossible under present conditions. Yellow fever contracted in the jungle or in farmlands adjacent to forests is called jungle (or sylvatic) yellow fever, but the urban and rural diseases are identical except for vectors. Occasionally the jungle fever is introduced into a town by an infected traveler (or monkey, perchance), and then we may have an outbreak of classic urban yellow fever if the *Aedes aegypti* (or other urban mosquitoes, in Africa) are prevalent in the town. Jungle yellow fever is still present in the Americas as is evident from the data shown in Table 39–3.

Until not long ago it would have been very serious indeed if an infected person or mosquito were introduced into one of the Gulf or other Southern states, since there were plenty of *Aedes* there. The mosquitoes are always under attack. Authorities exert the utmost care to see that airplanes arriving from areas where yellow fever is known to exist contain no mosquitoes and no person in the early (infective for mosquitoes) stages of yellow fever. A mosquito remains infectious for its lifetime (about two months).

YELLOW FEVER VACCINE.   A yellow fever *vaccine* (designated as 17D) is now available, and is one of the best known immunizing agents. A single dose confers a strong immunity of long, probably lifelong, duration. It is prepared in much the same way as influenza vaccine but differs in the following important respects: The entire chick embryo is ground up, filtered, and the fluid constitutes the vaccine. No preservative is added. It is an active-virus vaccine. The 17D virus is yellow fever virus that has been modified or attenuated by cultivation in tissue cultures and by animal passage. Injections of convalescent serum (antibodies) are of no demonstrated value in therapy, though they are effective in prophylaxis. Treatment consists of the administration of tetracyclines, often in combination with sulfonamide; penicillin and chloramphenicol are probably less effective. None is antiviral.

There are two special problems in prevention of yellow fever. The first is that of excluding mosquitoes. The second problem is the febrile blood (first four or five days), which is highly infectious for man, mosquitoes, and personnel of the health team.

ARTHROPOD-BORNE VIRAL ENCEPHALITIDES[3]

Encephalitis is a pathologic term meaning inflammation of the brain. It may be caused by a variety of agents, both physical and chemical, as well as by infectious agents, among which are so-called neurotropic viruses. These include poliomyelitis and rabies (previously discussed). Many of the neurotropic viruses are arboviruses, as noted earlier in this chapter.

Mosquito-Borne Viral Encephalitides

Each disease is caused by a specific virus; these are classified in groups: e.g., group A includes Eastern equine and Western equine encephalitis; group B, Japanese B, St. Louis, Murray Valley; LaCrosse is in the California group. The vectors are mosquitoes like *Culiseta melanura*, several *Aedes* and at least seven *Culex* species.

EASTERN EQUINE ENCEPHALITIS (EEE).   This disease is quite representative of the viral encephalitides. It occurs mainly in the eastern parts of North, Central, and South America, but is not necessarily limited to these areas. Its chief incidence is in the later summer and early fall, partly because it is transmitted by mosquitoes from migratory birds, reservoirs of the virus.

Mortality from this disease, as from any of the viral encephalitides, may run as high as 55 per cent, or even 80 per cent in older people and children. As in other viral encephalitides, onset is sudden, with headache, fever, vomiting, drowsiness, and apathy, and nervous signs and symptoms, including disturbances of reflexes, speech difficulties, rigidities of neck and back muscles, and paralyses. As in polio and many other viral diseases, more inapparent infections than recognized cases occur.

The arthropod vectors of EEE are mosquitoes of the genus *Aedes* (e.g., *A. aegypti*), *Culex*, *Anopheles* (the malaria mosquito), *Culiseta melanura*, and others.

Diagnosis.   This is most reliably done by inoculation of infected arthropods, or of febrile blood from patients, into suckling mice or other susceptible animals, and observing the disease there. Retrospective diagnosis (during convalescence or after recovery) can be made by repeated complement fixation and other serologic tests to observe rise in antibody titer over a period of a week or more.

Control.   Control of the viral encephalitides depends on: control or immunization of the animal hosts, control or avoidance of the arthropod vectors, and use of vaccine, such as the inactivated-virus vaccine for

---

[3]The diseases of the central nervous system due to the so-called neurotropic viruses are collectively spoken of as the *viral encephalitides* or *encephalomyelitides* (inflammations of the brain or of the brain and spinal cord).

Japanese encephalitis, made from the brains of infected mice or from infected embryonated eggs. The efficacy of such vaccines for human protection is still under evaluation.

VENEZUELAN EQUINE ENCEPHALITIS (VEE). This disease is caused by an arbovirus, immunologically distinct from others found in the United States. The recent outbreaks (1972) of equine encephalitis (VEE) in Mexico and Texas resulted in deaths of many horses and of a number of persons.

TICK-BORNE VIRAL ENCEPHALITIDES

These diseases like Russian spring-summer encephalitis, diphasic milk fever or Central European tick-borne encephalitis and others occur in the USSR, in Eastern and Central Europe, the British Isles and in Scandinavia, but the Powassan virus also exists in Canada and in the United States. The ticks *Ixodes persulcatus* and *I. ricinus* transmit the viruses to sheep, deer, birds or rodents and fortunately only rarely to man.

Supplementary Reading

Burrows, W.: Textbook of Microbiology, 19th Ed. 1968, Philadelphia, W. B. Saunders Co.

Davis, B. D., Dulbecco, R., Eisen, H. N., Ginsberg, H. S., and Wood, W. B., Jr.: Microbiology. 1967, New York, Harper & Row (Hoeber Medical Division).

Follow-up on Venezuelan equine encephalitis—Texas. *Morbidity and Mortality*, 1971, *20*:275.

Hahon, N., and Zimmerman, W. D.: Intracellular survival of viral and rickettsial agents at −60° C. *Appl. Microbiol.*, 1969, *17*:775.

Henderson, J. R., Karabatsos, N., Bourke, A. T. C., Wallis, R. C., and Taylor, R. M.: A survey for arthropod-borne viruses in south-central Florida. *Amer. J. Trop. Med. & Hyg.*, 1962, *11*:800.

Human Venezuelan equine encephalitis—Florida. *Morbidity and Mortality*, 1971, *20*:411.

Hunter, G. W., III, Frye, W. W., and Swartzwelder, J. C.: A Manual of Tropical Medicine, 4th Ed. 1966, Philadelphia, W. B. Saunders Co.

Justin, O. J.: The epidemiology of murine typhus in Texas, 1969. *J.A.M.A.*, 1970, *214*:2011.

Klingberg, W., Klingberg, M. A., and Goldwasser, R. A.: Recrudescent typhus. *Scand. J. Infect. Dis.*, 1970, *2*:215.

McDade, J. E.: Determination of antibiotic susceptibility of *Rickettsia* by the plaque assay technique. *Appl. Microbiol.*, 1969, *18*:133.

McDade, J. E., Stakebake, J. R., and Gerone, P. J.: Plaque assay system for several species of *Rickettsia. J. Bacteriol.*, 1969, *99*:910.

Weinberg, E. H., Stakebake, J. R., and Gerone, P. J.: Plaque assay for *Rickettsia rickettsii. J. Bacteriol.*, 1969, *98*:398.

Yellow fever in 1970—Africa and South America. *Morbidity and Mortality*, 1971, *20*:332.

Arthropod-Borne Protozoal and Helminthic Diseases

40

PROTOZOAL DISEASES

Malaria

In the United States malaria as an epidemic or endemic disease has been virtually eliminated. Persons entering the United States from malarious areas reintroduce it, but it does not spread. In 1971 a total of 2375 new cases of malaria were reported in the United States, most of these imported from South East Asia, and the rest from seamen traveling in the tropics (Fig. 40–1). The temporary increase of this disease in the United States also accounted for a few transmissions by blood transfusions. It is typical of our fight against pathogens that every time we think a disease is practically eliminated, we find that our vigilance still cannot be relaxed. Malaria still remains widespread and death-dealing in many areas outside the United States, especially in tropical and subtropical zones around the world. In 1955 its ultimate elimination from this planet became a major concern of many international health agencies such as the World Health Organization and the Pan-American Sanitary Bureau. However, in 1968 the WHO revised its scheme for global malaria eradication, considering it unattainable as long as basic medical services necessary for the detection and treatment of residual malaria remain insufficiently developed in many countries. Prior to the work of the WHO an estimated 1,692 million people were continuously endangered by malaria throughout the world; of these about two-thirds live now in regions entirely free of this disease, and other areas are making progress. Still, malaria will be with us for some time to come.

THE MALARIAL PARASITE. The disease is caused by a protozoan parasite belonging to the class *Sporozoa*. Its life history is quite complicated. It has two stages of development: the asexual stage, called *schizogony*, takes place in the human body; the sexual stage, called *gametogony* and *sporogony*, occurs in the mosquito. This is a good example of the phenomenon called *alternation of generations*. Both man and the mosquito are hosts of the parasite and both are necessary for its life and reproduction.

552

MALARIA — Cases* by Date of Report, United States, 1933-1970

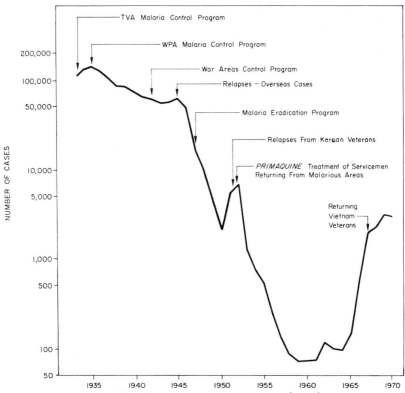

*The reported number differs from the more complete count from the case surveillance system.

Figure 40–1

Incidence of malaria in the United States 1933–1970. (From Morbidity and Mortality, Annual Supplement, 1970. U.S. Dept. of Health, Education, and Welfare.)

Unless it can pass from man to mosquito, and from the latter back again to man, it will die out.

LIFE IN MAN. The mosquito introduces the parasites as *sporozoites* into the blood of its victim with its saliva when it bites (Fig. 40–2). The parasites undergo a period of multiplication (one to five weeks, depending on species) in cells of the liver. This is called the *exoerythrocytic* (or *pre-erythrocytic*) *stage*. The sporozoites have now become *merozoites*. Very soon these enter erythrocytes and grow within them. This stage of the parasite is called the *trophozoite* stage. Each parasite multiplies asexually within its red cell, forming a *schizont* with many small, nucleated segments. Finally the affected red cell breaks up, and the segments escape into the circulating blood. Each segment is a new, active *merozoite* that is released into the plasma and immediately attacks another red blood cell, in order to multiply again. In this way the blood is soon teeming with the parasites (*parasitemia*), and the patient becomes anemic and weakened by the loss of so many red cells and possibly also suffers from poisonous products, especially fever-producing agents (*pyrogens*), formed by the parasites.

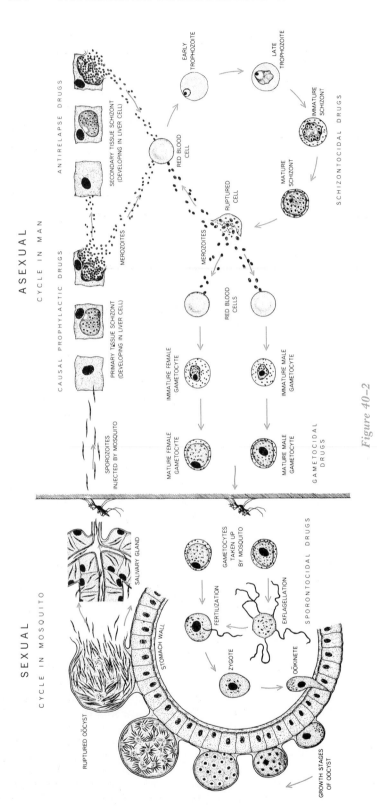

Figure 40-2

Life cycle of *Plasmodium*, the malaria parasite, in mosquito and in man. Various drugs can attack the parasite at different stages as indicated. (From Alvarado and Bruce-Chwatt: *Sci. Amer.*, Vol. *206*.)

The parasites appear in the blood in successive generations, all the individuals of which divide and burst out of the blood cells at about the same time. Each such process causes the chill and fever so characteristic of malaria. A chill means that a fresh crop of parasites has matured and entered the circulation.

After passing through several cycles of asexual development as just described, round, distinctive, male and female gametes begin to appear in the blood of the patient. They are called *gametocytes.* These are larger than the asexual forms and are easily recognized in smears of the blood examined under the microscope. These undergo no further development in the human erythrocytes. They die if not taken up by a mosquito.

LIFE IN THE MOSQUITO. When a female mosquito of the proper genus *(Anopheles)* bites a person who has malarial gametocytes in the blood, she takes these in with the blood she sucks. The gametocytes then become mature sex cells *(gametes),* and the sexual stage begins.

After fertilization of the female gamete by the male gamete in the stomach of the mosquito, the parasites invade the cells lining the mosquito's stomach and multiply there. The parasites undergo further development in a sac in the wall of the mosquito's stomach (an *oocyst*), a stage of development impossible in man but necessary for the continued existence of the parasite. Here the fertilized parasite multiplies by fission. The oocyst ruptures, liberating numerous new, young parasites *(sporozoites).* These, after moving about for some days inside the mosquito, reach the mosquito's salivary glands, and from there are injected into man when the insect bites. The life cycle is thus complete. Because of the necessary period of sexual reproduction of the parasite, a mosquito that has bitten a malaria patient cannot transmit the disease to another person until after ten to 21 days, depending on temperature and species. This period is spoken of as the *extrinsic incubation* period. A mosquito, once infected, remains so for the rest of its life, which may be two months or more.

SPECIES. There are four species of the human malarial parasite. One of the most widely distributed in tropical and temperate zones is called *Plasmodium vivax,* from the vivacious activity of its trophozoite stage. It usually requires about 48 hours to complete its development within the red cells. The chills therefore commonly, but not invariably, occur at intervals of 48 hours (Fig. 40–3), or every third day. This type of malaria is called *tertian (third) fever.*

A second, less common species, called *Plasmodium malariae,* requires about 72 hours for development, and groups of parasites mature about every fourth day. This species causes *quartan (fourth) fever.* Both species commonly cause prolonged infections with relapses unless treated.

Figure 40–3

Malaria fever chart in man during height of infection. (Taken from Encyclopaedia Britannica, 1967 Ed. Vol. 14.)

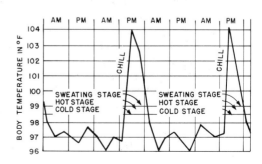

A third form, *Plasmodium falciparum* (the word falciparum is derived from the curved or sickle-shaped [falciform] sexual cells), causes "malignant tertian" or *aestivo-autumnal fever*, and requires from 24 to 48 hours for development. The temperature curve of this fever is irregular, and chills may occur every day or be entirely absent. It is called *aestivo-autumnal* because in temperate climates it frequently occurs in the late summer and fall. It is most prevalent in tropical zones. It is more severe than the other forms of malaria. Most of the fatal cases of malaria are caused by *p. falciparum*. *Plasmodium ovale*, a fourth species resembling *P. vivax*, causes a disease much like tertian malaria but milder.

Excepting acute falciparum malaria, malaria is usually a self-limiting disease. If the infected individual harbors the parasite in the tissues, attacks occur frequently at first, over the years less often, and finally not at all. One can never be sure that this disease is fully overcome; blood transfusions from people who have a history of malaria (however remote) must always be avoided.

Within the last decade, studies of tropical malaria have shown that species of *Plasmodium* formerly thought entirely confined to monkeys (simian malaria) are transmissible to man by various jungle mosquitoes. These are typical zoonoses and are probably much more common in man than previously supposed.

The Mosquito Vector.   There are numerous species of mosquitoes, but only a few carry the parasites of human diseases. All species that transmit malaria parasites of the four human types belong to the genus *Anopheles*. Only the female bites mankind, and she does so only because blood is necessary for egg-laying. One of the most dangerous is *Anopheles gambiae*.

Mosquitoes, like most other two-winged insects *(Diptera)*, pass through four stages of development (Fig. 40–4): the egg, the larva or "wiggler," the pupa, and the fully developed insect (imago). The first three stages develop in water.

The *Anopheles* mosquito may be recognized as she bites. First, she stands in a position like that indicated in Figure 40–4, with her hindlegs raised high in the air. Second, she usually has spots of silver or gray on the wings and often gray bands on the legs. The nonmalaria-bearing varieties are usually brownish or brown-gray and stand as shown in Figure 40–4.

Diagnosis of Malaria.   The laboratory diagnosis of malaria is commonly made by spreading a small drop of the patient's blood on a slide and either examining it in the fresh state or staining it with Wright's stain or any special stain used for blood smears. The parasites can be seen in or upon the blood cells and may have various appearances, depending on species and the stage of their development in the red cells.

Control of Malaria.   As in other arthropod-borne diseases, control is directed primarily against the vector arthropod. The control of mosquitoes in swamps and other breeding places is an engineering problem. Mosquitoes may be kept out of homes and away from sleepers by screens and insect repellents. The use of residual DDT or dieldrin or other residual sprays has been effective, since it kills the infected females in the house. Treatment of infected persons to kill the parasites in their blood is very important. Then the mosquitoes, even though they bite, do not become infected. Drugs now available include chloroquine, pyrimethamine, amodiaquin, and primaquine. Quinine was mainly of historical interest until recent outbreaks of the falciparum form in Southeast Asia, where

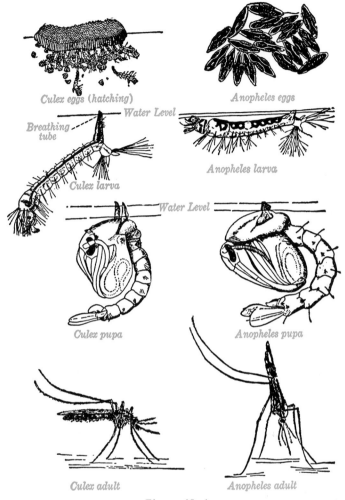

Culex eggs (hatching)

Anopheles eggs

Water Level

Breathing tube

Culex larva

Anopheles larva

Water Level

Culex pupa

Anopheles pupa

Culex adult

Anopheles adult

Figure 40–4

Stages in the life cycle of a common house mosquito of the genus *Culex* at the left and of a malaria mosquito, *Anopheles*, at the right. Note the distinctive biting positions of the adult mosquitoes, *Anopheles* with its hindlegs up in the air. (Courtesy of U.S. Bureau of Entomology.)

treatment with newer drugs was often unsuccessful until quinine was administered together with pyrimethamine. Treatment regimens differ in the different types and stages of malaria. Difficulties arise in control because of the development of strains of *Anopheles* that are resistant to the insecticides, and strains of *Plasmodium* that are resistant to drugs.

PREVENTION. The problem of prevention is primarily concerned with segregating and screening infectious patients to prevent their being bitten by *Anopheles* mosquitoes, and using insecticides and repellents. In addition, prophylactic doses of antimalarial drugs are used in populations heavily infected with the parasites.

The blood of malarious persons can be infectious via improperly sterilized syringes, and certainly through transfusions of freshly drawn blood.

Trypanosomiasis

THE TRYPANOSOMES.   The trypanosomes, of which there are several important species, are flagellate protozoa, some of which inhabit the blood and tissues of man and animals. They are transmitted in various ways. One, *Trypanosoma equiperdum*, is transmitted by sexual contact among horses. This species causes dourine or "equine syphilis." It does not infect man.

Other species, as *Trypanosoma gambiense* and *Trypanosoma rhodesiense*, are transmitted among African domestic and wild animals and to man in the saliva of any of six species of *Glossina*, the sanguivorous tsetse flies. Either the male or female of the tsetse fly may be infected by ingested blood of an infected person or animal. These trypanosomes cause infection of the blood and tissues of man, often producing encephalitis, which results in torpor called African sleeping sickness.

A species of trypanosomes in South and Central America and the southern United States, *Trypanosoma cruzi*, causes an infection of blood and tissues called Chagas' disease, in some respects similar to African sleeping sickness but without the marked brain involvement. The South American trypanosomes are transmitted in the feces of several blood-sucking bugs, often called "barberios" or "kissing bugs,"[1] represented by the species *Panstrongylus megistus*. These bugs are distantly related to the "squash bug" (Fig. 40–5).

DEVELOPMENTAL STAGES.   Trypanosomes generally pass through two or more of a series of developmental stages, some of which, like the malaria parasites, may appear only in the arthropod vector, the others in an animal host. As seen in Figure 40–6, at least four developmental forms are differentiated: leishmanial, the leptomonad, the crithidial, and the adult trypanosome. Progressive elongation, change in position of the parabasal body, and longitudinal development of the flagellum and undulating membrane characterize this cycle. The first two stages do not occur in *T. rhodesiense* and *T. gambiense*.

Adult trypanosomes are wavy, spindle-shaped organisms, with pointed ends, about 20 μm in length (without the flagellum), and an undulant, keel-like membrane extending from tip to tip. A flagellum is attached like an edging along the margin. The flagellum extends free for perhaps 15 μm anteriorly. There are a well-defined nucleus and other functional granules typical of eucaryotic cells (Fig. 40–6).

---

[1] So called because they often bite the lips of sleeping children, giving the appearance of kissing them: a true "kiss of death."

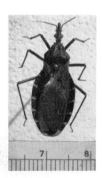

Figure 40–5

Triatoma gerstakeri (♀), from Texas. This formidable bug closely resembles *Panstrongylus megistus* and *Triatoma infestans*, vectors of Chagas' disease (South American trypanosomiasis). The scale is in cm and mm. (Courtesy of Dr. A. Packchanian, The University of Texas Medical Branch at Galveston.)

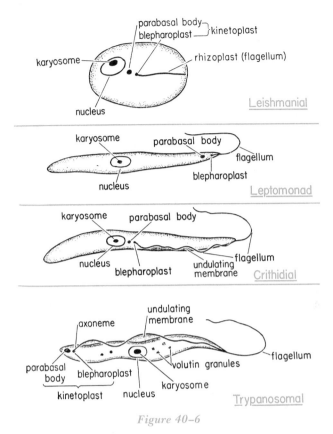

Figure 40–6

Forms of flagellate protozoa related to trypanosomes and to leishmanias. Note that from the first form (leishmanial) to the most highly developed form (trypanosomal) the flagellum becomes longer and more externally placed and that the location of the parabasal body changes rather systematically. Most leishmanias lack the two lower stages. (Hunter, Frye, and Swartzwelder: A Manual of Tropical Medicine, 4th Ed. 1966, Philadelphia, W. B. Saunders Co.)

Figure 40–7

Trypanosoma gambiense in a droplet of blood (the large, round objects are erythrocytes). This is one of the species of trypanosomes causing African trypanosomiasis (African "sleeping sickness"). Note the prominent flagellum along the edge of the wavy, keel-like membrane on each trypanosome (× 1525). (Courtesy of Dr. A. Packchanian, The University of Texas Medical Branch at Galveston.)

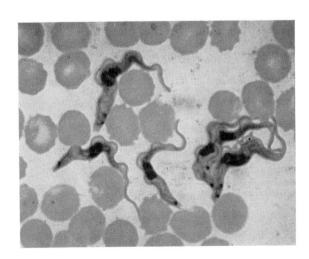

DIAGNOSIS.   Blood-infecting species, such as *Trypanosoma gambiense*, when plentiful in the blood, are easily visible in blood smears stained with Wright's or other polychrome stain. This is one of the principal means of diagnosis (Fig. 40–7). In Chagas' disease, and also in African sleeping sickness, the tissues, such as muscle in the former and lymph nodes in the latter, often contain the parasites. In trypanosomal sleeping sickness the spinal fluid also often contains the trypanosomes, and diagnosis may be made by microscopic examination of the fluid. In Chagas' disease, the trypanosome form is present in the blood for only a short period. The parasites soon enter tissue cells and assume the leishmanial form.

In tsetse flies and in *Triatoma, Panstrongylus*, and other vectors, the trypanosomes undergo a developmental cycle, passing through various phases in which they assume leishmanial form, leptomonad, crithidial or trypaniform shapes.

The Leishmaniases

The organisms causing these diseases are species of protozoa of the genus *Leishmania*, named for William Leishman, discoverer of an important species. These appear to represent a somewhat less highly evolved group than do the trypanosomes. They undergo a similar developmental cycle, but it proceeds only to the leptomonad stage. The leishmanial stage is found in the tissues of animal hosts, the leptomonad stage in arthropods. These protozoa characteristically cause ulcers or sores in which the leishmanias may be demonstrated microscopically and from which they may be transmitted.

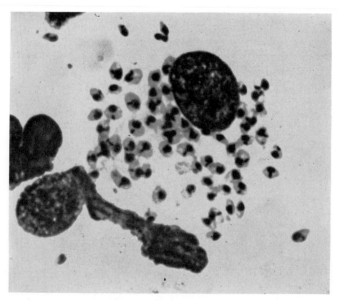

Figure 40–8

Leishmania donovani in stained smear from spleen puncture. Compare with top diagram in Figure 40–6 (× 1000). The large, deeply stained masses are cells of the spleen. (Hunter, Frye, and Swartzwelder: A Manual of Tropical Medicine, 4th Ed. 1966, Philadelphia, W. B. Saunders Co.)

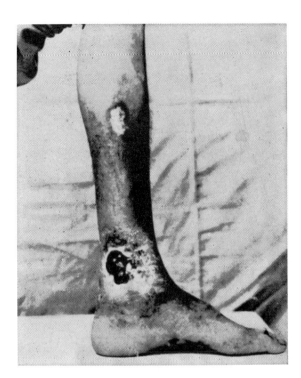

Figure 40–9

Cutaneous leishmaniasis, with ulcer near malleolus, and above, scar from healed ulcer. Metastases from healing ulcer are characteristic. (Culbertson: Medical Parasitology. Columbia University Press.)

KALA-AZAR.   This is caused by *Leishmania donovani*. It occurs in broad areas of Africa, South America, the Orient, India, and the Mediterranean countries, especially in children and in dogs and rodents. The liver, spleen, and bone marrow contain large numbers of the organisms (Fig. 40–8). Skin lesions are not prominent.

Because the parasite invades the internal organs, the disease is also called *visceral leishmaniasis*. Kala-azar is transmitted mainly by the bites of sandflies *(Phlebotomus)*. The organisms appear in nasal secretions and possibly in urine and feces of patients. Transmission may be by these means as well as by sandflies. The disease is often (95 per cent) fatal unless treatment is instituted. Somehow a more resistant parasite is involved in the Mediterranean areas and in the Sudan, than in India.

Prevention.   Since sandflies are the most important vector, they should be eliminated and avoided (screens, repellents, sprays). Care should be exercised in handling articles that have been in contact with any cutaneous lesions and oral and nasal secretions, as well as feces and urine. The usual precautions for bedding and fomites are recommended. Treatment is with antimony compounds. Dogs and cats in endemic zones may harbor the infection and can infect sandflies.

ORIENTAL SORE OR DELHI BOIL.   In the old world this disease is caused by *Leishmania tropica* and is found in India, the Middle East, and parts of Africa. In South and Central America it is caused by *L. brasiliensis* and *L. mexicana*. The lesions are large ulcers that tend to heal with scar formation (Fig. 40–9). Unlike kala-azar, these are entirely cutaneous or in the mucous membranes, and the organisms occur in the superficial ulcers. The disease is therefore often called *cutaneous leishmaniasis*. As in kala-azar, dogs and rodents are susceptible and are sources of infection via

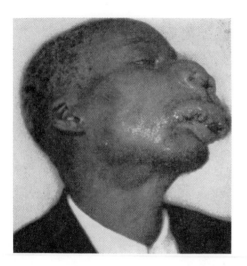

Figure 40–10

Granulomatous lesions in patient suffering from espundia. This lesion requires differentiation from South American blastomycosis. This variety of leishmaniasis is common in negroid populations. (Courtesy of Dr. M. Barretto, São Paulo, Brazil. From Craig and Faust: Clinical Parasitology. Philadelphia, Lea & Febiger.)

bites of sandflies. The organisms in the ulcers may be transmitted by direct contact if the skin is scratched or abraded. Recovery and vaccines immunize.

Prevention. Bandages, dressings, clothing, and bedding contaminated by the sores must be handled carefully and disinfected. As in kala-azar, transmission is mainly by means of sandflies and anti-sandfly measures are indicated. Antimony compounds are effective in treatment.

Espundia. This is also called *American leishmaniasis* and *uta*. It is caused by *Leishmania brasiliensis*, an organism almost indistinguishable from *Leishmania tropica*. The disease is a severe and tissue-destructive (sometimes invasive) form of cutaneous leishmaniasis that involves particularly the tissues of the nasopharyngeal mucosa, nose, and adjacent tissues of the face (Fig. 40–10). The organisms occur in the ulcerous lesions and are present in the discharges from the sores. Unless the patient is treated with antimony, the disease often progresses to a fatal termination. Dogs, cats, and rodents become infected and act as carriers. Sandflies transmit the organisms, but transmission may also occur as in other forms of cutaneous leishmaniasis. Preventive precautions are the same as in other cutaneous leishmaniases.

ARTHROPOD-BORNE HELMINTHS

Filarial Worms

These worms cause the disease *filariasis*, which is found in many tropical and some subtropical areas, depending on the distribution of certain vector arthropods. In some types of filariasis the notorious swellings about the legs and genitalia, called *elephantiasis*, occur. Many infections are subclinical. Several species of filarial parasites are known, *Wuchereria bancrofti, Onchocerca volvulus, Brugia malayi*, and *Loa loa* being especially common. Filarial worms are transmitted among human beings by various biting arthropods: mosquitoes, black flies ("coffee flies"), midges, and so on.

Filariasis. Details concerning the clinical features of the various forms of filariasis and life histories of the parasites differ among the various species, but all follow a generally similar pattern. In an infected person

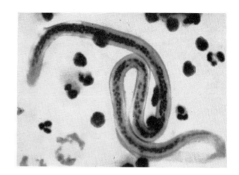

Figure 40–11

Microfilaria of *Wuchereria bancrofti* in a droplet of blood (the dark, rounded objects in the background are blood cells). *W. bancrofti* is one of the worms involved in the production of elephantiasis (× 1140). (Courtesy of Dr. F. Hawking. In *Sci. Amer.*, Vol. *199*.)

the adult male and female worms live in deep tissues, where they reproduce. The female produces the young in the larval stage. The larvae are long and thin (ranging in dimensions around 275 μm by 7 μm), actively motile roundworms and are called *microfilarias* (Fig. 40–11). They move out of the deep tissues and accumulate in the peripheral blood vessels during the hours when the arthropod vector for that particular species of microfilaria bites. They seem to know when the arthropods are to take a blood meal and they make a point of being on the spot to get a free ride![2]

In the arthropod vector they undergo a series of transformations toward maturation and they eventually migrate to the biting parts of the

[2] Of course, no intelligence is involved. The reaction is entirely one of instinct or biochemical response and can be utterly frustrated and even reversed by various experimental procedures.

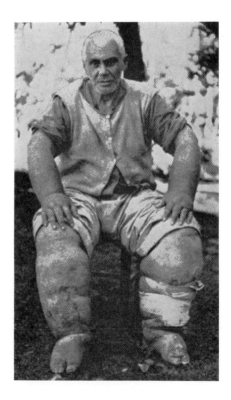

Figure 40–12

Elephantiasis in a patient 63 years of age. Symptoms of swelling were first noted in both legs at the age of 15 years and were seen in both arms at age 33. The patient also had scrotal elephantiasis. (Photograph from William A. Robinson, Papeete, Tahiti, and John F. Kessel, Medical School, University of Southern California. In Culbertson and Cowan: Living Agents of Disease. New York, G. P. Putnam's Sons.)

arthropod. From there they enter the blood of the next person bitten. The microfilarias themselves appear to do little damage. In the human host, however, they undergo further maturation, during which they move about or congregate in masses, causing various painful swellings, the location depending on species. Among these swellings is the notorious but not inevitable condition known as elephantiasis (Fig. 40–12), caused mainly by adults of *Wuchereria bancrofti*, which obstruct lymph channels.

CONTROL. Chemotherapy is used to eliminate the worms from human hosts. Any person contemplating working in the tropics will do well to keep this in mind. Screening and insect repellents are used to prevent reinfection. Unless persons are constantly exposed to the infectious arthropods, the worms eventually die out in the infected person. Elimination of sources of the arthropod vectors involves various problems in applied entomology.

Supplementary Reading

Faust, E. C., Beaver, P. C., and Jung, R. C.: Animal Agents and Vectors of Disease, 3rd Ed. 1968, Philadelphia, Lea & Febiger.

Hawking, F.: Filariasis. *Sci. Amer.*, 1958, *199*:94.

Horsfall, W. R.: Medical Entomology. 1962, New York, The Ronald Press Co.

Hull, T. G. (Editor): Diseases Transmitted from Animals to Man, 5th Ed. 1962, Springfield, Ill., Charles C Thomas.

Kerr, J. A.: Lessons to be learned from failure to eradicate. *Amer. J. Public Health*, 1963, *53*:27.

Soper, F. L.: The epidemiology of a disappearing disease. *Amer. J. Trop. Med. & Hyg.*, 1960, *9*:357.

Williams, L. L., Jr.: Malaria eradication in the United States. *Amer. J. Public Health*, 1963, *53*:17.

*Allied Health Personnel,
Assistants to the Physician*

41

In all areas of health consideration, the professional person has responsibilities for aiding the physician in diagnosis, treatment, and prevention of disease. The responsibilities for these aspects of transmissible diseases are as great as (and in some instances greater than) they are in other pathologic conditions. Many of the general statements made in this chapter refer not only to transmissible diseases but also to other diseases. This summary is necessarily very brief and does not include all the numerous activities of health personnel.

ASSISTING THE PHYSICIAN IN DIAGNOSIS

The Collection of Specimens

It is important for anyone responsible for collecting specimens for diagnostic examination to know the correct methods. Whoever has this responsibility should have an intelligent understanding of the nature and purpose of the procedure.

The value of a specimen depends entirely on the care with which it is taken. Poorly taken specimens waste the laboratory worker's time. Furthermore, it may be impossible to make any diagnosis on such a specimen. Worst of all, a wrong diagnosis may be made.

LABELING. The first consideration about a specimen is the label. Each label should have on it the patient's name, date, the place from which the specimen is taken (e.g., blood, throat, cervix, abscess), the physician's name and the ward or service. If the label is pasted on (undesirable), a rubber band wrapped around it is a necessary additional precaution because the gum often dries and the label drops from the smooth glass surface or flask or tube. Adhesive tape makes very good labels for specimens. Transparent tape over a label provides added protection.

If specimens are taken from a number of patients at the same time, each one must be labeled as soon as it is taken or immediately before it is taken. Finish entirely with one specimen before going on to the next. Do not let the specimen out of the hand until the label is complete. If there is the faintest suspicion that two specimens have been mixed, both must be discarded and a new start made; or both may be tested, and if one is found "positive," both must be retested. A mix-up in throat cultures or syphilis serology tubes could have serious consequences. Petri plates should be labeled on the bottom because the tops may be transposed.

TRANSMISSION TO LABORATORY.   Specimens should be sent to the laboratory at the earliest possible moment. This prevents the specimen from drying and bacteria from dying, makes possible an earlier report, is a convenience to the laboratory worker in planning his work, and may be a matter of life or death to the patient, who after all is the person around whom all these activities are centered.

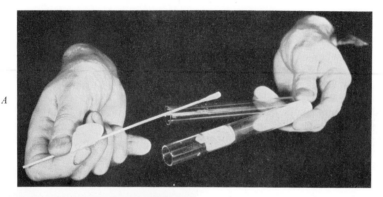

A

Figure 41–1

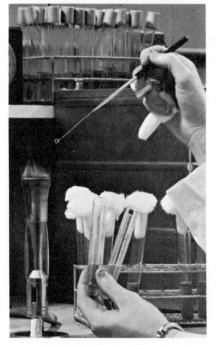

B

A, Method of inoculating a tube of medium by means of a swab. The plugs are held between the fingers in such a way that the ends that go into the tubes do not touch anything. The swab carrying the bacteria (e.g., a throat swab) is inserted into the tube of medium without coming into contact with anything. It is then wiped gently over the surface of the medium, being rotated between finger and thumb so as to bring all surfaces into contact with the medium. It is then put back into its tube in the same careful way before replacing the plugs. The worker in dispensary and community health field is often asked to inoculate tubes. Note that the tube of medium is labeled and is tilted downward to exclude dust. Tubes of fluid medium can be held almost horizontally without spilling.

B, Method of inoculating cultures by means of platinum loop. Note the Bunsen burner for sterilizing the loop and singeing shreds of cotton from the tubes. In making an inoculation, the loop is first heated to redness in the burner. The sterilized loop is cooled. The cotton plugs (or metal or plastic caps) are then withdrawn and held as shown. The loop is dipped into the broth culture (or used to take up a portion of the growth on an agar slant). It is then withdrawn from the tube and the material on the loop is quickly transferred to whatever culture it is desired to inoculate. The plugs or caps are promptly replaced in or on their respective tubes. The platinum loop is then heated to redness in the flame before laying it down. (*B* Courtesy of Rohm & Haas Company, Chemists, Philadelphia, Pa.)

SWABS.   Material for bacteriologic examination is often conveniently collected on *swabs*. These are put in some container (test tubes are very convenient) and the whole sterilized before use (Fig. 41–1). If preparing swabs, use only a small wisp of material, just enough to wrap firmly around about one inch of the end of a moist applicator to make a hard-tipped, slightly rounded, cigar-shaped padding. A "mop" is not needed; it often becomes loosened and comes off in the patient's nose or throat. It absorbs unnecessarily large amounts of fluid and is difficult to use with accuracy in small spaces. Making good swabs is an art. Excellent swabs for all purposes are now commercially available, in convenient sterile packings. Swabs are used for throat cultures, pus, smears from the cervix, eyes, ulcers, and so on. For use in the operating room, culture tubes containing swabs are wrapped so that the outside of the tube is sterile and can be handled by the surgeon at the operating table.

Swabs made of calcium alginate are preferable to cotton for many purposes; they are free from substances like fatty acids that may be inimical to microorganisms. Further, the alginate swab can be dissolved in physiological solution like Locke's with hexametaphosphate, thus releasing the entrapped organisms into the solvent.

Nurses or other health personnel are often required to use the swab to inoculate culture medium. This may be broth, or it may be agar medium slanted in a tube, or flat in a Petri plate. In inoculating agar, the tip of the swab, after it has touched the desired lesion or infected place, is passed back and forth over the surface of the solid medium with gentle pressure, making a series of numerous, closely spaced zigzag paths on the surface. The important point in taking a swab culture is to touch the swab only on the spot from which the culture is desired, and nowhere else, and to send it immediately to the laboratory or use it right away to inoculate media.

THROAT CULTURES.   These should be taken only with a clear view of the throat, in a good light, and using a tongue depressor. A swab is used. Material to be examined for diphtheria bacilli should be taken directly from the tonsil, or from any white or inflammed spots in the throat. The same is true of cultures for scarlet fever or other infections of the throat.

Figure 41–2

Method of taking a culture from the nasopharynx by means of a special swab: *W*, Flexible wire holder of swab (S); *P*, soft palate; *D*, tongue depressor. Sometimes a swab is passed back through the nostril as shown at *X*.

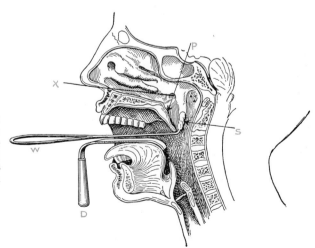

Cultures from the nasopharynx are made particularly for meningococci, sometimes by means of a special instrument (Fig. 41–2). Meningococci, when present, are often located high up behind the soft palate. An ordinary swab may be used by passing it back gently through the nostril (X, Fig. 41–2). The swab should be cultured and the culture incubated immediately because meningococci are very fragile and die quickly outside the body.

Although pharyngeal swabs often yield positive cultures in whooping cough, it is sometimes also advantageous to make "cough plates." These have been mentioned previously in connection with whooping cough but are equally applicable in other upper respiratory tract infections. A Petri plate containing medium suitable for the growth of the organism desired is held before the mouth of the patient when he coughs. The spray of sputum raised by the coughing inoculates the medium. The plate is immediately covered and placed in the incubator in an inverted position. Use of the cough plate with infants is often impracticable because of the difficulty of eliciting a productive cough.

SPUTUM.   If the examination is to be of value, the specimen must be obtained in the proper way. The sputum collected by patients in the ordinary sputum cup consists to a large extent of material from the mouth and throat, mucus, saliva, and bits of food. To collect a sputum specimen correctly, a sterile container should be obtained from the laboratory. If the patient is able, he should brush his teeth and rinse the mouth thoroughly with water. Sputum may be collected in wide-mouthed ointment jars of 1 to 2 oz capacity, or in other suitable water-tight containers with tight covers. The sputum should be collected directly after a cough that brings secretions up from the lungs (not just from the throat) and the specimen should be sent immediately to the laboratory. Sputum is obtained from infants by swabbing the throat, or better, by gastric lavage, as infants usually swallow their sputum.

URINE.   Except in cases of acute cystitis with obvious massive bacteriuria, specimens of urine for *bacteriologic* examination are of value only when they are collected with extreme care. There are innumerable bacteria on the skin and mucous membrane of the genitalia, and unless the mouth of the urethra is cleansed thoroughly, the culture is sure to be contaminated. The first part of the urine is allowed to run off, in order to wash out any bacteria that may be present in the urethra, and 20 ml of the middle and last portions are collected in separate sterile containers. A frank cystitis is usually evidenced by the large numbers of bacteria (over 100,000 per ml) in the urine. Contamination may originate from vaginal or prostatic discharges or other internal lesions. Specimens for *chemical* and other *microscopic* examination need not be sterile.

Specimens from the kidneys are collected by catheterization of the ureters, which is a surgical procedure. A very important point about specimens from the kidneys is to be absolutely sure that the tubes from the right and left kidneys are correctly designated. A mistake may prove fatal for the patient and disastrous for doctor and nurse.

FECES.   Laboratory examination of the feces for living organisms is undertaken most often for pathogenic Enterobacteriaceae, cholera vibrios, and so on, or for the eggs of animal parasites like hookworms or tapeworms, or for protozoal cysts. Stools for bacteriologic examination should be fresh. If blood or pus is present, it should be selected for the culture. A sterile tongue blade, knife, or spoon may be used to transfer a portion of stool about the size of a walnut to the desired container. If the stool is liquid, about a teaspoonful is sufficient. Fifty milliliter plastic sputum containers with screw covers are used by many hospitals, physicians, and community health agencies.

Carriers of pathogenic Enterobacteriaceae are found by making cultures from the feces. The finding of typhoid and dysentery bacilli in the stools or urine of carriers is often difficult, since the organisms may be absent at times, and are usually present in comparatively small numbers. Many health departments provide a special outfit for stool cultures from suspected typhoid cases or carriers. This may contain a solution of bile and an aniline dye, e.g., brilliant green. The solution is tubed in 5 ml amounts and sealed with a rubber stopper. To regulate the amount of feces added, a sterile swab is sent with each tube. The bile and brilliant green are favorable to the growth of the typhoid bacillus and unfavorable to other bacteria so that in some cases the bacilli may be found after the tube has been in transit for two, three, and even four days. A solution of 30 per cent glycerin in normal salt solution is often used as a preservative for stool specimens during shipment to the laboratory. It is not very effective. Other preservative solutions, such as mixtures of sodium citrate and sodium desoxycholate, are more valuable. The important point is not to use too much specimen in proportion to the volume of preservative solution. A ratio of 1:5 is about right. "Preservative" solutions leave much to be desired. It is better to rush the specimen to the laboratory and culture it immediately. The stools from patients suspected of having bacillary dysentery should be cultured as soon after evacuation as possible. Dysentery bacilli die out very rapidly in feces.

BLOOD CULTURES.   Bacteria are present in the circulating blood in septicemia associated with various diseases. Streptococci may be found during the severe stages of any streptococcal disease (Fig. 41–3). Pneumococci often enter the blood in pneumonia. In typhoid fever, typhoid bacilli are always present in the blood in the early stage of the disease. Septicemia

Figure 41–3

Petri plate with blood culture from patient with severe septicemia due to beta hemolytic streptococci (³⁄₄ life size). The use of an agar pour plate for a measured blood culture gives some idea of the number of organisms per ml of blood, thus furnishing a guide to prognosis and treatment, as well as permitting prompt isolation of the organism if tests for sensitivity to various antibiotics are desired. A broth blood culture permits the use of a larger blood sample and is therefore a more sensitive diagnostic procedure but is not quantitative. (Preparation by Dr. Elaine L. Updyke. Photo courtesy of U.S. Public Health Service, Communicable Disease Center, Atlanta, Ga.)

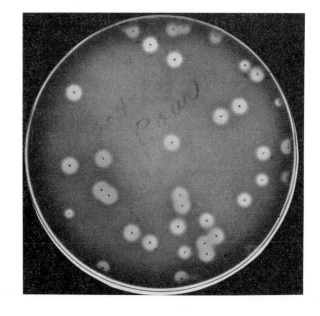

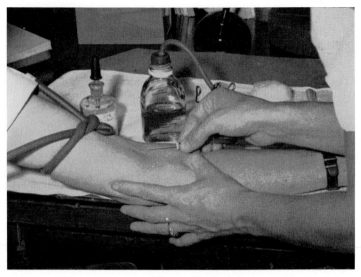

Figure 41–4

Method of taking blood for culture. A tourniquet consisting of plastic tubing is tightened moder-ately about the patient's upper arm. It is important that before introducing the needle the skin around the site of the puncture be well cleansed with alcohol and wiped with a disinfectant, such as very weak iodine solution. A sterile needle is inserted into a convenient vein in the bend of the elbow. The blood may be drawn into any sterile receptacle, such as a syringe, for transfer immedi-ately to culture media. In this picture the needle is attached, by means of a previously prepared sterile rubber tube, to a bottle with a diaphragm-type rubber stopper and containing culture me-dium. The tube is clamped shut until the needle enters the vein. A sterile needle attached to the distal end of the tube pierces the rubber bottle cap; vacuum of the specially prepared bottle draws in the blood. After the proper quantity of blood is drawn, the tourniquet is released, the tube is pinched shut and the distal needle is withdrawn from the culture flask. Immediately afterward, the needle is withdrawn from the arm. Drops of blood remaining in the tube and needle may be used to make blood cell counts, smears for microscopic examination, and so on. A pledget of sterile cotton is pressed against the puncture in the skin till bleeding stops. Note the clamp for closing the tube, the sterile towel, and bottle of disinfectant. (Courtesy of U.S. Public Health Service, Communi-cable Disease Center, Atlanta, Ga.)

of any sort is always a serious condition. The diagnosis is made by cultivat-ing the bacteria in the blood, usually taken from one of the large veins of the arm.

The skin over the vein is prepared by painting with alcoholic solution of iodine (1 per cent) or other approved disinfectant. Excess iodine is removed in a minute or two with a bit of sterile gauze moistened with ethyl alcohol (70 per cent). This procedure is followed whenever the skin is to be punctured and is of great importance in obtaining the blood uncontaminated with staphylococci from the skin, and avoiding infection of the patient.

A bandage or short length of flexible tubing is wound snugly around the upper arm in order to make the veins stand out prominently (Figs. 41–4, 41–5). The pressure should be sufficient to close the veins but not the arteries. About 10 ml of blood is removed with a syringe or by other methods. The site for puncture should be located by palpation *before* applying the disinfectant, or by means of a sterile-gloved finger *after* disinfection.

A vacuum tube (Fig. 41–6), of which there are many modifications, is

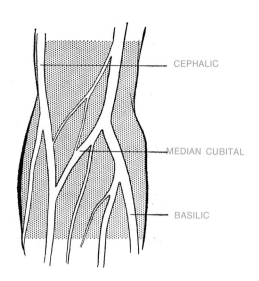

Figure 41–5

Location of the principal veins at the elbow suitable for drawing blood samples and for intravenous therapy. (U.S. Civil Defense Administration, Instructor's Guide, 1G-11-1: Venipuncture and Intravenous Procedures. Washington, D.C.)

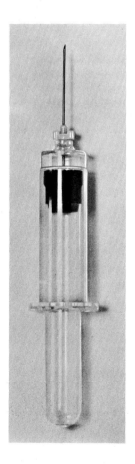

Figure 41–6

The B-D Vacutainer, a disposable, combined blood-letting syringe and collecting tube. It is manipulated like a syringe and yet cannot inject, since the vacuum already exists in the collecting tube. The rubber-diaphragm closure of the vacuum tube is pierced by forcing the butt of the needle through it after the point has entered the vein. (Becton, Dickinson & Co., Rutherford, N.J.)

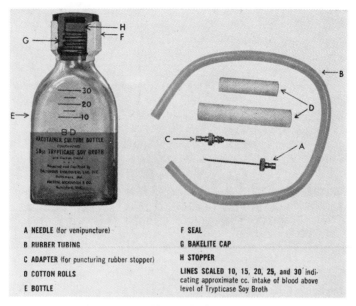

Figure 41–7

The B-D Vacutainer Culture Bottle. (Becton, Dickinson & Co., Rutherford, N.J.)

often used instead of a syringe for withdrawing blood. Good examples of modern blood-culture equipment are shown in Figures 41–7 and 41–8.

TRYPTICASE SOY BROTH[1] IN B-D VACUTAINER CULTURE BOTTLES. Trypticase soy broth has been tested for its ability to support early and rapid growth of most bacteria likely to be encountered in blood infections. Furthermore, since many pathogens prefer an atmosphere with increased carbon dioxide, the space in the culture bottle contains air with about 10 per cent CO_2. Because blood contains natural antibacterial substances the volume used for the inoculum should not be too large—about one tenth the volume of culture fluid, which may be broth or melted agar medium for plating.

The bacteriologist may bring his culture tubes to the bedside and inoculate them on the spot, before the blood has clotted. If the blood must be carried some distance to the laboratory before it can be inoculated, it is

---

[1]Originated by the Baltimore Biological Laboratory, Inc., now BBL, a division of Bio-Quest.

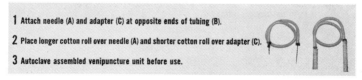

Figure 41–8

How to assemble venipuncture unit. In the physician's unit the venipuncture unit is supplied completely assembled and sterilized. (Becton, Dickinson & Co., Rutherford, N.J.)

drawn into a sterile solution of sodium citrate, which prevents it from clotting. If the blood is being collected for chemical examination only, sodium oxalate is often used to prevent clotting.

BLOOD FOR SEROLOGIC TEST.   This may be obtained in the same way as for a blood culture. It is generally withdrawn with a sterile syringe instead of a vacuum tube. If a syringe is to be used, blood may be drawn at the one puncture for culture, serology, and microscopic examination. After withdrawing the blood from the vein, the blood for serology is put into a clean, dry test tube. The tube containing this blood should be set upright and not moved until the blood has clotted. Health departments furnish outfits consisting of a sterile closed test tube and a sterile needle for collecting serum.

In infants, blood for various tests may be taken from the longitudinal sinus, a great vein that lies immediately under the anterior fontanel. The blood is withdrawn in a syringe after shaving and cleansing the skin.

For some serologic tests, blood grouping and leucocyte counts, only a few drops of blood are needed. Unless these are taken from the syringe when blood is drawn for a serologic test or blood culture, it is necessary to puncture the finger or the lobe of the ear. The latter has the advantage that the patient cannot watch the procedure. The ball of the index or middle finger is generally used. Before the puncture, the finger or ear should be wiped with cotton moistened in alcohol. The needle used for making the puncture must be sterile. An excellent type of device is the small, sterile, individually packaged, disposable lancet available under the name of "Hemolet." Previously, more elaborate instruments, with a hidden needle activated by a spring and trigger, were used. Such needles have sometimes been very effective vectors of syphilis, various bacterial infections, homologous serum hepatitis, and other conditions when not properly heat-sterilized.

Blood for films to be examined microscopically is taken from the finger or ear, and spread in a thin uniform layer on an absolutely clean slide. The slides are prepared by washing with detergent and water, rinsing, then washing with alcohol, and drying with gauze.

It is possible to make good films of blood as shown in Figure 41–9. It is also common to make these smears on glass coverslips. A drop of blood is placed on a clean glass coverslip and covered by a second clean coverslip at an angle so that all four corners of the two coverslips protrude on all sides. The two coverslips are separated by moving them sideways as quickly as possible, and each provides a slide that can be examined microscopically.

FLUID FROM THE PERITONEAL AND PLEURAL CAVITIES.   This is either withdrawn in a syringe or allowed to run from the puncture needle

Figure 41–9

Glass slides arranged for making a film of blood for microscopic examination. A small drop of blood is first placed on the horizontal slide under the small arrow. The edge of the tilted slide is then drawn from the left into contact with the drop and the blood spreads across the slide in the angle. We are looking at the slides edgewise. The arrow shows how to move the tilted slide after the blood touches it.

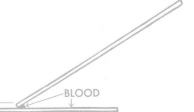

BLOOD

directly into sterile test tubes or centrifuge tubes. The site of the needle puncture must be carefully disinfected before insertion and protected with sterile gauze after the needle is withdrawn. If tuberculosis is suspected, some of the fluid may be inoculated intraperitoneally into a guinea pig or onto suitable culture medium, or both. It is advisable also to examine a stained smear. These specimens are usually taken by the physician, but assisting personnel often prepare the sterile needles and flasks and are responsible for proper labeling and getting the specimen promptly to the laboratory.

CEREBROSPINAL FLUID.   This is examined for the diagnosis of the different kinds of meningitis, for acute poliomyelitis, and for syphilis of the nervous system. The fluid is obtained by *lumbar puncture* and is allowed to run from the needle directly into sterile test tubes or centrifuge tubes. The puncture is always made by a physician. The site should be carefully disinfected beforehand and covered with sterile gauze after the needle is withdrawn.

In acute meningitis caused by the meningococcus, pneumococcus, streptococcus, or other organisms, the appearance of the fluid may range from slightly cloudy to very turbid with leucocytes, or bacteria, or both. Smears and cultures are made to determine what bacteria and cells are present. The tube containing such fluid must be kept warm, and the culture should be made as soon as possible (within a few minutes) after the puncture. In most such cases diagnosis is attempted on the basis of a gram- or Ziehl-Neelsen-stained smear of sediment from the centrifuged specimen. In acute meningitis cultural methods are usually too slow to be of immediate value for instituting therapy.

In a clear or cloudy fluid the number of white cells is counted, using the same technique as in counting leucocytes in the blood. A differential count is made from a smear of the sediment. The amounts of albumin and globulin are determined chemically. Both the number of cells and the amount of protein may be much increased although the fluid remains clear. This is of special value in differentiating paresis from other forms of neurosyphilis.

Cultures are not made on fluids from suspected cases of syphilis, but a serologic test is carried out.

Reporting the Results of Laboratory Tests

As soon as the results of laboratory tests are received, the nurse or other appropriate personnel (if the patient is in a hospital), should read them and note any discrepancies from the normal range of the particular tests. Most reports contain a listing of general standards of test values; this permits the person receiving the report to evaluate the patient's deviation from the normal range. A nurse or other assistant is, of course, expected to know, even without these charts, what constitutes expected values in healthy individuals. Because the doctor usually visits patients in a hospital only once or twice a day, the attendant persons are responsible for keeping the doctor informed of unusual events that may occur between visits. The nurse or other assistant must be able to identify these unusual events. The doctor also expects that they will not call him unnecessarily and will know when a call is indicated. Reports of laboratory tests that show abnormal findings frequently provide the clues necessary for better diagnosis and immediate therapy for the patient. Failure to transmit this information to the physician may delay essential treatment, which may delay or in other ways influence the recovery of the patient. The student will rarely be held responsible for exercising the judgment necessary in determining when the physician is to be notified about abnormalities found in the reports from the laboratory, but this responsibility will be expected after graduation. It is essential, therefore, that during training the knowledge necessary for making such decisions be acquired.

ASSISTING THE PHYSICIAN IN TREATMENT

Part of the responsibility of every nurse or assistant is to carry out the orders that the physician gives for treatments and medications. Although it is important to give all medications on time, it is imperative when the substances to be given are antibiotics or chemotherapeutic drugs. As has been explained in Chapter 14, drug-fastness and antibiotic-resistant microorganisms may develop from too low a blood level of these therapeutic agents. Current problems with the highly resistant *Staphylococcus aureus* may have resulted from insufficient use of an antibiotic in an infection, its indiscriminate or ineffective use, or from failure to give it on time, thus reducing the blood level to a point where the more resistant individuals of that particular group of staphylococci could survive and multiply. If untoward symptoms seem to result from any treatment or medication, the nurse or assistant should report this to the physician as soon as possible.

ASSISTING IN THE PREVENTION
OF TRANSMISSIBLE DISEASES

The responsibilities of the health team in the prevention of transmissible diseases fall into two categories: inhibition, destruction, and removal of pathogenic microorganisms; and assisting with programs that increase the immunity of a population. In the earlier parts of this book,

Figure 41–10

Hypospray jet injector. It is used for subcutaneous, intramuscular and intradermal injections without a needle. (Courtesy The Texas State Department of Health.)

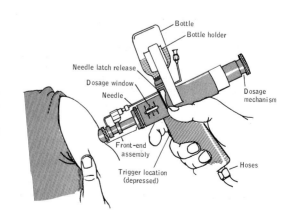

Table 41–1.   Body Fluids and Discharges Commonly Carrying Pathogenic Organisms, and Important Fomites Likely to Be Infectious

BODY FLUIDS AND DISCHARGES COMMONLY CARRYING PATHOGENIC ORGANISMS	ARTICLES IN CONTACT WITH PATIENT TO WHICH HEALTH WORKERS SHOULD GIVE SPECIAL ATTENTION
Feces and Urine: Salmonellosis Dysentery (feces only) Cholera Undulant fever Infectious (epidemic) hepatitis Leptospirosis (urine only) Anterior poliomyelitis (feces) Hookworm and some other helminthic diseases	Bed linen, clothing, eating utensils, bed pans; anything likely to be contaminated by feces or urine. **The health worker's hands.**
Sputum, Nose and Throat Discharges: Pneumonia (due to any organism) Diphtheria Scarlet fever Septic or any other form of infectious sore throat Whooping cough Epidemic meningitis Syphilis (with open lesions of mouth or respiratory tract) Colds, influenza, etc. Anterior poliomyelitis Measles; chickenpox; mumps Certain mold and yeast infections, such as thrush Smallpox Tuberculosis	Bed linen, clothing, handkerchiefs, towels, washcloths, toothbrushes, eating utensils, books, toys, pencils, dust from patient's room, sputum boxes or bottles, thermometers, tongue depressors, throat swabs; drinking fountains, medicine spoons, spray from coughing, sneezing, and talking; the health worker's mask, gown, shoes, gloves, apron, etc. **The health worker's hands.**

the values and applications of prophylactic vaccinations have been discussed in detail. One very useful device for injections of large numbers of people (e.g., in the army) has been used very successfully; it is illustrated in Figure 41–10. Theoretically, it would be possible to prevent outbreaks of transmissible diseases if the first case in a given community could be immediately recognized and completely isolated from all other people, and if all the pathogens that leave the body of the patient were completely destroyed. Obviously this is not feasible because the early symptoms of many transmissible diseases are not easily recognizable, unknown carriers for many diseases are present in the population, and not all of the methods of transfer for each disease are known or can be controlled at the present time. Nonetheless, health personnel should exert every effort to isolate patients who have transmissible diseases, particularly from any segment of the population known to have high susceptibility or high risk of complications.

Members of the health team are key figures in the control and destruction of microorganisms as they leave the body. The information on body fluids and discharges is summarized in Table 41–1. The articles

Table 41–1.   Body Fluids and Discharges Commonly Carrying Pathogenic Organisms, and Important Fomites Likely to Be Infectious (*Continued*)

BODY FLUIDS AND DISCHARGES COMMONLY CARRYING PATHOGENIC ORGANISMS	ARTICLES IN CONTACT WITH PATIENT TO WHICH HEALTH WORKERS SHOULD GIVE SPECIAL ATTENTION
Pus or Exudate from Local Lesion: Gonorrhea Syphilis Ulcers or abscesses of any kind "Pink-eye" Erysipelas Tuberculosis Blastomycosis "Trench mouth" (Vincent's angina) Any infection of eye, ear, nose, or genitalia Smallpox Plague Tularemia Undulant fever Staphylococcal and streptococcal infections	Bandages and dressings, swabs, clothing, bed linen, towels, washcloths; if the lesions are in the mouth, watch especially eating utensils, books, pencils, toys, and other articles mentioned above; toilet seats, wash water. **The health worker's hands.**
Blood: Typhoid fever (first week only) Undulant fever Malaria Leptospirosis Syphilis (not common) Generalized streptococcal and pneumococcal infections associated with "blood poisoning," scarlet fever, pneumonia and related diseases. Generalized staphylococcal infections Epidemic meningitis (early stages) Pneumonia Arthropod-borne viral diseases (early stages) Arthropod-borne bacterial diseases Rickettsial infections (early stages) Homologous serum hepatitis Infectious (epidemic) hepatitis	Any instrument used in taking blood, syringes, needles, gauze or cotton used to absorb blood; sheets or clothing or wash water contaminated with blood; obstetric instruments, dressings, etc. Arthropod vectors of the disease in question in arthropod-borne diseases. **The health worker's hands.**

designated in the right hand column of Table 41–1 should be thoroughly disinfected or sterilized by the procedures most effective for the causative organism and most feasible for the article that is likely to be contaminated.

Supplementary Reading

Bailey, W. R., and Scott, E. G.: Diagnostic Microbiology, 3rd Ed. 1970, St. Louis, The C. V. Mosby Company.

Benenson, A. S. (Editor): The Control of Communicable Disease in Man, 11th Ed. 1970, New York, The American Public Health Association.

Du Gas, R. W.: Introduction to Patient Care, 2nd Ed. 1972, Philadelphia, W. B. Saunders Co.

French, R. M.: Nurses Guide to Diagnostic Procedures, 2nd Ed. 1967, New York, McGraw-Hill Book Co., Inc.

Fuerst, E. V., and Wolff, L.: Fundamentals of Nursing, 4th Ed. 1969, Philadelphia, J. B. Lippincott Co.

Hopps, H. C.: Principles of Pathology, 2nd Ed. 1964, New York, Appleton-Century-Crofts, Inc.

Isenberg, H. D., and Berkman, J. I.: Microbial diagnosis in a general hospital. *Ann. N.Y. Acad. Sci.*, 1962, *98* (Art. 3):647.

Lepper, M. H.: Collection of Specimens. *In*: Manual of Clinical Microbiology (Blair, J. E., Lennette, E. H., and Truant, J. P., Editors). 1970, Bethesda, Md., American Society for Microbiology.

Simon, H. J.: Saprophytes in infection and the laboratory bedside interaction. *Ann. N.Y. Acad. Sci.*, 1962, *98* (Art. 3):745.

APPENDIX

A Proposed New Classification and Nomenclature of Bacteria for Bergey's Manual of Determinative Bacteriology*

PROCARYOTES

DIVISION I. THE CYANOBACTERIA†
DIVISION II. THE BACTERIA

PART 1.   PHOTOTROPHIC BACTERIA
   ORDER   I. RHODOSPIRILLALES
      FAMILY   I. RHODOSPIRILLACEAE
        Genus   I. *Rhodospirillum*
        Genus   II. *Rhodopseudomonas*
        Genus   III. *Rhodomicrobium*
      FAMILY II. CHROMATIACEAE
        Genus   I. *Chromatium*
        Genus   II. *Thiocystis*
        Genus   III. *Thiosarcina*
        Genus   IV. *Thiospirillum*
        Genus   V. *Thiocapsa*
        Genus   VI. *Lamprocystis*
        Genus   VII. *Thiodictyon*
        Genus VIII. *Thiopedia*
        Genus   IX. *Amoebobacter*
        Genus   X. *Ectothiorhodospira*
      FAMILY III. CHLOROBIACEAE
        Genus   I. *Chlorobium*
        Genus   II. *Prosthecochloris*
        Genus   III. *Chloropseudomonas*
        Genus   IV. *Pelodictyon*
        Genus   V. *Clathrochloris*

PART 2.   GLIDING BACTERIA
   ORDER   I. MYXOBACTERALES
      FAMILY   I. MYXOCOCCACEAE
        Genus   I. *Myxococcus*
      FAMILY II. ARCHANGIACEAE
        Genus   I. *Archangium*
      FAMILY III. CYSTOBACTERACEAE
        Genus   I. *Cystobacter*
        Genus   II. *Melittangium*
        Genus   III. *Stigmatella*
      FAMILY IV. POLYANGIACEAE
        Genus   I. *Polyangium*

---

*This material constitutes Chapter 6 of the forthcoming eighth edition of *Bergey's Manual of Determinative Bacteriology*. The Williams & Wilkins Co., Baltimore (in press). Although this was the arrangement of material as this edition went to press, it may not be the final form in Bergey's eighth edition.

†Blue-green algae; also sometimes called Schizophyceae, Cyanophyceae or Myxophyceae.

PART 19. THE MYCOPLASMAS

CLASS I. MOLLICUTES

ORDER   I. MYCOPLASMATALES

FAMILY   I. MYCOPLASMATACEAE

Genus   I. Mycoplasma

FAMILY II. ACHOLEPLASMATACEAE

Genus   I. Acholeplasma

GENUS OF UNCERTAIN AFFILIATION

Genus   Thermoplasma

MYCOPLASMA-LIKE BODIES IN PLANTS

Classification
of Representative Viruses[1]

B

PHYLUM VIRA......

SUBPHYLUM: RIBOVIRA (GENETIC MATERIAL—RNA)
CLASS: RIBOCUBICA
ORDER: GYMNOVIRALES

FAMILY (-VIRIDAE)	SUBFAMILIES (-VIRINAE)	GENUS	TYPE SPECIES[2]	COMMON NAME
Napoviridae . .	A. Napovirinae (nominative subfamily)	Napovirus (type genus).	flavicans.	Turnip yellow mosaic.
	B. Picornavirinae	1. Picornavirus (type genus).	aphthae.	Foot and mouth disease.
		2. Poliovirus.	primus.	Polio 1.
		3. Coxsackievirus.	(A) primus.	Coxsackie A1.
		4. Echovirus.	(hominis) primus.	ECHO 1.
		5. Rhinovirus.	(hominis) primus.	Rhinovirus 1.
		6. Cardiovirus.	ratti.	EMC.
	C. Androphagovirinae	Androphagovirus (type genus).	bacteri.	RNA phage.
Reoviridae . .		1. Reovirus (type genus).	(mammalis) primus (type genus).	Reovirus 1.
		2. Neovirus.	neoformans.	Wound tumor virus.

CLASS: RIBOCUBICA.
ORDER: TOGAVIRALES.

FAMILY (-VIRIDAE)	GENUS	TYPE SPECIES[2]	COMMON NAME
Arboviridae	Arbovirus (type genus).	occidentalis (type genus)	WEE.

SUBPHYLUM: RIBOVIRA (GENETIC MATERIAL—RNA)

CLASS: RIBOHELICA

FAMILY (-VIRIDAE)	GENUS (-VIRUS)	TYPE SPECIES[2]	COMMON NAME
Dolichoviridae	Dolichovirus (type genus).	brassicae.	Cabbage mosaic.
Protoviridae	Protovirus (type genus).	tabaci.	Tobacco mosaic.
Pachyviridae	Pachyvirus (type genus).	crotalum.	Rattle mosaic.
Leptoviridae	Leptovirus (type genus).	solanum.	Potato X.
Mesoviridae	Mesovirus (type genus).	pisum.	Pea mosaic.
Adroviridae	Adrovirus (type genus).	trifolii.	White clover mosaic.
Myxoviridae	1. Myxovirus (type genus).	(influenzae) A.	Influenza A.
	2. Rabiesvirus.	canis.	Rabies.
	3. Sigmavirus.	drosophilae.	Virus of L'Héritier.
Paramyxoviridae	1. Paramyxovirus (type genus).	(parainfluenzae) primus.	Myxovirus parainfluenzae 1.
	2. Bronchovirus.	syncytialis.	Respiratory syncytial.
Stomatoviridae	Stomatovirus (type genus).	bovis.	Vesicular stomatitis.

SUBPHYLUM: DEOXYVIRA (GENETIC MATERIAL—DNA)

CLASSES: DEOXYHELICA, DEOXYCUBICA, DEOXYBINALA

FAMILY (-VIRIDAE)	GENUS (-VIRUS)	TYPE SPECIES[2]	COMMON NAME
Poxviridae	1. Poxvirus (type genus).	variolae.	Variola.
	2. Dermovirus.	orfi.	Contagious pustular dermatitis.
	3. Pustulovirus.	ovis.	Sheep pox.
	4. Avipoxvirus.	galli.	Fowl pox.
	5. Fibromavirus.	myxomatosis.	Rabbit myxoma.
	6. Molluscovirus.	hominis.	Molluscum contagiosum.
Microviridae	1. Microvirus (type genus).	monocatena.	Phage φX 174.
Parvoviridae	1. Parvovirus (type genus).	ratti.	Kilham rat virus.
Papillomaviridae	1. Papillomavirus (type genus).	sylvilagi.	Shope papilloma virus.
	2. Polyomavirus.	neoformans.	Polyoma virus.
Adenoviridae	1. Adenovirus (type genus).	(hominis) quintus.	Adenovirus 5.
Iridoviridae	1. Iridovirus (type genus).	tipulae.	Tipula iridescens.
Inophagoviridae	1. Inophagovirus (type genus).	bacterii.	fd phage (Hoffmann-Berling).
Herpesviridae	1. Herpesvirus (type genus).	hominis.	Herpes simplex virus.
	2. Cytomegaliavirus.	hominis.	Human cytomegalovirus.
Phagoviridae	1. Phagovirus (type genus).	(coli) T secundus.	Phage T2.

[1]Adapted from Lwoff, A., and Tournier, P.: The classification of viruses. Am. Rev. Microbiol., 1966, 20:45.

[2]Names in parentheses correspond to subgenera.

APPENDIX C
Sterilization Charts

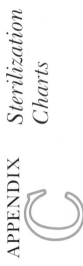

Hospital Equipment and Materials Sterilizable by Ethylene Oxide*

TELESCOPIC INSTRUMENTS	PLASTIC GOODS	RUBBER GOODS	INSTRUMENTS AND EQUIPMENT	MISCELLANEOUS
Bronchoscopes	Catheters	Tubing	Cautery sets	Dilators
Cystoscopes	Nebulizers	Surgical gloves	Eye knives	Electric cords
Electrotomes	Vials	Catheters	Lamps	Hair clippers
Endoscopes	Syringes	Drain and feed sets	Needles	Miller–Abbott tube
Esophagoscopes	Gloves	Sheeting	Neurosurgical instruments	Pumps
Ophthalmoscopes	Test tubes		Scalpel blades	Motors
Otoscopes	Petri dishes		Speculae	Books
Pharyngoscopes	I.V. sets		Syringes	Toys
Proctoscopes	Infant incubators		Dental instruments	Pottery
Resectoscopes	Heart-lung machines		Oxygen tents	Blankets
Sigmoidoscopes	Heart pacemakers			Sheets
Thoracoscopes	Artificial kidney machines			Furniture
Urethroscopes				Sealed ampules
				Sutures
				Medicine droppers

*Chemical Gas Sterilization. From: Ethylene Oxide Sterilization. The Journal of Hospital Research, 7:1, 1969. American Sterilizer Company.

Ethylene Oxide Mixtures Used in Gaseous Sterilization Procedures*

MIXTURES	MANUFACTURER
Ethylene oxide-carbon dioxide	
CARBOXIDE	
10% Ethylene Oxide	Union Carbide Corp.
90% Carbon Dioxide	Linde Division, New York, N.Y.
OXYFUME STERILANT-20	
20% Ethylene Oxide	Union Carbide Corp.
80% Carbon Dioxide	Linde Division, New York, N.Y.
STEROXIDE-20	
20% Ethylene Oxide	Castle Ritter Pfaudler Corp.
80% Carbon Dioxide	Rochester, N.Y.
Ethylene oxide-fluorinated hydrocarbons	
CRY-OXCIDE	
11% Ethylene Oxide	Ben Venue Laboratories
79% Trichloromonofluoromethane	Bedford, Ohio
10% Dichlorodifluoromethane	
BENVICIDE	
11% Ethylene Oxide	The Matheson Co.
54% Trichloromonofluoromethane	East Rutherford, N.J.
35% Dichlorodifluoromethane	
PENNOXIDE	
12% Ethylene Oxide	Pennsylvania Engineering Co.
88% Dichlorodifluoromethane	Philadelphia, Pa.
STEROXIDE-12	
12% Ethylene Oxide	Castle Ritter Pfaudler Corp.
88% Dichlorodifluoromethane	Rochester, N.Y.

*Chemical Gas Sterilization. From: Ethylene Oxide Sterilization. The Journal of Hospital Research, 7:1, 1969. American Sterilizer Company.

Sterilization of Apparatus and Supplies

ARTICLE	METHOD[1]	TIME IN MINUTES		
		at 165 C	at 121 C	at 132 C
Bronchoscopes	Autoclave		10	2–3
Bonewax	Hot Air	90		
Bougies	Chemical only			
Brushes	Autoclave		10	2–3
Catheters (Gum Elastic or Woven Silk Base)[2]	Chemical only			
Cellophane	Autoclave		30	15
Cystoscopes	Chemical only			
Diapers	Autoclave		30	15
Drains (Gutta Percha—Rubber)[2]	Autoclave		15	3
Drums—Dressing Loosely packed Full but not compressed	Autoclave		30 45	15
Electric Cords	Autoclave		10	2–3
Ether Cones	Autoclave		10	2–3
Glassware—Test Tubes, Tubing, Petri Dishes, etc.	Hot Air	120		
Glycerin	Hot Air	90		
Hard Rubber Details	Chemical only			
Instruments (In general) Routine Emergency Extreme Emergency Scalpels and Scissors Cataract Knives Tenotomes Urethrotomes	Autoclave Autoclave Autoclave Same as above Chemical only Chemical only Chemical only		10 5 3	2–3

[1] Sterilization by any approved sporicidal gas, such as ethylene oxide or beta-propiolactone, may be used in those situations in which heat and/or moisture would destroy the objects sterilized.

[2] Many supplies listed here, which were formerly assembled and sterilized as separate items, are now purchasable as complete kits or outfits, assembled for use, packaged, and properly sterilized; many are disposable.

12% Ethylene Oxide and 88% Freon-12 of the American Sterilizer Company, Erie, Pennsylvania should be used in this manner; 650 to 750 mg/liter of chamber space for 1¾ to 4 hours, at a total cycle time of 2½ to 5½ hours, temperature 125 to 135 F (52 to 57 C) and a relative humidity of 40 to 80%.

Dry heat sterilization in the oven is recommended at 340 F (171 C) for one hour, at 320 F (160 C) for two hours, or at 250 F (121 C) for six hours or longer. Common use is 165 C for two hours.

Sterilization of Apparatus and Supplies—Continued

ARTICLE	METHOD	TIME IN MINUTES		
		at 165 C	*at 121 C*	*at 132 C*
Intravenous Sets[2]	Autoclave		20	10
Iodoform	Do not sterilize			
Iodoform Drainage Material. Assemble previously sterilized parts under strict aseptic conditions, or purchase sterile.				
Jars—Enamelware	Autoclave		30	15
Lamb's Wool	Autoclave		30	15
Lamps, Diagnostic	Chemical only			
Maternity Packs[2]	Autoclave		30	15
Miller-Abbott Tubes	Chemical only			
Nebulizers	Chemical only			
Needles—Suture and Hypodermic	Hot Air	90		
Oils—Various	Hot Air	60		
Operating Motors—*See Manufacturer's Specifications*				
Paraffin Gauze	Hot Air	120		
Plastic Ware—*See Manufacturer's Specifications*[2]				
Proctoscopes	Chemical only			
Rubber Goods[2] Catheters Gloves Sheeting Tubing	Autoclave		20 15 20 20	10 3 10 10
Scalpel Blades Spares—in Medicine Bottles	Autoclave		30	15
Sigmoidoscopes	Chemical only			
Solutions—Aqueous, in: 2,000 ml Erlenmeyer Flask (Pyrex)[3] thin glass 2,000 ml Florence Flask (Pyrex) thin glass 1,800 ml Fenwal Flask (Pyrex) thick glass 1,000 ml Erlenmeyer Flask (Pyrex) thin glass 1,000 ml Florence Flask (Pyrex) thin glass	Autoclave		20 20 30 15 15	10 10 15 3 3

[3] Or Kimble products called *KIMAX*.

Sterilization of Apparatus and Supplies—Continued

ARTICLE	METHOD	TIME IN MINUTES		
		at 165 C	*at 121 C*	*at 132 C*
1,000 ml. Fenwal Flask (Pyrex)[3] thick glass	Autoclave		20	10
500 ml thin glass			12	3
250 ml thin glass			10	2–3
125 ml thin glass			8	2–3
2–4 ounce bottles, thick glass			10	2–3
Test Tubes, 150 x 18 mm.			8	2–3
Sulfa Drugs: Powder: At 300–315 F (150–155 C) only	Hot Air	90		
In solution	Autoclave		20	10
Surgical Packs—Major Packs[2]	Autoclave		30	15
Cotton filled Dressing Combines, Cotton Napkins, Cellulose Napkins, Gauze Sponges, etc.			20–30	10–15
Sutures Nonboilable Tubes	Chemical only			
Boilable Tubes	Autoclave		10	2–3
Silk, Cotton, Linen, Nylon	Autoclave		10	2–3
Syringes—Unassembled[2]	Hot Air	90		
	Autoclave		20	10
Talcum Powder	Hot Air	2 hours		
Thermometers	Chemical only			
Tongue Depressors	Autoclave		30	15
Transfusion Sets[2]	Autoclave		20	10
Trays—All kinds	Autoclave		20	10
Urethral Catheters[2]	Autoclave		10	2–3
Urethroscopes	Chemical only			
Utensils	Autoclave		15	3
Vaseline Petroleum Jelly (Petrolatum)	Hot Air	120		
Vaselinized Gauze	Hot Air	120		
Zinc Peroxide (Hold temperature at 280 F—135 C)	Hot Air	4 hours		

Packaging Materials for Articles to be Sterilized

MATERIAL	NATURE	TYPE OF PRODUCT	THICKNESS OR GRADE	SUITABLE FOR		
				Steam	*Dry Heat*	*EtO Gas*
Muslin	Textile	Wrappers	140 thread count	Yes	Yes	Yes
Jean Cloth	Textile	Wrappers	160 thread count	Yes	No	Yes
Broadcloth	Textile	Wrappers	200 thread count	Yes	No	Yes
Canvas	Textile	Wrappers	—	— Do Not Use —		
Kraft Brown	Paper	Wrappers Bags	30–40 lb	Yes	No	Yes
Kraft White	Paper	Wrappers Bags	30–40 lb	Yes	No	Yes
Glassine	Coated Paper	Envelopes Bags	30 lb	Yes	No	Yes
Parchment	Paper	Wrappers	Patapar 27-2T	Yes	No	Yes
Crepe	Paper	Wrappers	Dennison-Wrap	Yes	No	Yes
Cellophane	Cellulose Film	Tubing Bags	Weck Sterilizable	Yes	No	Yes
Polyethylene	Plastic	Bags Wrappers	1–3 mills	No	No	Yes
Polypropylene	Plastic	Film	1–3 mils	*	No	Yes
Polyvinyl Chloride	Plastic	Film Tubing	1–3 mils	No	No	Yes
Nylon	Plastic	Film Bags	1–2 mils	*	No	Yes
Polyamide	Plastic	Film Wrappers	1–2 mils	*	No	Yes
Aluminum	Foil	Wrappers	1–2 mils	No	Yes	No

*Not recommended. Difficult to eliminate air from packs.

From: Principles and Methods of Sterilization, 2nd Edition. by John J. Perkins. Permission to reproduce this table has been granted by Charles C Thomas, Publisher, Springfield, Illinois.

Disinfection of Miscellaneous Objects and Substances

OBJECT OR SUBSTANCE	METHODS OF DISINFECTION	ALTERNATE METHODS
Bedpans from noninfected patient.	Wash thoroughly after each use and return to patient unit. When patient is discharged, bedpan should be cleaned thoroughly and steamed or boiled for 2 minutes.	
Bedpans from patient who has an enteric disease, brucellosis, poliomyelitis, viral hepatitis, or tuberculosis of the intestinal or urinary tract.	Disinfect in special equipment for steaming bedpans at 95 to 100 C for 30 minutes after contents have been emptied into covered pail for disinfection or otherwise disposed of in an approved manner. After steaming, wash thoroughly with soap and water and return to patient.	If bedpan steaming equipment is not available, empty contents into covered pail for disinfection, or otherwise dispose of in an approved manner. Immerse bedpan in tub of chlorinated lime (5%) or saponated solution of cresol or iodophore (5%) for 1 hour or in boiling water at 95 to 100 C for 30 minutes. Wash thoroughly and return to the patient unit.
Dishes and eating utensils from a noninfected patient.	Scrape to remove uneaten food, wash thoroughly with soap and hot water (preferably in a mechanical dishwasher so that the temperature of the water can be near boiling temperature), rinse, allow dishes to drain dry, and store in clean closed cabinets.	Where mechanical dishwashers are not available, use plenty of soap, friction and hot water. After washing, soak in clear, cool water containing at least 50 parts per million of free chlorine. Drain dry.
Dishes and eating utensils from a patient who has an infection transferable via respiratory or gastrointestinal tract.	Completely immerse and boil for 10 minutes before washing. Wash as stated above.[4]	Where feasible, use paper plates, cups and other dishes that can be burned after use.
Gowns used in care of a communicable disease.	When gown technique is indicated, gowns should be used once and discarded with contaminated linen. Reuse of gowns by the same person or others has little justification bacteriologically or esthetically.	In the home, it is usually impossible to have enough gowns for each time that a gown is needed. Care must be taken to avoid contaminating the inside of the gown when it is removed. Gowns must remain in the sickroom until removed to be disinfected every eight hours or at least daily (see Linen).
Gowns used in assisting with surgery.	Sterilize in the autoclave at 121 C for 30 minutes or at 132 C for 15 minutes.	
Hands of personnel caring for patients who have communicable diseases.	Wash thoroughly with soap and water, after the care of each patient, after emptying a bedpan or urinal, before preparing medications, before serving meals, before going off duty or to the dining room for their own meals. Cover each area of the hands and to the middle of the forearm twice. Be sure to pay special attention to the fingernails and areas between the fingers. Apply soothing hand lotion several times each day to prevent rough and chapped hands.	

[4] If epidemic hepatitis, autoclave.

Disinfection of Miscellaneous Objects and Substances—Continued

OBJECT OR SUBSTANCE	METHODS OF DISINFECTION
Hands of nurse preparing to assist with surgery.	Wash thoroughly with hexachlorophene or soap and water, covering each area of the hands and to the elbow three times. Use good friction, enough soap to make a good lather, and be sure to give special attention to the fingernails, fingertips, and areas between the fingers. Rinse hands thoroughly with water and immerse or rinse with ethyl alcohol (70%) or aqueous iodophore 1:1,000. Dry with sterile towel and put on sterile rubber gloves. Use of hexachlorophene should be limited to relatively short exposures of small areas of the body. It should be thoroughly removed.
Infectious paper, gauze or linen handkerchiefs or "wipes" from patients with respiratory diseases.	See *Infectious dressings from wounds or lesions.*
Infectious dressings from wounds or lesions.	Wrap carefully in newspaper or other wrapping so that the outside of the package is not contaminated and with enough thicknesses of wrapping so that drainage will not soak through. Burn this package completely.
Infectious feces and urine from patients who have enteric infections, brucellosis, poliomyelitis, or viral hepatitis.	In some hospitals and communities the bedpan is emptied directly into existing sewerage or hoppers. If this is not done, empty into a vessel that can be tightly covered. Break up large particles of feces with a wooden tongue blade. Do not spatter! Leave the tongue blade with the infectious material. Add an approximately equal amount of chlorinated lime (5%), laundry bleach (full strength), organic iodine disinfectant like Wescodyne, or saponated solution of cresol (5%). Do not spatter! Place cover on the vessel and secure with Scotch tape or adhesive. Allow a minimum of 1 hour contact with the disinfectant. Remove the tongue blade with a forceps, wrap in paper and burn. Boil the forceps. Do not let blade or forceps drip. Empty into the toilet or hopper.
Instruments used on infected wounds.	Boil before washing unless the infection is gas gangrene or anthrax. Wash, wrap, and resterilize by autoclaving. If the infection is gas gangrene or anthrax, handle with forceps, place in tray, and autoclave before washing. Wash and resterilize in the autoclave.

OBJECT OR SUBSTANCE	METHODS OF DISINFECTION	ALTERNATE METHODS
Linen from the bed, and bedclothing, of a patient having a communicable disease.	Collect in a bag or pillowcase, keeping the outside of the bag or pillowcase uncontaminated. Autoclave or send to laundry room if automatic washers are available. (Laundry water temperature should be close to 100 C.) If linen is from a patient who has gas gangrene or anthrax, the linen must be autoclaved.	Completely immerse in boiling water in a large container and boil for 10 minutes, or soak overnight in 5% saponated cresol solution or strong chlorine laundry bleach or iodophore (follow manufacturer's directions).

Disinfection of Miscellaneous Objects and Substances—Continued

OBJECT OR SUBSTANCE	METHODS OF DISINFECTION	ALTERNATE METHODS
Sputum and other respiratory secretions.	Collect with paper gauze or old linen handkerchiefs or in covered paper cup, wrap carefully to prevent contamination of the outside of the package, and burn. (If sputum collected in the sputum cup is copious, it is desirable to add sawdust or shredded paper to absorb the moisture.)	If burning is not feasible, soak paper handkerchiefs or container with sputum in a covered vessel with a saponated solution of cresol (5%), iodophore or chlorinated lime (5%) for a minimum of 1 hour. Discard in toilet or hopper. Covered glass containers can be reused after they have been sterilized.

OBJECT OR SUBSTANCE	METHODS OF DISINFECTION
Stethoscopes, otoscopes.	After use on a patient with a communicable disease cover the bell of a stethoscope with gauze moistened with saponated solution of cresol (5%) or ethyl alcohol (70%) for 5 minutes. The rest of the stethoscope should be washed thoroughly with soap and water and scrubbed with cresol or alcohol. Before use on a patient with a communicable disease the battery part of an otoscope can be wrapped with a small towel or strips of muslin to protect it. The otoscope tip can be boiled for 5 minutes if it is metal. If the tip is plastic, follow instructions of manufacturer. Wash off cresol with soap and water.
Thermometers—oral.	There should be sufficient supply of thermometers so that there is one available for each patient on the ward. Thermometers should be taken to patients in a clean dry container. After use: (1) Wipe clean with pledget of cotton or gauze wet with tincture of green soap mixed in equal volumes with 95 per cent ethyl alcohol. (2) Rinse thoroughly with clear water. (3) Completely immerse thermometer in 70% ethyl or rubbing alcohol, preferably containing 0.5 to 1% iodine, for 10 minutes. Rinse and dry. Store in a clean, dry, covered container. If necessary the disinfectant can be returned to the stock bottle to conserve supplies and facilitate the work of the public health worker in the field. The thermometer should be returned to its container clean and dry.
Thermometers—rectal.	Rectal thermometers should be lubricated with water-soluble lubricant. If this is not available, soap is a better lubricant bacteriologically than petrolatum or oil. Cleaning and disinfection are the same as for oral thermometers.
Toys, books, mail from a patient who has a communicable disease.	Where possible, disposable toys and books should be used for the patient who has a communicable disease. Some toys can be autoclaved, or washed with soap and water and exposed to the sun, or washed with disinfectant and sunned. Expensive books can be autoclaved if stood on end but the steam will deteriorate the bindings and covers. Outgoing mail can be autoclaved if it is written in pencil. Stamps are placed on and flaps gummed with Scotch tape after autoclaving.
Urinal from patient who has a urinary communicable disease.	See instructions for bedpan.

Portals of Exit and Types of Pathogens Usually Associated with Them

I. Oral and respiratory tracts:

A. BACTERIA:
1. Gram-positive cocci (pneumonia, *Diplococcus pneumoniae;* scarlet fever, *Streptococcus pyogenes;* etc.)
2. Gram-negative cocci (epidemic meningitis, *Neisseria meningitidis*)
3. Gram-positive rods:
   a. diphtheria (*Corynebacterium diphtheriae*)
   b. tuberculosis (*Mycobacterium tuberculosis*)
4. Gram-negative rods (laryngitis, *Haemophilus influenzae;* whooping cough, *Bordetella pertussis;* etc.)
5. Spirochetes (Vincent's angina, syphilis)
6. Psittacosis organisms

B. VIRUSES:
1. Smallpox
2. Mumps
3. Measles
4. Chickenpox
5. Rabies
6. Myxoviruses
7. Adenoviruses, rhinoviruses, etc.
8. Poliovirus

C. FUNGI: (See Group V.)

II. Intestinal and/or urinary tracts:

A. BACTERIA
1. Enterobacteriaceae (typhoid, dysentery, etc.) (gram-negative rods)
2. *Brucella* (undulant fever)
3. *Leptospira* (leptospirosis)
4. *Clostridium* (gas gangrene and tetanus) (gram-positive rods) (See group V.)

B. VIRUSES
1. Poliomyelitis
2. Coxsackie
3. ECHO
4. Hepatitis A (epidemic hepatitis)

C. PROTOZOA
1. *Entamoeba histolytica* (dysentery, etc.)
2. *Trichomonas hominis* (enteritis, etc.)
3. *Giardia lamblia* (enteritis, etc.)

D. HELMINTHS
1. Hookworm
2. *Ascaris*
3. Pinworms
4. Whipworm
5. Flukes
6. Tapeworms

III. Genital tract:

A. BACTERIA
1. *Treponema pallidum* (syphilis)
2. *Neisseria gonorrhoeae* (gonorrheal infection)
3. *Haemophilus ducreii* (chancroid) ⎫
4. *Calymmatobacterium granulomatis* (granuloma inguinale) ⎬ gram-negative rods
5. Lymphogranuloma venereum organisms (*Chlamydiaceae*)

B. PROTOZOA
1. *Trichomonas vaginalis* (vulvovaginitis, etc.)

IV. Pathogens of man usually transmitted in blood:

A. MAINLY BY SANGUIVOROUS ARTHOPODS:
1. BACTERIA
   a. *Yersinia pestis* (bubonic plague) ⎫
   b. *Pasteurella tularensis* (tularemia) ⎬ gram-negative rods
   c. *Borrelia* (relapsing fever)
2. RICKETTSIAS (Rocky Mountain spotted fever, typhus, etc.)
3. VIRUSES
   a. Yellow and dengue fevers
   b. Other arboviruses
4. PROTOZOA
   a. *Plasmodium* (malaria)
   b. *Trypanosoma* (trypanosomiasis)
   c. *Leishmania* (leishmaniasis)
5. HELMINTHS
   a. Filarias (filariasis)

B. MAINLY BY ARTIFICIAL VECTORS (e.g., hypodermic needles, syringes, autopsy instruments, surgical instruments, etc., and by some blood derivatives—plasma, serum, whole blood, etc.):
1. VIRUSES (notably those of epidemic hepatitis and of homologous serum hepatitis, i.e. hepatitis viruses A and B), which may be circulating in the blood at the time the blood is drawn or the instruments used
2. BACTERIA WHICH FREQUENTLY CAUSE BACTERIEMIA: *Brucella, Salmonella, Streptococcus, Staphylococcus, Neisseria, Pasteurella, Diplococcus, Leptospira, Treponema*

V. Pathogens commonly found in the soil:

A. BACTERIA
1. Genus *Clostridium:* (anaerobes) ⎫
   a. Gas gangrene group ⎪
   b. *Cl. tetani* (tetanus) ⎬ gram-positive rods
   c. *Cl. botulinum* (food poisoning) ⎪
2. Genus *Bacillus:* (aerobes) ⎪
   a. *B. anthracis* (anthrax) ⎭

B. FUNGI
1. *Coccidioides immitis* (coccidiodomycosis)
2. *Histoplasma capsulatum* (histoplasmosis)
3. *Sporotrichum* (sporotrichosis)
4. *Blastomyces*, etc.

C. HELMINTHS (See Group II.)

APPENDIX *Some Films and Filmstrips Useful in Teaching Microbiology for Health Personnel*

CHAPTER	TITLE	LENGTH OF TIME	SOUND OR SILENT*	COLOR OR BLACK AND WHITE	AVAILABILITY	SOURCE
1	Career: Medical Technologist	24 min	Sound	Black and White	Loan-Free	National Medical Audiovisual Center Attention: Videotape Duplicating Service Atlanta, Ga. 30333
1	Health Heroes: The Battle Against Disease	11 min	Sound	Both	Loan	Modern Talking Pictures 160 E. Grand Ave. Chicago, Illinois 60611
1	Nursing in the Tropics	29 min	Sound	Black and White	Loan–Free	National Medical Audiovisual Center Attention: Videotape Duplicating Service Atlanta, Ga. 30333
2	Anatomy of the Cell	20 min	Sound	Black and White	Loan–Free	E. R. Squibb & Sons 909 Third Avenue New York, N.Y. 10022
2	What is a Cell?	30 min	Sound	Color	Loan	Department of Audiovisual Services University of Texas at Arlington Arlington, Texas 76010
2	The Origin of Life – Chemical Evolution	11 min	Sound	Both	Loan	EBE Corporation Preview/Rental Libraries 1822 Pickwick Ave. Glenview, Illinois 60025
2	The Cell – Structural Unit of Life	11 min	Sound	Color	Loan	Modern Talking Pictures 160 E. Grand Ave. Chicago, Illinois 60611
2	The Nature of Life: The Living Cell	14 min	Sound	Both	Loan	Modern Talking Pictures 160 E. Grand Ave. Chicago, Illinois 60611
2	Cell Biology: Life Functions	19 min	Sound	Both	Loan	Modern Talking Pictures 160 E. Grand Ave. Chicago, Illinois 60611
2, 4	Simple Plants: Bacteria	14 min	Sound	Both	Loan	Modern Talking Pictures 160 E. Grand Ave. Chicago, Illinois 60611

2	Laws of Heredity	15 min	Sound	Color	Loan	EBE Corporation Preview/Rental Libraries 1822 Pickwick Ave. Glenview, Illinois 60025
2	Genetics: Mendel's Laws	14 min	Sound	Both	Loan	Modern Talking Pictures 160 E. Grand Ave. Chicago, Illinois 60611
2	Genetics: Chromosomes and Genes (Meiosis)	16 min	Sound	Both	Loan	Modern Talking Pictures 160 E. Grand Ave. Chicago, Illinois 60611
2	Genetics: Functions of DNA and RNA	14 min	Sound	Both	Loan	Modern Talking Pictures 160 E. Grand Ave. Chicago, Illinois 60611
2	Gene Action	16 min	Sound	Both	Loan	EBE Corporation Preview/Rental Libraries 1822 Pickwick Ave. Glenview, Illinois 60025
2	DNA: Molecule of Heredity	16 min	Sound	Color	Loan	Department of Audiovisual Services University of Texas at Arlington Arlington, Texas 76010
2	Chemistry of the Cell. I: The Structure of Proteins and Nucleic Acids	21 min	Sound	Color	Loan	McGraw-Hill Films 330 West 42nd Street New York, N.Y. 10036
2	Chemistry of the Cell. II: Function of DNA and RNA in Protein Synthesis	16 min	Sound	Color	Loan	McGraw-Hill Films 330 West 42nd Street New York, N.Y. 10036
3	Microscopic Fungi	15 min	Sound	Color	Loan	McGraw-Hill Films 330 West 42nd Street New York, N.Y. 10036
3	Fungi	30 min	Sound	Color	Loan	Department of Audiovisual Services University of Texas at Arlington Arlington, Texas 76010
3	Simple Plants: Algae and Fungi	14 min	Sound	Both	Loan	Modern Talking Pictures 160 E. Grand Ave. Chicago, Illinois 60611

*Films are 16 mm; those marked with an asterisk are also available in 8 mm from National Audiovisual Center, Suitland, Md. 20405.

CHAPTER	TITLE	LENGTH OF TIME	SOUND OR SILENT	COLOR OR BLACK AND WHITE	AVAILABILITY	SOURCE
3	Life of the Molds	21 min	Sound	Both	Loan	McGraw-Hill Films 330 West 42nd Street New York, N.Y. 10036
3	Molds and How They Grow	11 min	Sound	Both	Loan	Modern Talking Pictures 160 E. Grand Ave. Chicago, Illinois 60611
3	Life in a Drop of Water	11 min	Sound	Both	Loan	Modern Talking Pictures 160 E. Grand Ave. Chicago, Illinois 60611
3	The Fresh Water Pond	13 min	Sound	Both	Loan	EBE Corporation Preview/Rental Libraries 1822 Pickwick Ave. Glenview, Illinois 60025
3	Plankton and the Open Sea	19 min	Sound	Both	Loan	EBE Corporation Preview/Rental Libraries 1822 Pickwick Ave. Glenview, Illinois 60025
3	Movements of *Endamoeba histolytica*	2 min	Silent	Color	Loan	Audiovisual Section Clendening Medical Library University of Kansas Medical Center Kansas City, Kansas 66103
3	Life Story of the *Paramecium*	11 min	Sound	Both	Loan	EBE Corporation Preview/Rental Libraries 1822 Pickwick Ave. Glenview, Illinois 60025
3	The Single-Celled Animals—Protozoa	17 min	Sound	Both	Loan	EBE Corporation Preview/Rental Libraries 1822 Pickwick Ave. Glenview, Illinois 60025

3	Protozoa (One-Celled Animals)	11 min	Sound	Both	Loan	EBE Corporation Preview/Rental Libraries 1822 Pickwick Ave. Glenview, Illinois 60025
4	Bacteria	19 min	Sound	Color	Loan	Department of Audiovisual Services University of Texas at Arlington Arlington, Texas 76010
4	The Enemy Bacteria	29 min	Sound	Color	Loan–Free	National Medical Audiovisual Center Attention: Videotape Duplicating Service Atlanta, Ga. 30333
4	Studies in Bacteriology. Part 2: Motility	4 min	Silent	Black and White	Loan–Free	National Medical Audiovisual Center Attention: Videotape Duplicating Service Atlanta, Ga. 30333
4	Studies in Bacteriology. Part 3: Cell Division	4 min	Silent	Black and White	Loan–Free	National Medical Audiovisual Center Attention: Videotape Duplicating Service Atlanta, Ga. 30333
4	Mycoplasma pneumoniae Pneumonia	31 min	Sound	Color	Loan–Free	The Pfizer Laboratories Division Film Library 267 West 25th Street New York, N.Y. 10001
5	Rickettsia—Laboratory Procedure for Their Isolation and Identification	47 min	Sound	Color	Loan–Free	National Medical Audiovisual Center Attention: Videotape Duplicating Service Atlanta, Ga. 30333
5	Embryonated Egg Techniques, Part 1	5.5 min	Sound*	Black and White	Loan	National Audiovisual Center Suitland, Md. 20405
5	Embryonated Egg Techniques, Part II	7 min	Sound*	Black and White	Loan	National Audiovisual Center Suitland, Md. 20405
6	Viruses: Threshold of Life	14 min	Sound	Both	Loan	Modern Talking Pictures 160 E. Grand Ave. Chicago, Illinois 60611
6	The Virus: Living or Non-Living	29 min	Sound	Black and White	Loan–Free	National Medical Audiovisual Center Attention: Videotape Duplicating Service Atlanta, Ga. 30333

*Films are 16 mm; those marked with an asterisk are also available in 8 mm from National Audiovisual Center, Suitland, Md. 20405.

CHAPTER	TITLE	LENGTH OF TIME	SOUND OR SILENT	COLOR OR BLACK AND WHITE	AVAILABILITY	SOURCE
6	The HeLa Cell Strain	11 min	Sound	Black and White	Loan	Audiovisual Section Clendening Medical Library University of Kansas Medical Center Kansas City, Kansas 66103
6	The Effect of Viruses on a Cell Line of Human Origin	28 min	Sound	Color	Loan	Audiovisual Section Clendening Medical Library University of Kansas Medical Center Kansas City, Kansas 66103
6	Influenza Virus Isolation	7 min	Sound*	Color	Loan – Free	National Medical Audiovisual Center Attention: Videotape Duplicating Service Atlanta, Ga. 30333
7	World of Microbes	30 min	Sound	Color	Loan – Free	National Medical Audiovisual Center Attention: Videotape Duplicating Service Atlanta, Ga. 30333
7	World of Microbes	30 min	Sound	Color	Loan	McGraw-Hill Films 330 West 42nd Street New York, N.Y. 10036
7	Air Sampling for Micro-biological Particulates	11 min	Sound	Color	Loan – Free	National Medical Audiovisual Center Attention: Videotape Duplicating Service Atlanta, Ga. 30333
8	Methods for Obtaining Anaerobiosis	12 min	Sound*	Color	Loan – Free	National Medical Audiovisual Center Attention: Videotape Duplicating Service Atlanta, Ga. 30333
8	The Health Fraud Racket	28 min	Sound	Color	Loan – Free	U.S. Food & Drug Administration Public Health Service Audio Visual Facility Atlanta, Georgia 30333
8	Cleanliness and Health	11 min	Sound	Both	Loan	Modern Talking Pictures 160 E. Grand Avenue Chicago, Illinois 60611

9	The Microscope	11 min	Sound	Both	Loan	McGraw-Hill Films 330 West 42nd Street New York, N.Y. 10036
9	The Compound Microscope	12.5 min	Sound	Color	Loan—Free	Film Distribution Service Bausch & Lomb 635 St. Paul Street Rochester, N.Y. 14602
9	The World of the Microscope	12 min	Sound	Color	Loan—Free	Film Distribution Service Bausch & Lomb 635 St. Paul Street Rochester, N.Y. 14602
9	Phase Microscopy of Normal Living Blood Cells	28 min	Sound	Color	Loan	Audiovisual Section Clendening Medical Library University of Kansas Medical Center Kansas City, Kansas 66103
9	Electron Microscopy: An Introduction	24 min	Sound	Color	Loan	Audiovisual Section Clendening Medical Library University of Kansas Medical Center Kansas City, Kansas 66103
9	Microscopic Life: The World of the Invisible	14 min	Sound	Black and White	Loan	EBE Corporation Preview/Rental Libraries 1822 Pickwick Ave. Glenview, Illinois 60025
9	Gram's Stain—A Demonstration of the Technique		Sound	Color	Loan	American Society for Microbiology Washington, D.C. 20006
9	Cultures of Normal and Cancer Cells; Reel 2: Cancer Cells	16 min	Silent	Black and White	Loan	Audiovisual Section Clendening Medical Library University of Kansas Medical Center Kansas City, Kansas 66103
10	The Third Pollution	23 min	Sound	Color	Loan—Free	National Medical Audiovisual Center Attention: Videotape Duplicating Service Atlanta, Ga. 30333
10	A Visit to the Waterworks	11 min	Sound	Both	Loan	EBE Corporation Preview/Rental Libraries 1822 Pickwick Ave. Glenview, Illinois 60025

*Films are 16 mm; those marked with an asterisk are also available in 8 mm from National Audiovisual Center, Suitland, Md. 20405.

CHAPTER	TITLE	LENGTH OF TIME	SOUND OR SILENT	COLOR OR BLACK AND WHITE	AVAILABILITY	SOURCE
10	Sewage Treatment	5 min	Sound	Black and White	Loan	Audiovisual Section Clendening Medical Library University of Kansas Medical Center Kansas City, Kansas 66103
10	Introduction to Swimming Pool Sanitation	24 min	Sound	Color	Loan – Free	National Medical Audiovisual Center Attention: Videotape Duplicating Service Atlanta, Ga. 30333
10	Food Storage	12 min	Sound	Black and White	Loan – Free	National Medical Audiovisual Center Attention: Videotape Duplicating Service Atlanta, Ga. 30333
10	Bacteria – Friend and Foe	11 min	Sound	Both	Loan	EBE Corporation Preview/Rental Libraries 1822 Pickwick Ave. Glenview, Illinois 60025
10	Dental Health: How and Why	11 min	Sound	Both	Loan	Modern Talking Pictures 160 E. Grand Ave. Chicago, Illinois 60611
10	Your Teeth	6 min	Sound	Both	Loan	EBE Corporation Preview/Rental Libraries 1822 Pickwick Ave. Glenview, Illinois 60025
10	Teeth Are to Keep	11 min	Sound	Color	Loan	EBE Corporation Preview/Rental Libraries 1822 Pickwick Ave. Glenview, Illinois 60025
10	Save Those Teeth	11 min	Sound	Black and White	Loan	EBE Corporation Preview/Rental Libraries 1822 Pickwick Ave. Glenview, Illinois 60025
10	The Sneeze	3 min	Silent	Black and White	Loan – Free	National Medical Audiovisual Center Attention: Videotape Duplicating Service Atlanta, Ga. 30333

	Title	Length	Sound	Color	Loan	Source
12	Pressure Steam Sterilization	25 min	Sound	Color	Loan	American Sterilizer Company, Erie, Pennsylvania
14	Antibiotics	14 min	Sound	Black and White	Loan—Free	National Medical Audiovisual Center, Attention: Videotape Duplicating Service, Atlanta, Ga. 30333
14	The Action of Antibiotics on Bacteria	7 min	Sound	Black and White	Loan—Free	National Medical Audiovisual Center, Attention: Videotape Duplicating Service, Atlanta, Ga. 30333
14	Penicillin in Medicine and Surgery	40 min	Sound	Color	Loan—Free	National Medical Audiovisual Center, Attention: Videotape Duplicating Service, Atlanta, Ga. 30333
14	Birth of a Drug	35 min	Sound	Black and White	Loan—Free	National Medical Audiovisual Center, Attention: Videotape Duplicating Service, Atlanta, Ga. 30333
14	An Aid to Therapy: Bacterial-Antibiotic Susceptibility Testing	26 min	Sound	Color	Loan	Audiovisual Section, Clendening Medical Library, University of Kansas Medical Center, Kansas City, Kansas 66103
14	I Dress The Wound	30 min	Sound	Black and White	Loan—Free	National Medical Audiovisual Center, Attention: Videotape Duplicating Service, Atlanta, Ga. 30333
15	Operating Room Procedures	20 min	Sound	Color	Loan—Free	National Medical Audiovisual Center, Attention: Videotape Duplicating Service, Atlanta, Ga. 30333
15	Aseptic Procedure in Oral Surgery	18 min	Sound	Color	Loan—Free	National Medical Audiovisual Center, Attention: Videotape Duplicating Service, Atlanta, Ga. 30333
15	Hospital Housekeeping: Mopping, Two-Bucket Method	9 min	Sound*	Black and White	Loan	National Audiovisual Center, Suitland, Md. 20405
15	First Aid. Part 3: Burns	14 min	Sound	Color	Loan—Free	National Medical Audiovisual Center, Attention: Videotape Duplicating Service, Atlanta, Ga. 30333
15	Bacterial Infection	35 min	Sound	Color	Loan—Free	National Medical Audiovisual Center, Attention: Videotape Duplicating Service, Atlanta, Ga. 30333

*Films are 16 mm; those marked with an asterisk are also available in 8 mm from National Audiovisual Center, Suitland, Md. 20405.

CHAPTER	TITLE	LENGTH OF TIME	SOUND OR SILENT	COLOR OR BLACK AND WHITE	AVAILABILITY	SOURCE
15	Chain of Asepsis	29 min	Sound	Black and White	Loan–Free	National Medical Audiovisual Center Attention: Videotape Duplicating Service Atlanta, Ga. 30333
15	Chemical Disinfection	30 min	Sound	Color	Loan–Free	National Medical Audiovisual Center Attention: Videotape Duplicating Service Atlanta, Ga. 30333
15	Disinfection of the Skin	23 min	Sound	Color	Loan–Free	National Medical Audiovisual Center Attention: Videotape Duplicating Service Atlanta, Ga. 30333
15	Keeping Clean and Neat	11 min	Sound	Black and White	Loan	EBE Corporation Preview/Rental Libraries 1822 Pickwick Ave. Glenview, Illinois 60025
16	The Blood	16 min	Sound	Color	Loan	Department of Audiovisual Services University of Texas at Arlington Arlington, Texas 76010
16	White Blood Cells	12 min	Sound	Both	Loan–Free	National Medical Audiovisual Center Attention: Videotape Duplicating Service Atlanta, Ga. 30333
16	White Blood Cells	12 min	Sound	Both	Loan	McGraw-Hill Films 330 West 42nd Street New York, N.Y. 10036
16	Normal and Abnormal Platelets	20 min	Sound	Black and White	Loan–Free	E. R. Squibb & Sons 909 Third Avenue New York, N.Y. 10022
16	Work of the Blood	14 min	Sound	Both	Loan	EBE Corporation Preview/Rental Libraries 1822 Pickwick Ave. Glenview, Illinois 60025

16	Emergency Medical Care—Control of Bleeding	20 min	Sound	Color	Loan—Free	National Medical Audiovisual Center Attention: Videotape Duplicating Service Atlanta, Ga. 30333
16	Control of Hemorrhage	20 min	Sound	Color	Loan—Free	National Medical Audiovisual Center Attention: Videotape Duplicating Service Atlanta, Ga. 30333
16	The Theory of Blood Coagulation	28 min	Sound	Black and White	Loan—Free	National Medical Audiovisual Center Attention: Videotape Duplicating Service Atlanta, Ga. 30333
16	Blood Transfusion Today	60 min	Sound	Black and White	Loan—Free	National Medical Audiovisual Center Attention: Videotape Duplicating Service Atlanta, Ga. 30333
16	The Cross-Matching of Blood	42 min	Sound	Color	Loan—Free	National Medical Audiovisual Center Attention: Videotape Duplicating Service Atlanta, Ga. 30333
16	Blood Fractions in Clinical Medicine	33 min	Sound	Color	Loan—Free	National Medical Audiovisual Center Attention: Videotape Duplicating Service Atlanta, Ga. 30333
16	Blood Grouping	21 min	Sound	Color	Loan—Free	National Medical Audiovisual Center Attention: Videotape Duplicating Service Atlanta, Ga. 30333
16	Circulation of the Blood	7 min	Sound	Color	Loan—Free	National Medical Audiovisual Center Attention: Videotape Duplicating Service Atlanta, Ga. 30333
17	Circulation	16 min	Silent	Color	Loan—Free	American Heart Association Post Office Box 9928 Austin, Texas 78766
17	Infectious Hazards of Bacteriological Techniques	13 min	Sound	Color	Loan—Free	National Medical Audiovisual Center Attention: Videotape Duplicating Service Atlanta, Ga. 30333
18	The Inflammatory Reaction	26 min	Sound	Color	Loan	Lederle Laboratories Pearl River, New York
18, 20	The Development of the Immune Capacity in the Newborn	26 min	Sound	Color	Loan—Free	The Pfizer Laboratories Division Film Library 267 West 25th Street New York, N.Y. 10001

CHAPTER	TITLE	LENGTH OF TIME	SOUND OR SILENT	COLOR OR BLACK AND WHITE	AVAILABILITY	SOURCE
18	Dynamics of Phagocytosis	28 min	Sound	Black and White	Loan – Free	The Pfizer Laboratories Division Film Library 267 West 25th Street New York, N.Y. 10001
18	Dynamics of Phagocytosis	29 min	Sound	Black and White	Loan	Audiovisual Section Clendening Medical Library University of Kansas Medical Center Kansas City, Kansas 66103
18	Phagocytosis and Degranulation: Studies in Neutrophil Leucocytes	14 min	Silent	Black and White	Loan	Audiovisual Section Clendening Medical Library University of Kansas Medical Center Kansas City, Kansas 66103
18	Your Protection Against Disease	8 min	Sound	Both	Loan	EBE Corporation Preview/Rental Libraries 1822 Pickwick Ave. Glenview, Illinois 60025
18	How Our Bodies Fight Disease	8 min	Sound	Black and White	Loan	EBE Corporation Preview/Rental Libraries 1822 Pickwick Ave. Glenview, Illinois 60025
18	Control of *Pseudomonas* Burn Wound Sepsis	17 min	Sound	Color	Loan – Free	National Medical Audiovisual Center Attention: Videotape Duplicating Service Atlanta, Ga. 30333
18	Nutrition in Wound Healing	20 min	Sound	Color	Loan – Free	National Medical Audiovisual Center Attention: Videotape Duplicating Service Atlanta, Ga. 30333
18	Debridement. Part 1: Multiple Soft Tissue Wounds	12 min	Sound	Color	Loan – Free	National Medical Audiovisual Center Attention: Videotape Duplicating Service Atlanta, Ga. 30333
18	Debridement. Part 2: Wounds of the Extremities	33 min	Sound	Color	Loan – Free	National Medical Audiovisual Center Attention: Videotape Duplicating Service Atlanta, Ga. 30333

18	Cellular and Molecular Aspects of the Immune Response	43 min	Sound	Black and White	Loan—Free	National Medical Audiovisual Center Attention: Videotape Duplicating Service Atlanta, Ga. 30333
19	The Specificity of Antigen-Antibody Reactions	33 min	Sound	Black and White	Loan—Free	National Medical Audiovisual Center Attention: Videotape Duplicating Service Atlanta, Ga. 30333
19	Microtechniques in Serology	7.5 min	Sound*	Black and White	Loan	National Audiovisual Center Suitland, Md. 20405
19	Flocculation Test for Parasitic Disease	7 min	Sound*	Color	Loan—Free	National Medical Audiovisual Center Attention: Videotape Duplicating Service Atlanta, Ga. 30333
20	Infectious Diseases and Man-Made Defenses	11 min	Sound	Both	Loan	Modern Talking Pictures 160 E. Grand Ave. Chicago, Illinois 60611
20	Infectious Diseases and Natural Body Defenses	11 min	Sound	Both	Loan	Modern Talking Pictures 160 E. Grand Ave. Chicago, Illinois 60611
20	Body Defenses Against Disease	11 min	Sound	Black and White	Loan	EBE Corporation Preview/Rental Libraries 1822 Pickwick Ave. Glenview, Illinois 60025
20	Physical Chemistry and Immunohematology	30 min	Sound	Black and White	Loan—Free	National Medical Audiovisual Center Attention: Videotape Duplicating Service Atlanta, Ga. 30333
20	Immunization (2nd Edition)	11 min	Sound	Black and White	Loan	EBE Corporation Preview/Rental Libraries 1822 Pickwick Ave. Glenview, Illinois 60025
20	Military Immunization: General Procedures	25 min	Sound	Black and White	Loan—Free	National Medical Audiovisual Center Attention: Videotape Duplicating Service Atlanta, Ga. 30333
20	Military Immunization: Smallpox Vaccination	10 min	Sound	Color	Loan—Free	National Medical Audiovisual Center Attention: Videotape Duplicating Service Atlanta, Ga. 30333

*Films are 16 mm; those marked with an asterisk are also available in 8 mm from National Audiovisual Center, Suitland, Md. 20405.

CHAPTER	TITLE	LENGTH OF TIME	SOUND OR SILENT	COLOR OR BLACK AND WHITE	AVAILABILITY	SOURCE
20	Smallpox	33 min	Sound	Color	Loan—Free	National Medical Audiovisual Center Attention: Videotape Duplicating Service Atlanta, Ga. 30333
20	Antibody Specificity and Antigen Heterogeneity	29 min	Sound	Black and White	Loan—Free	National Medical Audiovisual Center Attention: Videotape Duplicating Service Atlanta, Ga. 30333
21	Active Anaphylaxis in the Mouse Sensitized with Bovine Albumin-Adjuvant Emulsion	6 min	Sound	Color	Loan	Audiovisual Section Clendening Medical Library University of Kansas Medical Center Kansas City, Kansas 66103
21	Active Anaphylaxis in the Mouse Sensitized with Bovine Albumin-Adjuvant Emulsion	10 min	Sound	Color	Loan—Free	National Medical Audiovisual Center Attention: Videotape Duplicating Service Atlanta, Ga. 30333
22	Microorganisms That Cause Disease	11 min	Sound	Both	Loan	Modern Talking Pictures 160 E. Grand Ave. Chicago, Illinois 60611
22	Disease and Personal Hygiene	17 min	Sound	Black and White	Loan—Free	National Medical Audiovisual Center Attention: Videotape Duplicating Service Atlanta, Ga. 30333
22	Hygiene for Women: Protecting Health	26 min	Sound	Color	Loan—Free	National Medical Audiovisual Center Attention: Videotape Duplicating Service Atlanta, Ga. 30333
22	Hospital Housekeeping: Wet Pick Up	7 min	Sound*	Color	Loan—Free	National Medical Audiovisual Center Attention: Videotape Duplicating Service Atlanta, Ga. 30333
22	The Dental Assistant: A Career of Service	13 min	Sound	Color	Loan—Free	National Medical Audiovisual Center Attention: Videotape Duplicating Service Atlanta, Ga. 30333

22	Stress and the Adaptation Syndrome	35 min	Sound	Color	Loan—Free	The Pfizer Laboratories Division Film Library 267 West 25th Street New York, N.Y. 10001
23	Cholera Can Be Conquered	11 min	Sound	Color	Loan	Audiovisual Section Clendening Medical Library University of Kansas Medical Center Kansas City, Kansas 66103
23	Cholera Epidemic in South Vietnam	10 min	Sound	Black and White	Loan—Free	National Medical Audiovisual Center Attention: Videotape Duplicating Service Atlanta, Ga. 30333
23	Cholera Today—Bedside Evaluation and Treatment	19 min	Sound	Color	Loan—Free	National Medical Audiovisual Center Attention: Videotape Duplicating Service Atlanta, Ga. 30333
23	Cholera Today—Practical Laboratory Diagnosis	15 min	Sound	Color	Loan—Free	National Medical Audiovisual Center Attention: Videotape Duplicating Service Atlanta, Ga. 30333
23	The Enterobacteriaceae	12 min	Sound	Color	Loan	Analytab Products, Inc. 919 Third Avenue New York, N.Y. 10022
23	The Epidemiology of Salmonellosis in Man and Animals	15 min	Sound	Color	Loan—Free	National Medical Audiovisual Center Attention: Videotape Duplicating Service Atlanta, Ga. 30333
23	An Outbreak of *Salmonella* Infection	12 min	Sound	Color	Loan—Free	National Medical Audiovisual Center Attention: Videotape Duplicating Service Atlanta, Ga. 30333
23	Methods for the Isolation of *Salmonella* from Human Foods and Animal Feeds	12 min	Sound	Color	Loan—Free	National Medical Audiovisual Center Attention: Videotape Duplicating Service Atlanta, Ga. 30333
23	Isolation and Identification of *Salmonella*	24 min	Sound	Black and White	Loan—Free	National Medical Audiovisual Center Attention: Videotape Duplicating Service Atlanta, Ga. 30333
23	Isolation and Identification of *Shigella*	24 min	Sound	Black and White	Loan—Free	National Medical Audiovisual Center Attention: Videotape Duplicating Service Atlanta, Ga. 30333

*Films are 16 mm; those marked with an asterisk are also available in 8 mm from National Audiovisual Center, Suitland, Md. 20405.

CHAPTER	TITLE	LENGTH OF TIME	SOUND OR SILENT	COLOR OR BLACK AND WHITE	AVAILABILITY	SOURCE
23	Isolation of *Salmonella* and *Shigella* Cultures	9 min	Sound*	Color	Loan – Free	National Medical Audiovisual Center Attention: Videotape Duplicating Service Atlanta, Ga. 30333
23	F. A. Detection of Enteropathogenic *Escherichia coli*	14 min	Sound	Color	Loan – Free	National Medical Audiovisual Center Attention: Videotape Duplicating Service Atlanta, Ga. 30333
23	The Infectious Diarrheas	15 min	Sound	Color	Loan – Free	National Medical Audiovisual Center Attention: Videotape Duplicating Service Atlanta, Ga. 30333
24	Polio – Diagnosis and Management	60 min	Sound	Black and White	Loan – Free	National Medical Audiovisual Center Attention: Videotape Duplicating Service Atlanta, Ga. 30333
24	Nursing Care in Poliomyelitis	67 min	Sound	Color	Loan – Free	National Medical Audiovisual Center Attention: Videotape Duplicating Service Atlanta, Ga. 30333
24	Jonas Salk: Science of Life	26 min	Sound	Color	Loan	McGraw-Hill Films 330 West 42nd Street New York, N.Y. 10036
25	Worms: Flat, Round and Segmented	16 min	Sound	Both	Loan	Modern Talking Pictures 160 E. Grand Ave. Chicago, Illinois 60611
25	Parasitism (Parasitic Flatworms)	17 min	Sound	Color	Loan	Department of Audiovisual Services University of Texas at Arlington Arlington, Texas 76010
25	Ascariasis (Infestation with Ascarids)	13 min	Sound	Black and White	Loan – Free	National Medical Audiovisual Center Attention: Videotape Duplicating Service Atlanta, Ga. 30333
25	Intestinal Obstruction Due to *Ascaris lumbricoides*	14 min	Silent	Color	Loan – Free	National Medical Audiovisual Center Attention: Videotape Duplicating Service Atlanta, Ga. 30333

25	Intestinal Parasites. Part I: Introduction and Techniques of Handling Specimens	29 min	Sound	Black and White	Loan—Free	National Medical Audiovisual Center Attention: Videotape Duplicating Service Atlanta, Ga. 30333
25	Intestinal Parasites. Part II: Intestinal Amebiasis	24 min	Sound	Black and White	Loan—Free	National Medical Audiovisual Center Attention: Videotape Duplicating Service Atlanta, Ga. 30333
25	Intestinal Parasites. Part III: Extraintestinal Amebiasis	19 min	Sound	Black and White	Loan—Free	National Medical Audiovisual Center Attention: Videotape Duplicating Service Atlanta, Ga. 30333
25	Schistosomes in the Primary Host	7 min	Silent	Black and White	Loan—Free	National Medical Audiovisual Center Attention: Videotape Duplicating Service Atlanta, Ga. 30333
25	Schistosomiasis	27 min	Sound	Color	Loan—Free	National Medical Audiovisual Center Attention: Videotape Duplicating Service Atlanta, Ga. 30333
25	Schistosomiasis—Snail Fever	10 min	Sound	Black and White	Loan—Free	National Medical Audiovisual Center Attention: Videotape Duplicating Service Atlanta, Ga. 30333
25	Asiatic Schistosomiasis	22 min	Sound	Color	Loan—Free	National Medical Audiovisual Center Attention: Videotape Duplicating Service Atlanta, Ga. 30333
25	Biology and Control of Schistosomiasis in Puerto Rico	19 min	Sound	Color	Loan—Free	National Medical Audiovisual Center Attention: Videotape Duplicating Service Atlanta, Ga. 30333
25	The Pathology of Schistosomiasis	2 min	Silent	Black and White	Loan—Free	National Medical Audiovisual Center Attention: Videotape Duplicating Service Atlanta, Ga. 30333
25	Sporocysts and Cercariae of *Schistosoma mansoni*	6 min	Silent	Black and White	Loan—Free	National Medical Audiovisual Center Attention: Videotape Duplicating Service Atlanta, Ga. 30333
25	Miracidia of *Schistosoma japonicum*	4 min	Silent	Color	Loan—Free	National Medical Audiovisual Center Attention: Videotape Duplicating Service Atlanta, Ga. 30333

*Films are 16 mm; those marked with an asterisk are also available in 8 mm from National Audiovisual Center, Suitland, Md. 20405.

CHAPTER	TITLE	LENGTH OF TIME	SOUND OR SILENT	COLOR OR BLACK AND WHITE	AVAILABILITY	SOURCE
25	Cholesterol-Lecithin Flocculation Test for Schistosomiasis	8.5 min	Sound*	Black and White	Loan	National Audiovisual Center Suitland, Md. 20405
25	Life Cycle of *Entamoeba histolytica* in Dysenteric and Nondysenteric Amoebiasis	18 min	Silent	Color	Loan–Free	National Medical Audiovisual Center Attention: Videotape Duplicating Service Atlanta, Ga. 30333
25	Motility of *Entamoeba histolytica*	4 min	Silent*	Color	Loan–Free	National Medical Audiovisual Center Attention: Videotape Duplicating Service Atlanta, Ga. 30333
25	Excystation of *Entamoeba histolytica*	3 min	Silent	Black and White	Loan	Audiovisual Section Clendening Medical Library University of Kansas Medical Center Kansas City, Kansas 66103
25	The Problem of Hookworm Infection	8 min	Sound	Color	Loan–Free	National Medical Audiovisual Center Attention: Videotape Duplicating Service Atlanta, Ga. 30333
25	Ancylostoma: Life History of Hookworms	25 min	Sound	Color	Loan	Audiovisual Section Clendening Medical Library University of Kansas Medical Center Kansas City, Kansas 66103
25	Infective Larvae of *Ancylostoma caninum*	5 min	Sound	Black and White	Loan–Free	National Medical Audiovisual Center Attention: Videotape Duplicating Service Atlanta, Ga. 30333
25	Infective Larvae of *Wuchereria bancrofti*	4 min	Silent	Color	Loan–Free	National Medical Audiovisual Center Attention: Videotape Duplicating Service Atlanta, Ga. 30333
25	Microfilariae of *Wuchereria bancrofti*	4 min	Silent	Color	Loan	Audiovisual Section Clendening Medical Libarary University of Kansas Medical Center Kansas City, Kansas 66103
25	Microfilariae of *Wuchereria bancrofti*	4 min	Silent	Color	Loan–Free	National Medical Audiovisual Center Attention: Videotape Duplicating Service Atlanta, Ga. 30333

	Title	Length	Sound	Color	Loan	Source
25	A Fifty-Fifty Chance	28 min	Sound	Color	Loan–Free	National Medical Audiovisual Center Attention: Videotape Duplicating Service Atlanta, Ga. 30333
25	Filariasis in British Guiana	17 min	Sound	Color	Loan–Free	National Medical Audiovisual Center Attention: Videotape Duplicating Service Atlanta, Ga. 30333
25	Control of Filariasis in Tahiti	15 min	Sound	Color	Loan–Free	National Medical Audiovisual Center Attention: Videotape Duplicating Service Atlanta, Ga. 30333
25	Manson's Blood Fluke	16 min	Sound	Black and White	Loan	Audiovisual Section Clendening Medical Library University of Kansas Medical Center Kansas City, Kansas 66103
25	Hemagglutination Test for Echinococcosis	20 min	Sound*	Color	Loan–Free	National Medical Audiovisual Center Attention: Videotape Duplicating Service Atlanta, Ga. 30333
26	Leptospirosis	16 min	Sound	Color	Loan–Free	National Medical Audiovisual Center Attention: Videotape Duplicating Service Atlanta, Ga. 30333
27	Hospital Food Service Personnel Training. Part 1: Introduction	16 min	Sound	Black and White	Loan–Free	National Medical Audiovisual Center Attention: Videotape Duplicating Service Atlanta, Ga. 30333
27	Hospital Food Service Personnel Training. Part 2: The Individual	13 min	Sound	Black and White	Loan–Free	National Medical Audiovisual Center Attention: Videotape Duplicating Service Atlanta, Ga. 30333
27	Hospital Food Service Personnel Training. Part 3: Equipment	12 min	Sound	Black and White	Loan–Free	National Medical Audiovisual Center Attention: Videotape Duplicating Service Atlanta, Ga. 30333
27	Hospital Food Service Personnel Training. Part 4: Serving Food	15 min	Sound	Color	Loan–Free	National Medical Audiovisual Center Attention: Videotape Duplicating Service Atlanta, Ga. 30333
27	Hospital Food Service Safety	15 min	Sound	Color	Loan–Free	National Medical Audiovisual Center Attention: Videotape Duplicating Service Atlanta, Ga. 30333

*Films are 16 mm; those marked with an asterisk are also available in 8 mm from National Audiovisual Center, Suitland, Md. 20405.

CHAPTER	TITLE	LENGTH OF TIME	SOUND OR SILENT	COLOR OR BLACK AND WHITE	AVAILABILITY	SOURCE
27	Kitchen Habits	12 min	Sound	Color	Loan – Free	National Medical Audiovisual Center Attention: Videotape Duplicating Service Atlanta, Ga. 30333
27	Preventing the Spread of Disease	10 min	Sound	Black and White	Loan – Free	National Medical Audiovisual Center Attention: VideotapeDuplicating Service Atlanta, Ga. 30333
27	Poultry Processing Inspection	22 min	Sound	Color	Loan – Free	National Medical Audiovisual Center Attention: Videotape Duplicating Service Atlanta, Ga. 30333
27	Practical Production of Grade A Milk	31 min	Sound	Color	Loan-Free	National Medical Audiovisual Center Attention: Videotape Duplicating Service Atlanta, Ga. 30333
27	Milk and Public Health	12 min	Sound	Black and White	Loan – Free	National Medical Audiovisual Center Attention: Videotape Duplicating Service Atlanta, Ga. 30333
27	Surface Sampling for Microorganisms	8 min	Sound*	Black and White	Loan	National Audiovisual Center Suitland, Md. 20405
28	Hospital Sepsis: Communicable Disease	28 min	Sound	Color	Loan – Free	Audiovisual Section Clendening Medical Library University of Kansas Medical Center Kansas City, Kansas 66103
28	Hospital Sanitation	14 min	Sound	Black and White	Loan – Free	National Medical Audiovisual Center Attention: Videotape Duplicating Service Atlanta, Ga. 30333
28	Epidemiology of Staphylococcal Infections	13 min	Sound	Color	Loan – Free	National Medical Audiovisual Center Attention: Videotape Duplicating Service Atlanta, Ga. 30333
28	An Outbreak of *Staphylococcus* Intoxication	12 min	Sound	Color	Loan – Free	National Medical Audiovisual Center Attention: Videotape Duplicating Service Atlanta, Ga. 30333

28	Prevention and Control of Staphylococcal Infections	14 min	Sound	Black and White	Loan—Free	National Medical Audiovisual Center Attention: Videotape Duplicating Service Atlanta, Ga. 30333
28	The Coagulase and Clumping Factor Tests for *Staphylococcus aureus*	5 min	Sound†	Black and White	Loan	National Audiovisual Center Suitland, Md. 20405
28	The Catalase Test	6 min	Sound†	Black and White	Loan	National Audiovisual Center Suitland, Md. 20405
28	The Oxidase Test	5 min	Sound†	Black and White	Loan	National Audiovisual Center Suitland, Md. 20405
28	Solubility and Optochine Tests for *Streptococcus pneumoniae*	8 min	Sound†	Black and White	Loan	National Audiovisual Center Suitland, Md. 20405
28	Isolation and Identification of Beta Hemolytic Streptococci	16 min	Sound*	Color	Loan—Free	National Medical Audiovisual Center Attention: Videotape Duplicating Service Atlanta, Ga. 30333
28	Hemolytic Streptococcus Control	13 min	Sound	Black and White	Loan	Audiovisual Section Clendening Medical Library University of Kansas Medical Center Kansas City, Kansas 66103
28	Stop Rheumatic Fever	13 min	Sound	Black and White	Loan—Free	National Medical Audiovisual Center Attention: Videotape Duplicating Service Atlanta, Ga. 30333
28	Common Heart Disorders and Their Causes	17 min	Sound	Black and White	Loan—Free	American Heart Association Post Office Box 9928 Austin, Texas 78766
28	Rheumatic Heart Disease	7 min	Silent	Color	Loan—Free	American Heart Association Post Office Box 9928 Austin, Texas 78766
28	Bronchitis and Bronchiectasis	29 min	Sound	Color	Loan—Free	The Pfizer Laboratories Division Film Library 267 West 25th Street New York, N.Y. 10001

*Films are 16 mm; those marked with an asterisk are also available in 8 mm from National Audiovisual Center, Suitland, Md. 20405.
†Available in 8 mm only.

CHAPTER	TITLE	LENGTH OF TIME	SOUND OR SILENT	COLOR OR BLACK AND WHITE	AVAILABILITY	SOURCE
28	Tests for Bronchitis and Emphysema	7 min	Sound†	Black and White	Loan	National Audiovisual Center Suitland, Md. 20405
28	Meningococcal Disease—Early Diagnosis, Intensive Treatment	26 min	Sound	Color	Loan—Free	National Medical Audiovisual Center Attention: Videotape Duplicating Service Atlanta, Ga. 30333
28	Gail's Awakening (Teeth)	12 min	Sound	Color	Loan—Free	National Medical Audiovisual Center Attention: Videotape Duplicating Service Atlanta, Ga. 30333
29	Microscopic Study and Isolation of *C. diphtheriae*	13 min	Sound	Black and White	Loan—Free	National Medical Audiovisual Center Attention: Videotape Duplicating Service Atlanta, Ga. 30333
29	Determination of Types of *C. diphtheriae*	11 min	Sound	Black and White	Loan—Free	National Medical Audiovisual Center Attention: Videotape Duplicating Service Atlanta, Ga. 30333
29	In Vitro Pathogenicity Test for *C. diphtheriae*	6.5 min	Sound*	Black and White	Loan	National Audiovisual Center Suitland, Md. 20405
29	In Vitro Toxigenicity Test for *Corynebacterium diphtheriae*	7 min	Sound	Color	Loan—Free	National Medical Audiovisual Center Attention: Videotape Duplicating Service Atlanta, Ga. 30333
29	In Vivo Toxigenicity Tests for *C. diphtheriae*	10 min	Sound*	Black and White	Loan	National Audiovisual Center Suitland, Md. 20405
29	Treatment of Chronic Obstructive Respiratory Diseases	40 min	Sound	Color	Loan—Free	The Pfizer Laboratories Division Film Library 267 West 25th Street New York, N.Y. 10001
29	Diagnosis of Chronic Obstructive Respiratory Diseases	40 min	Sound	Color	Loan—Free	The Pfizer Laboratories Division Film Library 267 West 25th Street New York, N.Y. 10001

29	Emergency Airway	21 min	Sound	Color	Loan—Free	The Pfizer Laboratories Division Film Library 267 West 25th Street New York. N.Y. 10001
29	Tracheotomy and Cricothyreotomy	23 min	Sound	Color	Loan—Free	The Pfizer Laboratories Division Film Library 267 West 25th Street New York. N.Y. 10001
31	Airborne Transmission of Tubercle Bacilli	7 min	Sound*	Color	Loan—Free	National Medical Audiovisual Center Attention: Videotape Duplicating Service Atlanta. Ga. 30333
31	Dynamics of the Tubercle	28 min	Sound	Color	Loan—Free	The Pfizer Laboratories Division Film Library 267 West 25th Street New York. N.Y. 10001
31	Tuberculin Testing	10 min	Sound‡	Color	Loan—Free	National Medical Audiovisual Center Attention: Videotape Duplicating Service Atlanta. Ga. 30333
31	Tuberculosis Laboratory Procedures: Drug Susceptibility Testing. Part I, Direct Method	5 min	Sound*	Color	Loan—Free	National Medical Audiovisual Center Attention: Videotape Duplicating Service Atlanta. Ga. 30333
31	Tuberculosis Laboratory Procedures: Drug Susceptibility Testing. Part II, Indirect Method	5 min	Sound*	Color	Loan—Free	National Medical Audiovisual Center Attention: Videotape Duplicating Service Atlanta. Ga. 30333
31	Tuberculosis Laboratory Procedures: Fluorescent Staining	5 min	Sound*	Color	Loan—Free	National Medical Audiovisual Center Attention: Videotape Duplicating Service Atlanta. Ga. 30333
31	Tuberculosis Laboratory Procedures: Ziehl-Neelsen Staining Procedures	5 min	Sound*	Color	Loan—Free	National Medical Audiovisual Center Attention: Videotape Duplicating Service Atlanta. Ga. 30333
31	Tuberculin Testing, Part 1: Tuberculins	6.5 min	Sound*	Black and White	Loan	National Audiovisual Center Suitland. Md. 20405

*Films are 16 mm; those marked with an asterisk are also available in 8 mm from National Audiovisual Center, Suitland, Md. 20405.
†Available in 8 mm only.
‡Also available in 35 mm.

CHAPTER	TITLE	LENGTH OF TIME	SOUND OR SILENT	COLOR OR BLACK AND WHITE	AVAILABILITY	SOURCE
31	Tuberculin Testing, Part II: Administration Techniques	5.5 min	Sound*	Black and White	Loan	National Audiovisual Center Suitland, Md. 20405
31	Dynamics of the Tubercle: in vivo Observations of Pathogenesis and Effect of Chemotherapy in the Clark Rabbit Ear Chamber	28 min	Sound	Color	Loan	Audiovisual Section Clendening Medical Library University of Kansas Medical Center Kansas City, Kansas 66103
31	Colony Characteristics of Mycobacteria in 7H-10 Agar Medium	7 min	Sound	Color	Loan—Free	National Medical Audiovisual Center Attention: Videotape Duplicating Service Atlanta, Ga. 30333
31	The Combined Niacin-Nitrate Reduction Test for *M. tuberculosis*	6 min	Sound	Color	Loan—Free	National Medical Audiovisual Center Attention: Videotape Duplicating Service Atlanta, Ga. 30333
31	Niacin-Nitrate Reduction Test	5.5 min	Sound*	Black and White	Loan	National Audiovisual Center Suitland, Md. 20405
31	Steps to Recovery: Rehabilitation of the Patient with Pulmonary Tuberculosis	30 min	Sound	Black and White	Loan—Free	National Medical Audiovisual Center Attention: Videotape Duplicating Service Atlanta, Ga. 30333
31	Recognition of Leprosy	13 min	Sound	Color	Loan—Free	National Medical Audiovisual Center Attention: Videotape Duplicating Service Atlanta, Ga. 30333
32	Human Rabies	16 min	Silent	Black and White	Loan—Free	National Medical Audiovisual Center Attention: Videotape Duplicating Service Atlanta, Ga. 30333
32	Rabies Control in the Community	11 min	Sound	Black and White	Loan—Free	National Medical Audiovisual Center Attention: Videotape Duplicating Service Atlanta, Ga. 30333
32	Rabies: F-A Staining	8 min	Sound*	Color	Loan—Free	National Medical Audiovisual Center Attention: Videotape Duplicating Service Atlanta, Ga. 30333

32	Rabies in Man	Silent	Black and White	Loan—Free	National Medical Audiovisual Center Attention: Videotape Duplicating Service Atlanta, Ga. 30333
32	Laboratory Diagnosis of Rabies in Animals	Sound	Color	Loan—Free	National Medical Audiovisual Center Attention: Videotape Duplicating Service Atlanta, Ga. 30333
32	The Taming of a Virus	Sound	Black and White	Loan—Free	National Medical Audiovisual Center Attention: Videotape Duplicating Service Atlanta, Ga. 30333
32	The Diagnosis of Viral Meningitis: What the Practitioner Will Know, Think, and Do	Sound	Color	Loan	Audiovisual Section Clendening Medical Library University of Kansas Medical Center Kansas City, Kansas 66103
32	Stop Rubella	Sound	Color	Loan—Free	National Medical Audiovisual Center Attention: Videotape Duplicating Service Atlanta, Ga. 30333
32	The Epidemiology of Influenza	Sound	Black and White	Loan—Free	National Medical Audiovisual Center Attention: Videotape Duplicating Service Atlanta, Ga. 30333
32	Eaton Agent Pneumonia	Sound	Color	Loan—Free	National Medical Audiovisual Center Attention: Videotape Duplicating Service Atlanta, Ga. 30333
34	Pinta	Sound	Color	Loan	Audiovisual Section Clendening Medical Library University of Kansas Medical Center Kansas City, Kansas 66103
34	A Lecture on the Spirochetes	Silent	Black and White	Loan	Audiovisual Section Clendening Medical Library University of Kansas Medical Center Kansas City, Kansas 66103
34	The Invader (Syphilis)	Sound	Black and White	Loan—Free	National Medical Audiovisual Center Attention: Videotape Duplicating Service Atlanta, Ga. 30333
34	Identification of Early Syphilis	Sound	Color	Loan—Free	National Medical Audiovisual Center Attention: Videotape Duplicating Service Atlanta, Ga. 30333

*Films are 16 mm; those marked with an asterisk are also available in 8 mm from National Audiovisual Center, Suitland, Md. 20405.

CHAPTER	TITLE	LENGTH OF TIME	SOUND OR SILENT	COLOR OR BLACK AND WHITE	AVAILABILITY	SOURCE
34	A Practical View of Syphilis	30 min	Sound	Color	Loan—Free	National Medical Audiovisual Center Attention: Videotape Duplicating Service Atlanta, Ga. 30333
34, 35	Treatment of Venereal Disease	30 min	Sound	Color	Loan—Free	The Pfizer Laboratories Division Film Library 267 West 25th Street New York, N.Y. 10001
34	Introduction to the Fluorescent Treponemal Antibody Test	9 min	Sound	Color	Loan—Free	National Medical Audiovisual Center Attention: Videotape Duplicating Service Atlanta, Ga. 30333
34	VDRL Slide Qualitative Test With Serum	6 min	Sound	Color	Loan—Free	National Medical Audiovisual Center Attention: Videotape Duplicating Service Atlanta, Ga. 30333
34	VDRL Tests for Syphilis	22 min	Sound	Black and White	Loan—Free	National Medical Audiovisual Center Attention: Videotape Duplicating Service Atlanta, Ga. 30333
35	VD—Stopping the Spread	18 min	Sound	Black and White	Loan—Free	National Medical Audiovisual Center Attention: Videotape Duplicating Service Atlanta, Ga. 30333
35	VD—"A Plague on Our House"	34 min	Sound	Color	Loan—Free	The Pfizer Laboratories Division Film Library 267 West 25th Street New York, N.Y. 10001
35	Non-Syphilitic Venereal Diseases	23 min	Sound	Color	Loan—Free	E. R. Squibb & Sons 909 Third Avenue New York, N.Y. 10022
36	Detection of *Clostridium botulinum* in Food. Part 1: Preparation of Food Samples and Direct Cultures	11 min	Sound*	Color	Loan—Free	National Medical Audiovisual Center Attention: Videotape Duplicating Service Atlanta, Ga. 30333

	Title	Length	Sound	Color	Loan	Source
36	Detection of *Clostridium botulinum* in Food. Part II: Mouse Toxin Neutralization Test	13 min	Sound*	Color	Loan – Free	National Medical Audiovisual Center Attention: Videotape Duplicating Service Atlanta, Ga. 30333
36	Detection of *Clostridium botulinum* in Food. Part III: Isolation from Mixed Culture	7 min	Sound*	Color	Loan – Free	National Medical Audiovisual Center Attention: Videotape Duplicating Service Atlanta, Ga. 30333
37	Coccidioidomycosis	7 min	Sound	Color	Loan – Free	National Medical Audiovisual Center Attention: Videotape Duplicating Service Atlanta, Ga. 30333
37	Coccidioidomycosis, Its Epidemiologic and Clinical Aspects	19 min	Sound	Color	Loan – Free	National Medical Audiovisual Center Attention: Videotape Duplicating Service Atlanta, Ga. 30333
37	Isolation of *C. immitis*	6.5 min	Sound*	Black and White	Loan	National Audiovisual Center Suitland, Md. 20405
37	An Epidemic of Histoplasmosis	17 min	Sound	Color	Loan – Free	National Medical Audiovisual Center Attention: Videotape Duplicating Service Atlanta, Ga. 30333
37	Histoplasmosis, Mason City, Iowa	16 min	Sound	Color	Loan – Free	National Medical Audiovisual Center Attention: Videotape Duplicating Service Atlanta, Ga. 30333
37	Mississippi Valley Disease: Histoplasmosis	30 min	Sound	Black and White	Loan	Audiovisual Section Clendening Medical Library University of Kansas Medical Center Kansas City, Kansas 66103
37	Isolation of *Blastomyces dermatitidis*	4 min	Sound*	Color	Loan – Free	National Medical Audiovisual Center Attention: Videotape Duplicating service Atlanta, Ga. 30333
37	North American Blastomycosis	8 min	Sound	Color	Loan – Free	National Medical Audiovisual Center Attention: Videotape Duplicating Service Atlanta, Ga. 30333

*Films are 16 mm; those marked with an asterisk are also available in 8 mm from National Audiovisual Center, Suitland, Md. 20405.

CHAPTER	TITLE	LENGTH OF TIME	SOUND OR SILENT	COLOR OR BLACK AND WHITE	AVAILABILITY	SOURCE
37	Mycosis Fungoides	16 min	Sound	Color	Loan – Free	National Medical Audiovisual Center Attention: Videotape Duplicating Service Atlanta, Ga. 30333
37	Phase Microscopy in the Diagnosis of Thrush	6 min	Sound	Color	Loan – Free	National Medical Audiovisual Center Attention: Videotape Duplicating Service Atlanta, Ga. 30333
38	Plague Control	21 min	Sound	Color	Loan	Audiovisual Section Clendening Medical Library University of Kansas Medical Center Kansas City, Kansas 66103
38	Plague in Sylvatic Areas	26 min	Sound	Color	Loan – Free	National Medical Audiovisual Center Attention: Videotape Duplicating Service Atlanta, Ga. 30333
38	Insect-Borne Diseases	17 min	Sound	Color	Loan – Free	National Medical Audiovisual Center Attention: Videotape Duplicating Service Atlanta, Ga. 30333
38	Biology and Control of the Cockroach	14 min	Sound	Color	Loan – Free	National Medical Audiovisual Center Attention: Videotape Duplicating Service Atlanta, Ga. 30333
38	The Biology and Control of Domestic Flies	15 min	Sound	Color	Loan – Free	National Medical Audiovisual Center Attention: Videotape Duplicating Service Atlanta, Ga. 30333
38	Life Cycle of the Fly	13 min	Sound	Black and White	Loan	McGraw-Hill Films 330 West 42nd Street New York. N.Y. 10036
38	Flies and Mosquitoes – Their Life Cycle and Control	10 min	Sound	Both	Loan	EBE Corporation Preview/Rental Libraries 1822 Pickwick Ave. Glenview, Illinois 60025
38	Fly Control Through Basic Sanitation	9 min	Sound	Color	Loan – Free	National Medical Audiovisual Center Attention: Videotape Duplicating Service Atlanta, Ga. 30333

	Title	Duration	Sound	Color	Loan	Source
38	The Rat Problem	25 min	Sound	Black and White	Loan–Free	National Medical Audiovisual Center Attention: Videotape Duplicating Service Atlanta, Ga. 30333
38	Hemorrhagic Fever: Clinical Features	45 min	Sound	Color	Loan–Free	National Medical Audiovisual Center Attention: Videotape Duplicating Service Atlanta, Ga. 30333
39	The Task We Face	17 min	Sound	Black and White	Loan	Audiovisual Section Clendening Medical Library University of Kansas Medical Center Kansas City, Kansas 66103
39	Unconditional Surrender	14 min	Sound	Black and White	Loan	Audiovisual Section Clendening Medical Library University of Kansas Medical Center Kansas City, Kansas 66103
39	Control of Louse-Borne Diseases	15 min	Sound	Black and White	Loan	Audiovisual Section Clendening Medical Library University of Kansas Medical Center Kansas City, Kansas 66103
39	The Life History of the Rocky Mountain Wood Tick	35 min	Silent	Color	Loan–Free	National Medical Audiovisual Center Attention: Videotape Duplicating Service Atlanta, Ga. 30333
39	Life History of the Rocky Mountain Wood Tick	18 min	Sound	Color	Loan–Free	National Medical Audiovisual Center Attention: Videotape Duplicating Service Atlanta, Ga. 30333
39	The Story of Rocky Mountain Spotted Fever	29 min	Sound	Color	Loan–Free	National Medical Audiovisual Center Attention: Videotape Duplicating Service Atlanta, Ga. 30333
39	The Removal of Biting Ticks	3.5 min	Sound†	Black and White	Loan	National Audiovisual Center Suitland, Md. 20405
39	Epidemiology of Murine Typhus	18 min	Sound	Black and White	Loan–Free	National Medical Audiovisual Center Attention: Videotape Duplicating Service Atlanta, Ga. 30333
39	Tsutsugamushi – The Scrub Typhus Mite	21 min	Sound	Black and White	Loan–Free	National Medical Audiovisual Center Attention: Videotape Duplicating Service Atlanta, Ga. 30333

†Available in 8 mm only.

CHAPTER	TITLE	LENGTH OF TIME	SOUND OR SILENT	COLOR OR BLACK AND WHITE	AVAILABILITY	SOURCE
39	Typhus in Naples	11 min	Sound	Color	Loan	Audiovisual Section Clendening Medical Library University of Kansas Medical Center Kansas City, Kansas 66103
39	Epidemic Encephalitis	Two Reels	Silent	Black and White	Loan	Audiovisual Section Clendening Medical Library University of Kansas Medical Center Kansas City, Kansas 66103
39	Venezuelan Equine Encephalitis Epidemic in Colombia	20 min	Sound	Color	Loan – Free	National Medical Audiovisual Center Attention: Videotape Duplicating Service Atlanta, Ga. 30333
39	Disease Recognition: Japanese B Encephalitis	18 min	Sound	Color	Loan – Free	National Medical Audiovisual Center Attention: Videotape Duplicating Service Atlanta, Ga. 30333
39	Breakbone Fever, "Dengue"	8 min	Sound	Color	Loan – Free	National Medical Audiovisual Center Attention: Videotape Duplicating Service Atlanta, Ga. 30333
39	Organized Mosquito Control	16 min	Sound	Color	Loan – Free	National Medical Audiovisual Center Attention: Videotape Duplicating Service Atlanta, Ga. 30333
39	Malaria – Cause and Control	30 min	Sound	Color	Loan – Free	National Medical Audiovisual Center Attention: Videotape Duplicating Service Atlanta, Ga. 30333
39	Malaria Prevention (Short Version)	14 min	Sound	Color	Loan – Free	National Medical Audiovisual Center Attention: Videotape Duplicating Service Atlanta, Ga. 30333
39	Clinical Malaria	26 min	Sound	Black and White	Loan – Free	National Medical Audiovisual Center Attention: Videotape Duplicating Service Atlanta, Ga. 30333

No.	Title	Length	Sound	Color	Loan	Source
39	Erythrocytic Stages of *Plasmodium vivax*	4 min	Sound	Black and White	Loan–Free	National Medical Audiovisual Center Attention: Videotape Duplicating Service Atlanta, Ga. 30333
39	Mosquito Stages of *Plasmodium falciparum*	11 min	Sound	Black and White	Loan–Free	National Medical Audiovisual Center Attention: Videotape Duplicating Service Atlanta, Ga. 30333
39	The Dissection of a Mosquito for Malaria Parasites	10 min	Sound	Color	Loan–Free	National Medical Audiovisual Center Attention: Videotape Duplicating Service Atlanta, Ga. 30333
39	Staining Blood Films for Detection of Malaria Parasites	8 min	Sound*	Black and White	Loan	National Audiovisual Center Suitland, Md. 20405
39	Preparation of Thick and Thin Blood Films	5.5 min	Sound*	Black and White	Loan	National Audiovisual Center Suitland, Md. 20405
39	Biology and Control of Domestic Mosquitoes	22 min	Sound	Color	Loan–Free	National Medical Audiovisual Center Attention: Videotape Duplicating Service Atlanta, Ga. 30333
39	Let's Finish the Job (Mosquito)	11 min	Sound	Color	Loan–Free	National Medical Audiovisual Center Attention: Videotape Duplicating Service Atlanta, Ga. 30333
39	Mosquito Prevention in Irrigated Areas	7 min	Sound	Black and White	Loan–Free	National Medical Audiovisual Center Attention: Videotape Duplicating Service Atlanta, Ga. 30333
39	The *Aedes aegypti* Inspector	23 min	Sound	Color	Loan–Free	National Medical Audiovisual Center Attention: Videotape Duplicating Service Atlanta, Ga. 30333
39	Life History of the Yellow Fever Mosquito	10 min	Silent	Black and White	Loan–Free	National Medical Audiovisual Center Attention: Videotape Duplicating Service Atlanta, Ga. 30333
40	The Mosquito and Its Control	11 min	Sound	Both	Loan	Modern Talking Pictures 160 E. Grand Ave. Chicago, Illinois 60611

*Films are 16 mm; those marked with an asterisk are also available in 8 mm from National Audiovisual Center, Suitland, Md. 20405.

CHAPTER	TITLE	LENGTH OF TIME	SOUND OR SILENT	COLOR OR BLACK AND WHITE	AVAILABILITY	SOURCE
40	Sandfly Control	32 min	Sound	Color	Loan	Audiovisual Section Clendening Medical Library University of Kansas Medical Center Kansas City, Kansas 66103
40	Disseminated Anergic Leishmaniasis	7 min	Sound	Color	Loan—Free	National Medical Audiovisual Center Attention: Videotape Duplicating Service Atlanta, Ga. 30333
40	Early Cutaneous Leishmaniasis	7 min	Sound	Color	Loan—Free	National Medical Audiovisual Center Attention: Videotape Duplicating Service Atlanta, Ga. 30333
40	Late Cutaneous Leishmaniasis	7 min	Sound	Color	Loan—Free	National Medical Audiovisual Center Attention: Videotape Duplicating Service Atlanta, Ga. 30333
40	African Trypanosomiasis	16 min	Sound	Color	Loan	Audiovisual Section Clendening Medical Library University of Kansas Medical Center Kansas City, Kansas 66103
40	Disease Recognition: American Trypanosomiasis (Chagas' Disease)	12 min	Sound	Color	Loan—Free	National Medical Audiovisual Center Attention: Videotape Duplicating Service Atlanta, Ga. 30333
40	Eggs and Miracidia of Schistosoma mansoni	3 min	Silent	Black and White	Loan—Free	National Medical Audiovisual Center Attention: Videotape Duplicating Service Atlanta, Ga. 30333
40	Preparation of Wright's Stain	11 min	Sound	Color	Loan—Free	National Medical Audiovisual Center Attention: Videotape Duplicating Service Atlanta, Ga. 30333
41	Technique of Parenteral Injection	22 min	Sound	Color	Loan	Becton, Dickinson and Co. Rutherford, New Jersey 07070
41	Needle Injections. Part 1: Equipment and Medications	15 min	Sound	Black and White	Loan—Free	National Medical Audiovisual Center Attention: Videotape Duplicating Service Atlanta, Ga. 30333

	Title	Length	Sound	Color	Loan	Source
41	Needle Injections. Part 2: Intradermal, Subcutaneous and Intramuscular Injection Techniques	8 min	Sound	Black and White	Loan—Free	National Medical Audiovisual Center Attention: Videotape Duplicating Service Atlanta, Ga. 30333
41	Needle Injections. Part 3: Intravenous Needle Injection Technique	5 min	Sound	Black and White	Loan—Free	National Medical Audiovisual Center Attention: Videotape Duplicating Service Atlanta, Ga. 30333
41	The Inoculating Needle	10 min	Sound	Black and White	Loan—Free	National Medical Audiovisual Center Attention: Videotape Duplicating Service Atlanta, Ga. 30333
41	Programmed Approach to Disposable Hypodermic Equipment	8 min	Sound	Color	Loan	Becton, Dickinson and Co. Rutherford, New Jersey 07070
41	Modern Technics of Collecting Blood Samples	44 min	Sound	Color	Loan—Free	National Medical Audiovisual Center Attention: Videotape Duplicating Service Atlanta, Ga. 30333
41	Collecting Blood Samples: The Vacutainer Technique	20 min	Sound	Color	Loan	Audiovisual Section Clendening Medical Library University of Kansas Medical Center Kansas City, Kansas 66103
41	The Vacutainer System	21 min	Sound	Color	Loan	Becton, Dickinson and Co. Rutherford, New Jersey 07070
41	Serological Technique: Venipuncture	7 min	Sound	Color	Loan—Free	National Medical Audiovisual Center Attention: Videotape Duplicating Service Atlanta, Ga. 30333
41	Normal And Pathological Red Cells of Human Blood (A study by Phase Contrast and Electron Microscope)	22 min	Sound	Black and White	Loan—Free	National Medical Audiovisual Center Attention: Videotape Duplicating Service Atlanta, Ga. 30333
41	Surface Sampling for Microorganisms	5 min	Sound*	Black and White	Loan	National Audiovisual Center Suitland, Md. 20405
41	In A Medical Laboratory	28 min	Sound	Color	Loan—Free	Audiovisual Section Clendening Medical Library University of Kansas Medical Center Kansas City, Kansas 66103

*Films are 16 mm; those marked with an asterisk are also available in 8 mm from National Audiovisual Center, Suitland, Md. 20405.

CHAPTER	TITLE	LENGTH OF TIME	SOUND OR SILENT	COLOR OR BLACK AND WHITE	AVAILABILITY	SOURCE
41	Preparation of Sputum Specimens	16 min	Sound	Black and White	Loan – Free	National Medical Audiovisual Center Attention: Videotape Duplicating Service Atlanta, Ga. 30333
41	Collection and Processing of Specimens for Respiratory Virus Isolation	4 min	Sound†	Black and White	Loan	National Audiovisual Center Suitland, Md. 20405
41	Fecal Smears for Parasitological Examination	7.5 min	Sound†	Black and White	Loan	National Audiovisual Center Suitland, Md. 20405
41	Formalin-Ether Concentration of Fecal Parasites	13 min	Sound	Color	Loan – Free	National Medical Audiovisual Center Attention: Videotape Duplicating Service Atlanta, Ga. 30333
41	Techniques of Laboratory Diagnosis of Influenza	17 min	Sound	Black and White	Loan – Free	National Medical Audiovisual Center Attention: Videotape Duplicating Service Atlanta, Ga. 30333
41	Ox Cell Hemolysin Test (Infectious Mononucleosis)	9.5 min	Sound*	Black and White	Loan	National Audiovisual Center Suitland, Md. 20405
41	Mycological Slide Culture Technique	7 min	Sound*	Color	Loan – Free	National Medical Audiovisual Center Attention: Videotape Duplicating Service Atlanta, Ga. 30333
41	The Communicable Disease Center	22 min	Sound*	Black and White	Loan	National Audiovisual Center Suitland, Md. 20405
41	Health in our Community	14 min	Sound	Both	Loan	EBE Corporation Preview/Rental Libraries 1822 Pickwick Ave. Glenview, Illinois 60025

41	First Aid on the Spot	10 min	Sound	Black and White	Loan	EBE Corporation Preview/Rental Libraries 1822 Pickwick Ave. Glenview, Illinois 60025
41	Key to Cleanliness	18 min	Sound	Color	Loan	Sound Services Ltd. 269 Kingston Road London S.W.19, England
41	A Career in Bacteriology	20 min	Sound	Color	Loan	Becton, Dickinson and Co. Rutherford, New Jersey 07070
41	B-D Controls—The Conscience of a Company	10 min	Sound	Color	Loan	Becton, Dickinson and Co. Rutherford, New Jersey 07070
	Dance Little Children	25 min	Sound	Color	Loan—Free	National Medical Audiovisual Center Attention: Videotape Duplicating Service Atlanta, Ga. 30333

*Films are 16 mm; those marked with an asterisk are also available in 8 mm from National Audiovisual Center, Suitland, Md. 20405.
†Available in 8 mm only.

INDEX

Boldface page numbers indicate main topic; *italic* numbers refer to illustrations; (t) indicates tables.

635